LANDESMAN'S

PUBLIC HEALTH MANAGEMENT OF DISASTERS

THE PRACTICE GUIDE

Fourth Edition

LANDESMAN'S

PUBLIC HEALTH MANAGEMENT OF DISASTERS

THE PRACTICE GUIDE

Fourth Edition

Linda Young Landesman, DrPH, MSW
Rita V. Burke, PhD, MPH

APHA PRESS
AN IMPRINT OF AMERICAN PUBLIC HEALTH ASSOCIATION

American Public Health Association
800 I Street, NW
Washington, DC 20001-3710
www.apha.org

Georges C. Benjamin, MD, FACP, FACEP (Emeritus), FNAPA, Executive Director

Printed and bound in the United States of America
Book Production Editor: Maya Ribault
Typesetting: The Charlesworth Group
Cover Design: Abduallahi Abdulgader
Printing and Binding: Sheridan Books

Library of Congress Cataloging-in-Publication Data

Names: Landesman, Linda Young, author. | Burke, Rita V., author. | American Public Health Association, issuing body.
Title: Landesman's public health management of disasters : the practice guide / authors, Linda Young Landesman, Rita V. Burke.
Other titles: Public health management of disasters
Description: Fourth edition. | Washington, DC : American Public Health Association, [2017] | Preceded by Public health management of disasters / Linda Young Landesman. 3rd ed. c2012. | Includes bibliographical references and index.
Identifiers: LCCN 2017003895 (print) | LCCN 2017005632 (ebook) | ISBN 9780875532790 (softcover: alk. paper) | ISBN 9780875532806 (ebook)
Subjects: | MESH: Disaster Planning | Public Health Administration | Disasters
Classification: LCC RA645.9 (print) | LCC RA645.9 (ebook) | NLM WA 295 | DDC 363.34/8–dc23
LC record available at https://lccn.loc.gov/2017003895

Dedicated to Paul Landesman for 40 great years and to Jacob Benjamin Burke for being a true source of inspiration and motivation to make the world safer for the next generation.

TABLE OF CONTENTS

CHAPTERS

APPENDICES

BASICS

STANDARDS, CAPABILITIES, AND RESPONSIBILITIES

MANAGEMENT STANDARDS

MORBIDITY

BEHAVIORAL HEALTH

FIRST AID

AT-RISK POPULATIONS

INFECTIOUS DISEASE AND CBRNE

WORKER HEALTH AND SAFETY

RESOURCES AND REFERENCES

LIST OF TABLES AND FIGURES

CHAPTER 5

CHAPTER 6

CHAPTER 7

CHAPTER 8

CHAPTER 13

CHAPTER 14

CHAPTER 15

FOREWORD

The first edition of *Public Health Management of Disasters: A Practice Guide* was published in 2001 in the wake of 9/11 and the anthrax attacks. At the time, it was difficult to imagine that preparing for and responding to the public health consequences of disasters would become a core component of public health practice. Nor was it likely that most public health practitioners could imagine the frequency, diversity, and complexity of disasters that would ensue.

Fast forward to 2017. The world has changed dramatically. Well over half of its population lives in dense, urban environments, and many of these places are vulnerable when it comes to phenomena such as sea-level rise or earthquakes. Other environments amplify their own vulnerabilities through poverty and overcrowding, creation of heat islands, air pollution, dependence on fragile electrical grids, and other factors. New and emerging infectious disease outbreaks continue; not long before the publication of the third edition, the world experienced an influenza pandemic, which fortunately was not as severe as initially feared. Since then, we have confronted other scary, new and re-emerging diseases, including Ebola virus disease and Zika virus. Laboratory accidents and deliberate bioterrorism are continual threats. Environmental disasters, often man-made, also occur with distressing frequency; some impact generations, as was the case with the Fukushima power plant disaster and the Flint water crisis. Terrorist-related events also continue to occur, and while thankfully not on the scale of the World Trade Center attack, terrorists continue to kill, maim, and evoke epidemics of fear. Mass shootings, which are largely not caused by foreign terrorists, have become so frequent in the United States that there is now an informal network of health officers that support and share lessons learned with one another, particularly regarding the mental health sequelae, after the events.

One way or another, crises with public health implications happen in communities every day. Most are handled locally and do not grab national or international headlines. Those that are catastrophic in size and scope also continue to occur, perhaps with increasing frequency. The only questions are what form they will take, when and where they will occur, and whether they will occur without warning.

With such diversity of events, the task of preparing for and responding to public health aspects of disasters could seem daunting. Yet, when something happens, we must respond with the day-to-day systems we have in place at the time, not the ones we imagine or would like to have. That reality highlights the importance of building and maintaining strong day-to-day health systems; if disease surveillance and detection systems or laboratory capacity is degraded, or if we fail to modernize them, the ability of public health systems to respond to a crisis will be limited. If a hospital is understaffed and boarding patients for 24 hours in the emergency department is the norm not the exception, the hospital will struggle to handle a surge of patients in a mass casualty event.

Further, as different as they seem, all disasters require public health agencies to respond using a core set of capabilities. For example, all events require good situational awareness, superb risk communication, and attention to public fear and behavioral health. Recovery is recognized as central to response. Public health agencies that can fulfill those core capabilities, which are well outlined by both the Office of the Assistant Secretary for Preparedness and Response (*2017–2022 Health Care Preparedness and Response Capabilities)* and the Centers for Disease Control and Prevention (*Public Health Preparedness Capabilities: National Standards for State and Local Planning)* and are the subject of many chapters in this book, will have the agility to adjust to the differences between events. Those that struggle with core capabilities will likely struggle in managing an event.

Following the events of 2001, many policy makers, including those responsible for federal, state, and local public health and preparedness budgets, were of the view that preparedness was a one-time investment, that if made would cover us for years. Emergency preparedness and response have become a new normal. In the last decade, funding for preparedness at all levels of government has seen dramatic cuts. Yet, the people who do the work, day in and day out, continue to change. They need to be trained, to know their intersectoral colleagues, and to drill and exercise together. And, systems and equipment become outdated and need to be refreshed.

Finally, preparedness system professionals must be continually learning. This means that they need to be capable of conducting scientific research before, during, and after events and that they should strive never to make the same mistakes or confront an event with the same knowledge gaps as the ones they have already addressed. We must not just keep on learning but must put into practice what we have learned. That is exactly what this edition has sought to do and what subsequent editions must continue to do.

Nicole Lurie, MD, MSPH

FOREWORD TO THE THIRD EDITION

Recent history has shaped our understanding of the health and medical impact of natural disasters, especially lessons learned from the December 2004 Indian Ocean Southeast Asian tsunami event and the powerful 9.0-magnitude earthquake that hit Japan on March 11, 2011, at 2:46 p.m. local time (0546 GMT), unleashing massive tsunami waves that crashed into the northeastern coast of Honshu—the largest and main island of Japan, resulting in widespread damage and destruction—then raced across the Pacific at 800 miles per hour before hitting Hawaii and the West Coast of the United States. According to the government of Japan, at least 25,000 people are confirmed dead. All search, rescue, and relief operations, evacuations, and international humanitarian assistance were conducted within the framework of the possibility of significant radiation release and a nuclear meltdown resulting from the fires and explosions at a coastal nuclear facility.

This past spring, in the United States, we have had record flooding along the Mississippi River, with displacement of tens of thousands, and the worst year on record for tornado-related deaths (both for an outbreak [375 deaths] and for a single event [130 deaths]), with most of the tornado season yet to come. With the incidence of such catastrophes of nature—and the number of people affected by such events—on the increase, the importance of disasters as a public health problem has captured the attention of the world.

This situation represents an unprecedented challenge to public health practitioners.

Ten years have now passed since the landmark first edition of *Public Health Management of Disasters: A Practice Guide* was published by the American Public Health Association in the wake of the catastrophic events of September 11, 2001. The first edition was so successful in part because it was able to serve as a quick reference for public health practitioners or public safety personnel who required quickly available information in an easy to access "practice guide" format. The third edition of *Public Health Management of Disasters: The Practice Guide* was confronted with the daunting task of both summarizing the many important new findings that have now become available through extensive research and the experience of public health practitioners and yet maintain the convenience of a manual. Dr. Landesman has succeeded in accomplishing this magnificently.

The third edition of *Public Health Management of Disasters* has increased the number of pages, with the addition of both new chapters and appendices that summarize in tabular form all of the new elements included in the Centers for Disease Control and Prevention standards for public health capabilities in preparedness and planning, as well as the important changes at the federal level that have occurred since 9/11 and Hurricane Katrina, such as those resulting from Presidential Decision Directive-8, the National Response Framework (NRF), National Incident Management System, and key elements of emergency planning: disaster prevention, mitigation, preparedness, response, recovery, reconstruction, and community resiliency. The influenza section has been expanded to include our experience with the 2009 novel H1N1 influenza response and includes global considerations, including World Health Organization guidance. Chapters on surveillance have been updated to include global positioning system technology, social media, smartphones, and all of the new alerting systems the U.S. government has put in place; updated and expanded occupational and health guidance; cultural considerations; all of the new functional needs as outlined in NRF, community planning networks for vulnerable population groups, standards and indicators for disaster shelter care for children, ethical issues in disaster response; and the evolving priorities of the U.S. Department of Homeland Security.

As this book goes to print, Japan's social, technical, administrative, political, legal, health care, and economic systems are being tested to their limits by the nature, degree, and extent of the socioeconomic impacts of the earthquake, the tsunami, and the looming possibility of a "nightmare nuclear disaster." This unfolding tragedy more than ever illustrates the enduring value of this publication by the American Public Health Association. *Public Health Management of Disasters: A Practice Guide* will continue to serve as both a timely and comprehensive text for public health officials and for educating the next generation of public health practitioners.

Eric K. Noji, MD, MPH
Centers for Disease Control and Prevention (Retired)

PUBLISHER'S NOTE

A disaster is defined by Merriam-Webster as "a sudden calamitous event bringing great damage, loss, or destruction." Disasters are often unpredictable and complex events that the public health and emergency management community increasingly has to prepare for. Recent events have ranged from man-made ones such as the 2016 mass shooting in an Orlando, Florida, nightclub that resulted in 49 deaths and 53 injuries; severe weather storms like Hurricane Sandy, the most destructive and deadliest storm of the 2012 hurricane season; a major epidemic (2014–2016) from a mutated Ebola virus; and multiple earthquakes worldwide.

A decade and a half after the September 11, 2001, terror attacks and the subsequent anthrax letters, this updated edition is being released to help public health professionals further strengthen their disaster response. It is a practical guide that has been updated to recognize the newest thinking around public health and emergency preparedness.

Updates to the fourth edition take into account the most current federal preparedness guidance from the National Preparedness Goal, the National Health Security Strategy, and the National Response Framework. Additional updates to emerging approaches for public health surveillance, laboratory and disaster information systems, and hospital surveillance in hospitals are included. New threat and hazard identification and alerting and warning systems are profiled along with the use of new electronic technologies to communicate, such as smartphone apps and social media (e.g., texting and Twitter). Environmental health and occupational health are now discussed in 2 separate chapters that include updates on environmental standards and common food-borne diseases.

New federal guidance is profiled around engaging health care coalitions, the National Planning System, the National Disaster Recovery Framework, and the National Planning Framework. The Ebola epidemic that started in West Africa and was designated as a public health emergency by the World Health Organization created new challenges for both public health and medical care systems. Lessons learned about preparedness and response from this major epidemic have been included in this text. The Ebola informed material on infection control, worker protections, and personal protective equipment is particularly relevant to today and makes this book a must-have reference. A comprehensive discussion on the Zika virus, the first mosquito-borne disease to cause birth defects and other disabilities, has been included. The chapter on at-risk populations is now focused on people with disabilities and others with access and functional needs, with an updated section on communicating with people who are deaf or hard of hearing. The section on children has been updated, and new material has been included on access to primary care and radiation emergencies. Several new and updated tables and appendices have been added as well.

The strength of this text is in its delivery of the core approach to disaster management. It is also a reminder that we in the public health community play an important role in preparing individuals, families, and communities to be resilient. Resiliency is the essential capacity that helps with recovery and reconstruction.

In this fourth edition, public health professionals can learn not only about the structure of health management in disasters but also about hazard assessment, delivery of care under extreme conditions, ways to put a preparedness plan into practice, vulnerability analysis, key considerations in surge capacity, and other important preparedness methods. Professionals can explore behavioral health strategies, an often overlooked area during crises. The diagnostic criteria for post-traumatic stress disorder (*Diagnostic and Statistical Manual of Mental Disorders*, Fifth Edition) have been updated in this edition. The text also addresses updated concepts pertaining to ethical issues in disaster management. Although emergency responders make many life and death decisions during a disaster, none are as sensitive as those around changing the standard of care from the norm. This often occurs when decisions have to be made concerning who should get limited resources such as ventilators or medications. Those ethical considerations have been explored once more in this new edition.

This book is an essential resource for those who find that their work must contain more than a minimal understanding of public health disaster management.

Georges C. Benjamin, MD, MACP, FACEP (Emeritus), FNAPA
Executive Director, American Public Health Association

AUTHORS' REFLECTIONS AND ACKNOWLEDGMENTS

Evolution of the Field

Public health preparedness is now a recognized field; this is far different from the early 1980s to late-1990s when colleagues would ask Linda Landesman, "What does public health have to do with disasters?" Disasters disrupt the usual operations of public health agencies, health care organizations, and emergency response groups, and thus it is critical that those who work in those systems understand how to effectively work together to integrate their response efforts. Now, as in any established field, there is a large body of specialized technical information critical to this function. The preparedness practitioner must know where to gather information about a broad range of public health problems in order to make decisions quickly.

The first edition, published just after September 11, 2001, established foundational principles and consolidated important information into one source. The second edition incorporated the many improvements that were made after the 9/11 terrorist attacks. The numerous difficulties following Hurricane Katrina in 2005 highlighted the need for a reorganization of our country's response and the provision of services to at-risk populations. These advancements were reflected in the third edition. The fourth edition continues to bring together both that essential knowledge and the sustained progress that followed Hurricane Sandy in 2012, Ebola virus disease in 2014, and Zika virus in 2016. Like the previous editions, this book reflects the many advances since its predecessor was published.

Along with the evolution of the field, the concept of *preparedness* has changed. In the third edition, being prepared had become the responsibility of everyone—government at all levels, the private sector, nonprofit organizations, and residents of communities across the United States. In 2017, with the national push for communities to develop resilience, we now understand that those communities and individuals who are resilient are better prepared when they plan more effectively by anticipating potential impacts (rather than planning only to respond to what happens). The concept of resilience has influenced the entire lifecycle of disasters. The Office of the Assistant Secretary for Preparedness and Response, recognizing the importance and far-reaching implications of self-reliant communities, has made resilience its first goal in the latest health care capabilities. The push for heightened resilience has spurred the creation of health care coalitions in every state to boost self-sufficiency for each community.

The science of understanding the effects of disasters has also shifted. Those in the field are well aware of the challenges inherent in conducting disaster research. These challenges have historically and consistently included obtaining approval from institutional review boards in a timely manner and identifying and assembling available experts necessary to conduct studies in the immediate aftermath of a disaster. The science preparedness framework, discussed in Chapter 14, will streamline the process, allowing for the conduct of timely investigation, something that has been almost impossible to do up to this point. Timely research will better inform decision making about public health impacts by obtaining critical information earlier.

Future preparedness will include preparing for the spread of novel diseases that we may not be aware of today. Reducing the potential impact of the next pandemic requires an in-depth understanding of the threat. Global surveillance for these emerging exposures is occurring through USAID's Emerging Pandemic Threats program. Their PREDICT project, which identifies and tracks potential zoonotic disease where pathogens can spillover from animal hosts to people, has detected over 800 novel viruses in animals and humans. Identifying dangerous pathogens found in animals before they can become significant threats to humans is a key to future emergency public health.

Lessons Learned

With each edition of this book, new and often more devastating disasters are experienced worldwide. In 2016 and in the first 2 months of 2017, 26 major disasters were declared for incidents of flooding in the United States with Louisiana experiencing some of the worst inundation in its history, resulting in 13 deaths and thousands of evacuations. Hurricane Matthew resulted in a major disaster declaration in 5 states—Florida, Georgia, North Carolina, South Carolina, and Virginia. Sadly, Hurricane Matthew restruck neighborhoods in North Carolina that had chosen to rebuild after having been devastated by Hurricane Floyd in 1999. New Zealand experienced a powerful magnitude 7.8 earthquake that caused massive damage to infrastructure, triggered between 80,000 and 100,000 landslides, and resulted in a tsunami causing billions in damage. More than 180,000 people were forced to evacuate from Oroville, California, in mid-February 2017 when their dam threatened to overflow following severe erosion of the dam's spillway.

Similar catastrophes due to infrastructure failure are likely to surge as the foundations of our cities age without repair or replacement. The impacts of these disasters and the key principles in this book are not new. What has changed are the weaknesses identified in the response to the most recent major disasters. These lessons lead to subsequent guidance that is applied at the state and local levels to lessen the impact and devastation of future disasters.

To apply the lessons, we first have to believe that catastrophic events can happen to *us*. It is common to think of catastrophic events as the *perfect storm*, where a rare combination of conditions results in calamitous experiences. Another term—*Black Swan* events—is used to characterize the rare events that have a significant impact upon society. The Black Swan theory, popularized by Nassim Nicholas Taleb, has 3 main components: rarity, extreme impact, and retrospective predictability. Many think of the Black Swans as the low-probability, high-consequence events that happen to someone else. Thinking that catastrophes are rare prevents us from taking the kinds of actions needed to be better prepared.

The devastations from the 2011 earthquake and tsunami in Japan and from the 2010 Gulf of Mexico oil spill remind us that the importance of preparedness cannot be taken for granted. The Black Swan experience of Japan, when it was struck by a devastating earthquake followed by a historic tsunami and radiation leak, continues to be a great teacher. Despite the ancient markers along the Japanese coastline warning future generations about the dangers of tsunamis, high-risk areas were developed significantly. The most recent Black Swan event in the United States was the explosion of the Deepwater Horizon oil platform and subsequent spill that spread to 1,600 miles of shoreline and spoiled over 800 miles of beach and marsh Gulf of Mexico shoreline.

In both cases, the events were predicted but were not adequately prepared for. In Japan, the Japanese government had anticipated that similar catastrophic events would occur in their country, though in a different location, and had taken steps to mitigate and manage them. The extensive planning for massive tremors was focused on caring for innumerable casualties and injuries typically found following earthquakes. Despite being well prepared, the Japanese government did not do enough to protect the population along the coastline and failed to heed the message of the markers: "Remember the calamity of great tsunamis." The response was further hindered by the failure to recognize and communicate the severity of a secondary disaster—the nuclear accident—in a timely manner. In the case of the Deepwater Horizon incident, poor preparation, lack of training, poor management in the response, and ineffective communication systems exacerbated the disaster. Both events had all 3 elements of a Black Swan event: they were rare, had a devastating impact on their region and beyond, and in retrospect, could have been anticipated. Hopefully we have learned the lessons about better preparedness for future Black Swans.

World leaders were given warning about the need for public health systems to be robust when Ebola virus disease spread beyond a few villages in West Africa in 2014. The most calamitous disaster of our lifetime may come with the next pandemic of a novel virus, which has a high mortality rate or to which no one has immunity. If public health laboratories do not have sufficient staff and resources to test specimens, if departments of health are decimated and lack adequate staff for even routine surveillance, and if the fiscal status of health care systems is so fragile (because of not being fully compensated for the care provided)—that hospitals lack additional capacity, the next novel virus could devastate communities across our country and the globe.

How to Use this Book

This practice guide has 2 purposes: to educate public health workers and students about the areas where they will intervene as professionals and to be a resource for anyone involved in preparing for or responding to disasters where public health problems are confronted. Using the material in this book, public health professionals will be better able to carry out the capabilities expected of them.

The principles in this book are applicable to disasters around the world. Although governmental systems may vary, similar disasters have common problems and similar outcomes—only more dramatic in countries lacking a robust infrastructure. All large-scale catastrophes require a coordinated response across many professional agencies and disciplines. This guide includes guidance from both the U.S. and world health experience.

Emerging technologies continue to transform the field of emergency management. People have revolutionized disaster communication by finding creative uses for social media. Chapter 7 and Appendix Y identify some of the tools currently available in disaster operations. Public health agencies can make an important contribution in assessing how well these tools impact outcomes in all phases of a disaster.

Finally, the chapters of the fourth edition, although organized by general content area, have some overlap in application and the reader will see references to relevant chapters. For crosscutting emergencies, such as the response to Ebola virus disease, the reader may wish to review relevant sections of several chapters to have a comprehensive understanding of the issues. Further, the appendices have continued to grow in importance in the fourth edition as more technical resources have become available. The field has experienced enormous growth and has leveraged many of the technologies of other fields to improve preparedness. We look forward to seeing how public health preparedness continues to grow and innovate.

Appreciation

Our colleagues have been a wonderful source of knowledge, resources, and tips. As always, we are indebted to them for their help and guidance:

Bridger Berg, Brenna Carlson, and Mary Virgalitto, Children's Hospital Los Angeles, provided their expertise on the latest Ebola guidance.

Michael Colleta, Paula Yoon, Umed Ajani, Emory Meeks, and Lesliann Helmus, Centers for Disease Control and Prevention, helped shape the surveillance chapter with their review and shared the latest in disaster surveillance.

Natalie Demeter, Children's Hospital Los Angeles, graciously provided her expert research.

Marisa Derman, New York State Department of Mental Health, carefully reviewed the chapter on behavioral health, supplying critical information.

Malcolm Hardy, FEMA Region II, shared the latest material about disaster recovery.

Pamela Young Holmes, member of the National Council on Disability, provided insightful comments for the chapter on at-risk populations and ensured that the content was current on services for those who are deaf or hard of hearing.

June Issacson Kailes, pioneer in disabilities and disasters, graciously shared her updated guidance for at-risk populations and provided invaluable feedback to ensure that the fourth edition included the necessary information for individuals with disabilities and access and functional needs.

Melani Kaplan, leading advocate for the deaf and hard of hearing, shared valuable resources for individuals who are deaf or hard of hearing.

Michael Lowy, USEPA Region 2, was the source for the application of the revised drinking water standards.

Jenna Mandel-Ricci, Greater New York Hospital Association, shared both the response of New York City hospitals during Hurricane Sandy and the new regulations promulgated by the Centers for Medicare & Medicare Services.

Chris Mangal, Association of Public Health Laboratories, ensured that the description of laboratory testing for infectious agents is current.

Michael Primeau, New York State Office of Health Emergency Preparedness, provided both a helpful review of the chapter discussing the Threat and Hazard Identification and Risk Assessment process and insights about current disaster planning.

Mitchel Rosen, Office of Public Health Practice, Rutgers School of Public Health, provided an expert review of the environmental and occupational chapter, which led to the content being split into 2 chapters.

L. Vance Taylor provided invaluable perspective and feedback from the Office of Access and Functional Needs for the California Governor's Office.

Jeffrey Upperman and Henri Ford provided Rita Burke with unwavering support, trust, and encouragement.

David Abramson, Oscar Alleyne, Scott Becker, Eric Noji, and Kathleen Wright wrote much appreciated endorsements for the fourth edition.

Nicole Lurie, former Assistant Secretary of Preparedness and Response, philosophically laid out why this book is important and what the field is currently facing in her thoughtful foreword for this edition.

Much appreciation to Georges Benjamin, Ashell Alston, David Hartogs, and especially Maya Ribault for their roles in making this fourth edition the book that it is.

Finally, thanks to all those who protect the public's health and make our world more resilient.

Linda Young Landesman, DrPH, MSW
Rita V. Burke, PhD, MPH

ABOUT THE AUTHORS

Dr. Linda Young Landesman is a nationally recognized expert in emergency preparedness with a long and distinguished career in public health working as a clinician, administrator, educator, policy maker, and author. In 2012, she retired from her Assistant Vice President position at the Office of Professional Services and Affiliations, New York City Health and Hospitals Corporation (HHC). There, Dr. Landesman was responsible for managing over $870 million in workforce contracts between HHC and 5 medical schools and 4 professional medical groups, and she was responsible for the oversight, restructuring, negotiation, implementation, monitoring, and evaluation of these affiliation contracts. She was also responsible for the oversight of Graduate Medical Education and the approval of Research. Dr. Landesman was recognized for innovative work when she received an award for Business Process Improvement from the Technology Managers Forum.

At the onset of her career, Dr. Landesman practiced clinical social work in academic medical centers in Southern California. She worked with alcoholic women, families, and children who had cystic fibrosis; women with high-risk pregnancies; and families whose babies required care in the neonatal intensive care unit. Dr. Landesman was the Principal Investigator for the first national curriculum on the public health management of disasters published in 2001. This earliest curriculum was developed through a cooperative agreement with the Association of Schools of Public Health and sponsored by the Centers for Disease Control and Prevention. She developed national standards for Emergency Medical Services response and taught at the Federal Emergency Management Agency's Emergency Management Institute.

Appointments to numerous committees and community boards have included the Rye Brook Airport Advisory Committee; Regional Advisory Committee, New York Health Benefit Exchange, New York City/Metro Region; Regional Advisory Committee for the New York State Commission on Health Care Facilities for the Twenty-First Century; Commissioners' Advisory Committee, New York City Department of Health and Mental Hygiene; Advisory Committee, World Trade Center (WTC) Evacuation Study; Weapons of Mass Destruction Advisory Council, New York City Department of Public Health; Emergency Preparedness Council, HHC; Research Subcommittee, Advisory Group Subcommittee, Office of Emergency Management Subcommittee, Curriculum Subcommittee, and WTC Subcommittee at the Center for Public Health Preparedness, Mailman School of Public Health of Columbia University; Violence Prevention Subcommittee, Albert Einstein College of Medicine; Environmental Subcommittee, New York Academy of Medicine; F30 accelerated writing groups and content expert, ASTM International;

Masters of Public Health Program Community Advisory Board at Long Island University; and the Disabled in Disaster Advisory Group, Orange County, California.

Dr. Landesman is a member of the Publications Board of the American Public Health Association, a fellow at the New York Academy of Medicine, and a member of the Regional Board of the Anti-Defamation League. She has edited or authored ten books, including the landmark book *Landesman's Public Health Management of Disasters: The Practice Guide* now in its fourth edition. She has written dozens of journal articles and book chapters. Dr. Landesman earned her BA and MSW degrees from the University of Michigan. She received her DrPH in health policy and management from the Columbia University Mailman School of Public Health. Her doctoral dissertation focused on hospital preparedness for chemical accidents and won the Doctoral Dissertation Award from the Health Services Improvement Fund in 1990. She also received the Excellence in Health Administration from the Health Administration Section, American Public Health Association. Dr. Landesman is currently on the faculty of the Public Health Practice Program at the University of Massachusetts–Amherst where she teaches research methods and public health emergency management online.

Dr. Rita V. Burke is an Assistant Professor of Research Surgery and Preventive Medicine at the Keck School of Medicine at the University of Southern California and the Division of Pediatric Surgery at Children's Hospital Los Angeles. Dr. Burke leads all research efforts and provides training in both quantitative and qualitative analysis and evaluation. Previously, she worked at the Los Angeles Department of Public Health for the Acute Communicable Control Program and was part of the newly created Bioterrorism Unit. While there, she was integral in creating pandemic influenza plans for Los Angeles County and led the development of their bioterrorism detection systems.

Dr. Burke has authored over 40 peer-reviewed publications and book chapters and placed over 50 abstracts with local, state, and national conferences. She is the former co-chair of the Research Committee for the Pediatric Trauma Society, the current co-chair for the Los Angeles Children in Disaster Working Group, and the co-chair of the Disaster and Emergency Response Subcommittee of the Injury Control and Emergency Health Services section of the American Public Health Association. She is a member of the American Public Health Association, the Society for Epidemiologic Research, the American College of Epidemiology, and the Resuscitation Subcouncil for the American Red Cross Scientific Advisory Council. She is the Associate Editor for the peer-reviewed journal *Disaster Medicine and Public Health Preparedness*. She is the Principal Investigator to examine the gaps in preparedness for families with children with access and functional needs and has another grant that allows her to examine the role of faith-based organizations in disaster preparedness.

Dr. Burke received her MPH and PhD in epidemiology from the University of California, Los Angeles where she also received several competitive grants and fellowships while earning her doctorate. She currently teaches the Public Health Leadership and Management course in the masters of public health program at the University of Southern California.

CHAPTER 1

TYPES OF DISASTERS AND THEIR CONSEQUENCES

A disaster can be defined as an emergency of such severity and magnitude that the combination of deaths, injuries, illnesses, and property damage cannot be effectively managed with routine procedures or resources. These events can be caused by nature, equipment malfunction, human error, intentional acts, or biological hazards and disease. Public health agencies must be concerned about the universal risk for disaster, the increase in natural disasters across the United States, the negative impact of disasters on public health, and the likely increase of actual and potential effects of man-made disasters.[1]

A significant proportion of Americans are at risk from only 3 classes of natural disasters: floods, earthquakes, and hurricanes. An estimated 25 million to 50 million people live in floodplains that have been highly developed as living and working environments. More than 110 million people live in coastal areas of the United States, including the Great Lakes region. While most people are familiar with the San Andreas fault in California, the New Madrid fault line runs through the central part of the country and could affect more than 15 million people in 8 states (Alabama, Arkansas, Illinois, Indiana, Kentucky, Mississippi, Missouri, and Tennessee). A category 4 hurricane has an 80% chance of hitting the coastal area from Maine to Texas.

The population in America's 10 largest cities is growing faster than the population in nonurban areas, putting more people at risk if disaster strikes those urban centers. Further, using the definition of "at-risk" individuals discussed later in Chapter 11, more than 50% of the U.S. population is vulnerable to the effects of disaster. Of the 308.7 million people (2010) living in the United States, 56 million (almost 20%) have a disability, 74.2 million are children (2%), and 40.3 million (12.4%) are 65 years old or older.

Disasters pose a number of unique problems not encountered in the routine practice of emergency health care. Examples include the need for warning and evacuation; widespread urban search and rescue; triage and casualty distribution; and coordination among multiple jurisdictions, government offices, and private-sector organizations. The effective management of these concerns requires special expertise. However, public health agencies, hospitals, and other health care agencies must be able to address these situations quickly and effectively to meet the standards of federal agencies, The Joint Commission, and the regulations of the Occupational Safety and Health Administration.

1. The National Response Framework uses the terms "disaster," "emergency," and "incident." See Appendix C for an explanation of the different terms used.

Natural and Technological Disasters

Natural disasters can be categorized as either acute or gradual in their onset. They are predictable because they cluster in specific geographic areas. Natural hazards are unpreventable and, for the most part, uncontrollable. Even if quick recovery occurs, natural disasters can have long-term effects. Natural disasters with acute onsets include events such as extreme cold or blizzard; cyclone, hurricane, and typhoon; drought; earthquake; flood; heat wave; thunderstorm; tornado; tsunami; volcanic eruption; and wildfires. Some natural events can lead to technological disasters, such as the 2011 earthquake and subsequent tsunami in Japan that led to an accident at the Fukushima Daiichi Nuclear Power Plant. Natural hazards with a slow or gradual onset include drought, famine, desertification, deforestation, and pest infestation.

To keep the public informed of such disasters, the Federal Emergency Management Agency (FEMA) offers an app that sends smartphone users local alerts, weather warnings, safety tips on surviving a natural disaster, and the location of local shelters. The FEMA app is available at: https://www.fema.gov/mobile-app. The most important natural disasters and examples of their environmental effects are listed in Table 1-1.

Technological or man-made disasters include incidents such as nuclear accidents, blasts and explosions, bioterrorism, and epidemics. Increasingly, agencies involved in disasters and their management are concerned with the interactions between man and nature, which can be complex and can aggravate disasters. The severity of damage caused by natural or technological disasters is affected by population density in disaster-prone areas, local building codes, community preparedness, and the use of public safety announcements and education on how to respond correctly at the first signs of danger. Recovery following a disaster varies according to the public's access to pertinent information (such as sources of government and private aid), preexisting conditions that increase or reduce vulnerability (such as economic or biological factors), prior experience with stressful situations, and availability of sufficient savings and insurance.

Extreme Cold or Blizzard

A major winter storm can be lethal. Winter storms bring ice, snow, cold temperatures, and, often, dangerous driving conditions in the northern parts of the United States. Even small amounts of snow and ice can cause severe problems for southern states where storms are infrequent. Familiarity with winter storm warning messages such as *wind chill, winter storm watch, winter storm warning,* and *blizzard warning* can facilitate quick action by public health professionals. *Wind chill* is a calculation of how cold it feels outside when the effects of temperature and wind speed are combined. The National Weather Service uses the wind chill temperature (WCT) index to calculate potential dangers from

Table 1-1. Natural Disasters and Their Environmental Effects

Disaster	Environmental Effects
Extreme cold or blizzard	Avalanche, erosion, snow melt (flooding), loss of plant and animal life, river ice jams (flooding)
Cyclone, hurricane, and typhoon	Flooding, landslide, erosion, loss of plant and animal life
Drought	Fire, depletion of water resources, deterioration of soil, loss of plant and animal life
Earthquake	Landslide, rock fall, avalanche
Flood or thunderstorm	Heavy rainfall, fire, landslide, erosion, destruction of plant life
Heat wave	Fire, loss of plant and animal life, depletion of water resources, deterioration of soil, snow melt (flooding)
Tornado	Loss of plant and animal life, erosion, water disturbance
Tsunami	Flooding, erosion, loss of plant and animal life
Volcanic eruption	Loss of plant and animal life, deterioration of soil, air and water pollution
Wildfires	Destruction of ground cover, erosion, flooding, mudslides, long-term smog, tainted soil

winter winds and freezing temperatures. The WCT uses meteorology, biometeorology, and computer modeling as the basis of its predictions.

A *winter storm watch* indicates that severe winter weather may affect an area. A *winter storm warning* indicates that severe winter weather conditions are definitely on the way and emergency preparedness plans should be activated. A *blizzard warning* means that large amounts of falling or blowing snow and sustained winds of at least 35 miles per hour are expected for several hours.

Risk of Morbidity and Mortality

Transportation accidents are the leading cause of death during winter storms. Keys to safe winter driving include preparing vehicles for the winter season, knowing how to drive on ice and in snow, and how to react if stranded when caught in a storm or lost on the road. Morbidity and mortality associated with winter storms includes frostbite, hypothermia, carbon monoxide poisoning from using gas-powered heaters or engines in poorly ventilated areas, blunt trauma from falling objects, penetrating trauma from the use of mechanical snowblowers, and cardiovascular events usually associated with snow removal. Frostbite is a severe reaction to cold exposure that can permanently damage its victims. A loss of feeling and a white or pale appearance of fingers, toes, the nose, or earlobes are symptoms of frostbite. Hypothermia is a condition brought on when the body temperature drops to less than 90°F. Symptoms of hypothermia include uncontrollable shivering, slow speech, memory lapses, frequent stumbling, drowsiness, and exhaustion.

Water expands as it freezes, which puts tremendous pressure on whatever contains it, including metal or plastic pipes. No matter the "strength" of a container, expanding water can burst pipes and cause flooding. Flooding creates a risk for drowning and electrocution. Pipes that freeze most frequently are those that are exposed to severe cold, like outdoor hose bibs, swimming pool supply lines, water sprinkler lines, and water supply pipes in unheated interior areas like basements and crawl spaces, attics, garages, or kitchen cabinets. Pipes that run against exterior walls that have little or no insulation are also subject to freezing. Pipe freezing is a particular problem in warmer climates, where pipes often run through uninsulated or under-insulated attics or crawl spaces. A secondary risk is the loss of heat as a result of frozen pipes.

Individuals who are particularly vulnerable to exposure from freezing temperatures, such as the elderly and those with disabilities, should schedule activities outside of their home for the warmest part of the day (usually noon to 2:00 p.m.). Those paralyzed from the chest or waist down and individuals who have difficulty sensing and maintaining heat in their extremities are at risk for severe frostbite and need to protect their feet, pelvic areas, and hands because of circulation problems. It is important to dress for the weather by wearing several layers of clothing, keeping one's head, neck, and chest covered with scarves, and wearing 2 pairs of thick socks inside lined boots. Wheelchair users should wrap a blanket over their pelvic regions and limit the amount of time outside.

To enable the full functioning of driving adaptation equipment in motor vehicles, these vehicles have to warm up before the person gets in them. Service animals should wear a coat or cape underneath their regular harness and should sit or lie on a blanket in the vehicle. Dogs' paws should be protected with boots and they should be prevented from licking the boots or trying to chew off any ice since the boots could be contaminated with rock salt or other caustic deicing agents.

Pneumatic tires provide better traction for wheelchairs on icy surfaces. As an alternative, tires for dirt bikes (sold in bicycle shops) can be used. Ramps should be cleared of ice by using standard table salt, cat litter, or ice melters that are safe for pets since rock salt is poisonous to service dogs. Rock salt can also be slippery for certain types of mobility aides. Freezing rain can stick to canes, walkers, forearm cuffs, and wheelchairs, making metal parts slippery and cold to the touch. Driving gloves that grip can be helpful. When returning wheelchairs to vehicles, it is important to remove the wheelchair tires and shake the debris and ice from them. Tire rims and other metal parts need to be wiped clean of any salt or other deicing chemicals, which may cause rust on the metal parts.

Public Health Interventions

Educating communities about preventive steps that can be taken both in advance of winter and once a storm has begun will help reduce the impact. Winter storm preparation activities should include:

- Winterize homes and other buildings (i.e., insulating pipes, installing storm windows).

- Collect winter clothing and supplies such as extra blankets, warm coats and clothes, water-resistant boots, hats, and mittens.
- Assemble a disaster supplies kit containing a first aid kit, battery-powered weather radio, flashlight, and extra batteries.
- Stock canned food, a nonelectric can opener, and bottled water.
- Winterize vehicles (i.e., keep gas tank full, assemble a disaster supplies car kit).

Finally, people should avoid downed power lines during shoveling, walking, and driving because the lines might be buried in heavy snow.

Cyclone, Hurricane, and Typhoon

Cyclones, hurricanes, and typhoons are large-scale storms characterized by low pressure in the center surrounded by circular wind motion (counterclockwise in the Northern Hemisphere, clockwise in the Southern Hemisphere). Severe storms arising in the Atlantic Ocean are known as hurricanes, while those developing in the Northwest Pacific Ocean and the China Seas are called typhoons. Cyclones occur in the South Pacific and Indian Ocean. The precise classification (e.g., tropical depression, tropical storm, hurricane) depends on the wind-force (Beaufort Wind Scale), wind speed, and manner of creation.

Hurricanes are powerful storms that form at sea with wind speeds of 74 miles per hour or greater. They are tracked by satellites from the moment they begin to form, so warnings can be issued 3 to 4 days before a storm strikes. A hurricane covers a circular area between 200 and 480 miles in diameter. In the storm, strong winds and rain surround a central, calm "eye," which is about 15 miles across. Winds in a hurricane can sometimes reach 200 miles per hour. However, the greatest damage to life and property is not from the wind but from tidal surges and flash flooding. Hurricanes are rated on a 1-to-5 scale, known as the Saffir-Simpson Hurricane Wind Scale (see Table 1-2). Category 3, 4, and 5 hurricanes are considered major storms.

Owing to its violent nature, its potentially prolonged duration, and the extensive area that could be affected, the hurricane is the most devastating of all storms. The Atlantic hurricane season lasts from June 1 through November 30, but most occur in August and September. Scientists have developed a relatively good understanding of the nature of hurricanes through observation, radar, weather satellites, and computer models.

A distinctive characteristic of hurricanes is the increase in sea level, often referred to as the storm surge. This increase in sea level is the result of the low-pressure central area of the storm creating a vacuum, the storm winds piling up water, and the tremendous speed of the storm. Rare storm surges have risen as much as 14 meters (almost 46 feet) above normal sea level. They occur when the storm pushes an abnormally large mass of seawater with great force. When it reaches land, the impact of the storm surge can be exacerbated by high tide, a low-lying coastal area with a gently sloping seabed, or a semi-enclosed bay facing the ocean.

Table 1-2. Saffir-Simpson Hurricane Wind Scale

Category	Damage	Winds	Storm Surge
1	Minimal	74–95 mph	4-5 feet
2	Moderate	96–110 mph	6-8 feet
3	Extensive	111–130 mph	9–12 feet
4	Extreme	131–155 mph	13–18 feet
5	Catastrophic	156 mph+	18 feet+

The severity of a storm's impact on humans is exacerbated by deforestation, which often occurs as the result of population pressure. When trees disappear along the coastlines, the winds and the storm surges can enter the land with greater force. Deforestation on the slopes of hills and mountains increases the risk of violent flash floods and landslides caused by the heavy rain associated with tropical cyclones. At the same time, the beneficial effects of the rainfall—replenishment of the water resources—may be negated because of the inability of a forest ecosystem to absorb and retain water.

Risk of Morbidity and Mortality

Deaths and injuries from hurricanes occur because victims fail to evacuate or take shelter, do not take precautions in securing their property despite adequate warning, and do not follow guidelines on food and water safety or injury prevention during recovery. Morbidity during the storm itself results from drowning, electrocution, lacerations or punctures from flying debris, and blunt trauma from falling trees or other objects. Heart attacks and stress-related disorders can also arise during the storm or its aftermath. Gastrointestinal, respiratory, vector-borne, skin disease, and accidental pediatric poisoning can all occur during the period immediately following the cyclone. Injuries from improper use of chainsaws or other power equipment, disrupted wildlife (e.g., bites from animals, snakes, or insects), and fires are common. Fortunately, the ability to detect and track storms has helped reduce morbidity and mortality in many countries.

Injury Prevention

Public health professionals work with local emergency management agencies to prepare people to evacuate and to turn off their utilities. To avoid injury, residents should be advised to use common sense and wear proper clothing, including long-sleeved shirts, pants, and safety shoes or boots. Furthermore, they should learn proper safety precautions and operating instructions before operating gas-powered or electric chainsaws.

People should use extreme caution when using electric chainsaws to avoid electrical shock and should always wear gloves and a safety face shield or eyeglasses when using any chainsaw. Evacuees should be advised against wading in water since there may be downed power lines, broken glass, metal fragments, or other debris beneath the surface.

When returning to their dwellings after a disaster, residents should check for structural damage and electrical or natural gas or propane tank hazards. They should return to homes during the daytime and only use battery-powered flashlights and lanterns to provide light rather than candles, gas or oil lanterns, or torches (i.e., anything with an open flame).

During the recovery period, public health and local emergency management officials must ensure an adequate supply of safe water and food for the displaced population. In addition to offering acute emergency care, community plans should provide for the continuity of care for homeless residents with chronic medical conditions.

Public Health Interventions

- Conduct a needs assessment for affected communities, including a review of public health infrastructure.
- Establish active and passive surveillance systems for deaths, illnesses, and injuries.
- Educate the public about maintaining safe and adequate supplies of food and water.
- Establish environmental controls.
- Monitor infectious disease and make determinations about needed immunizations (e.g., tetanus).
- Institute multifaceted injury control programs.
- Establish protective measures against potential disease vectors.
- Monitor potential release of hazardous materials.
- Ensure evacuation plans for people with functional needs in nursing homes, hospitals, and home care.
- Work with local communities to improve building codes (e.g., developing improved designs for wind safety).

Drought

Drought affects more people than any other environmental hazard, yet it is perhaps the most complex and least understood type of all environmental hazards. Drought is often seen as the result of too little rain and used synonymously with famine. However, fluctuation in rainfall alone does not cause a famine. Drought often triggers a crisis in arid and semiarid areas where rain is already sparse and irregular, although lack of rain alone does not cause desertification. The ecosystem changes leading to desertification are all attributed to human activities, such as overcultivation, deforestation, overgrazing, and unskilled irrigation. Each of these activities is exacerbated by increasing human populations. The first 3 activities strip the soil of vegetation and deplete its organic and nutrient content. This leaves the soil exposed to the eroding forces of the sun and the wind. The subsoil that is left can become so hard that it no longer absorbs rain, and the water flows over the surface and carries away any topsoil that might have remained.

Risk of Morbidity and Mortality

Displaced populations suffer high rates of disease caused by the stress of migration, crowding, and unsanitary conditions of relocation sites. Morbidity and mortality can result from diarrheal disease, respiratory disease, and malnutrition. Malnutrition retards normal growth and is a risk factor for illness and death. Low weight-to-height is identified through the percentage of children who are 2 or more standard deviations (z-score) from the reference median compared with mean z-scores; children with edema are severely malnourished. Mortality exceeding a baseline rate of 1 death per 10,000 people per day is the index of concern.

Public Health Interventions

- Monitor health and nutritional status by assessing weights and heights.
- Assess and ensure food security, including availability, accessibility, and consumption patterns.
- Monitor death rate.
- Ensure safe water, sanitation, and disease control.

Earthquake

Earthquakes are sudden slippages or movements in a portion of the earth's crust accompanied by a series of vibrations. Aftershocks of similar or lesser intensity can follow the main quake. Earthquakes can occur at any time of the year. An earthquake is generally considered to be the most destructive and frightening of all forces of nature. Earthquake losses, like those of other disasters, tend to cause more financial impacts in industrialized countries and more injuries and deaths in undeveloped countries. In fact, more than 200,000 people died in the earthquake that struck Haiti in 2010, but less than 30,000 were dead or missing following the massive magnitude 9.0 earthquake and subsequent tsunami that devastated northern Japan in early 2011.

The Richter magnitude scale, used as an indication of the force of an earthquake, measures the magnitude and intensity or energy released by the quake. This value is calculated based on data recordings from a single observation point for events anywhere on earth, but it does not address the possible damaging effects of the earthquake. According to global observations, an average of 2 earthquakes of a Richter magnitude 8 or slightly more occur every year. A 1-digit drop in magnitude equates with a tenfold increase in frequency. Therefore, earthquakes of magnitude 7 or more generally occur 20 times in a year, and those with a magnitude 6 or more occur approximately 200 times.

Earthquakes can result in a secondary disaster: a catastrophic tsunami (see "Tsunami" below). Geologists have identified regions where earthquakes are likely to occur. With the increasing population worldwide and urban migration trends, higher death tolls and greater property losses are more likely in many areas prone to earthquakes. At least 70 million people face significant risk of death or injury from earthquakes because they live in the 39 states that are seismically active. In addition to the significant risks in California, the Pacific Northwest, Utah, and Idaho, 6 Midwestern cities with populations greater than 100,000 are located within the seismic area of the New Madrid fault. Major South American cities in which large numbers are forced to live on earthquake-prone land in structures unable to withstand damage include Lima, Peru; Santiago, Chile; Quito, Ecuador; and Caracas, Venezuela.

Risk of Morbidity and Mortality

Deaths and injuries from earthquakes vary according to the type of housing available, time of day of occurrence, and population density. Common injuries include cuts, broken bones, crush injuries, and dehydration from being trapped in rubble. Stress reactions are also common. Morbidity and mortality can occur during the actual quake, the delayed collapse of unsound structures, or cleanup activity.

Injury Prevention

Public health officials can intervene both in advance of and after earthquakes to prevent post-earthquake injuries. The safety of homes and the work environment can be improved by building standards that require stricter codes and use of safer materials. Measures to prevent injuries include securing appliances, securing hanging items on walls or overhead, turning off utilities, storing hazardous materials in safe, well-ventilated areas, and checking homes for hazards such as windows and glass that might shatter.

Public health workers should follow the recommendations listed previously under "Cyclone, Hurricane, and Typhoon."

Public Health Interventions

- Encourage earthquake drills to practice emergency procedures.
- Recommend items for inclusion in an extensive first aid kit and a survival kit for home and automobile.
- Teach basic precautions regarding safe water and safe food.
- Ensure the provision of emergency medical care to those who seek acute care in the first 3 to 5 days after an earthquake.
- Ensure continuity of care for those who have lost access to prescriptions, home care, and other medical necessities.
- Conduct surveillance for communicable disease and injuries, including location and severity of injury, disposition of patient, and follow-up contact information.
- Prepare media advisories with appropriate warnings and advice for injury prevention.
- Establish environmental controls.
- Facilitate use of surveillance forms by search and rescue teams to record type of building, address of site, type of collapse, amount of dust, presence of fire or toxic hazards, location of victim, and the nature and severity of injuries.

Flood

Global statistics show that floods are the most frequently recorded destructive events, accounting for about 30% of the world's disasters each year. The frequency of floods is increasing faster than any other type of disaster. Much of this rise in incidence can be attributed to uncontrolled urbanization, deforestation, and the effects of the El Niño and La Niña climate patterns. Floods may also accompany other natural disasters, such as storm surges during hurricanes and tsunami following earthquakes.

Except for flash floods, flooding causes few deaths. Instead, widespread and long-lasting detrimental effects include mass homelessness, disruption of communications and health care systems, and heavy loss of business, livestock, crops, and grain, particularly in densely populated, low-lying areas. The frequent repetition of flooding means a constant, or even increasing, drain on the economy for rural populations.

Risk of Morbidity and Mortality

Flood-related mortality varies from country to country. Flash flooding, such as from excessive rainfall or sudden release of water from a dam, is the cause of most flood-related deaths. Most flood victims become trapped in their cars and drown when attempting to drive through rising or swiftly moving water. Other deaths have been caused by wading, bicycling, or other recreational activities in flooded areas.

The stress and exertion required for cleanup following a flood also cause significant morbidity (mental and physical) and mortality (e.g., myocardial infarction). Fires, explosions from gas leaks, downed live wires, and debris can all cause significant injury. Waterborne diseases (e.g., enterotoxigenic *Escherichia coli [E. coli]*, *Shigella,* hepatitis A, leptospirosis, giardiasis) and contaminated waters become a significant hazard, as do other vector-borne disease and skin disorders. Injured and frightened animals, hazardous waste contamination, disruption of sewer and solid waste collection systems, molds and mildew, and dislodging of graves pose additional risks in the period following a flood. Flooding and storm surges may result in food shortages caused by water-damaged stocks. Finally, extra-long shifts can make workers and volunteers susceptible to injury.

Injury Prevention

Educating the public about the dangers of floods and about avoiding risky behaviors may prevent deaths. Since most flood-related deaths are caused by drowning in motor vehicles, educational campaigns can discuss how cars do not provide protection from moving water and that as little as 2 feet of water is capable of carrying vehicles away.

Even more important to injury and disease prevention is education regarding cleanup procedures and precautions. Rubber boots and waterproof gloves should be worn during cleanup. Walls, hard-surfaced floors, and many other household surfaces should be cleaned with soap and water and disinfected with a solution of 1 cup of bleach to 5 gallons of water. Surfaces on which food may be stored or prepared and areas in which small children play must be thoroughly disinfected. Children's toys must be disinfected prior to use or discarded. All linens and clothing must be washed in hot water or dry-cleaned. Items that cannot be washed or dry-cleaned, such as mattresses and upholstered furniture, should be air-dried in the sun and then sprayed thoroughly with a disinfectant. All carpeting must be steam-cleaned. Household materials that cannot be disinfected should be discarded.

Residents must understand that floodwater may contain fecal material from overflowing sewage systems as well as agricultural and industrial byproducts. Although skin contact with floodwater does not by itself pose a serious health risk, there is some risk of disease from eating or drinking anything contaminated with floodwater. Anyone with open cuts or sores who could be exposed to floodwater must keep these areas as clean as possible by washing with soap to control infection. Wounds that develop redness, swelling, or drainage require immediate medical attention.

Routine sanitary procedures are essential for disease prevention. Hands must be washed with soap and water that has been boiled or disinfected before preparing or eating food, after toilet use, after participating in flood cleanup activities, and after handling articles contaminated with floodwater or sewage. Children's hands should be washed frequently, and children should not be allowed to play in previously flooded areas.

Public Health Interventions

- Conduct a needs assessment to determine the status of the public health infrastructure, utilities (water, sewage, electricity), and health, medical, and pharmaceutical needs.
- Conduct surveillance of drinking water sources, injuries, increases in vector populations, and endemic, waterborne, and vector-borne disease.
- Organize the delivery of health care services, supplies, and continuity of care.
- Educate the public regarding proper sanitation and hygiene.
- Educate the public regarding proper cleanup procedures.

Heat Wave

Over time, populations can acclimatize to hot weather. However, mortality and morbidity rise when daytime temperatures remain unusually high for several days in a row and nighttime temperatures do not drop significantly. Because populations acclimatize to summer temperatures, heat waves in June and July in the United States and Europe have more of an impact than do those in August and September. There is often a delay between the onset of a heat wave and adverse health effects. Deaths occur more commonly during heat waves where there is little cooling at night and taper off to baseline levels if a heat wave is sustained. Table 1-3 lists common terms associated with heat-related conditions.

Table 1-3. Heat Wave Terms

Heat Wave: A prolonged period of excessive heat often with high humidity. The National Weather Service steps up its procedures to alert the public during heat and humidity.

Heat Index: A number in degrees Fahrenheit that tells how hot it really feels when relative humidity is added to the actual air temperature. Exposure to full sunshine can increase the heat index.

Heat Cramps: Heat cramps are muscular pains and spasms caused by heavy exertion, usually involving the abdominal muscles or legs. It is generally thought that the loss of water from heavy sweating causes the cramps.

Heat Exhaustion: Heat exhaustion typically occurs when people exercise heavily or work in a warm place where body fluids are lost through heavy sweating. Blood flow to the skin increases, causing blood flow to decrease to vital organs. This results in a form of mild shock. If not treated, the victim's condition will worsen. Body temperature will keep rising and the victim may suffer heatstroke.

Heatstroke: Heatstroke is life-threatening. The victim's temperature control system, which produces sweating to cool the body, stops working. The body temperature can rise so high that brain damage and death may result if the body is not cooled quickly.

Sunstroke: Another term for heatstroke.

Risk of Morbidity and Mortality

Heat waves result in adverse health effects in cities more than in rural areas. Those at greatest risk of adverse health outcomes include older adults, infants, those with a history of prior heatstroke, and those who are obese. Drugs that may predispose users to heatstroke include neuroleptics and anticholinergics. Heat-related morbidity and mortality come from heat cramps, heatstroke, heat exhaustion, heat syncope, myocardial infarction, loss of consciousness, dizziness, cramps, and stroke.

Injury Prevention

Residents at greatest risk must be moved to air-conditioned buildings for at least a few hours each day. All residents must maintain adequate hydration and reduce outdoor activity levels. Education campaigns should concentrate on protecting older adults and helping parents of children younger than 5 years of age understand how to protect their children from heat and to prevent heat disorders.

Public Health Interventions

- Develop an early warning surveillance system that triggers the mobilization of prevention and intervention activities.
- Identify the location of residents who might be at risk as a result of age, preexisting conditions, lack of air-conditioning, and other environmental or health factors.
- Work with utilities to educate the public about preventive actions when energy blackouts are anticipated.

Thunderstorm

A thunderstorm is formed from a combination of moisture, rapidly rising warm air, and a force capable of lifting air such as a warm or cold front, a sea breeze, or a mountain. All thunderstorms contain lightning. Thunderstorms may occur singly, in clusters, or in lines. Thus, it is possible for several thunderstorms to affect one area in the course of a few hours. Some of the most severe weather occurs when a single thunderstorm affects one area for an extended time. Thunderstorms can bring heavy rains (which can cause flash flooding), strong winds, hail, lightning, and tornadoes. Severe thunderstorms can cause extensive damage to homes and property.

Lightning is a major threat during a thunderstorm. Lightning is an electrical discharge that results from the buildup of positive and negative charges within a thunderstorm.

When the buildup becomes strong enough, lightning appears as a "bolt." This flash of light usually occurs within the clouds or between the clouds and the ground. A bolt of lightning reaches a temperature approaching 50,000°F in a split second. The rapid heating and cooling of air near the lightning causes thunder.

Although thunderstorms and lightning can be found throughout the United States, they are most likely to occur in the central and southern states. The state with the highest number of thunderstorm days is Florida. Table 1-4 identifies the terms used to alert the public about weather conditions and defines each condition.

Risk of Morbidity and Mortality

In the United States, an average of 49 people are hit and killed each year by lightning, with July being the peak month. Those who die from lightning strikes were often participating in outdoor leisure activities (i.e., fishing, camping, boating, soccer, beach activities, and golfing), ranching/farming, riding, doing yardwork, and walking outdoors. While only 10% of those struck by lightning are killed, some are left with permanent disabilities.

Morbidity is reduced if, when caught outdoors, individuals avoid items that act as natural lightning rods, such as tall isolated trees in an open area or the top of a hill and metal objects such as wire fences, golf clubs, and metal tools. It is a myth that lightning never strikes twice in the same place. In fact, lightning may strike several times in the same place during the course of one discharge.

Injury Prevention

Before going outdoors, people should be advised to check the weather forecast and postpone any outdoor activity if thunderstorms are predicted. To avoid lightning, people and their pets should find indoor shelter when they hear thunder and stay inside for 30 minutes after the last rumble. Anyone caught in an open area should not lie down flat. Those caught should crouch down in a ball-like position and try to have minimal contact with the ground. People in groups during a thunderstorm should separate to reduce the number of injuries if lightning strikes the ground. If indoors, people should not bathe, shower, wash dishes, or have any other contact with water because lightning can travel through a building's plumbing. Lightning can also travel through electrical systems, radio and television reception systems, and any metal wires or bars in concrete walls or flooring. Homes should be equipped with whole-house surge protectors to protect appliances and residents should be advised to not use anything connected to an electrical outlet. While corded phones should not be used, it is safe to use cordless or cellular phones during a thunderstorm. Finally, people should be cautioned to avoid windows, doors, and porches.

Table 1-4. Severe Weather Watches and Warnings: Definitions

Flood Watch: High flow or overflow of water from a river is possible in the given time period. It can also apply to heavy runoff or drainage of water into low-lying areas. These watches are generally issued for flooding that is expected to occur at least 6 hours after heavy rains have ended.

Flood Warning: Flooding conditions are actually occurring or are imminent in the warning area.

Flash Flood Watch: Flash flooding is possible in or close to the watch area. Flash flood watches are generally issued for flooding that is expected to occur within 6 hours after heavy rains have ended.

Flash Flood Warning: Flash flooding is actually occurring or imminent in the warning area. It can be issued as a result of torrential rains, a dam failure, or ice jam.

Tornado Watch: Conditions are conducive to the development of tornadoes in and close to the watch area.

Tornado Warning: A tornado has actually been sighted by spotters or indicated on radar and is occurring or imminent in the warning area.

Severe Thunderstorm Watch: Conditions are conducive to the development of severe thunderstorms in and close to the watch area.

Severe Thunderstorm Warning: A severe thunderstorm has actually been observed by spotters, or indicated on radar, and is occurring or imminent in the warning area.

Tropical Storm Watch: Tropical storm conditions with sustained winds from 39 to 73 miles per hour are possible in the watch area within the next 36 hours.

Tropical Storm Warning: Tropical storm conditions are expected in the warning area within the next 24 hours.

Hurricane Watch: Hurricane conditions (sustained winds greater than 73 miles per hour) are possible in the watch area within 36 hours.

Hurricane Warning: Hurricane conditions are expected in the warning area in 24 hours or less.

Public Health Interventions

- Work with emergency management on weather alerts that include preventive actions that people can take.
- Educate people on how to protect themselves from being struck by lightning.
- Conduct surveillance on the impacts of lightning strikes.

Tornado

Tornadoes are rapidly whirling, funnel-shaped air spirals that emerge from a violent thunderstorm and reach the ground. Tornadoes can have a wind velocity of up to 200 miles per hour and generate sufficient force to destroy even massive buildings. The average circumference of a tornado is a few hundred meters, and it is usually exhausted before traveling as far as 20 kilometers (12.4 miles). Severity in the United States is rated on the Enhanced Fujita (EF) Scale, which estimates wind speed based on the damage caused. When using the EF-Scale to determine a tornado's EF-rating, investigators assess both the destruction caused by the storm against 28 Damage Indicators (e.g., 1 or 2 family residences, high-rise building) and the Degree of Damage (e.g., loss of roof covering, all walls collapsed). The EF-Scale uses a scoring system of EF-0 (no damage) to EF-5 (total destruction). The extent of damage depends on updrafts within the tornado funnel, the tornado's atmospheric pressure (which is often lower than the surrounding barometric pressure), and the effects of flying debris.

Risk of Morbidity and Mortality

Approximately 1,000 tornadoes occur annually in the United States, and none of the lower 48 states is immune. Certain geographic areas are at greater risk as a result of their recurrent weather patterns; tornadoes most frequently occur in the Midwestern and Southeastern states. Although tornadoes often develop in the late afternoon and more often from March through May, they can arise at any hour of the day and during any month of the year.

Injuries from tornadoes occur because of flying debris or people being thrown by the high winds (i.e., head injury, soft tissue injury, secondary wound infection). Stress-related disorders are more common, as are diseases related to loss of utilities, potable water, or shelter.

Injury Prevention

Because tornadoes can occur so quickly, communities should develop redundant warning systems (such as media alerts and automated telephone warnings), establish protective shelter to reduce tornado-related injuries, and practice tornado-shelter drills. In the event of a tornado, the residents should take shelter in a basement if possible, away from windows, while protecting their heads. Special outreach should be made to people with functional needs to assist them in making a list of their limitations, capabilities, and medications and in readying an emergency kit of needed supplies. People with functional needs should have a "buddy" who has a copy of the list and who knows of the emergency kit. For more information on functional needs, see Chapter 11.

Other precautions include those listed under "Cyclone, Hurricane, and Typhoon."

Public Health Interventions

- Work with emergency management on tornado shelter drills for vulnerable communities.
- Conduct a needs assessment using maps that detail preexisting neighborhoods, including landmarks, and aerial reconnaissance.
- Ensure the provision of medical care, shelter, food, and water.

- Establish environmental controls.
- Establish a surveillance system based at both clinical sites and shelters.

Tsunami

Tsunami, a series of waves of very great length and period, are usually generated by large earthquakes under or near the oceans and close to the edges of the tectonic plates. These waves may travel long distances, increase in height abruptly when they reach shallow water, and cause great devastation far away from the source. Submarine landslides and volcanic eruptions beneath the sea or on small islands can also be responsible for tsunami, but their effects are usually limited to smaller areas. Volcanic tsunami are usually of greater magnitude than are seismic ones; waves of more than 40 meters (131.2 feet) in height have been witnessed. The effects of a tsunami can vary greatly, ranging from being barely noticeable to total destruction. Tsunamis are often called tidal waves because they can act like a tide of violent rushing water rather than the surf that normally comes to shore. These waves are often powerful enough to move through any obstacle. Damage is caused by massive amounts of water that follow the initial wave and the powerful flooding that results from the quickly rising water.

While tsunamis are neither preventable or predictable, there are warning signs. Any of the following events may signal an approaching tsunami:

- A strong earthquake;
- Large quantities of gas rise to the surface of the ocean, giving it the appearance of "boiling";
- The ocean water is hot;
- The ocean water smells like "rotten eggs";
- The ocean water stings the skin;
- There is a sound of thunder followed by a roaring airplane, a helicopter, or a whistling;
- The ocean water may recede a great distance from the coast; and/or
- Red light might be visible near the horizon and, as the wave approaches, the top of the wave may glow red.

Risk of Morbidity and Mortality

The floods that accompany a tsunami result in potential health risks from both contaminated water and food supplies. Potential waterborne diseases that follow tsunamis include diarrheal or fecal oral diseases (i.e., cholera, amebiasis, *Campylobacter*, cryptosporidiosis, cyclosporiasis, giardiasis, hepatitis A and E, leptospirosis, parasitic diseases, rotavirus, shigellosis, typhoid and paratyphoid fevers). The risk of communicable diseases after flooding, such as occurs in tsunami, varies as follows:

- Person-to-person spread is medium risk.
- Food-borne illness (i.e., *E. coli*, infectious hepatitis, Salmonella) is medium risk.
- Waterborne illness is high risk.

In addition, tsunami victims can develop illness from exposure to animals or mosquitoes, (i.e., rabies, malaria, Japanese encephalitis, dengue, and dengue hemorrhagic fever), respiratory illness, and wound-associated infections and diseases (i.e., tetanus). Finally, the behavioral health consequences can be significant.

Most deaths from tsunamis are related to drownings, but traumatic injuries (i.e., cuts, abrasions, broken limbs, head injuries) are common due to the impact of people being washed into debris. Polymicrobial wound infections are not uncommon (i.e., Aeromonas species, *E. coli, Klebsiella pneumoniae, Pseudomonas aeruginosa*), some of which are resistant to all antibiotics.

With the loss of shelter, people are vulnerable to exposure to insects, heat, and other environmental hazards. Further, the lack of medical care may result in exacerbations of chronic illness, such as cardiac disease, hypertension, diabetes, and asthma.

Injury Prevention

Warning systems have been developed that can detect tsunamis before the wave hits land. Some systems advise residents where to evacuate to avoid an incoming tsunami. One of the earliest warnings comes from animals, who run to higher ground before the water arrives. Other mitigating actions include building high walls in front of populated coastal areas or redirecting the incoming water via floodgates and channels. However, the effectiveness of these strategies can be limited since tsunamis, such as the Indian Ocean tsunamis in 2005, can be higher than these barriers.

Public Health Interventions

In the immediate aftermath of a tsunami, primary concerns include the rescue of survivors, the provision of health care with an infusion of supplies and personnel, and the provision of behavioral health and social support services. The effects of tsunamis are prolonged and require extended surveillance of infectious and water- or insect-transmitted diseases. The prevention and control of disease includes the following actions:

- Provide food, clean water, and shelter.
- Ensure proper hand washing and sewage disposal.

- Ensure proper handling of water and food (see Appendix I for information on common food-borne diseases), including:
  - avoiding preparing food directly in areas surrounded by floodwater,
  - separating raw and cooked food,
  - cooking food thoroughly,
  - keeping food at safe temperatures, and
  - using safe water.
- Provide needed medical care, including oral rehydration therapy for diarrheal illnesses.
- Wear appropriate protective clothing during rescue and cleanup operations. Avoid entering contaminated water.
- Provide vaccinations where appropriate (i.e., hepatitis, Strep, pneumonia, measles, meningitis, dengue, Japanese encephalitis, and yellow fever).
- Ensure mosquito control by providing insecticide-treated nets, bedding, and clothing and by the emptying of containers with standing water.

Volcanic Eruption

Volcanic activity involves the explosive eruption or flow of rock fragments and molten rock in various combinations of hot or cold, wet or dry, and fast or slow. Extremely high temperature and pressure cause the mantle, located deep inside the earth between the molten iron core and the thin crust at the surface, to melt and become liquid rock or magma. When a large amount of magma is formed, it rises through the denser rock layers of the crust toward the earth's surface. Magma that has reached the surface is called lava. Volcanic hazards vary in severity depending on the size and extent of the eruption and whether the eruption is occurring in a populated area. Volcanoes are classified by similar characteristic behavior, with eruptions called "Strombolian," "Vulcanian," "Vesuvian," "Pelean," "Hawaiian," and more. When active, volcanoes may exhibit only one characteristic type of eruption or a sequence of types.

A volcano may begin to show signs of unrest several months to a few years before an eruption. Accurate long-term predictions that specify when and where an eruption is most likely to occur and what type and size eruption should be expected are not possible. Warnings that an eruption is hours to days away are possible because volcanic eruptions are preceded by such changes as earthquake activity, ground deformation, and gas emissions over a period of days to weeks.

In the United States, volcano warnings are made through a series of alert levels that correspond generally to increasing levels of volcanic activity. Each increase in the alert level helps authorities gauge and coordinate their response to a developing volcano emergency.

Depending on the location of the volcano (e.g., California, Alaska, Pacific Northwest, or Hawaii), different alert levels[2] are used to provide volcano warnings and emergency information regarding volcanic unrest and eruptions. Different alert levels are used because volcanoes exhibit different patterns of unrest in the weeks to hours before they erupt, differing volcano hazards require a warning scheme that addresses specific volcano hazards, and there is variability in the intensity of monitoring U.S. volcanoes. The Volcanic Explosivity Index (VEI) is the eruption magnitude scale used to rate the eruption. The VEI considers the plume height, volume of magma, classification, and how often the volcano in question erupts. The VEI ranges from VEI 0 to VEI 8. Any eruption that occurs anywhere will rate at least a VEI 0 on the scale, which is defined as having less than 10,000 cubic meters of ejecta, the combination of lava and ash. VEI 3 volcanoes have as much as 100 million cubic meters of ejecta. A VEI 8 volcano spews out a minimum of 1 trillion cubic meters of ejecta.

Risk of Morbidity and Mortality

Many kinds of volcanic activity can endanger the lives of people and property located both close to and far away from a volcano. The range of adverse health effects is quite broad and extensive. Immediate, acute, and nonspecific irritant effects have been reported in the eyes (e.g., corneal abrasions), nose, skin, and upper airways of persons exposed to volcanic dusts and ash particles. Victims can experience exacerbation of their asthma symptoms and can asphyxiate as a result of inhalation of ash or gases. There is the potential of injuries from blasts and projectile of rock fragments. Lacerations can occur if sound waves shatter windows and break glass. Volcanic flow can set homes on fire, causing thermal injuries including death. Victims can experience trauma from fallen trees or rocks or the collapse of buildings under the weight of the ash. Foraging animals may be unable to find adequate supply of food or water. Indoor air radon levels may be elevated. Flooding and pooling of water secondary to debris or obstruction of waterways can lead to spread of infectious disease. Finally, victims can experience anxiety, depression, or post-traumatic stress disorder.

Public Health Interventions

- Collaborate with emergency management specialists to develop effective warning schemes.
- Participate in volcano emergency planning workshops and emergency response exercises.
- Prepare educational materials, including fact sheets, booklets, video programs, and maps.

---

2. Also referred to as status levels, condition levels, or color code.

- Designate areas for evacuation and evacuate when indicated.
- Provide emergency air monitoring equipment for detecting toxic gases.
- Stockpile and distribute masks and eye shields or goggles where indicated.
- Prepare for the breakdown of water systems.
- Encourage people to remain inside sturdy houses with shuttered windows when evacuation is not indicated or possible.
- Encourage people to strengthen building roofs with supports or take shelter in the most resistant part of the building.
- Encourage people to stay indoors during the worst conditions.

Wildfires

More and more people are building their homes in woodland settings in or near forests, rural areas, or remote mountain sites. As residential areas expand into relatively untouched wildlands, these communities are increasingly threatened by forest fires. Protecting structures in the wildlands from fire poses special problems and can stretch firefighting resources to the limit. Wildfires often begin unnoticed and can spread quickly, igniting brush, trees, and homes.

There are 3 different classes of wildfires. A *surface fire* is the most common type and burns along the floor of a forest, moving slowly and killing or damaging trees. A *ground fire* is usually started by lightning and burns on or below the forest floor in the humus layer down to the mineral soil. *Crown fires* spread rapidly by wind and move quickly by jumping along the tops of trees. Depending on prevailing winds and the amount of water in the environment, wildfires can quickly spread out of control, causing extensive damage to personal property and human and animal life. If heavy rains follow a fire, other natural disasters can occur, including landslides, mudflows, and floods. Once ground cover has been burned away, little is left to hold soil in place on steep slopes and hillsides, and erosion becomes one of several potential problems. A major wildland fire can leave a large amount of scorched and barren land, and these areas often do not return to prefire conditions for decades. Danger zones include all wooded, brush, and grassy areas—especially those in Kansas, Mississippi, Louisiana, Georgia, Florida, the Carolinas, Tennessee, California, Massachusetts, and the national forests of the western United States.

Risk of Morbidity and Mortality

Morbidity and mortality associated with wildfires include burns, inhalation injuries, respiratory complications, and stress-related cardiovascular events (i.e., exhaustion and myocardial infarction from fighting or fleeing the fire).

Public Health Interventions

More than 4 out of every 5 wildfires are started by people. Negligent human behavior, such as smoking in forested areas or improperly extinguishing campfires, is the cause of many forest fires. Another cause of forest fires is lightning. Prevention efforts include working with the fire service to educate people to:

- Build fires away from nearby trees or bushes. Ash and cinders are lighter than air and may float or be blown into areas with a heavy fuel load and start wildfires.
- Be prepared to extinguish fires quickly and completely. If a fire becomes threatening, it needs to be extinguished immediately.
- Never leave any fire—even a lit cigarette—burning unattended. Fire can quickly spread out of control.
- Encourage the development of a family wildfire evacuation plan if your community is at risk for wildfire.

Summary of Effects

Table 1-5 summarizes the types of short-term effects that occur following major natural disasters, and Table 1-6 identifies common environmental impacts caused by natural disasters.

Man-Made and Technological Disasters

Man-made and technological disasters are unpredictable, can spread across geographic boundaries, may be unpreventable, and may have limited physical damage but long-term effects. Some disasters in this class are entirely man-made, such as terrorism. Other technological disasters occur because industrial sites are located in communities affected by natural disasters, equipment failures occur, or workers have inadequate training or fatigue and make errors. The threat of terrorism is categorized as a potential technological disaster and includes bombings, civil and political disorders, economic emergencies, and riots.

Technological disasters include a broad range of incidents. Some are accidental and unintentional such as airplane crashes, hazardous materials spills, nuclear accidents, oil spills, and train derailments. Others are intentional and deliberate, such as terrorist acts. Intentional disasters include biological, chemical, explosives, nuclear, and radiological attacks. Routes of exposure are through water, food and drink, airborne releases, fires

Table 1-5. Short-Term Effects of Major Natural Disasters

Effect	Earthquakes	High Winds (Without Flooding)	Tidal Waves/ Flash Floods	Slow-Onset Floods	Landslides	Volcanoes
Deaths[a]	Many	Few	Many	Few	Many	Many
Severe injuries requiring extensive treatment	Many	Moderate	Few	Few	Few	Few
Increased risk of communicable diseases	Potential risk following all major disasters (probability rising with overcrowding and deteriorating sanitation)					
Damage to health facilities	Severe (structure and equipment)	Severe	Severe but localized	Severe (equipment only)	Severe but localized	Severe (structure and equipment)
Damage to water systems	Severe	Light	Severe	Light	Severe but localized	Severe
Food shortage	Rare (may occur due to economic and logistic factors)		Common	Common	Rare	
Major population movements	Rare (may occur in heavily damaged urban areas)		Common (generally limited)			

Source: Reprinted with permission from Pan American Health Organization (PAHO). 2000. *Natural Disasters: Protecting the Public's Health*. Table 1.1. Washington, DC: PAHO.

[a]Potential lethal impact in absence of preventive measures.

Table 1-6. Most Common Effects of Specific Events on Environmental Health

	Earthquake	Hurricane	Flood	Tsunami	Volcanic Eruption
Water Supply and Wastewater Disposal					
Damage to civil engineering structures	1	1	1	3	1
Broken mains	1	2	2	1	1
Damage to water sources	1	2	2	3	1
Power outages	1	1	2	2	1
Contamination (biological or chemical)	2	1	1	1	1
Transportation failures	1	1	1	2	1
Personnel shortages	1	2	2	3	1
System overload (due to population shifts)	3	1	1	3	1
Equipment, parts, and supply shortage	1	1	1	2	1
Solid Waste Handling					
Damage to civil engineering structures	1	2	2	3	1
Transportation failures	1	1	1	2	1
Equipment shortages	1	1	1	2	1
Personnel shortages	1	1	1	3	1
Water, soil, and air pollution	1	1	1	2	1
Food Handling					
Spoilage of refrigerated food	1	1	2	2	1
Damage to food preparation facilities	1	1	2	3	1
Transportation failures	1	1	1	2	1
Power outages	1	1	1	3	1
Flooding of facilities	3	1	1	1	3
Contamination/degradation of relief supplies	2	1	1	2	1
Vector Control					
Proliferation of vector breeding sites	1	1	1	1	3
Increase in human/vector contacts	1	1	1	2	1
Disruption in vector-borne disease control programs	1	1	1	1	1
Home Sanitation					
Destruction or damage to structures	1	1	1	1	1
Contamination of water and food	2	2	1	2	1
Disruption of power, heating, fuel, water, or supply waste disposal services	1	1	1	2	1
Overcrowding	3	3	3	3	2

Source: Reprinted with permission from Pan-American Health Organization (PAHO). 2000. *Natural Disasters: Protecting the Public's Health.* Table 8.1. Washington, DC: PAHO.

Note: 1 = severe possible effect; 2 = less severe possible effect; 3 = least or no possible effect.

Table 1-7. Health Consequences of Exposure to Chemical Agents

Chemical Agent	Health Effects
Nerve agents	Miosis, rhinorrhea, dyspnea
Vesicants	Erythema, blisters, eye irritation, cough, dyspnea
Cyanide	Loss of consciousness, seizures, apnea
Pulmonary CG (phosgene)	Dyspnea, coughing

and explosions, and hazardous materials or waste released into the environment from a fixed facility or during transport. Building or bridge collapse, transportation crashes, dam or levee failure, nuclear reactor accidents, and breaks in water, gas, or sewer lines are other examples of unintentional technological disasters.

Risk of Morbidity and Mortality

Communities in which industrial sites are located or through which hazardous materials pass via highway, rail, or pipeline are at risk for technological disasters. Injuries can occur to workers at the site, responders bringing the incident under control and providing emergency medical care, and residents in the community. Those with preexisting medical conditions, such as lung or heart disease, could be at increased risk for negative health outcomes if exposed to toxic releases. Burns, skin disorders, and lung damage can result from exposure to specific industrial agents. Table 1-7 lists the health consequences of several classes of toxins.

Injury Prevention

Ensuring that local industry implements basic safety procedures can significantly reduce negative health outcomes from accidental releases of toxins. Emergency preparedness—including the ability of prehospital and hospital systems to care for patients exposed to industrial agents, the training of medical personnel to work in contaminated environments, and the stockpiling of personal protective equipment for responders—is key to providing care following industrial accidents or acts of bioterrorism. Government agencies, in coordination with hospitals and public health, should conduct computer simulations or field exercises to test the community's ability to evacuate those at risk and the ability of the health sector to provide care to those exposed to accidental releases. Information about the clinical management of exposure to toxins can be provided by poison control centers, CHEMTREC, and industry databases.

Following nuclear accidents involving radioactive iodine it is possible to protect the thyroid gland from radiation injury. The U.S. Food and Drug Administration approved both a tablet and liquid form of potassium iodide (KI) that people can take by mouth to help block radioactive iodine from being absorbed by the thyroid gland. The tablets come in 2 strengths, 130 milligram (mg) and 65 mg and are scored so that they may be cut into smaller pieces with lower doses. Each milliliter (mL) of the liquid solution contains 65 mg of KI.

Public Health Interventions

- Take a visible role in community planning.
- Provide emergency services and medical care to victims.
- Activate the health alert network.
- Conduct hazard assessments.
- Review material safety data sheets for industrial agents produced, stored, or used locally and regionally to evaluate the range of potential adverse health effects.
- Conduct vulnerability analyses to identify target populations and potential adverse public health consequences.
- Conduct a risk assessment to determine if specific industrial agents will reach toxic levels in the vicinity of vulnerable populations.
- Determine the minimal thresholds of exposure for specific industrial agents that would trigger an evacuation.
- Gather information on chemical neutralization, estimation models of plume dispersion, and appropriate antidotes.
- Work with local hospitals to stockpile appropriate antidotes, medications, and supplies.
- Stockpile KI in communities located within 10 miles of nuclear reactor sites and follow CDC guidelines (available at: https://emergency.cdc.gov/radiation/ki.asp#who). The FDA recommends the following doses after internal contamination with (or likely internal contamination with) radioactive iodine:
    - Newborns from birth to 1 month of age should be given 16 mg (¼ of a 65 mg tablet or ¼ mL of solution). This dose is for both nursing and nonnursing newborn infants.
    - Infants and children between 1 month and 3 years of age should take 32 mg (½ of a 65 mg tablet or ½ mL of solution). This dose is for both nursing and nonnursing infants and children.
    - Children between 3 and 18 years of age should take 65 mg (one 65 mg tablet or 1 mL of solution). Children who are adult size (i.e., those who weigh 150 pounds or more) should take the full adult dose, regardless of their age.

- Adults should take 130 mg (one 130 mg tablet or two 65 mg tablets or 2 mL of solution).
- Women who are breastfeeding should take the adult dose of 130 mg.

Blasts and Explosions

Explosions can inflict multisystem life-threatening injuries on many persons simultaneously. Multiple factors contribute to the injury patterns that result from blasts. Contributing factors include the composition and amount of the materials involved, the environment in which the event occurs, the method of delivery (e.g., a bomb), the distance between the victim and the blast, and the absence or presence of protective barriers or environmental hazards in the area of the blast. To predict subsequent demand for medical care and resources needed, it is useful to remember that post-blast, half of the initial casualties will seek medical care during the first hour. Those with minor injuries often arrive before the most severely injured because they go directly to the closest hospitals using whatever transportation is available. Furthermore, when the explosion has resulted in a structural collapse, victims will be more severely injured and their rescue can occur over prolonged time periods.

The 2 types of explosives, high-order explosives (HEs) and low-order explosives (LEs), cause different injury patterns. Injury patterns also differ whether the bombs are manufactured or improvised. HE devices, such as TNT, C-4, Semtex, nitroglycerin, dynamite, and ammonium nitrate fuel oil, produce a defining supersonic overpressurization shock wave. LE devices, such as pipe bombs, gunpowder, and pure petroleum-based bombs (e.g., Molotov cocktails), create a subsonic explosion and lack the overpressurization wave. Manufactured explosives are usually those used by the military, mass produced, and quality tested as weapons. Improvised explosives and incendiary (fire) bombs are often individually produced in small quantities and include devices used differently from their initial purpose.

Risk of Morbidity and Mortality

The most common injury for survivors of explosions is penetrating and blunt trauma. Blast lung is the most common fatal injury among initial survivors. Explosions in confined spaces (e.g., mines, buildings, or large vehicles) and structural collapse are associated with the greatest morbidity and mortality. Blast injuries can occur to any body system: auditory, digestive, circulatory, central nervous system, extremities, renal, and respiratory. Up to 10% of all blast survivors have significant eye injuries. These injuries can occur with minimal discomfort initially and patients can seek care days, weeks, or

Table 1-8. Mechanisms of Blast Injury

Category	Characteristics	Body Part Affected	Types of Injuries
Primary	Unique to HE, results from the impact of the overpressurization wave with body surfaces	Gas-filled structures are most susceptible—lungs, gastrointestinal tract, and middle ear	Blast lung (pulmonary barotrauma) Tympanic membrane rupture and middle ear damage Abdominal hemorrhage and perforation Globe (eye) rupture Concussion (traumatic brain injury without physical signs of head injury)
Secondary	Results from flying debris and bomb fragments	Any body part may be affected	Penetrating ballistic (fragmentation) or blunt injuries Eye penetration (can be occult)
Tertiary	Results from individuals being thrown by the blast wind	Any body part may be affected	Fracture and traumatic amputation Closed and open brain injury
Quaternary	All explosion-related injuries, illnesses, or diseases not due to primary, secondary, or tertiary mechanisms Includes exacerbation or complications of existing conditions	Any body part may be affected	Burns (flash, partial, and full thickness) Crush injuries Closed and open brain injury Asthma, chronic obstructive pulmonary disease, or other breathing problems from dust, smoke, or toxic fumes Angina, hyperglycemia, hypertension

Source: Reprinted from Centers for Disease Control and Prevention (CDC). 2006. *Explosions and Blast Injuries: A Primer for Clinicians*. Table 1. Mechanisms of blast injury. Atlanta, GA: CDC. Available at: http://www.cdc.gov/masstrauma/preparedness/primer.pdf. Accessed December 29, 2016.

even months after the event. Symptoms can include eye pain or irritation, foreign body sensation, altered vision, periorbital swelling, or contusions. Clinical findings in the gastrointestinal tract may be absent until the onset of complications. Victims can also experience tinnitus or temporary or permanent deafness from blasts.

Table 1-8 describes the 4 basic mechanisms of blast injury and Table 1-9 provides an overview of explosive-related injuries.

Public Health Interventions

- As part of a community preparedness plan, identify the medical institutions and personnel who can provide the emergency care that will be required, including otologic assessment and audiometry, burn and trauma centers, hyperbaric oxygen chamber, and so forth.

- Ensure that the community preparedness plan includes a structure for surge capacity. To estimate the "first wave" of casualties, double the number appearing for care in the first hour. Prepare written communications and instructions for victims who may experience temporary or permanent deafness.
- Work with the regional emergency management organization, police, fire, and emergency medical services to have a plan in place to identify potential toxic exposures and environmental hazards for which the health department will need to help protect responders in the field and the community.
- Establish a victim identification registry with the hospital community.
- Plan for the reception of and intervention with family and friends with the mental health community.

Epidemics

The spread of infectious disease depends on preexisting levels of the disease, ecological changes resulting from disaster, population displacement, changes in density of population, disruption of public utilities, interruption of basic public health services, and compromises to sanitation and hygiene. The risk that epidemics of infectious diseases will

Table 1-9. Overview of Explosive-Related Injuries

System or Area	Injury or Condition
Auditory	Tympanic membrane rupture, ossicular disruption, cochlear damage, foreign body
Eyes, orbits, face	Perforated globe, foreign body, air embolism, fractures
Respiratory	Blast lung, hemothorax, pneumothorax, pulmonary contusion and hemorrhage, arterioventricular fistulas (source of air embolism), airway epithelial damage, aspiration pneumonitis, sepsis
Digestive	Bowel perforation, hemorrhage, ruptured liver or spleen, sepsis, mesenteric ischemia from air embolism
Circulatory	Cardiac contusion, myocardial infarction from air embolism, shock, vasovagal hypotension, peripheral vascular injury, air embolism-induced injury
Central nervous system	Concussion, closed and open brain injury, stroke, spinal cord injury, air embolism-induced injury
Renal	Renal contusion, laceration, acute renal failure due to rhabdomyolysis, hypotension, and hypovolemia
Extremities	Traumatic amputation, fractures, crush injuries, compartment syndrome, burns, cuts, lacerations, acute arterial occlusion, air embolism-induced injury

Source: Adapted from Centers for Disease Control and Prevention (CDC). 2006. *Explosions and Blast Injuries: A Primer for Clinicians*. Table 2. Overview of explosive-related injuries. Atlanta, GA: CDC. Available at: http://www.cdc.gov/masstrauma/preparedness/primer.pdf. Accessed December 29, 2016.

occur is proportional to the population density and displacement. A true epidemic can occur in susceptible populations in the presence or impending introduction of a disease agent compounded by the presence of a mechanism that facilitates large-scale transmission (e.g., contaminated water supply or vector population).

Quick response is essential because epidemics, which result in human and economic losses and political difficulties, often arise rapidly. An epidemic or threatened epidemic can become an emergency when the following characteristics of the events are present:

- Risk of introduction to and spread of the disease in the population
- Large number of cases may reasonably be expected to occur
- Disease involved is of such severity as to lead to serious disability or death
- Risk of social or economic disruption resulting from the presence of the disease
- Authorities are unable to cope adequately with the situation because of insufficient technical or professional personnel, organizational experience, and necessary supplies or equipment (e.g., drugs, vaccines, laboratory diagnostic materials, vector-control materials)
- Risk of international transmission

Not all of these characteristics need be present and must be assessed with regard to relative importance locally.

The categorization of "emergency" differs from country to country, depending on 2 local factors: whether the disease is endemic and a means of transmitting the agent exists. Table 1-10 describes epidemic emergencies for particular diseases listed in nonendemic areas.

Public Health Interventions

- Control or prevent epidemic situations.
- Conduct surveillance to identify when an epidemic is likely to occur.
- Ensure that items requiring refrigeration, such as vaccines, are kept refrigerated throughout the chain of distribution.
- Monitor the maintenance of immunization programs against childhood infectious diseases (e.g., measles, mumps, polio).

Table 1-10. Epidemic Emergencies Defined

Disease	Nonendemic Areas	Endemic Areas
Cholera	One confirmed indigenous case	Significant increase in incidence over and above what is normal for the season, particularly if multifocal and accompanied by deaths in children younger than 10 years old
Giardiasis	A cluster of cases in a group of tourists returning from an endemic area	A discrete increase in incidence linked to a specific endemic place
Malaria	A cluster of cases, with an increase in incidence in a defined geographic area	Rarely an emergency; increased incidence requires program strengthening
Meningococcal meningitis	An incidence rate of 1 per 1,000 in 1 week in a defined geographic area	The same rate for 2 consecutive weeks is an emergency
Plague	One confirmed case apparently linked by domestic rodent or respiratory transmission or by a rodent epizootic	A cluster of cases
Rabies	One confirmed case of animal rabies in a previously rabies-free locale	Significant increases in animal and human cases
Salmonellosis	A large cluster of cases in a limited area, with a single or predominant stereotype (e.g., specific event or restaurant), or a significant number of cases occurring in multiple foci, apparently related by a common source (such as a specific food product)	
Smallpox	Any strongly suspected case	N/A
Typhus fever/ rickettsia	One confirmed case in a louse-infested, nonimmune population	Significant increase in number of cases in a limited period of time
Viral encephalitis	Cluster of time- and space-related cases in a nonimmune population (a single case should be regarded as a warning)	Significant increase in the number of cases with a mosquito-borne single, identified etiological agent in a limited period
Viral hemorrhagic fever	One confirmed indigenous or imported case with an etiological single agent with which person-to-person transmission may occur in a limited period of time	Significant increase in the number of cases with an identified etiological agent
Yellow fever	One confirmed case in a community	Significant increase in the number of cases in a population and an adequate/limited period of time for vector population to increase

CHAPTER 2

ROLE AND RESPONSIBILITY OF PUBLIC HEALTH

Public health professionals take responsibility for community health in both disaster preparedness and response. The Homeland Security Presidential Directive 21 (HSPD-21) defines public health and medical preparedness as "the existence of plans, procedures, policies, training, and equipment necessary to maximize the ability to prevent, respond to, and recover from major events, including efforts that result in the capability to render an appropriate public health and medical response that will mitigate the effects of illness and injury, limit morbidity and mortality to the maximum extent possible, and sustain societal, economic, and political infrastructure." Since HSPD-21 was issued in 2007, the implementation of these responsibilities has evolved as our country learned from each subsequent catastrophic disaster. Future disasters are likely to provide unforeseen lessons. This chapter discusses the role and responsibility of public health professionals, public health and health care capabilities, carrying out public health responsibilities, incident action plans, personnel requirements, applicable laws, and the functional model of public health response.

Public Health Role

Prevention

- Provide education regarding what to expect in a disaster and how to deal with effects of a disaster.

Protection

- Coordinate, plan, and administer public health response.
- Develop an all-hazards public health emergency response plan.
- Collaborate with and participate in the exchange of health information both prior to and during a disaster.

Mitigation

- Assure that primary health, public health, mental health, and social impacts are adequately addressed in disaster planning.
- Identify the potential hazards, vulnerabilities, risks, and necessary community resources applicable to the physical, social, and psychosocial effects of disaster.
- Identify groups most at risk from disaster (e.g., children, older adults, homeless, chronically ill, homebound, physically or mentally disabled).
- Consult with health care systems and facilities to determine the magnitude and extent of public health and medical problems and the assistance needed.
- Develop and advocate public policies designed to reduce the public health impact.
- Disseminate critical health and safety information to alert about potential health risks and ways to reduce the risk of exposure to ongoing and potential hazards.
- Disseminate information in languages and formats that account for demographics, at-risk populations, economic disadvantages, limited language proficiency, and cultural or geographical isolation.

Response

- Take responsibility for the health of a community following a disaster.
- Prevent disease by providing health advisories on injury prevention, food and water safety, and vector control.
- Coordinate public health interventions, including dispensing of antibiotics, vaccinations, and issuing social distancing requirements (e.g., quarantine, isolation).
- Conduct and oversee data collection, analysis, interpretation, and management of public health-related data for surveillance, epidemiological, and environmental investigation.
- Use such resources as assessment, epidemiology, and data analysis to make and implement recommendations for limiting morbidity and mortality following a disaster.
- Use public health laboratories to assess biological, chemical, and radiation samples and determine threats.
- Assure that health services continue postimpact, including acute care, continuity of care, primary care, and emergency care.
- Provide information on cleanup and contamination.
- Communicate with government officials about the public health effects of potential disasters and provide expert assistance during and after disasters.

Recovery

- Assess the impact of an incident on the public health system to determine and prioritize the recovery needs of the public health, medical, or mental/behavioral health systems.
- Provide access to health services, medication and consumable medical supplies (e.g., hearing aid batteries and incontinence supplies), and durable medical equipment.
- Carry out responsibilities delineated in Emergency Support Function (ESF) #6: Mass Care, Emergency Assistance, Temporary Housing, and Human Services, including an environmental health and safety assessment of congregate shelters and feeding operations.
- Request, recruit, and credential health and medical volunteers through established programs.
- Work with local authorities on the management of fatalities.
- Collaborate with other health and human service professionals to rigorously evaluate intervention outcomes.

Local public health authorities, working with their hospital-based colleagues, have the primary responsibility for the health of a community following a disaster. Health departments are usually not the lead in responding to a disaster and function as part of the community's emergency response effort, as part of the emergency operations plans, procedures, guidelines, and incident management system used by your community. This requires collaboration with federal partners—such as the U.S. Department of Health & Human Services' Office of the Assistant Secretary for Preparedness and Response (ASPR) and the Centers for Disease Control and Prevention (CDC)—nongovernmental organizations, state and governmental offices, utilities, and others.

These professionals bring unique resources to the emergency management community that can limit morbidity and mortality caused by both natural and technological disasters. In fact, the contributions of public health authorities to community disaster preparations and response represent an extension of their normal activities. Public health officials are knowledgeable about the prevention of infectious disease and injury, routinely conduct surveillance for infectious disease, maintain working relationships with other agencies within the health sector, have governmental jurisdiction for overseeing the public's health, can draw from the expertise of multidisciplinary members, and use triage skills that can easily be adapted for use following a disaster.

Public health workers can conduct assessments and epidemiological studies and can make and implement appropriate recommendations based on data analysis. Such data collection is critical to identify potential vulnerabilities before disaster occurs to ensure that potential social impacts are adequately addressed in disaster planning and that emergency, public, and mental health needs are met in the community.

Maintenance of continuity of care is especially important for older adults, those with chronic disease, and those in long-term care facilities. Health advisories on injury prevention, food and water safety, and disaster-specific precautions should be developed in advance and available for immediate distribution when needed. Public health officials should regularly communicate with elected officials about the likely impact of potential disasters for which the community is at risk and should help develop policies and regulations that can prevent or reduce morbidity and mortality following disaster. Communication is accomplished, in part, through community engagement tools such as public health emergency preparedness Web sites and online portals which allow partners to easily communicate in preparation for and in response to public health emergencies.

Public Health and Health Care Capabilities

The National Preparedness Goal (NPG; see Chapter 3) described 5 key domains or duties that are required in the United States' preparing for and responding to a disaster. These are often referred to as missions. In addition, the NPG identified capabilities, which are the means necessary to accomplish these critical duties in order to achieve the NPG. While this national framework is focused on the responsibilities of the emergency management community, public health professionals respond as part of this broader structure. In the NPG framework, "prevention" is focused specifically on terrorist threats, while the other mission areas are designed to address an all-hazards approach.

The 5 mission areas in the NPG and the focus of the capabilities for each are:

- Prevention Capabilities: "to avoid, prevent, or stop a threatened or actual act of terrorism"
- Protection Capabilities: "to secure the homeland against acts of terrorism and manmade or natural disasters"
- Mitigation Capabilities: "to reduce loss of life and property by lessening the impact of disasters"
- Response Capabilities: "to save lives, protect property and the environment, and meet basic human needs after an incident has occurred"
- Recovery Capabilities: "to assist communities affected by an incident to recover"

To aid public health and health care professionals in understanding their role and responsibilities and to facilitate and guide joint planning to carry out ESF #8 (see Chapter 3), the ASPR and the CDC developed profession-specific capabilities. ASPR's *Healthcare Preparedness Capabilities: National Guidance for Healthcare System Preparedness* (available at https://www.phe.gov/Preparedness/planning/hpp/reports/Documents/2017-2022-healthcare-pr-capablities.pdf) and CDC's *Public Health Preparedness Capabilities: National Standards for State and Local Planning* (see Appendix E for the complete

Table 2-1. Public Health and Health Care Capabilities

Public Health Capabilities	Health Care Capabilities
Community Preparedness	Foundation for Health Care and Medical Readiness
Community Recovery	Health Care and Medical Response Coordination
Emergency Operations Coordination	Continuity of Health Care Service Delivery
Emergency Public Information and Warning	Medical Surge
Fatality Management	
Information Sharing	
Mass Care	
Medical Countermeasure Dispensing	
Medical Materiel Management and Distribution	
Medical Surge	
Nonpharmaceutical Interventions	
Public Health Laboratory Testing	
Public Health Surveillance and Epidemiological Investigation	
Responder Safety and Health	
Volunteer Management	

Source: Based on Centers for Disease Control and Prevention (CDC). 2011. *Public Health Preparedness Capabilities: National Standards for State and Local Planning*. Washington, DC: CDC. Available at: http://www.cdc.gov/phpr/capabilities/dslr_capabilities_july.pdf. Accessed December 29, 2016; Office of the Assistant Secretary for Preparedness and Response (ASPR). 2016. *2017–2022 Health Care Preparedness and Response Capabilities*. Washington, DC: ASPR. Available at: https://www.phe.gov/Preparedness/planning/hpp/reports/Documents/2017-2022-healthcare-pr-capablities.pdf. Accessed March 16, 2017.

guidelines) provide operational guidance for state and local public health and health care systems.

Table 2-1 lists the public health and health care capabilities.

Carrying Out Public Health Responsibilities

The responsibilities of public health agencies in disaster preparedness and response are more complicated than in a typical public health activity. In preparedness activities, public health professionals must participate as part of a multiagency team, some members of which have little or no knowledge of public health. Public health and other human service departments (e.g., aging, disability, behavioral health) are often organized as separate governmental units. As such, careful advance coordination of preparedness efforts is an essential part of community planning. Further, public health practitioners must work with multiple bureaucratic layers of infrastructure in a condensed time frame, as well as interact with personnel with whom they may not have contact as part of their daily work activities and whose lexicon and methods may be different. In some communities, public health may not be integrated into the jurisdictional Incident Command System and must find a way to work cohesively with this established response, particularly where there is a unified command.

Public health organizations involved in delivering services during a disaster response and recovery must also ensure that their agencies have administrative preparedness. An agency's preparedness plan should include processes to ensure that fiscal and administrative practices (e.g., funding, procurement, contracting, hiring, and legal capabilities) are well defined and can be quickly operationalized in a disaster. These processes include emergency procurement, contracting, and hiring and must define how the emergency processes differ from normal operations.

Incident Action Plan

The health sector is responsible for ensuring the continuity of health care services. Resource problems following disasters in the United States have resulted from poor planning in the use or distribution of assets rather than a deficiency of those assets. The public health system works with health sector agencies in the community to coordinate planning for the continued delivery of services both during and after the disaster. This interagency coordination includes the development of an incident action plan to address community health needs. Action plans for the public health response ensure the continuity of health care services (e.g., acute emergency care, continuity of care, primary care, and preventive care), monitoring environmental infrastructure, assessing the needs of the elderly and other vulnerable populations, initiating injury prevention programs and surveillance, and ensuring that essential public health sector facilities will be able to function postimpact (e.g., ambulatory care centers, hospitals, health departments, pharmacies, physicians' offices, storage sites for health care supplies, dispatch centers, paging services, and ambulance stations). When a disaster occurs, public health agencies establish an action plan based on their assessment of the situation. The action plan should be based on objectives for the initial health response that are specific and achievable, can be measured, and have a definite time frame. Once the action plan is in place, agency staff are assigned responsibilities.

Components of the plan include the following:

- Incident goals (where the organization wants to be at the end of response)
- Operational period objectives (major tasks to be addressed during the specified time to meet the goals)
- Response strategies (priorities and the general approach to accomplish the goals)
- Response tactics (methods to achieve the goals)
- Organizational chart indicating roles and relationships in agency's Incident Command System
- List of assignments with specific tasks

- Resources needed with status updates
- Health and safety plan to prevent responder injury or illness
- Communications
- Logistics (e.g., procedures to support operations with equipment, supplies)

Personnel

The responsibility of disaster preparedness should be assigned to someone who has the organizational authority to ensure an adequate level of preparation. Otherwise, the effort may be less than optimal because the designated individual lacks authority to delegate tasks to the proper offices and personnel. In addition, such a decision creates the false impression that an effective program exists because someone has been assigned to disaster preparedness.

Both the lead individual and all those involved in disaster preparedness and response must have a well-grounded understanding of both the public health consequences of disaster and human response to disaster on the part of both victims and responders. Public health practitioners must recognize how the health sector fits into the emergency management model of disaster preparedness and response, including components of a typical response and team-based, interdisciplinary problem-solving. Those involved in disaster response must have both the expertise and ability to access state-of-the-art resources to provide technical assistance to communities and to collect and analyze data as quickly as possible. Through such data collection, epidemiological methods can be applied to develop the best disaster response both to prevent morbidity and mortality and to mitigate medical or public health problems. Public health officials also help blend public health approaches with clinical practice. Likewise, they provide direction to the American Red Cross (Red Cross) to ensure the provision of appropriate care and resources and inspect Red Cross shelters and feeding operations.

Public Health Law and Emergencies

As part of public health disaster preparedness, health departments must review state and local laws to understand the nuances of their authority in these circumstances and to prepare a legal plan of action for times of emergency. Although universal generalities form the underpinnings of emergency authority, operational authority will vary among jurisdictions. Indeed, the CDC has developed a public health law program whose mission is to articulate the connection between law and public health for public health practitioners, including during emergencies.

The authority to protect the health of the public in emergencies is not assigned in a single law, but generally requires a chain of events. For example, a Board of Health could declare an emergency, allowing the commissioner of health to modify requirements set forth in the health code. A mayor could declare an emergency, which would in turn allow the mayor's office to modify provisions of local laws and regulations or the health code. Similarly, if a governor declares an emergency, the governor can modify applicable provisions of state and local laws and regulations, including the health code. However, again, each public health department must research in advance which procedures for declaring emergencies and altering health codes apply to each jurisdiction.

Functional Model of Public Health Response

The functional model summarizes a typical disaster response within the public health field and categorizes the cycle of activities. The model identifies tasks assigned to each of the core areas of public health in the context of emergency management activities. The functional model expands traditional public health partnerships with other disciplines and agencies and emphasizes collaboration to ensure competence in disaster preparedness and response.

The functional model outlined below and on the following pages comprises the 5 phases identified in the NPG that correspond to the type of activities involved in preparing for and responding to a disaster: prevention, protection, mitigation, response, and recovery.

Prevention

Primary Prevention (Before Event)

- Conduct biosurveillance to discover, identify, and locate biological threats.
- Provide immunizations.
- Control and prevent outbreaks.
- Protect against risks identified in hazards, vulnerability, and needs assessments.
- Protect and distribute safe food and water.

Protection

Primary Prevention

- Provide immunizations.
- Control and prevent outbreaks.
- Protect against risks identified in hazards, vulnerability, and needs assessments.
- Conduct community education in first aid, personal hygiene, and injury prevention.
- Protect and distribute safe food and water.
- Protect or reestablish sanitation systems.

Mitigation

Community Preparedness

- Be integrated into the community's disaster plans that define how the community will provide public health, medical, and mental/behavioral health services as directed under the ESF #8 definition at the state or local level.
- Have input in the community's risk assessment and disaster plan. These should identify and prioritize the potential hazards, health vulnerabilities, and risks related to any interruption to public health, environmental, medical, or mental/behavioral health systems, as well as disruptions to infrastructure in the community.

Secondary Prevention (Response to Event)

- Organize and deploy teams for immunization of the general public or selected populations.
- Coordinate public health interventions, including dispensing of antibiotics or vaccines and ordering social distancing.
- Provide advice to the public regarding personal protection.
- Ensure responder health and safety.
- Determine need for and coordinate the delivery of medical and pharmaceutical supplies.
- Organize services and treatment.
- Conduct case identification and surveillance and recommend, monitor, and analyze mitigation actions.
- Establish infectious disease control.
- Control contamination.
- Conduct short-term counseling and intervention.

Response

Operational Coordination

- Initiate agency's Emergency Operations Center and Incident Command System.
- Staff the local/state Emergency Operations Center, Disaster Recovery Centers, and Disaster Field Offices as requested.
- Coordinate with emergency management response structures (Incident Command System, federal response, international disaster relief, United Nations agencies, International Committee of the Red Cross, nongovernmental organizations, etc.).

- Determine whether public health operations or medical and health care facilities have been affected.
- Develop specific requests for assistance under ESF #8 (where federal assistance is being requested or has been approved), including medical personnel, equipment, and supplies.
- Ensure that the site health and safety plan is established, reviewed, and followed.
- Coordinate with the safety officer to identify hazards or unsafe conditions associated with the response.
- Initiate responder safety and health reports, updates, and briefings and ensure that medical staff are available to evaluate and treat response workers.
- Collaborate with poison centers, health care systems, and clinical laboratories on protocols for chemical exposures, symptom recognition (e.g., infectious disease), and reporting protocols.

Medical Surge

- Supporting triage and patient tracking efforts, monitor bed status and other issues across affected facilities and serve as a liaison between hospitals and response partners.
- Coordinate the evacuation and subsequent return of patients from health care facilities, including movement of patients to definitive care facilities that are part of the National Disaster Medical System.
- Develop a tracking mechanism to facilitate family reunification for hospitalized or long-term care patients transferred to alternate locations.
- Administer logistics of reception site(s) for medications and supplies from Strategic National Stockpile.
- Establish distribution site(s) for medical countermeasures (e.g., vaccine, medications) and provide technical assistance.
- Organize services (e.g., casualty management, behavioral health).
- Identify need for and provide emergency treatment, resources, and equipment.
- Identify at-risk populations and share information on health concerns and protective measures, such as evacuation routes, shelter-in-place guidance, and instructions for decontamination and obtaining medical care in disasters requiring such actions.
- Continue provision of primary care.

Surveillance, Hazard Identification, and Assessment

- Identify and determine the magnitude and extent of public health and medical problems associated with the disaster.

- Conduct "quick and dirty" assessments to identify affected individuals and to use as a base for initial decisions.
- Utilize geographic information system mapping of at-risk populations.
- Canvass households door-to-door to identify those in need of power, water, heat, and medical attention and make appropriate referrals.
- Establish syndromic information systems to identify potential outbreaks and identify appropriate data to collect for decision making.
- Conduct sentinel surveillance, using active or passive systems, of disease and public health conditions to determine incidence of disease and causal factors.
- Conduct public health epidemiological investigations (i.e., long-term monitoring of exposed individuals and environmental health impacts).
- Use data to recognize acute disease states and vulnerable populations.
- Identify potential medical, behavioral, social, and political effects of event.
- Identify infectious disease, establish treatment, and control.
- Assess potential effect of loss of infrastructure on health and mental health.
- Identify potential hazards and levels of acceptable exposure.
- Determine vulnerability, level of risk, and requirement for a rapid needs assessment.
- Summarize damage to health care infrastructure.
- Establish continuous data monitoring.

Nonpharmaceutical Interventions

- Recommend and enforce nonpharmaceutical intervention(s) where indicated.

Operational Communications, Public Information, and Warnings

- Assist officials by providing information on public health matters.
- Address requests for assistance and information, including health-related requests for assistance and information from other agencies, organizations, and the public.
- If a Joint Information Center (JIC) has been established, ensure that a public health representative has been assigned as part of a Joint Information System to establish communications and maintain close coordination with the JIC.
- Communicate results of surveillance and laboratory analyses to appropriate personnel in a timely manner through established operations plans, procedures, or guidelines.
- Establish a public health information "hotline."
- Communicate plans and needs (internal and external).

- Educate the public on how long foods can be stored in a refrigerator or freezer after the power goes off.
- Determine when water is or is not safe to drink.
- Educate the public on how long water should be boiled before it is safe for drinking.
- Determine when it is safe to reenter homes or eat food after a toxic cloud has dissipated.
- Determine the risks of delayed effects (e.g., cancer, birth defects) from a chemical or nuclear mishap to the average citizen and to those who are pregnant.

Environmental Response

- Understand the mechanics of hazardous agents (e.g., radiation, toxins, thermal and water pollution, landmines, weapons).
- Dispose of waste, debris, human and animal remains, and biologic hazards.
- Control disease vectors and manage pests.
- Monitor and provide information on water, sanitation, food, and shelter.
- Educate the public on health and safety during cleanup.
- Coordinate delivery of behavioral health services.

Laboratory

- Ensure that laboratories have the analytical capacity of specimen collection and analysis needed to meet the demand.

Fatality Management

- Coordinate in the provision of nonintrusive, culturally sensitive mental/behavioral health support services to family members of the deceased, incident survivors, and responders.
- Assist in gathering and disseminating antemortem data, when requested.

Recovery

- Ensure continuity of public health programs, services, and infrastructure.
- Provide long-term counseling and mental health intervention.
- Educate the public about injury prevention and safe cleanup.
- Determine the present level and extent of patient care capability.
- Reestablish health services.
- Work with community agencies to mitigate long-term impact on public health.

- Plan and direct field studies.
- Manage media relations.
- Use the principles of capacity building.
- Mobilize resources.
- Use techniques for supplemental and therapeutic food distribution and feeding.
- Organize and conduct large-scale immunization and deliver primary health care.
- Ensure maintenance of mental health programs.
- Work with the Red Cross to incorporate functional needs services in shelters.
- Provide basic medical care and referral services for those requiring medical attention in shelters through 24-hour staffing.
- Set up an emergency public health hotline staffed 24 hours a day for medical issues and another one for mental health issues with workers who speak the major languages of the community.
- Use information revealed through evaluation to make decisions about a community's emergency management needs or about improving future response.
- Conduct evaluations of emergency planning and disaster response to provide feedback that can improve an organization or community's preparedness.
- Facilitate interaction among community agencies and organizations to build a network of support services to minimize any negative public health effects of the disaster.

CHAPTER 3

STRUCTURE AND ORGANIZATION OF HEALTH MANAGEMENT IN DISASTER RESPONSE

The public health profession has become increasingly involved in national emergency management since the 1980s. The recognition of health effects from the volcanic eruption at Mount St. Helens motivated the beginning of formal public health and medical sector participation in preparedness and response activities. While the earlier efforts were not universal across the country, the catastrophic tragedies that resulted from the terrorist attacks in 2001 and Hurricane Katrina in 2005 led to the transformation of emergency preparedness and response from a mostly volunteer service to a highly professional corps and solidified the public health profession's inclusion as a permanent member of the emergency management team in the United States.

The requirements for preparedness and response in the United States have come from presidential policies and congressional action. The response to disasters is organized through multiple jurisdictions, agencies, and authorities. Effective preparedness and response to disasters requires both collaboration and partnerships across multiple levels of government working with a community's nonprofit and private sectors. As a result, local response to disaster situations requires extensive planning, organization, and coordination with other regional, state, and federal officials. The term *comprehensive emergency management* is used to refer to these activities.

Undertaking these activities with the participation of the whole community is the approach used in the United States today. This chapter discusses the legal authority, guidelines, structure of the federal response, structure of the state and local response, deployment of volunteers, and costs and reimbursement for disaster response and relief.

Public Health Role

- Participate with other professionals who engage in emergency preparedness and response.
- Activate public health emergency operations centers (EOCs) and participate in communitywide EOCs.

- Assess medical, public health, and mental health needs.
- Prepare recommendations on clinical aspects of emergency and working with the health care sector to ensure provision of services, including medical equipment and supplies, hospital care, movement of patients, care for chronic diseases, and blood services and products. Assess viability of health care infrastructure and provide additional support where needed.
- Conduct health surveillance; detect, identify, and verify individual cases through laboratory sciences; and institute measures to control infectious disease.
- Provide expert assistance in responding to chemical, radiological, or biological hazards.
- Staff public health clinics in emergencies.
- Supplement clinical backup to school health program sheltering activities.
- Assure potable water supply, food safety, and sanitation.
- Assure worker health and safety.
- Educate about vector control and implement appropriate measures.
- Provide public health information.
- Work with voluntary organizations, such as the American Red Cross (Red Cross) to provide emergency shelter.
- Identify victims and manage corpses.
- Provide mental health and substance abuse services.
- Provide veterinary services.
- Be able to respond 24 hours a day, 7 days a week.
- Coordinate with other sectors on long-term prevention and recovery.

Structure of the Federal Response

Federal activities in emergency preparedness and response are directed by both executive (presidential) and congressional guidance. This section begins with the legal authority, continues with federal preparedness and response guidance, and ends with a description of key federal agencies involved in the breadth of disaster- and emergency-related activities.

Legal Authority: Federal Disaster Assistance and Policy

Throughout this chapter, reference is made to the specific laws whose provisions specify legal authority for governmental actions in emergency preparedness and response. An overview of key laws follows. The first group concerns federal disaster assistance and policy, including the Stafford Act, Presidential Directives and Presidential Decision Directives, and the National Emergencies Act.

Stafford Act

The Robert T. Stafford Disaster Relief and Emergency Assistance Act (Public Law 100-707; amended by the Disaster Mitigation Act 2000 [Public Law 106-390] and by the Post-Katrina Emergency Management Reform Act of 2006 [Public Law 109-295]) was signed into law on November 23, 1988. The Stafford Act amended the Disaster Relief Act of 1974, which established the process of presidential disaster declarations and established the statutory authority for most federal disaster response activities, especially those of the Federal Emergency Management Agency (FEMA). The Stafford Act provides for both financial and resource assistance through FEMA following a presidential disaster declaration or an emergency declaration. The act assigns FEMA the responsibility of coordinating federal relief efforts, with contributions of numerous federal agencies and nongovernmental organizations, such as the Red Cross. (See "Organization of Response" below for more information.)

Under the Stafford Act, there are 2 types of declarations:

- An *emergency declaration*, which is more limited in scope than a major disaster declaration, provides fewer federal programs and is not usually followed by recovery programs. Federal assistance and funding are provided to meet specific needs associated with the emergency or to attempt to prevent a catastrophe from occurring. The president may issue an emergency declaration before an incident to reduce or prevent a catastrophe.
- A *major disaster declaration* provides the full range of federal programs for response and recovery. Unlike an emergency declaration, a major disaster declaration may only be issued after an incident.

Directives by the President

Presidents of the United States have issued executive orders, known as Presidential Directives (PDs), Presidential Policy Directives (PPDs), or Presidential Decision Directives (PDDs), which established national policy regarding disasters. PDD-39 (January 21, 1995) defined federal actions to be taken in response to threats or acts of terrorism, and PDD-62 (May 22, 1998) established the fight against terrorism as a top national security priority. Homeland Security Presidential Directive 5 (HSPD-5) (February 28, 2003) required that all responses to emergencies be conducted using a comprehensive National Incident Management System (NIMS) with a unified command. The development of a national strategy for public health and medical preparedness was mandated in HSPD-21 (October 18, 2007). HSPD-21 identified biosurveillance, countermeasure distribution, mass casualty care, and community resilience as essential components of public health and medical preparedness and called for planning by federal agencies in each of these areas. On March 30, 2011, President Barack Obama issued PPD-8, which required the development of a national domestic all-hazards preparedness goal and a national preparedness system with an evaluation component in which a report will be compiled annually to address (1) how we know whether we are prepared and (2) whether we are better prepared than we were the previous year. The methods in which these policies were implemented are described in this chapter.

National Emergencies Act, Sections 201 and 301

The National Emergencies Act (NEA) authorizes the president to declare a national emergency, activating emergency powers covered in other federal statutes while identifying which emergency powers will be applied. All emergencies expire 1 year after declared if not renewed by the president. After Hurricane Katrina in 2005, President George W. Bush declared a state of emergency under the NEA allowing him to waive federal wage laws. As a result, contractors rebuilding after the hurricane did not have to pay workers the local prevailing wage.

Legal Authority: Public Health Response

The second group of laws providing legal authority includes the Social Security Act and 1135 Waivers, Public Health Service Act, public health emergency declarations, Pandemic and All-Hazards Preparedness Act, Pandemic and All-Hazards Preparedness Reauthorization Act, and Public Readiness and Emergency Preparedness Act and concerns laws that specify the public health role and response and that extend insurance coverage.

Social Security Act and 1135 Waivers

The Social Security Act of 1935 established a system of benefits for retirees and others, including victims of industrial accidents, the blind, and the physically handicapped.

Through the Social Security Act (SSA), the secretary of the Department of Health and Human Services (HHS) can temporarily modify or waive certain Medicare, Medicaid, Children's Health Insurance Program (CHIP), and Health Insurance Portability and Accountability Act (HIPAA) requirements when a public health emergency has been declared and the president has declared an emergency or a major disaster under the Stafford Act or a national emergency under the NEA (discussed above) and the HHS secretary declares a public health emergency. Known as *1135 Waivers,* such waivers should be necessary to ensure that sufficient health care "items and services" are available to meet the needs of individuals enrolled in SSA programs. Further, the waiver ensures that providers who are unable to comply with statutory requirements when providing these services are reimbursed and exempted from sanctions for noncompliance in the emergency area during the emergency period.

Examples of what may be waived or modified include:

- certain requirements for participation certification or program participation for individual health care providers or types of health care providers;
- preapproval requirements;
- licensure requirements for purposes of Medicare, Medicaid, and CHIP reimbursement only—physicians and other health care professionals who are licensed to practice in another state and are not disqualified from practice can provide services in a state with a disaster or emergency where they are not licensed;
- sanctions under the Emergency Medical Treatment and Active Labor Act (EMTALA) for redirecting or reallocating individuals to another location to receive a medical screening. This transfer must be in accordance with a state's appropriate preparedness plan for the transfer of individuals who have not been stabilized, where the transfer is necessary due to the circumstances of the declared public health emergency. A waiver of EMTALA sanctions will be allowed only if actions under the waiver do not discriminate on the basis of a patient's source of payment or ability to pay;
- sanctions under SSA Section 1877(g) (Stark law) relating to limitations on physician referral as deemed appropriate by the Centers for Medicare & Medicaid Services;
- limitations on payments to permit Medicare Advantage Plan enrollees to use out-of-network providers in an emergency situation;
- sanctions and penalties arising from noncompliance with HIPAA privacy regulations relating to: (1) obtaining a patient's agreement to speak with family members or friends or honoring a patient's request to opt out of the facility directory, or (2) the patient's right to request privacy restrictions or confidential communications.

During the 2009 H1N1 influenza pandemic, waivers for Section 1135 of the Social Security Act and other Medicare and Medicaid regulations (e.g., ability to screen or treat an infectious illness off-site and waive medical privacy laws) were granted. The ability to waive these regulations were the outcome of the president's declaration of a national emergency under the NEA, combined with the determination by the secretary of HHS of a public health emergency. Further, following Hurricane Sandy in November 2012, Secretary of Health & Human Services Kathleen Sebelius declared a public health emergency for the entire state of New York, including New York City. With the declaration, the Centers for Medicare & Medicaid Services were able to provide waivers under

Section 1135 so health care providers could continue to provide services to beneficiaries of Medicare, Medicaid, and CHIP during the emergency. More information on requesting a 1135 Waiver is available at: https://www.cms.gov/About-CMS/Agency-Information/H1N1/Downloads/RequestingAWaiver101.pdf.

Public Health Service Act

The Public Health Service Act (PHS) was enacted in 1944 to establish the federal government's authority to engage in quarantine activities. The United States Public Health Service had initial responsibility for preventing the introduction, transmission, and spread of communicable diseases from foreign countries into the United States. Quarantine authority was transferred to the agency now known as the Centers for Disease Control and Prevention (CDC) in 1967. The PHS Act is foundational to many federal actions during emergencies, such as public health emergency declarations discussed below.

The PHS Act provides for:

- enabling the secretary of the HHS to lead the federal public health and medical response to public health emergencies and incidents covered by the 5 National Planning Frameworks (see Chapter 4);
- granting the ability to declare a public health emergency (PHE) and to take actions to respond;
- enabling agencies within the HHS to respond to a PHE;
- assisting states in their preparedness and response to health emergencies;
- controlling communicable diseases;
- maintaining the Strategic National Stockpile (SNS);
- providing for the operation of the National Disaster Medical System;
- establishing and maintaining a Medical Reserve Corps (MRC); and
- providing targeted immunity, when approved, for medical countermeasures to certain groups involved in the administration of covered treatments to patients and their employees.

Public Health Emergency Declaration. Public health emergency declarations are made by the secretary of HHS (under Section 319 of the PHS Act) when the office consults with public health officials as necessary and determines that (1) a disease or disorder presents a public health emergency or (2) that a public health emergency, including significant outbreaks of infectious disease or bioterrorist attacks, otherwise exists. The declaration is in place for the duration of the emergency or 90 days, but may be extended by the secretary. Declarations require notifying Congress within 48 hours and keeping relevant agencies informed, including the Department of Homeland Security (DHS), Department of Justice, and Federal Bureau of Investigation.

Public Readiness and Emergency Preparedness Act

The Public Readiness and Emergency Preparedness Act (PREP Act) of 2005 authorizes the secretary of the HHS to issue a declaration that provides immunity from liability for the manufacture, testing, development, distribution, administration, and use of medical countermeasures. This liability extends to diseases, threats, and conditions determined in the declaration to be a present or credible risk of a future public health emergency. Once a PREP Act declaration is made, eligible individuals can be compensated by the U.S. Department of the Treasury for serious physical injuries or deaths directly caused by administration or use of a countermeasure covered by the declaration. A list of PREP Act declarations can be found at: http://www.phe.gov/Preparedness/legal/prepact/Pages/default.aspx.

The Pandemic and All-Hazards Preparedness Act

The Pandemic and All-Hazards Preparedness Act (PAHPA; Public Law 109-417) amended the PHS Act, became law in December 2006, and was reauthorized in 2013 (see discussion below). PAHPA created mechanisms to improve public health preparedness and response at all levels of government and created clear lines of authority and accountability when responding to public health emergencies and incidents covered by the National Response Framework (NRF).

PAHPA sought to ensure that state and local public health departments met established standards in preparedness. PAHPA established numerous approaches to create surge capacity at the federal, state, and local levels. The approaches included enhancing the training of health care providers and volunteers, making it easier for qualified health care providers to volunteer during emergency situations, allowing treatment to be delivered at alternative health care facilities and mobile hospitals, providing liability protections as incentives for service, and funding grants to hospitals and other health care facilities. PAHPA also reinforced preparedness efforts for at-risk individuals by requiring that implementation of the National Preparedness Goal (NPG), state and local grant activities, and the SNS (discussed later in this chapter) must incorporate the public health and medical needs of at-risk individuals. Further, best practices had to be disseminated on outreach to and caring for at-risk individuals during any phase of a disaster (see Chapter 11 for discussion of at-risk populations).

The HHS was responsible for achieving the goals of this act. Within HHS, the Office of the Assistant Secretary for Preparedness and Response (ASPR) was created to provide both leadership in preventing, preparing for, and responding to the adverse health effects of public health emergencies and disasters. The ASPR also provides federal support to augment state and local capabilities (i.e., methods to accomplish the critical tasks of the NPG) during a disaster and is discussed later in this chapter.

At the state level, PAHPA established funding for the MRC and Emergency System for Advance Registration of Volunteer Health Professionals (ESAR-VHP). MRC is a state-administered, locally run program for medical volunteers who train together so they are ready to augment a medical response in the event of disasters involving many serious injuries, known as mass casualty incidents, in their community. For ESAR-VHP, a state registers health care volunteers before an incident to ensure that they are properly licensed and credentialed. Both are discussed in the section on volunteers later in this chapter.

The Pandemic and All-Hazards Preparedness Reauthorization Act

PAHPA was reauthorized through Public Law No. 113-5 in March 2013 to continue and expand "certain programs under the Public Health Service Act and the Federal Food, Drug, and Cosmetic Act with respect to public health security and all-hazards preparedness." The Pandemic and All-Hazards Preparedness Reauthorization Act (PAHPRA) provides funding through 2018. The 4 major sections of the law are:

- Strengthening national preparedness and response for public health emergencies,
- Optimizing an all-hazards preparedness and response at both the state and local levels,
- Enhancing the review of medical countermeasures, and
- Accelerating cutting-edge research and development for medical countermeasures.

PAHPRA advances national health security by funding the Hospital Preparedness Program (HPP) and the Public Health Emergency Preparedness (PHEP) cooperative agreements, which provide greater flexibility for state health departments to meet community needs in a disaster by dedicating staff resources and funding the purchase of medical countermeasures. PAHPRA also enhances the authority of the United States Food and Drug Administration (FDA) to support rapid responses to public health emergencies.

Preparedness and Response Guidance

The federal government has vast resources that are intended to guide the country's preparedness activities and response when the reserves of communities and states are exhausted. This section describes the federal guidance and the federal agencies that lead those efforts.

National Health Security Strategy

The creation of the first National Health Security Strategy (NHSS) was called for in the PAHPA to improve the nation's response to and coordination for health needs following a disaster. The NHSS is the "vision" that focuses national preparedness and response efforts to protect against threats or emergencies that could negatively affect health. The NHSS is established every 4 years by HHS, with input from governments at all levels, academia, and private and nonprofit organizations. The 2015-2018 NHSS, discussed further in this chapter, has 5 objectives:

- Build and sustain health resilience.
- Produce and use medical countermeasures and nonpharmaceutical interventions.
- Ensure that decision makers have comprehensive awareness of situations affecting health before, during, and after emergencies through better use of resources, improved data-sharing, and innovations in systems and tools.
- Enhance the integration and effectiveness of the public health, health care, and emergency management systems. These efforts require the strengthening of health care coalitions, regional planning, the "scaling- up" of personnel and resources to meet increased need, and creation and maintenance of a competent workforce and volunteer corps.
- Strengthen global health security.

National Preparedness Goal

Released 6 months after the issuance of PPD-8, the NPG defines a *whole community* approach to being prepared for the full range of disasters and emergencies. Whole community preparedness involves partnering with institutions, groups, and individuals actively engaged in preparedness and with communities dealing with the effects of a disaster. Planning for and implementing disaster strategies using a whole community approach incorporates population requirements based on both the community's composition and individual needs, including those related to age, economics, and/or accessibility requirements.

The implementation of whole community preparedness has fundamentally changed how the United States carries out disaster preparedness, response, recovery, and mitigation. The previous approach to disaster response was centered on government action. Whole community readiness involves all parts of a community (e.g., community and faith-based organizations, private sector, residents, volunteers) in a unified approach to preparedness and response. This approach necessitates knowing and meeting the preparedness needs of the entire community, engaging the full community in identifying those needs and arranging to fulfill them, and strengthening what works well in populations to improve their resilience (see Chapter 8 for a discussion of resilience).

The NPG is: "A secure and resilient nation with the capabilities required across the whole community to prevent, protect against, mitigate, respond to, and recover from the threats and hazards that pose the greatest risk." These risks include events such as natural disasters, emerging infections and pandemics, man-made and technological emergencies such as chemical spills, terrorist attacks, and cyber-attacks. Enhanced planning for these risks center on the competencies contained in the NPG and the key principles, or phases, of a disaster discussed in this book: prevention, protection, mitigation, response, and recovery. (For the complete NPG, see https://www.fema.gov/media-library/assets/documents/25959, and for a summary of changes in the 2015 NPG see http://www.fema.gov/media-library-data/1443703117389-27c542ca395218d3154e5c1dfa8bfcb6/National_Preparedness_Goal_Whats_New_2015.pdf.)

Core Capabilities

The NPG also identified 31 core capabilities, considered critical elements in achieving the goal. To meet the requirements of the NPG, DHS developed core capabilities for the emergency management community, but these are not public health focused. In March 2011, the CDC published national standards for 15 capabilities that apply to public health agencies, known as Public Health Preparedness Capabilities.[1] In addition, revised capabilities for health care systems were published in 2017 by the ASPR and are available at: https://www.phe.gov/Preparedness/planning/hpp/reports/Documents/2017-2022-healthcare-pr-capablities.pdf. (See Chapters 2 and 4 and Appendix E.)

National Preparedness System

The National Preparedness System provides guidance using a whole community approach to achieving the NPG and how the country should prepare. Using an all-hazards methodology, the National Preparedness System guides national planning, organization, equipment training and exercises in 6 areas:

- *Identifying and assessing risk* by collecting and analyzing historical and recent data on existing, potential, and perceived threats and hazards. These risk assessments inform the actions that follow.

1. The public health capabilities are being revised with an expected publication in 2017.

- *Estimating capability requirements* by determining the specific capabilities and activities needed to deal with the identified risks. Some capabilities may already exist and some may need to be built or improved.
- *Building and sustaining capabilities* by identifying the best way to use limited resources to build capabilities. The risk assessments will identify the threats with the highest probability or highest consequence and guide the prioritization of needed resources.
- *Planning to deliver capabilities* by using a whole community approach. Plans should be developed in coordination with all parts of the community (e.g., individuals, businesses, nonprofits, community and faith-based groups) and all levels of government.
- *Validating capabilities* through participation in exercises, simulations or other activities. These test runs help communities both identify gaps in plans and the capabilities defined to carry out those plans, and recognize progress toward meeting preparedness goals.
- *Regularly reviewing and updating* identified capabilities, resources, and plans ensures that communities are prepared for evolving risks and changing resources.

National Response Framework

To provide direction for the national preparation and response to all hazards, the DHS created the NRF and the National Incident Management System (NIMS) discussed below. Whereas the NRF provides the structure and mechanisms that guide national policy for emergency response, NIMS provides the template for managing emergencies regardless of size, scope, or cause. Together, these guidelines provide methods to implement and coordinate a comprehensive, unified, and consistent federal response in support of state and local officials.

The NRF defines the principles, roles, and structures that organize and unify how the United States responds to disasters and emergencies. Updated in June 2016, the NRF is implemented by FEMA. It provides the mechanism for coordinating the delivery of federal assistance and resources to augment efforts of state and local governments in support of the Stafford Act (discussed earlier in this chapter) or a federal response managed under the Economy Act of 1932.[2] Rather than detailing a specific plan for response, the NRF describes the planning process and directs federal agencies to participate in the entire spectrum of emergency management from preparedness to recovery. The NRF:

- Describes how communities, tribes, states, the federal government, private sectors, and nongovernmental partners work together in an engaged partnership to coordinate the national response.

2. The Economy Act provides a mechanism to avoid duplication of work by governmental agencies. It allows for interdepartmental procurement where one federal agency can request the assistance of another agency under the transfer of funds between agencies for the provision of goods and services.

- Describes specific authorities and best practices for managing incidents, including a tiered response that provides for disasters being managed at the lowest possible jurisdictional level and supported by additional capabilities only when needed.
- Builds upon NIMS; provides a common template and an operational structure based on the principles and standard methodology of the Incident Command System (ICS) for managing incidents. ICS is used because disasters, regardless of magnitude, require a coordinated response from a number of different agencies for organizing the delivery of services in disaster response. ICS is discussed later in the chapter.

It should be noted that some types of responses are generated by authorities other than the Stafford Act and are managed outside of the NRF. The 2010 Gulf of Mexico oil spill, the 2009–2010 influenza pandemic, and the U.S. response to Ebola in 2014–2015 exemplify disasters in which the national responses included a significant medical component yet were not managed through the NRF. As an example, the oil spill was managed through the authority of the National Contingency Plan. Authorization to respond to international incidents is provided through treaties and arrangements with the United States Department of State. Although these are the exceptions, they are not that uncommon. The key is that without a presidential declaration and the resources of the Stafford Act, funding for federal assistance is limited and unorganized.

Information on the NRF, including documents, annexes, references, briefings, and training courses, can be obtained from the NRF Resource Center (available at: http://www.fema.gov/media-library/assets/documents/32230).

National Incident Management System

The goal of HSPD-5 is to enhance the ability of the United States to oversee a coordinated response by establishing a single, comprehensive model for the national management of major domestic emergencies. The comprehensive model that provides the template for managing all emergencies is the NIMS. The NIMS is built upon the principle that effective preparedness involves many groups working together, including preparedness organizations, elected and appointed officials at all levels of government, nongovernmental and faith-based organizations, and the private and nonprofit sectors. NIMS is intended to be used by the whole community, including individuals, families, and communities with everyone using a standardized, common approach. Further, everyone involved in managing an emergency should understand the command reporting structures, common terminology, and roles and responsibilities inherent in a response operation.

NIMS is relevant to all jurisdictions and functional disciplines and is applicable across all emergencies, regardless of size, location, or complexity. NIMS was designed to improve coordination and cooperation and to provide a common standard for the broad range of personnel who interact to manage emergencies. Using NIMS principles, a diverse group of professionals can develop a shared understanding of the procedures and protocols that will be used and how equipment and personnel will be deployed. All involved in emergency response, whether career professionals, volunteers, or government officials, are required to complete federally approved NIMS training. Further, all recipients of federal funding for preparedness and response activities must be NIMS compliant. Finally, hospitals and health care systems receiving federal funds for preparedness must implement NIMS. As of this writing in 2016, NIMS is being revised. (See https://www.fema.gov/national-incident-management-system for updates.)

Emergency Support Functions

The emergency management community uses the term *function* to describe the responsibilities within the NRF that must typically be addressed in a disaster response. These responsibilities are grouped into 15 Emergency Support Functions (ESFs), each headed by a federal department or agency, with the support of the others, who organize their response to meet the functions defined in each ESF. Support partners include numerous and varied federal agencies (e.g., Departments of Agriculture, Transportation, Defense, Veterans Affairs, Homeland Security, Interior, and Labor; Environmental Protection Agency) and the Red Cross.

Many ESFs directly or indirectly affect efforts to protect the health and welfare of disaster victims. The federal response to supplement state, local, and tribal resources in meeting the medical and public health needs of disaster victims is specified in ESF #8: Public Health and Medical Services Annex to the NRF. The PAHPRA provides that the HHS is the lead agency for ESF #8, with coordination provided by the ASPR. The public health and medical areas of responsibility include the following:

- Assessment of public health/medical needs
- Public health surveillance
- Medical surge
- Health, medical, veterinary equipment and supplies
- Patient movement
- Patient care
- Safety and security of drugs, biologics, and medical devices
- Blood and tissues
- Food safety and defense
- Agriculture safety and security
- All-hazards public health and medical consultation, technical assistance, and support
- Behavioral health care

- Public health and medical information
- Vector control
- Guidance on potable water/wastewater and solid waste disposal
- Mass fatality management, victim identification, and decontaminating remains
- Veterinary medical support

The 14 ESFs and their responsible lead federal agencies are shown in Table 3-1.

National Terrorism Advisory System

Following HSPD-3 (March 11, 2002), the DHS established the DHS Advisory System (HSAS) to guide preventive actions taken in response to information about threats and vulnerability assessments. Most remember the color-coding alerts as key to the HSAS. In 2011, the National Terrorism Advisory System (NTAS) replaced the HSAS. The NTAS is also designed to communicate information about terrorist threats so that preventive actions can be taken. Under the new system, DHS with other federal entities issue alerts when the federal government receives information about a specific or credible terrorist threat. These alerts include a clear statement that there is an imminent or elevated threat. The alerts provide a summary of the potential threat, information about actions being taken to ensure public safety, and recommended steps that individuals and communities, businesses, and governments can take. Alerts are sent directly to the affected groups, such as law enforcement, the private sector, or to the general population. Multiple communication channels are used, including a designated DHS Web page (available at: http://www.dhs.gov/alerts) and social media (Facebook and Twitter @ NTASAlerts). Individual threat alerts are issued with a specified end date but can be extended if needed.

As the NTAS evolves, public health agencies should develop a checklist of activities that they would undertake with changing levels of threat. The checklist should include:

1. Information gathering—Check information from the CDC, state departments of health (DOH), local offices of emergency management, and others.
2. Surveillance system—Check emergency and ambulatory admissions for patients who may have conditions or illness suggestive of chemical, biological, nuclear, or radiological exposures.
3. Security—Enhance security measures with an increased level of threat.
4. Staffing—Assess staffing patterns and determine what to do for coverage.
5. Communications—Check availability of systems, including state information systems.
6. Supplies and equipment—Verify availability and functionality.

Table 3-1. Emergency Support Functions and Responsible Lead Federal Agency

ESF	ESF Title and Function	ESF Coordinator
1	Transportation–management of transportation systems and infrastructure	Department of Transportation
2	Communications–restoration of communications infrastructure, coordinates communications support to response efforts, facilitates the delivery of information to emergency management decision makers, and assists in the stabilization and reestablishment of systems and applications	DHS/National Protection and Programs Directorate/Office of Cybersecurity and Communication
3	Public Works and Engineering–coordinates and organizes the resources of the federal government to facilitate the delivery of multiple core capabilities	Department of Defense/U.S. Army Corps of Engineers
4	Firefighting–detection and suppression of wildland, rural, and urban fires resulting from, or occurring coincidentally with, an all-hazard incident	Department of Agriculture/Forest Service/ FEMA/U.S. Fire Administration
5	Information and Planning–collects, analyzes, processes, and disseminates information about a potential or actual incident, and conducts deliberate and crisis action planning activities	DHS/FEMA
6	Mass Care, Emergency Assistance, Temporary Housing and Human Services–coordinates and provides life-sustaining resources, essential services, and statutory programs when the needs of disaster survivors exceed government capabilities	DHS/FEMA
7	Logistics Management and Resource Support–comprehensive logistical planning and support	General Services Administration/DHS/FEMA
8	Public Health and Medical Services–federal assistance in response to a disaster, emergency, or incident that may lead to a public health, medical, behavioral, or human service emergency, including those that have international implications	HHS
9	Search and Rescue–lifesaving and search and rescue operations	DHS/FEMA
10	Oil and Hazardous Materials Response–response when there is release of oil or hazardous materials	Environmental Protection Agency
11	Agriculture and Natural Resources–nutrition assistance; respond to animal and agricultural health issues; provide technical expertise, coordination and support of animal and agricultural emergency management; ensure the safety and defense of the Nation's supply of meat, poultry, and processed egg products; and ensure the protection of natural and cultural resources and historic properties	Department of Agriculture
12	Energy–coordinating government capabilities, services, technical assistance, and engineering expertise during incidents when a federal response is needed for producing, storing, refining, transporting, generating, transmitting, conserving, building, distributing, maintaining, and controlling energy systems and system components	Department of Energy
13	Public Safety and Security–facility and resource security, security planning, response, and assistance	Department of Justice/Bureau of Alcohol, Tobacco, Firearms & Explosives
15	External Affairs–provides information to affected audiences, including governments, media, the private sector, and the local populace, including children; those with disabilities and others with access and functional needs; and individuals with limited English proficiency	DHS

Source: Based on Federal Emergency Management Agency (FEMA). 2016. *Emergency Support Function Annexes*. Washington, DC: FEMA. Available at: https://www.fema.gov/media-library/assets/documents/25512. Accessed February 9, 2017.

Note: DHS=Department of Homeland Security; ESF=Emergency Support Functions; FEMA=Federal Emergency Management Agency; HHS=Health & Human Services.

Federal Agencies

Homeland Security

The Department of Homeland Security was established by the president and Congress (in the Homeland Security Act of 2002) to coordinate federal programs and to assist state and local governments in responding to the full range of emergencies, disasters, and catastrophes. The lead federal department for emergency management is the DHS. By assuming primary responsibility in the event of a terrorist attack, natural disaster, or other large-scale emergency, DHS provides a unifying core for the vast national network of organizations and institutions involved in preparedness efforts. DHS is responsible for developing and implementing preparedness plans; developing procedures and policies to guide response to a terrorist attack; conducting training and exercises for first responders; enhancing partnerships with state and local governments, private-sector institutions, and other organizations; and funding the purchase of equipment for first responders, states, cities, and towns.

Central to the country's system of responding to emergencies, state and local resources are the first line of support in response to a disaster. This principle drives all preparedness at the state and local level, since states must pay a share of the costs of federal response and recovery, and an efficient use of local resources can reduce that additional cost. Once state resources and capabilities are exhausted, federal assistance may be provided to supplement state operations.

Health & Human Services

In disasters of the magnitude requiring a presidential declaration, HHS has lead responsibility for supporting local officials in their response to medical and public health needs. PAHPA provides that public health resources may also be deployed by HHS through its executive agent, the Assistant Secretary for Preparedness and Response.

Assistant Secretary for Preparedness and Response

In a health emergency or public health event, the secretary of HHS delegates to the ASPR the leadership role in carrying out the support function for health and medical services. The ASPR works with other federal agencies and with state and local governments to coordinate the planning and response, provides logistical support for any federal response, and oversees the development and procurement of medical countermeasures to pandemics and other hazards.

While the organizational structure may change with a new federal administration in 2017, historically 2 key functions within the ASPR organization are an operations office, currently called the Office of Emergency Management (OEM), and the Biomedical Advanced Research and Development Authority (BARDA). To ensure federal preparedness, the OEM develops operational plans, participates in training and exercises, and secures the systems and logistical support necessary for the ASPR to coordinate HHS's operational response. BARDA provides coordination and helps develop and procure medical countermeasures to speed the development and availability of vaccines and pharmaceuticals to treat highly infectious diseases in public health emergencies. BARDA has responsibility for establishing strategies for the deployment and use of medical countermeasures supplied through the SNS. BARDA acquires medical countermeasures for at-risk populations, such as vaccines for immunocompromised populations.

The Public Health Emergency Medical Countermeasures Enterprise (PHEMCE) is the federal body that provides federal agency coordination of what is referred to as the "lifecycle" of medical countermeasures in response to chemical, biological, radiological, nuclear, and emerging infectious diseases. Led by the ASPR, other federal agencies include the CDC, the FDA, and the National Institutes of Health, with BARDA providing expertise and leadership on the PHEMCE. Examples of activities include funding for pandemic influenza vaccine development, alternative techniques for vaccine production, and novel testing and treatments for bioterrorism agents. PAHPRA required that the FDA issue an annual report detailing its medical countermeasure activities, including the development and availability of measures to protect against emerging infectious disease threats, such as pandemic influenza, Ebola, or Middle East Respiratory Syndrome Coronavirus. More information about the strategy for preparing for emerging infections and other biological threats can be found at: http://www.phe.gov/Preparedness/mcm/phemce/Documents/2015-PHEMCE-SIP.pdf.

Centers for Disease Control and Prevention

The Centers for Disease Control and Prevention has a critical role in public health readiness. The CDC helps local and state DOHs strengthen their abilities to respond to all types of emergencies by providing funding and technical assistance. When local and state resources are not sufficient to respond to an emergency, the CDC provides scientific and logistical expertise and deploys personnel and critical medical assets to the site of an emergency. The CDC also helps DOH partners recover and restore public health functions after the initial response.

At the CDC, the Office of Public Health Preparedness and Response (PHPR) provides strategic direction, coordination, and support for all of the CDC's terrorism preparedness and emergency response activities. Support is provided through funding, building capacity, and technical assistance.

Specific tasks carried out by the CDC's PHPR include:

- providing preparedness, assessment, response, recovery, and evaluation services prior to and during public health emergencies;
- convening an EOC, which is staffed 24 hours a day, for monitoring and coordinating the CDC's emergency response to public health threats in the United States and abroad;
- managing the PHEP cooperative agreement, which supports preparedness nationwide in state, local, tribal, and territorial public health departments;
- delivering critical medical assets to the site of a national emergency;
- managing and maintaining the SNS;
- providing technical assistance to state and local sites to prepare for emergencies and when SNS resources are deployed; and
- overseeing the Federal Select Agent Program, which regulates all entities that possess, use, and/or transfer biological agents or toxins that could pose a severe threat to public health and safety; providing guidance to registered entities about select agent regulations; and conducting evaluations and inspections. Select agents include the bacteria that cause anthrax and plague and the virus that causes smallpox.

The CDC program focuses on a number of critical aspects of public health infrastructure. It seeks to improve disease surveillance and epidemiology; assure and support readiness at the state and local level; provide for the availability of key medical supplies, including pharmaceuticals and vaccines; expand laboratory capacity; strengthen the ability for risk and emergency communication; protect at-risk populations; improve the surge capacity of the public health workforce; enhance education and training programs; regulate entities that possess, use, and/or transfer biological agents or toxins (e.g., bacteria that cause anthrax and plague); and support planning for infectious disease, such as Ebola virus disease or pandemic influenza. During an emergency, the CDC provides information for clinical diagnosis and medical management; as guidance to first responders; to inform the public health response; to facilitate the utilization of clinical and reference laboratory protocols; and to educate the public. Federal assistance may be provided directly to the states by the Epidemic Intelligence Service officers from the CDC or by experts from the Agency for Toxic Substances and Disease Registry, among others. These federal public health personnel, stationed at regional offices of HHS, can quickly enter the field to conduct surveillance and rapid needs assessments.

Federal Emergency Management Agency

DHS delegates much of the strategic planning and response activities for emergency management to FEMA, which coordinates the federal government's role in preparing for, preventing, mitigating the effects of, responding to, and recovering from all domestic disasters, whether natural or man-made, including acts of terror. FEMA's responsibility for coordinating government-wide relief efforts was authorized in the Stafford Act. In addition to their Washington, D.C., headquarters, FEMA operates a number of regional offices (see Appendix AA for a list of offices and locations). The staff at the regional field offices help states and communities become better prepared through the development of all-hazards operational plans. These regional offices mobilize federal assets and evaluation teams to work with state and local agencies in response to a disaster. Other agencies, such as HHS and its National Disaster Medical System described later in the chapter, use the same geographic zones to organize personnel and resources throughout the nation. FEMA's role is discussed in more depth below.

Organization of Response

As the nation saw in the responses to Hurricanes Katrina and Sandy, a catastrophic disaster requires resources at every level of government and from every agency. The coordination of such an immense response is complicated and involves numerous levels of bureaucracy. When the resources of communities and states could be or are overwhelmed by the events that unfold from a disaster, federal resources, known as *assets*, can be requested. For natural disasters, the process is known as a disaster declaration.

Disaster Declarations and Federal Assistance

In the event of a natural disaster, the Stafford Act provides for "an orderly and continuing means of assistance by the federal government to state and local governments in carrying out their responsibilities to alleviate the suffering and damage which result from major disasters and emergencies." Under the Stafford Act, the president may provide federal resources, financial assistance, services, medicine, food, and other consumables through what is known as a presidential declaration. In a major disaster, the Post-Katrina Emergency Management Reform Act of 2006 authorized the president to order precautionary evacuations and provide accelerated federal support even before state and local governments have made a specific request.

Before the passage of the Homeland Security Act of 2002 (HSA), which established the DHS, federal assistance was initiated in 1 of 3 ways: (1) states request federal assistance in advance of the disaster to activate a declaration when the threat is imminent and warrants limited pre-deployment actions to lessen or avert a catastrophe; (2) governors submit requests after the disaster has struck; or (3) the president exercises primary authority, as was done following the bombing at Oklahoma City. With the passage of the

HSA, the secretary of DHS has a lot of discretion in the deployment of federal resources. DHS can activate the federal government's resources if and when any of the following four 4 conditions apply:

- A federal department or agency, acting under its own authority, requests the assistance of the secretary;
- The resources of state and local authorities are overwhelmed and federal assistance is requested by the appropriate state or local authorities (i.e., through the Stafford Act);
- More than one federal department or agency becomes substantially involved in responding to the incident; or
- The secretary is directed to assume responsibility for managing the incident by the president.

When there is a declaration, each affected state must take the initiative in requesting a declaration. States must individually request a separate declaration, even when affected by the same disaster. FEMA assigns a sequential number to each major disaster (DR) or emergency (EM). For the small number of declared disasters or emergencies, the events are of such magnitude that a subsequent major disaster declaration is requested (e.g., Hurricanes Katrina and Sandy).

Once there has been a presidential declaration, FEMA is responsible for coordinating the federal response for emergency management. FEMA performs many of the same functions as a local emergency management agency but can also direct federal resources and money toward the preparation for, response to, and recovery from larger emergencies and disasters. If communities and agencies provide mutual aid to one another and there is no presidential declaration, it is important that they execute interagency agreements. Mutual aid in response to a disaster will be voluntary without authorization under the Stafford Act. Table 3-2 outlines the declarations and assessment process.

The Federal Response

When a governor, or designee, of an affected state requests a presidential declaration under the Stafford Act, the NRF is activated. In anticipation of a catastrophic event, federal assets may also be mobilized and deployed in advance of a formal request for assistance. The Catastrophic Incident Supplement of the NRF establishes the procedures and mechanisms by which this occurs.

More than 28 federal agencies and the Red Cross provide personnel, technical expertise, equipment, and other resources to state and local governments, and they assume an active role in managing a national response. Within HHS, the lead federal agency, the CDC and National Institute of Occupational Safety and Health provide

Table 3-2. Disaster Declaration Process

Declaration Process/Action	Preliminary Damage Assessments	Primary Considerations for Declarations
After initial response by local groups, governor consults with local government officials and determines that combined resources of both the state and local governments are not sufficient	PDAs, conducted in affected counties, assist governor in determining if request for assistance is needed	Criteria used by FEMA: Amount and type of damage (number of homes destroyed/major damage) Impact on infrastructure or on critical facilities Imminent threats to public health and safety Impacts on essential government services and functions Unique capability of federal government Dispersion or concentration of damage Level of insurance coverage in place Other available assistance Previous state and local commitments for resources Frequency of disaster events over recent time period
Governor declares a state of emergency and invokes the state's emergency plan	FEMA, state's emergency management agency, county and local officials, and the U.S. Small Business Administration conduct assessments	
Governor: Submits written request to the president through FEMA regional office	Team reviews: Types of damage Emergency costs incurred Impact to critical facilities	

(Continued)

Table 3-2. (Continued)

Declaration Process/Action	Preliminary Damage Assessments	Primary Considerations for Declarations
Governor (continued):		
Requests supplemental federal assistance under the Robert T. Stafford Disaster Relief and Emergency Assistance Act, 42 U.S.C. §§ 5121–5206	Effect on individuals and businesses Number of people displaced Threats to health and safety	
Certifies that severity and magnitude of disaster exceed state and local capabilities	Any additional data from the Red Cross	
Certifies federal assistance is necessary to supplement state and local governments, disaster relief organizations, and compensation by insurance companies for disaster-related losses		
Confirms execution of the state's emergency plan		
Certifies adherence to cost sharing		
Request and findings of the PDAs are reviewed by FEMA regional and national offices	Team collects estimates of the expenses and damages	
FEMA provides an analysis of the situation and recommends a course of action to the president		
	Governor uses information to support declaration request, identify cost of response, and certify that damage exceeds state and local resources	

Source: Based on Federal Emergency Management Agency (FEMA). 2010. Disaster declaration process fact sheet. Washington, DC: FEMA. Available at: https://www.fema.gov/pdf/media/factsheets/dad_disaster_declaration.pdf. Accessed December 29, 2016; Association of State and Territorial Health Officials (ASTHO). 2016. Robert T. Stafford Disaster Relief and Emergency Assistance Act fact sheet. Arlington, VA: ASTHO. Available at: http://www.astho.org/Programs/Preparedness/Public-Health-Emergency-Law/Emergency-Authority-and-Immunity-Toolkit/Robert-T--Stafford-Disaster-Relief-and-Emergency-Assistance-Act-Fact-Sheet. Accessed December 29, 2016.

Note: FEMA = Federal Emergency Management Agency; PDA = Preliminary Damage Assessment.

technical personnel and logistical support, such as epidemiologists, environmental sampling equipment, and laboratory assistance. The Departments of Defense (DOD) and Veterans Affairs (VA) provide support in the event of a catastrophic disaster where many people require hospitalization. Agencies issue mission assignments, or work orders, which direct the agency to carry out and fund specified tasks in response to the disaster.

Federal Agencies and Staff

Under the NRF and NIMS, the president designates a principal federal official (PFO) to coordinate the activities of all federal agencies during a catastrophic disaster and to serve as the secretary of DHS's direct representative to the response. The PFO interfaces with all jurisdictional officials regarding the management of the incident and is the primary federal spokesperson. For major disasters, the president appoints a federal coordinating officer (FCO) who is responsible for coordinating the timely delivery of federal disaster assistance to the affected state and local governments and disaster victims. The FCO oversees the commitment of FEMA resources and the assignment of other federal departments or agencies. In many cases, the FCO also serves as the disaster recovery manager and administers the financial aspects of assistance authorized under the Stafford Act. Different individuals will serve as the PFO and FCO for a given response.

Federal and state personnel work together to carry out their response and recovery responsibilities. The FCO works closely with both the state coordinating officer (SCO), appointed by the governor to oversee disaster operations for the state, and the governor's authorized representative, empowered by the governor to execute all necessary documents for disaster assistance on behalf of a state. In accordance with the state's emergency operations plan, requests for assistance from local jurisdictions are channeled first to the SCO through the designated state agencies and then to the FCO or designee for consideration. When resources from the federal government are required, states must complete a purchase order, blanket purchase agreement, contract, or cooperative agreement to formalize the request. Additionally, DHS may use a mission assignment as discussed above. The Financial Management Support Annex of the NRF provides additional information about this process (available at: http://www.au.af.mil/au/awc/awcgate/frp/frpfm.htm).

FEMA maintains both a National Response Coordination Center (NRCC) and 10 Regional Response Coordination Centers (RRCCs) in the event that incidents require federal-level resources. Both the NRCC and the RRCCs are staffed round-the-clock to provide all necessary coordination. In the event of an incident requiring extensive federal support, both coordinating centers can augment their staffing with additional personnel from FEMA and other relevant federal agencies.

In the Field

For the response in the field, a federal Joint Field Office (JFO) coordinates federal and state activities and provides tactical-level direction. Before the establishment of a JFO, an Emergency Response Team-Advance (ERT-A) goes to the affected area to assess the requests for assistance and the capacity of the local and state agencies to meet the requirements of a response. The JFO, led by a Unified Coordination Group (UCG), uses a unified incident command structure. The UCG includes senior state and federal leaders who work with all of the potential stakeholders in a coordinated federal response. The UCG can also include a senior federal official from HHS when the events involve health care delivery or public health concerns. In the event of a terrorist act, the UCG will include a senior federal law enforcement officer. Liaisons from the affected governments, businesses, and the Joint Information Center are assigned to work with the coordinating staff.

Officials responsible for 4 functional areas within NIMS—planning, operations, logistics, and finance and administration—report to the coordinating staff. Planning and operations activities are closely coordinated with the same functional units at the state level. Figure 3-1 lists the participants and shows the reporting structure for the JFO.

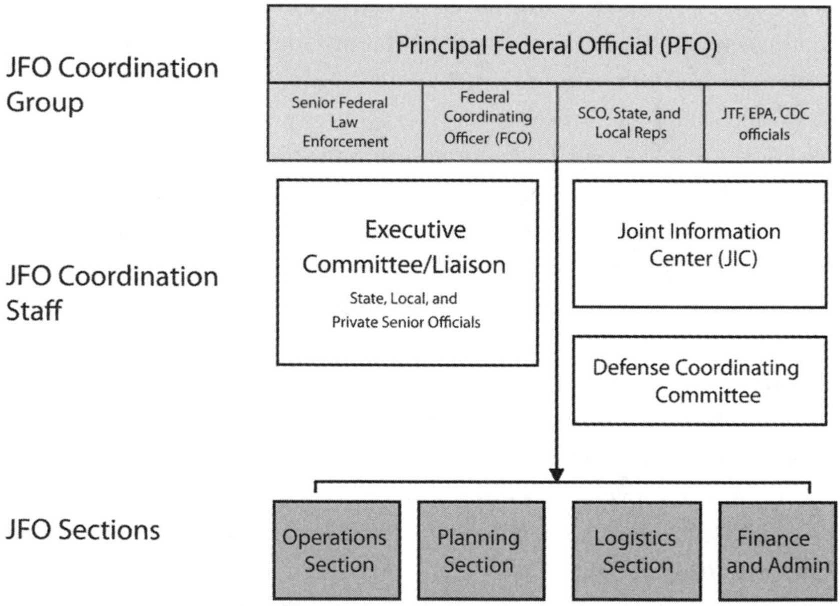

Source: Adapted from Department of Homeland Security (DHS). 2006. *Joint Field Office Activation and Operations: Interagency Integrated Standard Operating Procedure.* Washington, DC: DHS. Available at: https://www.fema.gov/pdf/emergency/nrf/NRP_JFO_SOPAnnexes.pdf. Accessed December 29, 2016.

Note: CDC=Centers for Disease Control and Prevention; EPA=Environmental Protection Agency; JTF=Joint Task Force; SCO=State Coordinating Officer.

Figure 3-1. Joint Field Office Organizational Chart

Local and state officials activate an EOC, which is the physical location where numerous agencies (e.g., emergency management, public health, and hospital groups) gather to manage the response. EOCs are staffed 24 hours a day while in operation. Depending on the scale of the disaster, the JFO will coordinate with the EOC and report to either the NRCC or RRCC.

Deployment and Operations

Requests for assistance (RFAs) from the federal government come through either the ERT-A or the JFO. RFAs can be submitted to the SCO, who sends the RFA to the ERT-A or to the JFO. Requests can also be submitted directly by the governor to senior DHS leadership or to the president. The FCO reviews RFAs and can approve all appropriate requests. Once approved, the JFO identifies what is required to meet the needs of the RFA. The federal agency with the identified capability validates the requirement and assigns a unit to meet the request. The funding for the assigned unit is provided through the Stafford or Economy Acts.

Once deployed, the assigned unit works either directly for a local or state agency or as part of a larger federal response. Regardless of assignment, response activities are conducted using the principles of NIMS. Coordination occurs among the local, state, and federal responders and each level develops and implements an incident action plan, which contains the specific action steps that will be taken to respond to the emergency. Federal involvement decreases when the incident no longer requires the most intensive level of response. Eventually, all resources are returned to their original location and are readied for future needs.

As the lead agency for ESF #8, HHS developed a Concept of Operations Plan (CONOPS) to provide a framework for its management of the public health and medical response. CONOPS, consistent with HSPD-5 and the NRF, provides strategies to ensure that there is a unified approach to all activities carried out by HHS. Table 3-3 describes federal actions that can be initiated under the provisions of the Stafford Act.

Figure 3-2 graphically shows the flow of federal activities following an incident.

Federal Public Health and Medical Response

At the national level, the management of information and strategic-level command and control for ESF #8 occur in the HHS Secretary's Operations Center (SOC). When states request federal assistance and FEMA issues mission assignments, the HHS mission assignments are directed to the Emergency Management Group (EMG) through the SOC. The OEM at ASPR then determines which resources within the department and external to the department are best suited to support the mission assignment. During an emergency, the HHS EMG coordinates the ESF #8 response out of their operations center.

Table 3-3. Federal Actions Under the Stafford Act

Pre-event	DHS National Operations Center monitors potential disasters
	With advance warning, DHS may deploy liaisons to state emergency operations centers
	An RRCC may be fully or partially activated
	Mobilization centers may be established
Immediately after	Local emergency personnel respond and assess
	Locals seek help through mutual aid and from state
	State reviews situation, mobilizes state resources, requests assistance through EMACs, and provides assessments to FEMA regional office
	Governor activates state emergency operations plan, declares state of emergency, and requests state/DHS PDA
	PDA conducted
	Governor requests presidential declaration based on PDA
Post-disaster declaration	The RRCC coordinates regional and field activities until the JFO is in place
	Regional teams assess needs and start setting up field facilities
	National-level Incident Management Assistance Team is deployed when regional resources are overwhelmed
Response activities	The National Response Coordination Center supports the RRCC
	Governor appoints State Coordinating Officer to coordinate state activities
	President appoints Federal Coordinating Officer to coordinate federal activities
	JFO established
	UCG leads JFO
	UCG develops objectives and action plan
	UCG coordinates field operations from JFO
	Emergency Support Functions assess and identify needs
	Federal agencies provide support under DHS/FEMA mission assignments or own authorities
	Stafford Act public assistance program provides assistance
	UCG releases federal resources as need indicates

Source: Adapted from Federal Emergency Management Agency (FEMA). 2008. *National Response Framework: Overview of Stafford Act Support to States.* Washington, DC: FEMA. Available at http://www.fema.gov/pdf/emergency/nrf/nrf-stafford.pdf. Accessed December 29, 2016.

Note: DHS=Department of Homeland Security; EMAC=Emergency Management Assistance Compacts; FEMA=Federal Emergency Management Agency; JFO=Joint Field Office; PDA=Preliminary Damage Assessment; RRCC=Regional Response Coordination Center; UCG=Unified Coordination Group.

Each level of government has designated responsibility in responding to a disaster. State, local, tribal, and territorial agencies are responsible for assessing the situation and identifying and prioritizing requirements, while activating available resources and capabilities. Many resources are available in both the assessments and response. In the coordination of public health and medical assistance under ESF #8, the ASPR has many available resources. The ASPR provides medical assistance through the National Disaster Medical System (NDMS), the SNS, and volunteers registered with the MRC as discussed under volunteers below.

An Incident Response Coordination Team (IRCT) is mobilized by the ASPR to coordinate all deployed ESF #8 assets. The IRCT, usually led by a regional emergency coordinator, serves as the link between the SOC/EMG and those responding in the field. The

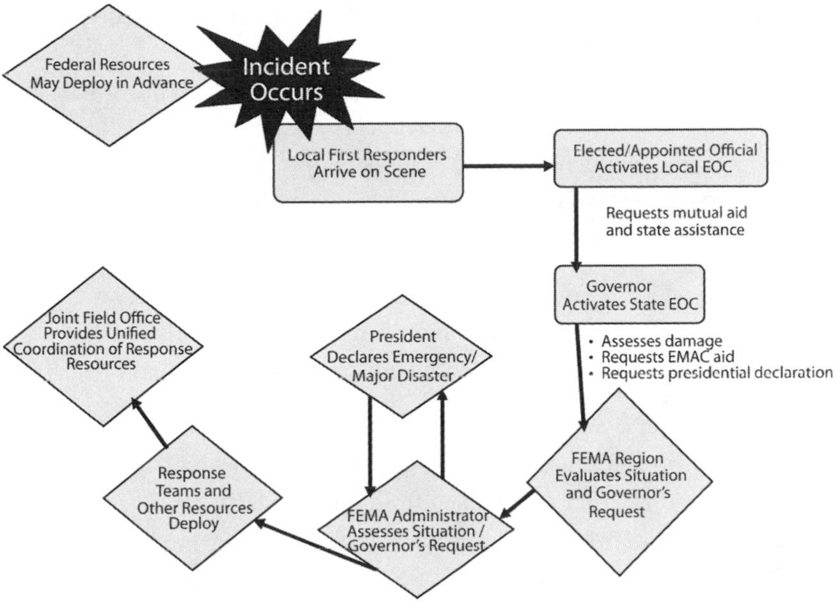

Source: Adapted from Federal Emergency Management Agency (FEMA). 2008. *Overview of Stafford Act Support to States.* Washington, DC: FEMA. Available at: http://www.fema.gov/pdf/emergency/nrf/nrf-stafford.pdf. Accessed December 29, 2016.

Note: EOC=Emergency Operations Center; EMAC=Emergency Management Assistance Compact; FEMA=Federal Emergency Management Agency.

Figure 3-2. Federal Actions in Disaster Response

IRCT team leader is accountable for executing field activities for the ASPR. During the response to Hurricane Sandy, an HHS IRCT in New York and New Jersey provided command-and-control to HHS teams requested in that state. Among other federal staff, regional emergency coordinators from the office of the ASPR were deployed to the Regional Response Coordination Centers and served as public health and medical services liaisons for the FEMA incident management assistance teams.

Other federal resources for medical assistance include the United States Public Health Service (USPHS) Commissioned Corps, Federal Medical Stations, and volunteers registered with ESAR-VHP. Through the federal programs, volunteer clinicians can be activated to augment federal assets and practice as federal providers.

National Disaster Medical System

NDMS, operating within the office of the ASPR, provides federal support, including health care professionals, to augment state and local capabilities to major emergencies and federally declared disasters under the NRF. NDMS works in partnership with the USPHS, FEMA, DOD, and VA.

NDMS provides a nationally integrated medical response to (1) help state and local authorities address the medical and health effects of major peacetime disasters and (2) provide support to the military and medical systems of the VA in caring for casualties evacuated to the United States from overseas armed conflicts.

NDMS has 3 components:

- Medical response to a disaster area in the form of teams, supplies, and equipment
- Patient movement from a disaster site to unaffected areas of the nation
- Definitive medical care at participating hospitals located in unaffected areas

When the mission assignment is received by NDMS headquarters, an Incident Management Team determines how best to meet the tasks and what resources are required. An operations group, assembled from an on-call list, works with the affected state(s) as they articulate what they need and will be requesting. Health care at the site of the disaster is provided by NDMS and USPHS teams with NDMS headquarters supporting the team coordination. NDMS also interacts with the JFO to meet the responsibilities of ESF #8.

Federal Coordinating Centers and Patient Movement

Federal Coordinating Centers (FCCs) recruit hospitals and maintain local nonfederal hospital participation in NDMS; assist in the recruitment, training, and support of Disaster Medical Assistance Teams (DMATs); coordinate exercises and emergency plans with participating hospitals and other local authorities to develop patient reception, transportation, and communication plans; and coordinate the reception and distribution of patients being evacuated to the area. FCCs are managed by the DOD and the VA.

Hospitals become part of NDMS by signing a memorandum of agreement between the chief executive of the hospital and the director of the FCC in their locale. As of this printing, NDMS reimburses participating hospitals up to 110% of Medicare and is the third-level payer after private insurance and Medicare. Hospitals should assume that comprehensive and complete documentation will be required to receive reimbursement and must establish the information systems necessary to comply.

FCCs contract with local emergency medical services (EMS) to transport patients in the communities where NDMS member hospitals are located. The contracts facilitate the availability of ambulances from outside the affected region to be able to transport patients from the disaster within 24 hours. Contracts are in place for ambulances, paratransit seats, and air ambulances. The FEMA regional ambulance contract also provides medical transport resources for deployment.

In the event of a federally declared natural or technological disaster, the DOD sets up a tracking system, the Global Patient Movement Requirements Center (GPMRC), to determine if patients need to be evacuated. When a mission assignment is issued to the DOD, the FCCs are activated. The FCCs partner with NDMS and NDMS member hospitals to identify and report available beds. While the number of beds is being assessed, patient information is gathered at the disaster site and forwarded to the GPMRC. The GPMRC determines the movement of patients to specific FCCs based on both the victims' needs and the availability of beds and transportation. In addition to the tracking done by the DOD tracking, NDMS tracks patients through the Joint Patient Assessment & Tracking System from the time that the status of patients is known at the FCCs until they are discharged.

Where the need for hospital beds exceeds local capacity, patients are stabilized at the site of the disaster by DMATs or other specialty teams and then evacuated by the DOD aeromedical system to hospitals that are part of NDMS. At the airport of the NDMS reception area, patients are met by a team from the local EMS. EMS assesses patients and transports them to participating hospitals according to procedures developed by local authorities and the local area's FCC.

National Disaster Medical System Teams

There are multiple teams within NDMS including DMATs, Disaster Mortuary Operational Response Teams (DMORTs), National Veterinary Response Teams (NVRTs), and the International Medical Surgical Response Teams (IMSURT). Members of these teams are required to maintain appropriate certifications and licensure within their discipline and are activated as federal employees with their licensure and certification recognized by all states. When activated, team members are paid as intermittent federal employees, retain rights to return to their full-time employment, are protected with workers' compensation insurance, and have the protection of the Federal Tort Claims Act in which the federal government becomes the defendant in the event of a malpractice claim. As federal employees, NDMS team members also have to comply with federal ethics and conflict of interest regulations.

Disaster Medical Assistance Teams. DMATs are squads of licensed, actively practicing multidisciplinary medical personnel who function as rapid-response medical teams to supplement local medical care during a disaster or other event. DMAT personnel include physicians, nurses, nurse practitioners, emergency medical technicians (EMTs), paramedics, pharmacists and pharmacy technicians, dentists, respiratory therapists, communication specialists, social workers, and other allied health personnel. During mass casualty incidents, their responsibilities include triaging patients, providing austere medical care, and preparing patients for evacuation. In other situations, they may provide primary health care or assist overloaded medical staffs. Additionally, they are prepared to provide patient care during evacuation to definitive care sites.

NDMS organizes reservists, recruits members, arranges training, and coordinates the dispatch of the team. NDMS registers and verifies the credentials of the members of DMATs in advance of activation.

Disaster Mortuary Operational Response Teams. DMORTs were developed to fulfill the responsibilities outlined for NDMS in ESF #8. DMORTs are composed of private citizens who, when activated into federal service, work under the guidance of local authorities and whose function is to augment the capacity of the local coroner. They provide technical assistance and personnel in the recovery, identification, and processing of deceased victims during an emergency response. Teams comprise funeral directors, medical examiners, coroners, pathologists, forensic anthropologists, medical records technicians and transcribers, fingerprint specialists, forensic odontologists, dental assistants, X-ray technicians, mental health specialists, computer professionals, administrative support staff, and security and investigative personnel. The team members are skilled in identifying victims and working with relatives of victims.

These responsibilities include the following:

- Temporary morgue facilities
- Victim identification
- Forensic dental pathology
- Forensic anthropology methods
- Processing
- Preparation
- Disposition of remains

Family Assistance Center Teams work with family members to gather information about identifying features such as jewelry, dental work, or tattoos and to collect items that may carry genetic markers, such as tooth or hair brushes. The DMORTs work to match the antemortem materials with the human remains for victim identification.

National Veterinary Response Teams. The NRF requires that NVRTs deliver veterinary medical treatment and address animal and public health issues resulting from disasters when the local veterinary community is overwhelmed. NVRTs are teams of veterinarians, animal health technicians, epidemiologists, toxicologists, safety officers, logisticians, communications specialists, and other support personnel. NVRTs can be deployed only if a state or the federal government requests an NVRT following a presidential disaster declaration. Once the state determines that its local veterinary community is overwhelmed, the state submits a request for federal assistance through FEMA and, once approved, the request is forwarded to USPHS for approval. If a state requests an NVRT without a presidential disaster declaration, the state may be required to fund the response. If a federal disaster is declared, the federal government covers a large part of the cost.

NVRT team members triage and stabilize animals such as search and rescue dogs at a disaster site and provide austere veterinary medical care. The veterinary teams are composed of private citizens hired as intermittent federal employees and activated in the event of a disaster. These mobile units can deploy within 12 to 24 hours when their assistance is requested by the state officials from the affected state. NVRT responsibilities during disasters include the following:

- Assessment of the veterinary medical needs of the community
- Medical support to working animals, which might include search and rescue dogs and animals (e.g., horses) used for law enforcement
- Treatment to injured and ill animals post-disaster
- Veterinary medical support for sheltered animals
- Health screening for any animal through response and recovery
- Assessment of environmental and zoonotic disease
- Support, assessment, and treatment where needed for animals in research laboratories
- Support, assessment, and treatment where needed for outbreaks in livestock and poultry (led by the U.S. Department of Agriculture)

International Medical Surgical Response Teams. This NDMS team provides medical and surgical care during a disaster or public health emergency. IMSURT personnel are federal employees deployed when there is a disaster or public health emergency to provide medical care when the community health care system is overwhelmed. As federal employees, IMSURT personnel are protected from liability, illness, and injury. To participate, team members must maintain their personal state licenses and certifications, which will be recognized both nationally and internationally when deployed as federal employees. IMSURT teams are normally deployed for a minimum of 14 days or until local medical resources are sufficiently recovered or have been supplemented by other organizations. The basic deployment configuration of an IMSURT consists of 50 personnel.

Federal Medical Stations

When health care systems cannot handle the number of patients who require medical care or nursing services because the systems are either damaged or overwhelmed, HHS can deploy a Federal Medical Station (FMS), or health care facility, to provide surge beds. Each FMS is equipped with a 3-day supply of medical and pharmaceutical resources for 50 to 250 stable primary or chronic care patients. An FMS can be staffed by local providers who are temporarily without a facility in which to practice because it is inoperable; by providers from other facilities within the region; through Emergency Management Assistance Compact (EMAC) agreements; or by the federal government through the

USPHS Commissioned Corps (discussed below). Potential roles for an FMS include the following:

- Provide surge capacity where local hospitals are overwhelmed through the temporary holding and provision of care for patients with disaster-related trauma or illness.
- Receive patients from nursing homes and skilled nursing facilities forced to evacuate due to the disaster.
- Provide low-acuity care for patients with chronic illnesses whose access to care has been lost or interrupted due to the disaster.

The FMS is not equipped with tents, thus each FMS requires an appropriate facility in which to operate. An FMS must be established in a structurally intact, accessible building with adequate hygiene facilities and functioning utilities (e.g., hot and cold potable water, electricity, heating, ventilation and air conditioning, and internet accessibility or capability). A 250-bed FMS requires approximately 40,000 square feet of open space, while a 50-bed FMS requires about 15,000 square feet. In addition, the community must arrange for a 10- to 12-person team to set up the FMS and arrange/contract for patient feeding, laundry, ice, medical oxygen, and biomedical waste disposal.

Once a request for an FMS has been approved, the cache of equipment and supplies will be delivered in 24–48 hours, after which 12 hours is needed to set up the FMS. The ASPR regional emergency coordinators for FMS preparedness or CDC's Division of Strategic National Stockpile can assist with site surveys and training for receipt and setup of FMSs.

Strategic National Stockpile

The SNS program, managed by the CDC, maintains a national repository of antibiotics and life-support medications, antitoxins, chemical antidotes, vaccines, and medical supplies and equipment used to supplement state and local resources during a large-scale public health emergency. The materials in the SNS are intended to be used after states and localities have depleted their own supplies.

Each state's emergency management office (SEMO), in partnership with the state DOH, is responsible for both the warehousing and logistics of the SNS distribution. Each state has a stockpile officer who is responsible for coordination with the SEMO. Relationships have also been worked out with private companies regarding warehousing and distribution. Requests for pre-deployment of full or modified "push packs" can be considered in advance if a community is anticipating a major event, such as the requests made in advance of the Democratic and Republican National Conventions.

The push packs are located in secure locations around the United States so that they can be delivered upon request within 12 or fewer hours. Each one weighs more than

50 tons and fills 7 53-foot trucks. The contents occupy 130 cargo containers and include pharmaceuticals, antibiotics, antitoxins, nerve agent antidotes, and other emergency medications, intravenous supplies, airway equipment, and so forth. Additional vendor-managed inventory is stored at pharmaceutical companies, which have the experience and manpower to deliver supplies quickly, and can be delivered within 24 to 36 hours. In addition, a state DOH can contact the CDC and request that only certain medications be delivered. Webinars on drug shortages, pharmaceutical regulations, and navigating and partnering with the supply chain during a disaster are available at: https://www.healthcareready.org/preparing-for-disasters.

During the Ebola response, the CDC monitored local supplies of personal protective equipment and helped hospitals, DOHs, and health care coalitions coordinate when the supply was insufficient for the demand. The CDC worked with industry to communicate expected delivery times of needed supplies and assisted in redirecting supplies where needed.

The SNS catalog is available at: http://health.mo.gov/emergencies/sns/pdf/snsformularyfinal.pdf. In an emergency, responsible personnel at the state DOH should refer to the CDC's response program for guidance.

United States Public Health Service Commissioned Corps

The United States Public Health Service Commissioned Corps is composed of more than 6,500 full-time officers and is one of the United States' 7 uniformed services. Commissioned Corps officers come from many professional backgrounds, including physicians, nurses, pharmacists, dentists, dietitians, engineers, environmental health officers, health service officers, scientists, therapists, and veterinarians. As part of their duties, Commissioned Corps officers are trained and equipped to respond to public health crises, natural disasters, disease outbreaks, and terrorist attacks and also to serve on humanitarian assistance missions. Strategic and policy direction for the Commissioned Corps is provided by the Assistant Secretary for Health and the Office of the Surgeon General (OSG) oversees its operations. Commissioned Corps emergency response teams are managed by the OSG. Specialized Service Access Teams (SAT) can also be deployed to supplement the local health care workforce in meeting the access and functional needs of at-risk individuals impacted by a disaster. The SAT can advise those making health care decision and help with discharge planning in health care institutions and general population shelters by connecting individuals to accessible housing, home health care, and personal assistant services.

The Patient Protection and Affordable Care Act, enacted March 23, 2010, created the Ready Reserve Corps (RRC) to provide surge capacity as part of the Commissioned Corps. The RRC was established to enable part-time personnel to volunteer on short notice to assist regular Commissioned Corps personnel during times of public health emergencies. When called up, RRC members perform duties for assigned periods of time. During these same emergencies, full-time Commissioned Corps members may be on extended active duty.

RRC officers participate in routine training, are available and ready for calls to active duty during national emergencies and public health crises or to backfill critical positions left vacant during deployment of regular Corps members, and are available for service assignments in isolated and medically underserved communities.

Operations/Deployment

Where the USPHS has preexisting agreements, the secretary of HHS or the ASPR considers requests for RRC assistance. Once the mission requirements and the category, discipline, and specialty of RRC members are determined, the director of the Readiness and Deployment Operations Group matches the requirements of the mission against the qualifications of officers on that month's rotational "ready roster." Table 3-4 summarizes the activation and deployment process.

Structure and Operation of the State and Local Response

Every state has an emergency management agency, alternately called an *office of emergency preparedness*. Under the authority of the governor's office, the emergency management agency coordinates the deployment of state resources used in an emergency or disaster. This includes the resources of the many agencies of state government, such as health, public safety, and social services.

Mutual Aid

When the resources of a local jurisdiction are insufficient to respond to a given disaster, additional resources are requested from the surrounding region, a process commonly referred to as *mutual aid*. States can receive aid from neighbors through regional mutual aid compacts, or they can request federal resources, as described earlier in this chapter. The request of additional resources from the state or federal governments is called *escalating a response*.

All 50 states, the District of Columbia, Puerto Rico, Guam, and the U.S. Virgin Islands have formed regional agreements through EMAC, which is a nonfederal, interstate

Table 3-4. Ready Reserve Corps Activation and Deployment Process

Activation Process	Request for Activation	Identification of Assets	Deployment
The secretary of HHS approves the activation of RCC officers.		The needs of the mission are matched with the skills and qualifications on the rotational ready roster.	Agencies are informed that officers from the roster are needed.
Requests can also be vetted through the ASPR EMG and are analyzed for the mission requirements, the RRC's ability to fill those requirements, and the ability to keep RCC officers safe.		Officers are identified.	Officers are contacted.
Once the secretary has given this approval, the Readiness and Deployment Operations Group director evaluates requests for RCC officers from any state, a federal government agency or department, tribal nations, or from a foreign government.	If the secretary of HHS or the ASPR EMG concur, RRC is activated.		Supervisory release is obtained.
			Travel orders and arrangements are prepared, and the officer is deployed.

Note: ASPR=Assistant Secretary for Preparedness and Response; EMG=Emergency Management Group; HHS=Health & Human Services; RRC=Ready Reserve Corps.

agreement for mutual aid. Member states that are geographically close to disaster sites can rapidly send response teams through EMAC. The deployment of assets, including expertise, services, and goods, is coordinated in conjunction with the NRF. In an emergency, states use EMAC's procedures to formally request assistance. States negotiate the costs and terms of providing assistance with the requesting state in formal written agreements. Intrastate and interstate mutual aid can be executed before a presidential disaster declaration or when a declaration is not necessary, providing both timely and cost-effective support.

While recognizing that EMAC may issue compact-specific rules and adopt additional processes and services, DHS issued guidelines for the credentialing of personnel through the NIMS. Whenever EMAC is requested:

- state and local officials are to provide assistance to ensure that a person deployed under EMAC can reach the check-in site or complete the process;
- individuals deployed for mutual aid under EMAC should not be unreasonably detained;

- the responding individuals, team, and resources are to be processed and directed to reach check-in sites or processes as quickly as possible when security and those controlling access control have the identity of the individual and the EMAC documentation has been authenticated;
- the identity of a person is established by documentation in the form of 2 government-issued photo IDs or a photo ID and an official EMAC Request for Assistance Form (known as REQ-A) or an EMAC Mission Authorization Form (known as a Mission Order), unless the incident/unified command or the jurisdiction having authority establishes different rules specific to the incident, disaster, or emergency.

A key lesson from the response to Hurricanes Katrina in 2005 and Sandy in 2012, which struck 13 states, was that although collaboration with one's neighbors is necessary, it may not be sufficient to respond to the most far-reaching disasters. Communities need to increase mutual aid by broadening their geographic and traditional partnerships through regional consortia and collaboration across jurisdictional boundaries to include agencies and organizations that were not previously linked. In some communities, there may be multiple agreements for mutual aid within the public health and medical community. Working with the local OEM, public health agencies can serve as a clearinghouse and help coordinate the mutual aid pacts that affect the health of the community.

Health Care Coalitions

Over the last decade there has been an emergence of *health care coalitions*, which is a group of health care organizations, public safety agencies, public health partners, and other relevant organizations that collaborate to prepare for and respond to emergencies. The composition of health care coalitions ideally reflects the unique needs and characteristics of local jurisdictions and may include hospitals, emergency medical service providers, emergency management associations, long-term care facilities, behavioral health organizations, public health agencies, and other public and private-sector partners. These alliances strengthen the preparedness of communities because working in a coordinated manner results in more efficient delivery of services, thus enhancing each partner's ability to respond to disasters. Although some communities had coalitions as early as 2001, the HPP of ASPR has promoted an extensive adoption of this model to increase the nation's capacity to respond to disasters and almost 95% of hospitals participate in a coalition.

With PPD-8 calling for a "whole-of-community" response, health care coalitions have worked to include other providers (e.g., long-term care, long-term acute care, dialysis, clinics, pharmacies, research institutes, home health care, private physician practices, ambulatory surgery centers, and diagnostic centers). Additionally, there has been a push to partner with other civic groups, such as local and regional business coalitions and not-for-profit organizations that provide services in times of crisis.

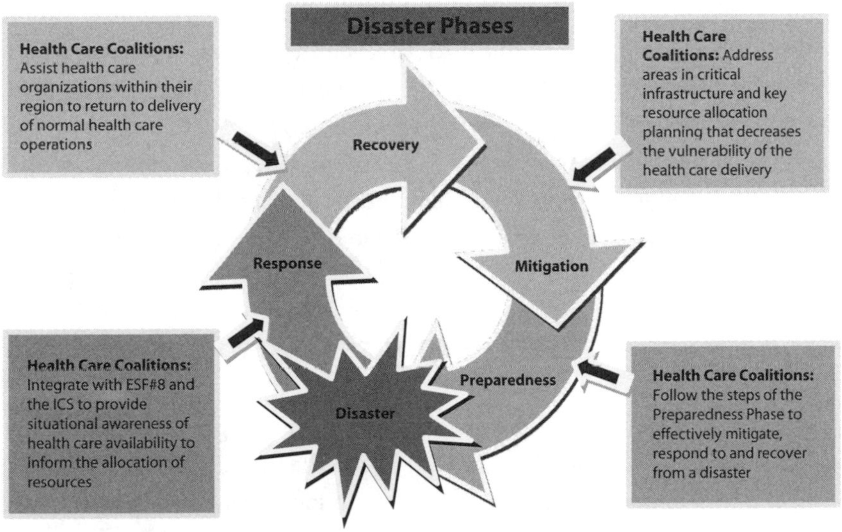

Source: Adapted from Office of the Assistant Secretary of Preparedness and Response (ASPR). 2012. *Healthcare Preparedness Capabilities: National Guidance for Healthcare System Preparedness.* Washington, DC: ASPR. Available at: http://www.phe.gov/preparedness/planning/hpp/reports/documents/capabilities.pdf. Accessed December 29, 2016.

Note: ESF=Emergency Support Functions; ICS=Incident Command System.

Figure 3-3. Role of Health Care Coalitions During Phases of a Disaster

Health care coalitions have a role at any phase of a disaster as demonstrated in Figure 3-3.

During the mitigation phase of a disaster, health care coalitions examine critical infrastructure and plan for the allocation of key resources in order to decrease the vulnerability of a community's health care delivery system. When planning how to respond, health care coalitions identify and coordinate resources, train and conduct emergency exercises, and develop warning systems. Once a disaster occurs and health care coalitions are involved in the response phase, they integrate with those carrying out the activities of ESF #8 and the responses' ICS. Being part of the response enables them to provide real-time information about health care delivery and community needs, known as *situational awareness*, in order to inform the decision making process used to allocate resources. Finally, during the recovery phase, these coalitions assist the health care organizations within their region to return to normal operations.

Health care coalitions may organize to address a particular recognized need or at-risk population. For example, the unique needs of children mandate specialized and appropriate planning for disasters. To protect children in the event of a disaster, dedicated coalitions where leaders decide together what actions are required is crucial. Many states and communities have developed coalitions to bring together diverse government agencies, nonprofit organizations, health care providers, and other groups or professionals to meet the needs of children. The AAP compiled a list of such coalitions (available at: https://www.aap.org/en-us/advocacy-and-policy/aap-health-initiatives/Children-and-Disasters/Pages/Disaster-Networks-Survey-Project.aspx).

The long-term sustainability of coalitions requires the support of a broad range of public and private stakeholders from within and outside the health care sector. Making the business case for coalitions to each of these stakeholder groups helps foster sustainability.

Emergency and Disaster Response Components

Based on response requirements identified by the state and approval by the FCO or designee, federal personnel responsible for ESF #8 coordinate with their counterpart state agencies. If directed, they may also coordinate with local agencies to provide the assistance required. Federal fire, rescue, and emergency medical responders arriving on the scene are integrated into the local response.

Although public safety agencies (e.g., emergency management, sheriff's office/police department, fire department) are usually the local lead for the overall disaster response, optimally the local or state DOH coordinates the many health-related agencies. The health department plans in advance how personnel will carry out their emergency response functions and assigns tasks to appropriate divisions within each department. Health departments work with the emergency management sectors, local hospitals, and other health care providers to develop an emergency response plan for public health systems. A well-designed preparedness program will include a hazard and vulnerability analysis, a risk assessment, a forecast of the probable health effects, a list of the resources needed, an analysis of resource availability, and the identification of at-risk individuals in the community who will require additional assistance (e.g., children, the elderly, homebound, or disabled).

Public health professionals work with many community agencies in a multidisciplinary effort. In a local operation, the Red Cross has a credentialing system for those who respond in the field. The Red Cross provides sheltering, feeding, emergency first aid, family reunification, and distribution of emergency relief supplies to disaster victims. They also feed emergency workers, handle inquiries from concerned family members outside the disaster area, provide blood and blood products to disaster victims, and help those affected connect with other resources. Faith-based affiliated groups provide meals, clothing, or assistance during recovery and reconstruction efforts. Public works departments manage the water supply and cleanup. Social services agencies work with the displaced, deliver psychosocial services, and ensure at-risk populations receive needed care. Importantly, if an agency's staff is not prepared, they will not be able to perform optimally. As part of any agency's preparedness, all staff should develop a preparedness plan for themselves and their families, so when they function as part of an organization's response during an emergency they will not need to begin putting personal plans in place.

Emergency Medical Services

Throughout most of the United States, EMS is provided by local agencies with oversight at the regional or state level. In most states, EMS is not provided directly by the state health department but is under its authority. The health department or other duly appointed governmental agency has training and regulatory jurisdiction over all EMS personnel regardless of their organizational affiliation. Some EMS systems are based in local fire departments, with ambulance and fire services operated side by side. Medics based in fire departments are often cross-trained in both firefighting and victim extrication. Some cities and counties operate independent EMS systems. In some parts of the United States, particularly the East Coast and in many rural areas, EMS is provided by volunteer independent rescue squads or volunteer ambulance squads, which may be connected with a volunteer fire department. Some EMS services are operated from local hospitals. It should be noted that volunteer EMS responders are being replaced with paid per diem employees in some communities, which may affect their agency's willingness and ability to respond to another community through mutual aid unless there is an arrangement to reimburse the agency for the services.

The EMS system includes both prehospital and in-hospital components. The prehospital components start with a public access system through which a resident notifies authorities that a medical emergency exists. Where available, the 911 emergency telephone system is used for this access. A dispatch communications system is then used to send ambulance personnel or other emergency first responders in response to the person(s) in need.

EMTs and paramedics, trained to identify and treat medical emergencies and injuries, provide medical support while transporting patients to hospitals or other sources of definitive care. The medical care delivered by EMS is classified as basic or advanced life support. Most EMS providers are trained to provide care at the basic life support level (e.g., noninvasive first aid, stabilization for a broad variety of emergency conditions, and defibrillation for cardiac arrest victims). Paramedics provide more sophisticated diagnosis through advanced life support, with treatment following medical protocols both in the field and while being transferred to the hospital. Ground ambulances are the vehicle of choice for most transports, but helicopters, boats, or snowcats may be used under specific circumstances.

When planning for the delivery of disaster care through EMS, officials must consider response patterns that commonly occur. Initially, units can be dispatched in an atypical fashion. Often they will hear about the disaster on police scanners or via the news media rather than through normal dispatch. Assuming that too much help is better than too little, emergency units may respond on an unsolicited basis, sometimes from tens or even hundreds of miles away. In widespread disasters such as earthquakes, floods, tornadoes, and hurricanes, there may be no single site to which trained emergency units can be sent. Similarly, hospitals may obtain their initial information about what has happened in an unplanned way from the first arriving casualties or the news media.

The National Association of State EMS Officials assembled evidenced-based and consensus-based practices into the *National Model EMS Clinical Guidelines*. These optional guidelines are intended to standardize EMS care and to assist EMS organizations in increasing safety and promoting positive outcomes in patient care. The guidelines are available at: https://www.nasemso.org/Projects/ModelEMSClinicalGuidelines/documents/National-Model-EMS-Clinical-Guidelines-23Oct2014.pdf.

Hospital Preparedness

While a comprehensive discussion of hospital preparedness is beyond the scope of this book, hospitals are a critical partner in public health preparedness and a preparedness system.

Previously, we discussed the prehospital component of an emergency medical system. The in-hospital system components include definitive care, delivered initially in the emergency department of a hospital and often continued when patients are admitted to specialized units within the hospital. The 2014 outbreak of Ebola in the United States demonstrated the importance of hospital preparedness, especially in taking travel histories, rapid identification of illness and patient isolation, and the proper use of and training on enhanced personal protective equipment. Hospitals face challenges similar to public health in becoming integrated within the community's emergency response system and with highly infectious disease, such as Ebola, that coordination is critical.

Hospitals must meet explicit standards for comprehensive emergency management as part of their accreditation by The Joint Commission. These standards mandate that hospitals marry the range of activities regularly conducted by the emergency management community with the traditional tasks of providing health care. Hospital disaster plans must be applicable to all hazards. Emergency management is a key standard for Joint Commission accreditation and is structured as a discrete chapter in the accreditation manual with 12 standards that include 112 performance elements.

The Joint Commission standards require that:

- hospitals engage in planning before developing an emergency operations plan (EM.01.01.01);
- hospitals develop an all-hazards emergency operations plan that coordinates communications, resources and assets, safety and security, staff responsibilities, utilities, and patient clinical and support activities during an emergency (EM.02.01.01);

- the emergency operations plan describes how they will communicate during emergencies (EM.02.02.01), manage resources and assets (EM.02.02.03), manage security and safety (EM.02.02.05), manage staff (EM.02.02.07), manage utilities (EM.02.02.09), and manage patients (EM.02.02.11);
- hospitals may grant privileges to volunteer licensed independent practitioners during a disaster (EM.02.02.13);
- in order to safeguard against inadequate care during a disaster, hospitals may assign disaster responsibilities to volunteer practitioners who are not licensed independent practitioners, but who are required by law and regulation to have a license, certification, or registration (EM.02.02.15); and
- hospitals must evaluate their emergency preparedness activities (EM.03.01.0) and the effectiveness of its emergency operations plan (EM.03.01.03).

Hospitals must follow federal procedures to be reimbursed for disaster-related response, and administrators should review the requirements of the Stafford Act, Joint Commission, and applicable state regulations. The Joint Commission has deeming authority, or the ability to determine compliance with regulations for the Centers for Medicare & Medicaid Services (CMS).

In 2016, CMS issued regulations to participate in the Medicare program (known as *conditions of participation*) that effect 17 types of health care facilities. These regulations (Emergency Preparedness Requirements for Medicare and Medicaid Participating Providers and Suppliers) laid out a framework for emergency preparedness that describes what should be done but not how and references the Joint Commission as a designated accrediting body. Major requirements include:

- Emergency plan—Providers develop an all-hazards plan based on a risk assessment specific to their location, which focuses on capabilities. Multi-facility systems that have a unified and integrated plan must include an all-hazards community-based risk assessment and a location-specific risk assessment for each individual facility.
- Policies and procedures—Policies and procedures are developed and implemented based on the risk assessment and emergency plan.
- Communication plan—A communication plan is developed and implemented that complies with federal and state law and includes the coordination of patient care within the facility and with health care providers, state and local DOHs, and emergency systems.
- Training and testing program—The training and testing program must include an initial and annual training, conducting of drills and exercises, or participation in an actual emergency that tests the plan.

CMS developed a Web site that provides resources, answers frequently asked questions, and provides guidance on compliance. It is available at: https://www.cms.gov/

Medicare/Provider-Enrollment-and-Certification/SurveyCertEmergPrep/Emergency-Prep-Rule.html.

Patient Movement

Repeatedly, hospitals or nursing homes are deemed unsafe following tornadoes, floods, or hurricanes and patients have to be evacuated. Many hospitals have Memorandums of Understanding with other institutions that enable the transfer of patients from one facility to another. However, disasters that strike an entire region can limit the ability to use those resources. In cases where regional capacity has been severely diminished, NDMS can be activated. However, some areas may be able to continue to care for patients using the resources within the community.

When facilities need to evacuate patients, key considerations include:

- Where are equivalent beds available? The task of matching a patient's needs with available beds is complicated. Critical care in one facility may not be at the same level as critical care in another. New York City (NYC) discovered this following Hurricane Sandy when quaternary level Tisch and Bellevue hospitals were flooded and had to be evacuated. NYC found that the key to caring for so many patients was cross-training highly skilled nurses.
- How will patients be transported? Having preexisting contracts in place with ambulance services was helpful in NYC. Dedicated transport centers can handle the transport arrangements, transfer of clinical information, etc.
- How will medical information be moved with patients to ensure continuity of quality of care? Regional planning groups can determine the minimum dataset that should travel with patients, preferably on 1 piece of paper. Inter-facility health care transfer forms can include the standard data elements common to the facilities in the region. Facilities can work with their electronic health record vendor to build transfer reports that can print when requested, even if requested from back-up systems in the cloud. Further, for hospitals using EPIC health care software, providers should be able to log-in from home and access medical records.
- What happens to homeless patients? Hospital social workers are critical in finding placements for the homeless or those who can't return to a damaged home.
- How will patients be tracked? Hospital Incident Command Systems (HICS), discussed below, often have a mechanism for tracking patients and notifying families. Bar codes have proven helpful when the equipment to use such a system is in place.
- The specifics of emergency credentialing are discussed below. Most regulations cover the first 72 hours. In NYC a large number of physicians worked in different facilities for months following Hurricane Sandy. The need for cross-credentialing

was highlighted after Sandy because doctors and nurses crossed borders and worked as volunteer staff to care for patients. One way of expanding care is to take care of patients in their homes.

- Other issues include ensuring patient privacy, returning patients to the original facility if the hospital will only be closed a few days, and the numerous liability- and revenue-related issues.

More on hospital preparedness and response is found in Chapters 9, 10, and 12.

Incident Command Systems

The emergency management field organizes its activities by sectors, such as fire, police, EMS, and health. All sectors use ICS for organizing their response to emergencies. Although ICS was originally developed in the 1970s as a way of responding to wildfires throughout California, this methodology now applies to all types of incidents, including hazardous material incidents, fires, transportation accidents, mass casualty incidents, search and rescue operations, and natural or technological disasters. ICS organizes its responses with a single person in charge and divides the tasks, functions, and resources into manageable components. Table 3-5 identifies some of the agencies involved in ICS and the resources that they bring.

Table 3-5. Agencies Involved in the Incident Command System

Agency	Resources
Red Cross	Shelter personnel
	Communications equipment
Electric company	Repair personnel
	Trucks
	Repair equipment
	Communications equipment
Emergency management	Emergency operations center
	Equipment
Fire	Firefighters
	Fire apparatus
Law enforcement	Police officers
	Flares, blockades
	Communications equipment
Public health	Surveillance systems
	Public health personnel
Public works/highway department	Repair personnel
	Trucks
	Repair equipment
	Communications equipment

The ICS organization is constructed with 5 major components: command, planning, operations, logistics, and finance/administration. Whether there is a routine emergency, a major event, or a catastrophic disaster, the management system employs all 5 components. The management system expands or contracts depending on the size of the event. An incident commander is responsible for on-scene management, regardless of the size or complexity of the event. Incident management encompasses the following:

- Establishing command
- Ensuring responder safety
- Assessing incident priorities
- Determining operational objectives
- Developing and implementing an incident action plan (IAP)
- Developing an appropriate organizational structure
- Maintaining a manageable span of control
- Managing incident resources
- Coordinating overall emergency activities
- Coordinating the activities of outside agencies
- Authorizing the release of information to the media
- Monitoring and recording costs

The sector responsible for public health services (including non-EMS health care providers, such as hospitals, urgent care centers, and health departments) faces several challenges when integrating their efforts into this coordinated response. Although NIMS requires all agencies to use ICS, until relatively recently in the evolution of emergency management, ICS was a preexisting management structure that may have planned and practiced for incidents without any input from the broader public health community. Public health agencies must continue to find a "fit" with this preexisting response structure. Additionally, health care systems draw patients from broader geographic areas than the political jurisdiction in which they are located. As a result, coordination is required between the prehospital system and the public health delivery system, which require a broader jurisdictional authority than in its day-to-day practice.

The DHS is sponsoring the development of a Next-Generation Incident Command System (NICS), which is a web-based command and control environment for incidents of all sizes and scope that facilitates collaboration across all levels of government. Key to NICS is facilitating situational awareness for responders who are widely dispersed. More information is available at: https://public.nics.ll.mit.edu/nicshelp/articles/frontpage.php.

Incident Command System Concepts and Principles. Many jurisdictions establish and maintain an EOC as part of their community's emergency preparedness program. ICS and EOC function together but at different levels of responsibility. ICS is responsible for on-scene activities, whereas the operations center is responsible for the communitywide response.

The organization of ICS response is modular and develops from a top-down structure at any incident. As incidents change in size, scope, and complexity, the ICS adapts by being able to scale up and down with flexible operational capabilities in order to meet the requirements under NIMS. The ICS/NIMS resources are requested, assigned, and deployed as needed and then demobilized when no longer necessary. Several communications networks may be established, depending on the size of the incident, but all communication is integrated. ICS employs a *unified command* whereby all agencies with responsibility for the incident, including public health, establish a common set of objectives and strategies. All involved agencies help to determine overall objectives, plan for joint operational activities, and maximize the use of assigned resources. Under unified command, the incident functions under a single, coordinated plan.

Effective response depends on all personnel using common terminology, as defined by ICS. The incident commander gives a specific name to the incident (such as "Ground Zero" for the bombing at the location). All of the response workforce uses the same name for all personnel, equipment, and facilities. Radio transmissions should not use agency-specific codes or terms but rather the language that everyone will understand.

An IAP for the local response to the emergency is organized by the planning section chief with tactical input from the operations section chief. In presidentially declared disasters where ESF #8 is being implemented, the IRCT described previously communicates the federal goals for the deployment of health and medical resources through a federal IAP. Figure 3-4 illustrates a typical organizational chart for an incident command system.

Public Health Incident Command

DOHs organize their internal emergency response structure using incident command principles. The cornerstone of a Public Health Incident Command System (PHICS) is to define the role, responsibility, chain of command, and job title of the person(s) carrying out each function that will be necessary to manage an incident. Table 3-6 lists the types of roles and responsibilities that might be predefined in DOHs. The goals are to (1) provide direct public health services as required by the emergency; (2) support the response of federal, state, local, and international health systems in public health emergencies; (3) support the deployment of health assets in response to or anticipation of a public health emergency; and (4) provide real-time situational information to and from federal, state, local, and international agencies, organizations, and field teams. The operationalization of PHICS includes the establishment of an agency EOC and each of the supporting units. The specific components of the EOC may vary from agency to agency. On a local level, typical units may include operations (including alert, notification, and escalation), epidemiology and surveillance, medical/clinical response teams, specialized laboratories and subject matter

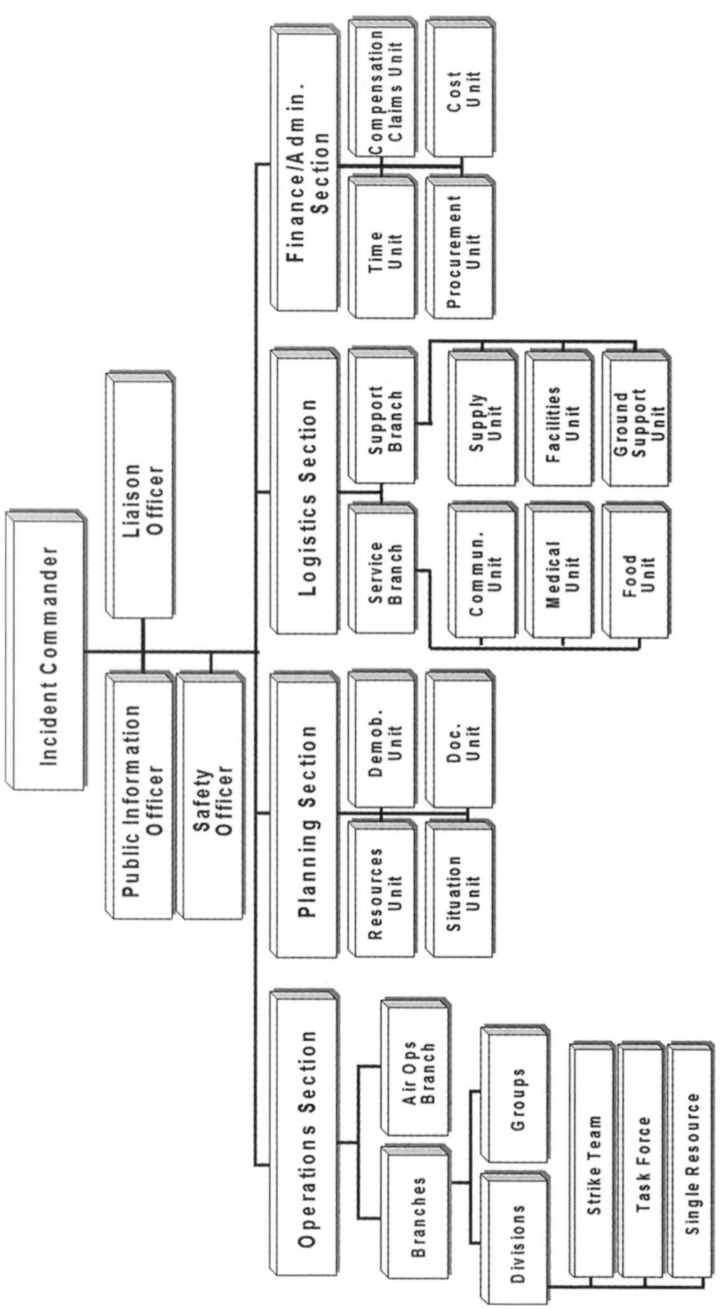

Source: Reprinted from Federal Emergency Management Agency. 2008. *ICS Review Material.* Washington, DC: ICS Resource Center. Available at: https://training.fema.gov/emiweb/is/icsresource/assets/reviewmaterials.pdf. Accessed December 29, 2016.

Figure 3-4. The Incident Command System

Table 3-6. Function, Roles, Responsibilities, and Chain of Command for Departments of Health

Function	Role	Responsibility	Chain of Command
Health commissioner or departmental director	Incident commander responsible for overall agency response	Declares emergency Authorizes DOH EOC activation Authorizes allocation of resources Communicates with mayor/governor and OEM EOC coordinator Principal departmental spokesperson to media Identifies need for consultants on technical issues Authorizes requests to the CDC for assistance Authorizes requests for mutual aid from other DOH jurisdictions	Reports to mayor/governor Reports to commissioner
Senior managers	Counsel and assist commissioner and/or DOH EOC members	Responds to request for assistance from commissioner and DOH EOC	
Deputy commissioner	Senior adviser to EOC coordinator on operational decisions	Senior adviser to commissioner on policy decisions Assumes commissioner's role in commissioner's absence	Reports to commissioner
Public affairs		Liaisons with press offices of mayor, OEM, and other agencies Coordinates press and public requests for information Drafts press releases Assists in creating and disseminating public information and educational messages Monitors press coverage of emergency Compiles/prepares material for Web site posting	Reports to commissioner or deputy commissioner
Governmental and community affairs		Liaisons with non-DOH governmental and community agencies/parties Notifies these agencies/parties of new developments or responses to emergency Assists in gaining cooperation of local officials for DOH activities	Reports to commissioner or deputy commissioner
Legal affairs		Monitors departmental activities and advises regarding legal issues Reviews documents related to emergency activities (e.g., declaration by commissioner)	Reports to commissioner

(Continued)

Table 3-6. (Continued)

Function	Role	Responsibility	Chain of Command
Incident-specific experts		Provide expertise and advice to guide policy making around emergencies: • Exposure, vector, and disease-specific knowledge • Training • Health and safety • Mental health	Report to commissioner or deputy commissioner
DOH EOC coordinator	Coordinates DOH response during emergency Responsible for all operational aspects of the response Oversees EOC during activation	Directs the DOH EOC Oversees emergency committees Oversees response to OEM activity requests Maintains documentation of key elements of the response and compiles final report Assesses need to request outside assistance (e.g., from the CDC) Responds to requests and needs of senior managers Synthesizes data from all sources Raises policy issues with commissioner	Reports to commissioner Receives input from senior emergency managers, committee representatives and senior managers
Senior emergency manager	Coordinates administrative and logistical operations of the DOH EOC	Communicates with DOH EOC coordinator Coordinates committee activities Communicates with DOH liaison at OEM EOC (e.g., report and job requests, transmits information and dispositions) Ensures ongoing rotation of staff at DOH EOC and OEM EOC Assists/coordinates mobilization of staff to carry out committee activities Compiles and distributes manual of operations (e.g., staffing schedule, contact numbers, protocols) to EOC participants	Reports to EOC coordinator Receives input from committee representatives and EOC liaison
EOC liaison	DOH representative at OEM EOC Liaisons between OEM EOC and DOH EOC	Staffs DOH workstation at OEM EOC Follows developments in emergency situation and in citywide response and provides briefing to DOH EOC Receives OEM requests for DOH activities and transmits to senior emergency manager (at DOH EOC) Informs OEM of DOH activities, responses, and recommendations Interacts with other agency representatives at OEM	Reports to senior emergency manager Receives input from OEM and senior emergency managers

(Continued)

Table 3-6. (Continued)

Function	Role	Responsibility	Chain of Command
Emergency committee representatives	Represent emergency committees at DOH EOC	Staff DOH EOC Provide policy guidance from OEM via senior emergency manager Accept action requests from OEM via senior emergency manager Accept request for data or activity orders from EOC coordinator Transmit information and requests for data or activity orders from EOC coordinator Report committee activities and information to EOC coordinator and senior emergency manager	Report to EOC coordinator and senior emergency manager Receive input from committee response coordinators
Committee response coordinators	Coordinate the emergency committee activities that comprise the DOH response to emergencies	Oversee activities of emergency committees Mobilize necessary workforce Receive information and job requests from committee representatives at DOH EOC Regularly report data and developments to committee representatives at DOH EOC Report needs to committee representatives at DOH EOC	Report to committee representatives at DOH EOC Receive input from committee members
Epidemiology surveillance		Research specific topic Provide background information Conduct field epidemiological investigations Identify and monitor existing surveillance and data systems Establish new surveillance systems Assemble field teams Develop questionnaires/abstraction forms/information sheets Liaison with hospital or other field personnel Collect data, establish databases, analyze data, develop recommendations for policy	

(Continued)

Table 3-6. (Continued)

Function	Role	Responsibility	Chain of Command
Medical clinical		Research specific topic Provide background information Prepare recommendations/advice on clinical aspects of emergency: • Public safety issues • Worker safety issues • Disinfection or decontamination issues • Clinical information and training of community physicians • Development of prevention and treatment messages Establish and staff prophylaxis or treatment distribution centers Staff DOH clinics engaged in clinical activities related to emergency Liaison with office of chief medical examiner Provide clinical backup to shelter committee activities	
Environmental		Research specific topic Provide background information Prepare advice/recommendations regarding public health threat, sample collection, evacuation, reoccupation Collect samples Collaborate with fire, hazmat, Department of Environmental Protection	
Shelter		Mobilize nurses to staff Red Cross clinics Provide medical backup to clinics	
Operations		Provide resources to facilitate emergency committee activities: • Transportation • Communication • Facility issues • Security • Human resources regarding mobilizing workforce • Printing	

(*Continued*)

Table 3-6. (Continued)

Function	Role	Responsibility	Chain of Command
Information management		Coordinate telephone hotlines for public and provider information Facilitate computing issues during emergency: • Web site posting • Field-to-HQ data transmission • Database management • Mapping and geographic information systems	
Laboratories		Provide recommendations regarding specimen types and handling Accept specimens for testing Ensure rapid transport to reference labs if testing not available at DOH lab Perform testing Coordinate with epidemiology/surveillance regarding data entry Liaison with outside labs regarding testing and data reporting	
DOH EOC	Integrated operations center for organizing and facilitating DOH response activities during emergencies	Provides accurate, timely information concerning the emergency to policy makers and public affairs officials Mobilizes DOH resources to respond to emergencies Communicates with and receives requests from OEM regarding data and activities Serves as a forum for integrating and synthesizing data as they come in from the emergency committees, OEM, EOC, senior managers	Staff: EOC coordinator, senior managers, emergency committee representatives Support staff as needed Senior managers and consultants as needed

Note: CDC=Centers for Disease Control and Prevention; DOH=department of health; EOC=emergency operations center; HQ=headquarters; OEM=office of emergency management.

experts, environmental consultation and response, management information services, and administration.

When a PHICS is activated, personnel must know what their role is and what they will be asked to do. Often, much of a disaster response is maintaining the daily functions of an agency. Most personnel will be doing their usual job, though possibly at a different time of day, in a different location, and with different people. The tasks and required skills will be more specific as the responsibilities become more administrative. Agency administration should ensure that each staff knows the task group they are assigned to, the responsibilities of that group, and how and where they get information about their responsibilities during an emergency. Although many skills are translatable (for example, clerical personnel can answer phones and provide directions as instructed and drivers can transport people and materials), some require additional training (such as chart abstractors who need specific skills in identifying disease-specific indicators).

Hospital Incident Command System

NIMS established 17 elements that hospitals must comply with, including a functioning ICS structure. Hospitals establish a system of incident command specific for their organizational structure known as HICS. Use of incident command improves a facility's ability to plan, respond, and recover from emergencies. HICS focuses on how a hospital organizes internally by establishing a chain of command with one person in charge and using job action sheets with predefined responsibilities. HICS requires that hospitals conduct a hazard analysis (as discussed in Chapter 6); establish mutual aid; coordinate with the local OEM; and maintain comprehensive documentation on how decisions were made, where patients went, how patients were tracked, and how reimbursement was obtained. These standards help to protect hospitals from claims of liability after a disaster.

Volunteers

The Citizen Corps is a national volunteer network that improves a community's resilience by involving citizens in all-hazards emergency preparedness. The Citizen Corps works to make communities better prepared by training and involving volunteers for response to public health disasters. Several teams are central to the Citizen Corp. FEMA's Community Emergency Response Team (CERT) program educates people about disaster preparedness and trains them in basic disaster response skills, such as fire safety, light search and rescue, team organization, and disaster medical operations. CERT members can assist others in their neighborhood or workplace following an event when professional responders are not immediately available to help. Other specialized partners with the Citizen Corps are the MRC and the ESAR-VHP. Following Hurricane Sandy, the New York and New Jersey Departments of Health requested medical support from federal HHS teams and more than 615 medical volunteers available through each state's ESAR-VHP and local MRC. These volunteers assisted in shelters (e.g., general, Red Cross, and special medical needs shelters), emergency departments, special needs registries, and call centers.

Medical Reserve Corps

The MRC is a federally sponsored program of the ASPR. The MRC provides an organized way for medical and public health volunteers from a community to supplement the manpower of existing local health and medical personnel by offering their skills and expertise during local emergencies. The MRC is designed to provide the appropriate training of these community volunteers and the needed organizational structure for deployment. The MRC can also be activated for nonemergency public health services, such as immunization or blood drives. MRC units are organized through governmental offices, faith-based groups, public health offices, hospitals, and other nongovernmental organizations.

There are 10 MRC regions in the United States, each with a variable number of local MRC units. Coordination occurs between the state and local MRCs and MRC regions. MRC units at the local level are responsible for recruiting and training volunteers to match specific community needs. Although MRC units are organized to supplement local response, they have been deployed outside their home areas in recent disasters.

Most MRCs are integrated with local health care, public health, or emergency management organizations. In communities that have established Citizen Corps Councils (which organize programs of volunteerism at a community level) it is important that the planners and managers of a local MRC unit have a working relationship with this council.

Nationally established criteria that guide the registration of MRC units include the following:

- Affiliation with an appropriate local organization
- Identification of MRC unit leader(s)
- Partnership with local and community stakeholder groups
- Verification of members' credential(s) (i.e., professional licenses/certificates)
- Plans for establishing, implementing, and sustaining the unit
- Participation in public health, preparedness, and emergency response activities
- Active involvement in the local, state, regional, and national MRC network

MRC units are funded from local and state resources, federal agencies such as the DHS Office of Domestic Preparedness and Citizen Corps, and through the CDC and the Health Resources and Services Administration.

Emergency System for Advance Registration of Volunteer Health Professionals

The ESAR-VHP is a federal program created to establish standardized volunteer registration programs when the impacts of disasters or public health emergencies require additional personnel. Each state or local organization verifies the identity and credentials of health professionals in advance so that they are ready to volunteer when their skills are needed. Once verified, ESAR-VHP volunteers are available to be deployed nationally through mutual aid mechanisms.

Currently licensed and credentialed health professionals can volunteer with ESAR-VHP. Registration varies from state to state. Some states use an online, electronic registration system, whereas other states may require volunteers to register via paper applications. Some states may accept both electronic and paper registrations. Volunteers may be entitled to workers' compensation if injured while participating in an emergency response and liability protections will vary by state. Check your state's ESAR-VHP Web site for information about the protections available in your state.

National Voluntary Organizations Active in Disaster

Through the National Voluntary Organizations Active in Disaster (VOAD), organizations share knowledge and resources about preparedness, response, and recovery to help disaster survivors and their communities. The VOAD has local chapters that participate in planning and includes individuals with disabilities and access and functional needs at all stages of the disaster cycle (see Chapter 11 for more information on disabilities and access and functional needs). Additional information can be found at: http://www.nvoad.org.

Tracking Volunteers

A mobile application (app) is available to help track both where volunteers are positioned and key locations during a deployment. Called "Deploy Pro," the app has a GPS-based interactive map that uses color-coded pins to track the whereabouts of team members. In addition, the platform can count the number of triage victims and has a reference guide for use in the field. Using the map in real time, team leaders can identify volunteers in different groups by color and visually see and locate each team. Further, other app users can see what has been noted, such as the location of victims. Available at: http://deploypro.net.

Liability

Liability is an issue that each locality must investigate thoroughly. Participation in a local MRC or registration with a state ESAR-VHP program does not result in the recognition of professional licensure by other states. All states have some form of "good Samaritan" legislation, although this legislation may be limited in its protections. Protection is also found through the Volunteer Protection Act (VPA; codified at 42 U.S.C. § 14501 et seq.). VPA, which provides qualified immunity from liability for volunteers, is helpful because it provides baseline legal protection where there is a wide variety of state laws. Further, during a declared emergency, the Uniform Emergency Volunteer Health Practitioners Act (UEVHPA) allows state governments to accept the licenses of providers from other states so that covered individuals may provide services without meeting the disaster state's licensing requirements. As of this writing, 17 states and territories had enacted UEVHPA: Arkansas, Colorado, the District of Columbia, Illinois, Indiana, Georgia, Kentucky, Louisiana, Nevada, New Mexico, North Dakota, Tennessee, Texas, Oklahoma, Oregon, Utah, and the U.S. Virgin Islands.

Hospital Credentialing of Volunteers

The RRC and DMATs are 2 systems in which the process of credentialing medical volunteers is "federalized," whereby the federal government waives state licensing procedures and also assumes liability. However, until those resources are in place, hospitals and public health agencies might have to credential staff in a rapid manner. Experience shows that following a disaster, the community is deluged with calls from volunteers, many of whom are physicians and nurses looking to help. As part of their overall disaster plan, hospitals and public health agencies should have a procedure to manage and verify the credentials of professional volunteer staff. (Coordinate planning with your state licensing boards, professional societies, and regional hospitals since they may have developed a uniform way to verify current licensure, specialty, and hospital status of professionals.) Medical staff bylaws should also be amended to allow for emergency credentialing in disaster situations and should designate who will be responsible for credentialing and overall clinical direction and supervision of volunteers. Practitioners should not be granted emergency privileges for procedures that they are not credentialed to perform at the hospitals where they are fully credentialed, and emergency privileges should terminate on their own when the disaster is under control and the hospital's emergency management plan is no longer activated. The 2015 Joint Commission standards (Volunteer Licensed Independent Practitioners, EM.02.02.13, and Volunteer Practitioners, EM.02.02.15) define the process for granting of emergency privileges when a hospital's emergency operations plan has been activated and the organization is unable to handle patient needs.

To grant emergency (or disaster) privileges to licensed independent practitioners who are not members of that hospital's medical staff, the following are necessary:

- The emergency operations plan is activated.
- The hospital is unable to manage its patients' immediate needs without outside assistance.
- Medical staff bylaws identify the individual(s) responsible for granting emergency privileges (i.e., chief executive officer or medical staff president or his or her designee[s]).
- Mechanisms are developed that allow medical staff to oversee the practice of and to readily identify individuals receiving emergency privileges.
- A privileging process, identical to the process established under the medical staff bylaws for granting temporary privileges, is established with a verification procedure.
- The chief executive officer or president of the medical staff or his or her designee(s) may grant emergency privileges upon presentation of a current valid photo identification issued by a state, federal, or regulatory agency and any of the following:
  - A current picture identification card from a health care organization that clearly identifies professional designation;
  - A current license to practice;
  - Primary source verification of licensure;
  - Identification indicating that the individual is a member of DMAT, MRC, ESAR-VHP, or other recognized state or federal response organization or group;
  - Identification indicating that the individual has been granted authority by a government entity to provide patient care, treatment, or services in disaster circumstances; or
  - Confirmation by a licensed independent practitioner currently privileged by the hospital or by a staff member with personal knowledge of the volunteer practitioner's ability to act as a licensed independent practitioner during a disaster.

The plan for credentialing physicians in an emergency should provide for clear identification of these practitioners. Identification should be easily legible and include a picture, their name and service, and the words "Disaster Privileges" in a different color. In the event of a power outage, a Polaroid camera and a label maker can be used, as can wristbands.

The management plan should provide precise record keeping of who was credentialed and their profession and specialty. Employees from the medical staff office should be identified to manage the emergency credentialing and to orient the volunteers and familiarize them with hospital operations and the nature of the emergency services needed.

Verify and check the following, or check similar agencies and databases that operate in your state:

- National Practitioner Data Bank
- State medical license
- Office of Professional Medical Conduct
- Office of Inspector General
- Photo identification

Finally, request that the hospital where the practitioner's current privileges are held confirms current active membership and privileges, check his or her American Medical Association or medical specialty profile, and require a signed statement from the non-staff physician who is attesting to the facts and allowing the hospital to obtain the necessary documents.

Costs, Funding, Reimbursement for Disaster Preparedness and Response

For public and nonprofit entities, the Stafford Act provides for federal reimbursement of some expenses associated with the effects of the disaster and disaster response. This funding is known as public assistance. FEMA's public assistance grant program provides assistance to state, tribal, and local governments and some nonprofit organizations to enable communities to respond and recover quickly from disasters receiving a presidential declaration. Through the public assistance program, FEMA provides disaster grants for removal of debris, emergency protective measures, and the repair, replacement, or restoration of disaster-damaged public or certain nonprofit facilities. The public assistance program also provides aid for hazard mitigation measures during the recovery process. These federal grants will pay at least 75% of the eligible cost and the grantee (usually the state) determines how the remaining share (up to 25%) is split among the subgrantees.

Disaster Assistance

Individuals, families, and businesses can receive direct assistance where property has been damaged or destroyed and losses are not covered by insurance. This money is intended to help pay for critical expenses that cannot be covered in other ways. Disaster assistance provides money for temporary housing, to repair damage to a primary residence, or to replace a destroyed home where these costs are not covered by insurance. In remote locations specified by FEMA where no other type of housing assistance is possible, disaster assistance provides money for the construction of a home. Some housing assistance funds are available through FEMA's Individuals and Households Program. However, most disaster assistance from the federal government is in the form of loans administered by the Small Business Administration. In addition, money is also available for necessary expenses or serious needs as determined by FEMA, such as disaster-related medical, dental, funeral, and burial costs.

Title 44 of the Code of Federal Regulations (CFR; Emergency Management and Assistance) contains the rules, policies, and procedures regarding the administration of federal disaster assistance programs by FEMA. Part 206 of the 44 CFR, contains the regulations applicable to FEMA's disaster assistance program. FEMA coordinates that process and provides the forms that must be submitted for reimbursement. When local governments receive the support of any federal assets, the federal government absorbs the costs in the initial hours of the response. However, local governments are expected to reimburse the federal government for assets provided thereafter through a cost-sharing formula. In extraordinary cases, the president may choose to adjust the cost share or waive it for a specified time period. The presidential declaration notes any cost-share waiver, and a DHS-State Agreement is signed further stipulating the division of costs among federal, state, and local governments and other conditions for receiving assistance.

The public assistance program reimburses for damage to infrastructure, for equipment, and for overtime for personnel. It does not reimburse for providing patient care as part of the normal course of doing business. The public assistance program does not reimburse for services eligible for funding under another federal program, such as the VA. All public health agencies should obtain a copy of the rules, including the details of documentation necessary for reimbursement. Local agencies should identify what aid is available through their state. Some have a state-funded reimbursement mechanism similar to the federal assistance program, which may reimburse local health departments for a percentage of costs for medical emergencies through public health law. However, total reimbursement from state and federal sources cannot exceed 100%. It is important to ensure that there is no duplication since disaster victims are responsible for repayment of federal assistance duplicated by private insurance or other federal programs. Finally, if an event is declared a terrorist attack, localities should realize that commercial insurance policies may deny reimbursement because care was required because of "an act of war."

Currently, there are a variety of funding opportunities to help communities prepare for disasters. Grant information was integrated at a DHS Web site (available at: https://www.dhs.gov/how-do-i/find-and-apply-grants) and the application process was streamlined. PAHPA provides for cooperative agreements and grants to state and local governments to improve health security. Grants can also be awarded to hospitals, clinical laboratories, and universities for improvements in real-time disease detection. The Catalog of Federal Domestic Assistance (available at: https://www.cfda.gov) links to a variety of federal funding programs.

The PHEP and HPP cooperative agreements are critical sources of funding for state, local, tribal, and territorial public health departments. HHS requires that health care organizations implement NIMS in order to be eligible to apply for preparedness funding through the ASPR HPP grant program (see http://www.phe.gov/Preparedness/planning/hpp/Pages/funding.aspx). PHEP efforts support the NRF. Administered by the CDC, PHEP funding is used to advance public health preparedness and response capabilities among state and local health departments (see http://www.cdc.gov/phpr/coopagreement.htm). By working collaboratively with federal health and preparedness programs in their jurisdiction to conduct joint planning and exercises and joint program operations, state and local DOHs can maximize resources and prevent duplicative efforts. Health departments use HPP funding, administered by the ASPR, to develop and expand health care preparedness capabilities through regional health care coalitions. Health care coalitions collaborate to ensure that each member has the necessary medical equipment and supplies, real-time information, communications systems, and trained health care personnel to respond to an emergency. Table 3-7 summarizes other federal funding opportunities..

Table 3-7. Federal Funding Opportunities

Source	Web Site
ASPR Hospital Preparedness Program	http://www.phe.gov/Preparedness/planning/hpp/Pages/funding.aspx
Government funding	http://www.grants.gov
CDC	http://www.cdc.gov/od/pgo/funding/grantmain.htm
CDC ATSDR Federal Assistance Funding Book	http://www.atsdr.cdc.gov/funding.html
Department of Homeland Security	https://www.dhs.gov/how-do-i/find-and-apply-grants
FEMA Fire Service	https://www.usfa.fema.gov/grants
Public Health Emergency Preparedness cooperative agreements	http://www.cdc.gov/phpr/coopagreement.htm

Note: ASPR=Assistant Secretary for Preparedness and Response; ATSDR=Agency for Toxic Substances and Disease Registry; CDC=Centers for Disease Control and Prevention; FEMA=Federal Emergency Management Agency.

CHAPTER 4

ESSENTIALS OF DISASTER PLANNING

Although the exact timing of disasters is often unforeseen, disaster planning can anticipate the common problems encountered and the tasks required following large-scale emergencies. This chapter highlights the federal requirements and federal guidance for planning, discusses the principles of disaster planning and the increased need for planning, identifies constraints on being able to plan, reviews planning for various types of disasters, describes common tasks of disaster response, highlights components of a disaster preparedness plan, examines key considerations in surge capacity and the delivery of care under extreme conditions, and considers exercises to practice the plan.

Public Health Role

- Use traditional planning principles in preparing for the delivery of public health and health care services during the impact and postimpact phases.
- Participate as full partners with the emergency management community and regional health care systems in planning for disaster response and recovery.
- Participate in the development of and serve as an integral part of a community's disaster preparedness plans.
- Participate in organizing health care coalitions and other health care partners in the community.
- Coordinate efforts with local, state, federal, and tribal partners.

Planning Is Required: Federal Guidance

Planning has been an essential component of the emergency management field for decades. The public health role was emphasized in 2005 when the devastating aftermath of Hurricane Katrina led to the passage of the Pandemic and All-Hazards Preparedness Act (PAHPA), which requires enhanced planning and the development of capabilities to improve the medical and public health response to future disasters. As defined in Chapter 3, capabilities are the operational capacity and ability to execute preparedness tasks. Planning based on capabilities both defines the specifics of how an organization's or agency's *assets* (i.e., staff, equipment, supplies, and space) can be utilized as part of the community's disaster plan and identifies the skills required to execute the needed preparedness tasks.

In addition to PAHPA, federal guidance on disaster planning discussed in this chapter includes the Pandemic and All-Hazards Preparedness Reauthorization Act (PAHPRA), the National Health Security Strategy (NHSS), National Planning Frameworks (NPF), and the National Planning System, as well as guidance from the Centers for Disease Control and Prevention (CDC) and the Office of the Assistant Secretary of Preparedness and Response (ASPR).

Pandemic and All-Hazards Preparedness Act

PAHPA requires that planning is fulfilled by both public health agencies and health care facilities. Through planning, these organizations are better able to meet the capabilities necessary to deliver services during and following a disaster. The process of planning based on capabilities can assist state and local organizations in their identification of gaps in a community's preparedness, determination of the priorities for designated jurisdictions, and development of a strategy for sustaining the jurisdiction's capabilities. This process also ensures more resilient and better prepared communities.

By requiring public health organizations to develop and sustain essential profession-specific capabilities for federal, state, local, and tribal governments, these agencies are better able to do the following:

- Monitor and contain disease:
    - Maintain situational awareness through detection, identification, and investigation domestically and abroad.
    - Contain disease through isolation, quarantine, social distancing, and decontamination.
    - Communicate about risks and preparedness.
- Rapidly distribute and administer medical countermeasures, products, and public health interventions (e.g., vaccines, antimicrobials, and antibody preparations; ventilators, devices, and personal protective equipment; and contact and transmission interventions, social distancing, and community shielding) used to prevent and mitigate the health effects of chemical, biological, radiological, or nuclear events.

PAHPA also requires that health care facilities (i.e., hospitals including trauma care, mental health facilities, and emergency medical service systems) develop plans to:

- strengthen the medical management of patients, treatment capabilities of facilities, medical evacuation following disasters, and management of fatalities;

- ensure the rapid distribution and administration of medical countermeasures;
- ensure effective utilization of public and private medical assets and successful integration with federal resources; and
- protect health care workers and first responders from workplace exposures and injuries during public health emergencies.

Pandemic and All-Hazards Preparedness Reauthorization Act

PAHPRA (as discussed in Chapter 3) expanded the role of the ASPR in planning for disasters by adding responsibilities, including:

- Develop federal preparedness and response policy coordination and strategic direction for public health emergencies covered by the National Response Plan.
- Delineate national and regional inefficiencies in medical and public health preparedness and response.
- Coordinate grants related to preparedness and response efforts.
- Conduct preparedness and response drills and exercises in collaboration with other federal departments and agencies.

National Health Security Strategy

The NHSS identifies capabilities for the provision of medical and public health services that are the underpinning to planning. The NHSS (as discussed in Chapter 3) includes 1 overarching goal and 5 objectives to meet the public health and medical requirements. Planning, by public health professionals, helps ensure that communities can maintain and sustain vital public health and medical services during a health emergency, which is key to achieving the NHSS. The implementation plan of the NHSS provides strategic direction for planning by establishing a common vision on how to carry out activities of prevention, protection, mitigation, response, recovery and health resilience.

The NHSS goal is "to strengthen and sustain communities' abilities to prevent, protect against, mitigate the effects of, respond to, and recover from incidents with negative health consequences." The NHSS for 2015–2018 is structured with a whole community approach, which incorporates the participation of many federal departments and agencies including the U.S. Department of Health & Human Services (HHS); governments at all levels; and the breadth of the whole community, including nongovernmental organizations, private sector businesses, the scientific and academic community, individuals, and families. These stakeholders work together to coordinate planning activities. Strong community and national planning requires strong leadership and commitment across all levels of government and communities.

Planning to Meet the 5 NHSS Objectives

The first objective focuses on building heath resilience in communities by encouraging individuals to be connected socially. Examples of planning activities that public health can do to meet the objective of building resilience include:

- Create templates and toolkits on community connectedness, social capital, and health resilience.
- Use social networking sites to strengthen neighbor-to-neighbor ties and explore uses of such sites for emergency response.
- Encourage people to get to know their neighbors.
- Create evidence-based, culturally sensitive guidance to encourage neighborhoods to increase their community's resilience.
- Identify individuals with access and functional needs and connect them with necessary support and supplies.
- Enhance coordination and partnerships among those providing health and human services.
- Build a culture of resilience through training of the general population in health-related areas such as first aid, cardiopulmonary resuscitation, and caring for self and family.

The second objective targets the expansion of the production and dispensing of medical countermeasures (MCM) and nonpharmaceutical interventions (NPI). Examples of planning activities include:

- Develop a plan to communicate to all stakeholders about the risks and benefits of implementing MCM and NPI during disaster events when they are needed.
- Work with state and local partners on a process of deciding when and how to use MCMs and NPIs.
- Develop a framework and capability to rapidly identify best practices and alternatives to control emerging infectious diseases.
- Draft guidance on dissemination and prioritization of MCMs for first responders and their families.
- Collaborate with academic and private partners to identify and evaluate novel ways of sustaining the Strategic National Stockpile.

The third objective focuses on the ability to have situational awareness through data to inform decisions about health threats, population health, health-related response assets, and other considerations such as emerging infectious diseases in animals that can impact human health. Examples of ways departments of health can plan for increased situational awareness on public health concerns include:

- Develop a list of chief environmental and zoonotic threats that should be tracked as part of a database.
- Work with state and local partners from the health, environmental, and agricultural sectors to expand the integration and sharing of surveillance data on outbreaks among both humans and animals.
- Partner with higher education and academic centers to develop a workforce that understands human, animal, and environmental health.
- Engage experts in industry to analyze and interpret data critical to comprehensive situational awareness about conditions related to health.
- Develop secure mechanisms to enable the exchange of information and intelligence products (e.g., technical systems that can collect the multiple types of data that are normally classified) and other relevant health information across agencies.

The fourth objective promotes the integration and effectiveness of the public health, clinical, and emergency management systems. Examples of related activities include:

- Work with coalitions to develop guidance for the development, implementation, and evaluation of emergency management programs for health systems.
- Collaborate with hospitals, providers, and academic institutions to explore how current telemedicine programs can address health care surge and access needs.
- Develop quality metrics to guide the delivery of service during events that disproportionately impact children.
- Work with stakeholders to develop guidance on the evacuation and sheltering of populations with specific privacy needs (e.g., victims of domestic violence).
- Encourage providers to discuss preparedness with at-risk populations.

The fifth objective strengthens global health security by supporting the implementation of the World Health Organization's International Health Regulations, which require 196 nations to develop and maintain the capacity to detect, assess, and respond to international public health threats. Examples include:

- Train frontline health care workers to improve the ability to recognize infectious disease threats.
- Develop mechanisms to identify, document, disseminate, and learn from the experience of international events that affected health security.
- Enhance early detection and alert systems that can identify public health threats through both traditional surveillance and innovative sources of information (e.g., social media).

- Expand emergency alert systems and risk communication strategies.
- Develop and perform interdisciplinary cross-training in health diplomacy.

National Planning Frameworks

The NPF, part of the National Preparedness System, provide information on how the whole community works together to build, sustain, and deliver the core capabilities needed to achieve the National Preparedness Goal (NPG; see Chapter 3). The planning frameworks have mutual elements and departments and agencies coordinate in carrying them out. There is 1 planning framework for each of the 5 preparedness areas: prevention, protection, mitigation, response, and recovery.

- The National Prevention Framework describes the core capabilities, aligns key roles and responsibilities, describes coordinating structures, and provides the basis for operational coordination and synchronized planning that may be needed to prevent an imminent act of terrorism or respond to natural disasters and other threats or hazards.
- The National Protection Framework examines the role of the whole community in protecting against acts of terrorism, natural disasters, and other threats.
- The National Mitigation Framework promotes the development of a culture of preparedness by mitigating risk and vulnerability in order to reduce the loss of life and damage to property following a disaster or other emergency.
- The National Response Framework is a guide for how the whole community responds to a disaster or other emergency. It describes the specific authorities which provide direction and best practices for managing the broadest range of incidents.
- The National Disaster Recovery Framework describes the core capabilities and recovery structure necessary to help state and local communities recover, especially from a catastrophic disaster. This framework structure for recovery is flexible to promote a unified and collaborative response.

National Planning System

As part of the National Preparedness System (see Chapter 3), the United States has a national planning approach which uses a common terminology and guidance. This structure encourages those at the national, state and local levels to complement the work of other jurisdictions in their development of all hazards plans in preparation for disasters. By involving many partners in a shared planning effort, including academic institutions and private and nonprofit organizations, this approach of complementary planning with the whole community is the foundation of a National Planning System. This approach enables the whole community to build, sustain, and deliver the core capabilities identified in the NPG.

This National Planning System is built upon 2 key elements: the Planning Architecture, which describes the strategic, operational, and tactical levels of planning and integration of those plans; and the Planning Process, which describes the steps necessary to develop a comprehensive plan. Here we describe each in more detail:

Planning Architecture

The National Planning System consists of 3 levels of planning:

- ***Strategic-level*** plans provide a framework for the implementation of long-term or ongoing processes to prevent, protect against, mitigate, respond to, and recover from all threats and hazards that might affect a jurisdiction. Strategic-level planning brings together multiple organizations each with their plans to develop a comprehensive approach. At the national level, planners would develop a national strategy for a specific threat, such as floods. At the local level, communities establish a strategy for addressing potential threats based on local assessments of risk such as those done in the Threat and Hazard Identification and Risk Assessment (as discussed in Chapter 6). These strategic level plans describe the mitigation goals and objectives for a given hazard and identify the existing and necessary capabilities and resources needed to meet those goals.
- ***Operational-level*** plans are developed once a community understands the hazards that it may confront. Operational plans provide a description of the roles and responsibilities, tasks, and actions required of a jurisdiction or its associated departments and agencies during disasters. These plans may also specify how a jurisdiction will meet the capabilities needed to respond to a given disaster. On a state level, operational plans detail those responsible for carrying out specific actions; identify what is needed in personnel, equipment, facilities, supplies, and other resources; and outline how the response will be coordinated.
- ***Tactical-level*** plans focus on managing resources, such as personnel and equipment, that are an integral part of a disaster response. Tactical planning is often used for special events or venues, such as when the Pope visited New York City in 2015 or the Democratic and Republican National Conventions during presidential election years. Here, the planners determine the assignment of resources, the routes, and designated staging areas. Tactical planning often provides "meat" about the detailed actions necessary to accomplish goals identified in an operational plan.

Planning Process

The process of planning involves 2 components: (1) ensuring support by those involved, and (2) conducting a unified planning process. The common planning process, as outlined in the *Comprehensive Preparedness Guide 101*, includes the following:

- ***Form a Collaborative Planning Team.*** Engage and integrate the whole community as part of the planning process
- ***Understand the Situation.*** Assess the risks of the community so that planning teams can make informed decisions about the management of risks and development of necessary capabilities
- ***Determine Goals and Objectives.*** Leverage the identified capabilities to establish priorities, goals and objectives. Priorities indicate a desired outcome. Goals are broad, general statements about the methods for achieving the desired results. Objectives are specific and identifiable actions.
- ***Plan Development.*** Develop and analyze possible solutions or courses of action for achieving the outcome and reaching the goals. Based on this analysis, select the preferred solution or course of action.
- ***Plan Preparation, Review, and Approval.*** The courses of action developed during plan development are used to draft a plan. Once drafted, the organizations responsible for implementation disseminate the plan for review and approval.
- ***Plan Implementation and Maintenance.*** Plans should be regularly reviewed and updated due to changes in assessed risk, statutes, policy, and better practices derived from lessons learned during the response to actual disasters.

Guidance From Centers for Disease Control and Prevention and Office of the Assistant Secretary of Preparedness and Response

In March 2011, the CDC published guidance for state and local planners preparing to meet the needs of their communities in a public health crisis. CDC identified 15 core capabilities grouped into 6 categories that describe the skills and capacity that each public health organization should have. The 6 categories are biosurveillance, community resilience, countermeasures and mitigation, incident management, information management, and surge management. The public health capabilities, definitions, and functions are identified in Appendix E. The complete standards include tasks, performance measures, and resource elements (available at: http://www.cdc.gov/phpr/capabilities/Capabilities_March_2011.pdf).[1]

1. The Public Health Capabilities are being revised with expected publication in 2017.

In 2016, the Office of the ASPR released its Healthcare Preparedness and Response Capabilities for 2017–2022. This directive developed 4 capabilities based on guidance provided in the previous 2012 Healthcare Preparedness Capabilities: National Guidance for Healthcare System Preparedness document. These health care capabilities were designed

> to describe what the health care delivery system, including health care coalitions (HCC), hospitals, and emergency medical services (EMS), have to do to effectively prepare for and respond to emergencies that impact the public's health. Each jurisdiction, including emergency management organizations and public health agencies, provides key support to the health care delivery system.

The ASPR guidance is intended to help any health care delivery system organization, HCC, or state or local agency that supports the provision of care during emergencies to identify gaps in preparedness, determine specific priorities, and develop plans specific to health care and public health. It is hoped that by identifying, building, and sustaining capabilities for health care and public health, communities will be better prepared, more resilient, and ultimately safer. The document is organized into a section for each capability, with a goal ("the outcome of developing the capability") and a set of objectives ("overarching component of the capability that, when completed, helps achieve the goal"); most objectives describe associated activities ("a task critical for achieving an objective"). The complete guidance is available at https://www.phe.gov/Preparedness/planning/hpp/reports/Documents/2017 2022 healthcare pr capablities.pdf.

ASPR identified the following 4 capabilities as basic skills and capacity needed for health care systems, coalitions, and organizations to be prepared:

- *Foundation for health care and medical readiness*: With a strong foundation, the health care delivery system and its partners are able to coordinate efforts before, during, and after disasters; continue operations; and surge their capacity to treat an increased number of patients when necessary.
  - Capability goal: The community's health care organizations and other stakeholders coordinate their efforts through a sustainable HCC in order to have strong relationships, identify hazards and risks, and prioritize and address gaps through planning, training, exercising, and managing resources.
  - Examples of the objectives and suggested activities to accomplish each include the following: (1) Establish and operationalize an HCC by defining HCC Boundaries, identifying HCC members, and establishing HCC governance; (2) identify risk and needs by assessing hazard vulnerabilities and associated risks, assessing health care resources in the region, and prioritizing resource gaps and mitigation strategies; (3) develop an HCC preparedness plan; (4) train and prepare the health care and medical workforce by promoting role-appropriate implementation of the National Incident Management System, educating and training on identified

preparedness and response gaps, and planning and conducting coordinated exercises with HCC members and other response organizations; and (5) ensure preparedness is sustainable by promoting the value of health care and medical readiness and engaging health care executives, clinicians, and community leaders.

- *Health care and medical response coordination*: Coordination of the medical response enables the health care delivery system and other organizations to share information, manage and share resources, and integrate their activities when carrying out their jurisdictional responsibilities under Emergency Support Functions (ESFs) #8 and #6 at both the federal and state levels.
  - Capability goal: Health care organizations, the HCC, their jurisdiction(s), and the HHS as the lead agency for ESF #8 plan and collaborate to share and analyze information, manage and share resources, and coordinate strategies to deliver medical care to all populations during emergencies and planned events.
  - Examples of the objectives and suggested activities to accomplish each include the following: (1) Develop and coordinate health care organization and HCC response plans by developing an emergency operations plan for health care organizations and for the HCC; (2) utilize information sharing procedures and platforms by developing procedures to share information, identifying procedures for accessing information and protecting data, and utilizing communications systems and platforms; and (3) coordinate response strategy, resources, and communications during an emergency by identifying and coordinating resource needs, coordinating Incident Action Planning, and communicating with health care providers, nonclinical staff, patients, and visitors.
- *Continuity of health care service delivery:* The ability to deliver optimal health care services is likely to be interrupted when utilities, electronic health records, and supply chains are disrupted. This capability aims to bolster the health care delivery system's ability to continue services during an emergency and return to normal operations more rapidly.
  - Capability goal: Health care organizations, with support from the HCC and the HHS as the lead agency for ESF #8, provide uninterrupted, optimal medical care to all populations in the face of damaged or disabled health care infrastructure. Health care workers are well trained, well educated, and well equipped to care for patients during emergencies. Simultaneous response and recovery operations result in a return to normal or, ideally, improved operations.
  - Examples of the objectives and suggested activities to accomplish each include the following: (1) Identify essential functions for health care delivery; (2) plan for continuity of operations by developing a plan for continuing operations for health care organizations and for the HCC and planning for each health care organization to shelter-in-place; (3) maintain access to nonpersonnel resources during an emergency by assessing the integrity of the supply chain and assessing and addressing

requirements for equipment, supplies, and pharmaceuticals; (4) develop strategies to protect health care information systems and networks; (5) protect responders' safety and health by distributing resources required to protect the health care workforce, training and conducting exercises to promote responders' safety and health, and developing health care worker resilience; (6) plan for and coordinate health care evacuation and relocation by developing and implementing plans for evacuating, relocating, and transporting those being evacuated; and (7) coordinate recovery of the health care delivery system by planning for and assessing the system's recovery after an emergency and facilitating recovery assistance and implementation.

- *Medical surge:* Medical surge is the ability to evaluate and care for a volume of patients that exceeds normal operating capacity. Providing an effective medical surge response is dependent on the 3 planning and response capabilities previously discussed.
    - Capability goal: While health care organizations are often able to deliver timely and efficient care to their patients even when the demand for health care services exceeds available supply, when an emergency overwhelms the HCC's collective resources, the HCC collaborates with the HHS (ESF #8 lead agency) in coordinating information and available resources for its members to maintain their conventional surge response. The HCC supports the health care delivery system's transition to a crisis surge response and promotes a timely return to conventional standards of care as soon as possible.
    - Examples of the objectives and suggested activities to accomplish each include the following: (1) Plan for a medical surge by incorporating medical surge planning into the Emergency Operations Plan for health care organizations, EMS, and the HCC response plan; and (2) respond to a medical surge by implementing the surge plan in the emergency department, inpatient units, and out-of-hospital facilities, developing an alternate care system, distributing medical countermeasures, and managing mass fatalities.

Principles of Disaster Planning

Along with their differences, disasters have similarities in that certain problems and tasks occur repetitively and predictably. On the other hand, disasters differ not only quantitatively but also qualitatively from common daily emergencies. Thus, effective disaster response involves much more than an extension of routine emergency response (i.e., mobilization of more personnel, facilities, equipment, or supplies). Understanding the planning process and the lexicon of emergency management increases the effectiveness of public health professionals.

Effective disaster plans are based on empirical knowledge of how people actually behave in disasters. Plans are easier to change than is human behavior, so disaster plans should be based on what people are likely to do rather than on the expectation that the public will behave "according to the plan." Plans must be flexible and easy to change as a result of the breadth and diversity of laws, organizations, populations, technologies, hazards, resources, and personnel involved in disaster response. When developing plans, it is crucial to establish partnerships within the community so that agencies formulate an interactive plan that maximizes the available resources.

Disaster planning should focus on a local response with federal and state support. In any major natural disaster, the main rescue effort will most likely be executed by local authorities during the first 48 to 72 hours to ensure a timely response for the severely injured (e.g., those trapped in a collapsed building). Thus, disaster plans must be acceptable to the elected officials who will execute the plans, to the departments that will implement the plans, and to those for whom the plans are designed. Plans should be widely disseminated among all those involved and should be exercised regularly, as discussed later in this chapter.

Because response to disasters is resource intensive and requires the broadest combination of skills, no single entity has the breadth needed for comprehensive planning. Planners should establish relationships with a variety of stakeholders who can contribute to the plan by understanding their agency's assets, capabilities, and limitations and their familiarity with the needs of the community. Groups and individuals who understand at-risk populations should be involved in all stages of the planning process so that the needs of those with disabilities and other access and functional needs (see Chapter 11) can be integrated into each component of the community's plan. The emergency plan can include an annex that specifically addresses the actions to be taken to protect those with functional needs. Community planning should include mutual aid agreements and memorandums of understanding regarding procedures for sharing resources during emergencies.

Similarly, disaster plans should provide for some authority at the lowest levels of the organization, since workers in the trenches must make many decisions during the impact and immediate postimpact phases. Disasters often present decision making demands that exceed the bureaucratic capacities and information-processing abilities of the day-to-day management structure. Disaster plans that require all decisions to be made from the top down do not optimize the resources of the organization.

Increased Need for Planning

With the rising occurrence and mounting damage associated with natural and technological events, the increasing threat of terrorism, and the federal regulations requiring the capabilities of public health professionals, public health agencies should give priority to planning for disasters. No region of the United States is free from disaster risk. In fact, the effects of natural disasters escalate each year as a result of increases in population and development in vulnerable areas (e.g., coastal areas, flood plains, seismic fault lines, wilderness areas). At the same time, emerging and resident infectious disease, immigration, imported goods, rapid international transportation, and terrorism increase the potential for technological disasters and epidemic spread of disease. Finally, the economic health of the United States affects both the number of persons displaced (e.g., the homeless, the working poor) and recovery following disaster.

Constraints on Ability to Respond

Trends in health care reimbursement and delivery interfere with efforts by health care facilities to prepare for disasters. First, while federal grants are available for some health care institutions, decreasing reimbursement reduces the likelihood that facilities and community providers will allocate funds for disaster preparedness. Even if the budgetary allocations are adequate, fewer resources are available for the delivery of unusual services. For example, fewer supplies may be available for disaster response because hospitals and other health facilities have eliminated the local warehousing of supplies and instead reorder as needed. The trend to outsource services (e.g., laundry, kitchen, security) reduces the availability of important resources that would be needed postimpact. With shorter inpatient lengths of stay and greater use of ambulatory care, hospitals have reduced the number of available, staffed beds; with fewer beds, there are fewer available staff. The availability of beds postimpact will be further complicated by the trend toward only hospitalizing sicker patients who require more intensive care, so fewer patients will be ready for discharge to create room for victims seriously injured in the disaster. Finally, while the focus on delivering care in nonhospital settings has increased, a parallel effort to ensure disaster readiness in nonhospital health care locations will be further improved due to the requirements of the Centers for Medicare & Medicaid Services regulations issued in 2016.

Planning for Various Disasters

Two strategies for disaster planning include the agent-specific and the all-hazards approaches. In agent-specific planning, communities only plan for threats most likely to occur in their regions (e.g., earthquakes, hurricanes, floods, tornadoes). For example, planning for earthquakes, floods, and wildfires will be more useful in California than would planning for hurricanes and tornadoes. Further, officials and taxpayers are more likely to be motivated by what are perceived locally as the most viable threats.

With the all-hazards approach to disaster planning, the level of preparedness is maximized for the effort and expenditures involved. Since many disasters pose similar problems and similar tasks, an all-hazards approach involves planning for the common problems and tasks that arise in the majority of disasters.

Table 4-1. National Planning Scenarios

Scenario	Description
1	Nuclear detonation–improvised nuclear device
2	Biological attack–aerosol anthrax
3	Biological disease outbreak–pandemic influenza
4	Biological attack–plague
5	Chemical attack–blister agent
6	Chemical attack–toxic industrial chemicals
7	Chemical attack–nerve agent
8	Chemical attack–chlorine tank explosion
9	Natural disaster–major earthquake
10	Natural disaster–major hurricane
11	Radiological attack–radiological dispersal devices
12	Explosives attack–bombing using improvised explosive devices
13	Biological attack–food contamination
14	Biological attack–foreign animal disease
15	Cyber-attack

Source: Based on Department of Homeland Security (DHS). 2007. *National Preparedness Guidelines.* Washington, DC: DHS; Federal Emergency Management Agency (FEMA). 2009. National planning scenarios. Washington, DC: FEMA. Available at: https://emilms.fema.gov/IS800B/lesson5/NRF0105060t.htm. Accessed January 2, 2017.

Federal Planning Scenarios

The federal agencies responsible for emergency preparedness have developed 15 all-hazards planning scenarios, known as the National Planning Scenarios for use at the national, state, and local levels. The scenarios are to be used as planning tools and represent the range of potential terrorist attacks and natural disasters that face our nation. The scenarios were developed to facilitate preparedness planning. The goal is that by planning for these scenarios, jurisdictions will be able to identify and develop the range of capabilities and resources needed to respond to the breadth of disasters. Table 4-1 lists the National Planning Scenarios. Additional information about the scenarios can be found at: http://cees.tamiu.edu/covertheborder/TOOLS/NationalPlanningSen.pdf.

Assistant Secretary for Preparedness and Response Playbooks

The office of the ASPR is developing playbooks so that states and localities will know how to integrate their planning with the federal response. The playbooks currently available include radiological dispersal devices and nuclear detonation. Additional playbooks are being developed. Each playbook addresses the core functions of the incident command system (ICS), logistics, planning, and response for each type of event. Further, each playbook describes the federal operational activities conducted under ESF #8. Such activities include providing for life-saving emergency medical care, restoration of the public health and medical infrastructure, evacuating and returning patients, providing veterinary medical assistance, managing fatalities, and providing for all human service needs, including those of vulnerable populations.

Each playbook contains the following 5 major sections:

- Scenario
- Concept of operations
- Action steps/issues
- Prescripted mission assignment subtasks
- Essential elements of information

These playbooks highlight the key decision points, actions, capabilities and assets that may be required to support a community's response to a specific type of emergency. Further, each playbook identifies how federal partners carry out their ESF #8 responsibilities when called upon to support a state response. The playbooks will be periodically updated as planners adopt new understanding about what is needed, or policy decisions evolve due to the consequences of future disasters. The playbooks are available at: http://www.phe.gov/preparedness/planning/playbooks/Pages/default.aspx.

Prior to the signing of PDD-8, HHS was also developing hazard-specific playbooks for each of the 15 National Planning Scenarios.[2] Following the nuclear events in Japan in March 2011, the ASPR highlighted a playbook to guide state and local planners in a medical response to a nuclear detonation (available at: http://www.phe.gov/Preparedness/planning/playbooks/stateandlocal/nuclear/Pages/default.aspx).

Common Tasks of Disaster Response

Twelve tasks address the problems that are likely to occur in most disasters, as summarized below.

- *Interorganizational coordination* is critical and is discussed in Chapters 2 and 3.
- *Sharing information among organizations* is complicated by the amount of equipment needed and the number of people involved. During the impact and postimpact phases, two-way radios (also known as *walkie-talkies*) might be the only reliable form of communication across distances. Even if landline, cellular, or wireless telephone systems are not damaged, they are generally congested or overloaded.

2. Planners should follow the policy development for PDD-8 to see whether there is an impact to the identified scenarios. Current updates are available at: https://www.fema.gov/ppd-8-news-updates-announcements.

- *Resource management*—the distribution of supplemental personnel, equipment, and supplies among multiple organizations—requires a process to identify which resources have arrived or are in transit and to determine where those resources are most needed. Once a security perimeter is established at the disaster site, a check-in or staging area is usually established outside this boundary. Each staging area has a manager who is in radio contact with the incident command post or emergency operations center. Law enforcement or security personnel are usually notified to refer all responders or volunteers to the closest check-in area. There, personnel are logged in, briefed on the situation, given an assignment, and provided with a radio, communications frequency, or hardware to link them to the broader response effort.
- When advance warnings are possible, *evacuation from areas of danger* can be the most effective lifesaving strategy in a disaster. The warning process is complex and requires precise communication among numerous agencies. A threat must be detected and analyzed to assess the specific areas at risk as well as the nature of that risk. Warnings should be delivered in such a manner that the population at risk will take the threat seriously and take appropriate action based on the warning. Detection and assessment are usually the responsibility of one agency (e.g., the National Weather Service, flood districts, dam officials). The decision to order an evacuation is the responsibility of other organizations (e.g., the sheriff's office), and the dissemination of the warning is the responsibility of a third group (e.g., commercial television or radio stations). The public tends to underestimate risks and downplay warnings if messages are ambiguous or inconsistent. Factors that enhance the effectiveness of warnings include the credibility of the warning source, the number of repetitions (especially if emanating from multiple sources), the consistency of message content across different sources, the context of the warning (e.g., a visible gas cloud or odor accompanying warnings about a hazardous substance leak), the inclusion of information that allows recipients to determine whether they are personally in danger (e.g., details on location or track), the inclusion of specific information on self-protective actions, and invitations from friends or relatives to take shelter.
- *Search and rescue* is an important aspect of the postdisaster response. In many disasters, casualties are initially treated in the field, and this process influences their entry into the health care system. To the extent that search and rescue is uncoordinated, the flow of patients through the EMS system and the health care system is also uncoordinated. Several characteristics of disaster search and rescue create problems amenable to improvement through organizational planning. Most disaster search and rescue, particularly in the immediate postimpact period, is not initiated by trained emergency personnel but by the spontaneous efforts of untrained bystanders who happen to be in the area. Care of patients also becomes complicated when the disaster occurs across jurisdictional boundaries or involves

emergency responders from many agencies (e.g., private ambulance providers; municipal first responders; and county, state, and federal agencies).

- *Using both mass and social media* to deliver warnings to the public and to educate the public about the avoidance of health problems in the aftermath of a disaster—such as food and water safety, injury prevention through education about chainsaw safety, avoidance of nail punctures, and monitoring carbon monoxide exposure from charcoal and unvented heaters—can be an effective public health tool.
- *Triage,* derived from the French verb *trier* or "to sort," is a method of assigning priorities for treatment and transport for injured citizens. Untrained personnel and bystanders who may do the initial search and rescue often bypass established field triage and first aid stations because they do not know where these posts are located or because they want to get the victims to the closest hospital.
- In most domestic disasters, several medical resources can handle the *casualty distribution.* Often, the closest hospitals receive the majority of patients, while other hospitals await casualties that never arrive. Transport decisions made by untrained volunteers are difficult to control. Established protocols between EMS and area hospitals will ensure the more even distribution of casualties.
- *Patient tracking* is complicated by the fact that most people evacuating their homes do not seek lodging in public shelters where their presence will be registered by the American Red Cross. Tracking the location of victims is further obfuscated because no single agency serves as a central repository of information about the location of victims from area hospitals, morgues, shelters, jails, or other potential locations. Tracking of the injured is also confounded because most patients get to hospitals by means other than ambulance, leaving EMS with an incomplete record of injuries. When hospitals themselves are damaged, the evacuation of hospitalized patients further complicates tracking where victims might be located.
- *Caring for patients* when the health care infrastructure has been damaged requires careful advance planning. Following natural disasters, hospitals should plan to care for greater numbers of minor injuries than for major trauma. Substantial numbers of patients seeking hospital care do so because of chronic medical conditions rather than trauma, caused in part by damage or loss of access to usual sources of primary medical care. People often evacuate their homes without prescription medications or underestimate how long they will be prevented from returning home. In addition, many injuries are sustained not during the disaster impact but during rescue or cleanup activities. Hospitals, urgent care centers, home health care agencies, pharmacies, and dialysis centers must make appropriate plans to ensure that their facilities will not be damaged or disabled in a disaster and that they have backup arrangements for the care of their patients postimpact. This includes providing backup supplies of power and water; building structures resistant to wind, fire, flood, and seismic hazards; maintaining

essential equipment and supplies that could be damaged by earthquakes or other disasters; supplying surge protection and data backup for computers with patient accounts, charts, or pharmacy information; making plans for alternative office, business, or clinical sites for displaced local health care resources (e.g., physicians, pharmacists, radiology); and developing plans to relocate the site of home health care to sites to which the patients have temporarily relocated.

- The *management of volunteers and donations* is a common problem in disasters. Disaster planning often focuses on the mobilization of resources, yet what frequently happens is that more resources arrive than are actually needed, requested, or expected. Procedures should be established to manage massive amounts of resources. First, planners should expect large numbers of donations and unsolicited volunteers (e.g., spontaneous civilian bystanders, family members, neighbors, coworkers, other survivors). Second, planners should channel public requests for aid to a locality outside the immediate disaster area where resources can be collected, organized, and distributed without disrupting ongoing emergency operations.
- Plan for *organized improvisation* in response to the disruption of shelter, utilities, communication systems, and transportation. Regardless of the level of preplanning, disasters will require some unanticipated tasks. Public health officials must develop the capacity, mutually agreed upon procedures, and training to participate in the community's coordinated, multiorganizational response to unexpected problems.

Components of a Plan

A regional plan will identify the potential jurisdictions that could be affected by a disaster and the corresponding agencies with assigned disaster response and recovery responsibilities. Such a plan will bring together the chief executives and operational leaders of these agencies, initiate a process of joint coordination and situational assessment, identify likely types of disasters, establish communication channels for sharing information, and create a standard protocol to assess the scope of damage, injuries, deaths, and secondary threats.

Baseline Assessment

To develop a regional plan, public health agencies must first work with the emergency management sector to determine the demographic profile of the community and assess:

- the health status and health risks of the community,
- the types of assistance required by various populations during an emergency,
- the condition of health care facilities,
- the protection of vital records,

- the potential requirements for public shelters,
- the available resources for alternative emergency and primary care, and
- the availability of and procedures for obtaining state and federal assistance.

Efforts to assess the health condition of the community must examine the following:

- Prevalent disease and people with functional needs who will need assistance related to evacuation and continuity of care
- Ability of the affected population to obtain prescription medications
- Building safety and ability to protect victims from injury, the elements, and hazardous material release
- Ability to maintain air quality, food safety, sanitation, waste disposal, vector control, and water systems

Hospitals, urgent care centers, physician offices, outpatient medical clinics, psychiatric clinics, dialysis centers, pharmacies, assisted living and residential facilities for the aged or disabled, and home health care services must have the capacity to meet patient needs and to ensure continuity of power, communications, water, sewer, and waste disposal during disaster situations. Data processing and exchange of patient information will be particularly important in the postimpact and recovery phases.

Disaster plans must take into account the availability of alternate treatment facilities when any or all of these locations are closed. Public health departments should work with hospitals and community providers to develop a plan for providing both routine care and continuity of care for victims experiencing acute exacerbations of chronic medical problems such as asthma, emphysema, diabetes, and hypertension. If the normal source of care for these individuals is not available and no alternative plan is communicated to the public, patients could be expected to seek care from overburdened hospital emergency departments. Following Hurricane Andrew, for example, more than 1,000 physician offices were destroyed or significantly damaged, greatly adding to hospital patient loads. Furthermore, provisions for alternative sources of care may continue long after responders from outside the area have returned home. Two years after Hurricane Katrina, 7 area hospitals were still not operating and 50% of the pre-hurricane hospital beds were no longer available.

In addition, plans should be developed for patients in hospitals, in residential care facilities (e.g., long-term care, assisted living, psychiatric treatment, rehabilitation), and living independently with functional needs who may need to be evacuated and placed elsewhere. Plans should also be made to maintain poison control hotlines and to continue home health care services (including dialysis, intravenous antibiotics, visiting nurse services, medical supply) at sites to which patients have been relocated.

Public health departments must collect background data on requirements for the medical needs, lodging, water, sanitation, and feeding arrangements for both victims and rescue and relief personnel. Plans for the management of resources—including directing incoming responders and volunteers to designated check-in or staging areas and determining what resources are present, available, or committed to the incident—should be established in advance. Assignments regarding which tasks will be coordinated or implemented by which agency or individual worker must be designated. This is particularly true for responsibilities that cross functional, geographic, or jurisdictional boundaries and for tasks for which no single person or agency has clear-cut statutory or contractual responsibility. Priorities for resource distribution, cost sharing, acquisition, training, and coordination must be set jointly and disseminated widely.

Finally, public health officials should ensure that the disaster preparedness plan identifies state and federal assistance programs (e.g., Robert T. Stafford Disaster Relief and Emergency Assistance Act of 1988 [Stafford Act], as explained in Chapter 3) for reimbursement and establishes procedures to verify that full reimbursement for disaster-related health care has been recovered.

Identifying Available Resources

Disaster response may call for the use of resources (e.g., personnel, equipment, supplies, information) that do not commonly reside in one location or under the jurisdiction of one agency. The ability to reduce morbidity and mortality in the early hours after disaster has struck may depend on locating resources that are not commonly used in response to routine emergencies or are in short supply. A comprehensive plan should establish procedures for locating specialty physicians, search dogs, specialized devices for locating trapped victims in the rubble of collapsed buildings, tools for cutting through and lifting heavy reinforced concrete blocks, dialysis centers or equipment to treat crush injury, laboratories to rapidly analyze hazardous chemicals or biological agents, radiation detection instruments, confined-space rescue teams, and hazardous materials response teams with appropriate protective gear.

Surge Capacity

Surge capacity is the ability to treat a large increase in the number of people requiring treatment and specimens for analysis, or to conduct the necessary assessments following an emergency event. As a primary tenet, governments at all levels must first ensure that public health agencies have the manpower and resources to handle their core mission and responsibilities on a daily basis, or they will not have the capacity to provide services when a surge is needed during emergencies.

The principles of *capacity planning management* are used in industry to determine how much production capacity is needed, under which conditions and where capacity needs to be increased, and how that increase will be structured. In response to a disaster, health care systems often have to expand their configuration to care for those affected by the incident. Dr. Boaz Tadmor, former chief medical officer for the Home Front Command in Israel, has said that in times of disaster, the organization of the response is more important than the delivery of patient care. Surge capacity requires regional systems that are resilient and flexible to respond effectively to an emergency.

Increasing the capacity of a community's public health and health care system requires the connectedness of health departments, hospitals, and community agencies. For example, in an event involving infectious disease, the burden on the public health system is dependent on many factors, including the nature of the event, the demography and prevalence or incidence of disease in the local population, and the projected spread of the infection. The ability to care for patients will vary according to demand for services and the available staff, equipment, space, antibiotics, and other medical supplies. Community organizations and institutions may need to provide services such as housing for quarantine. Some state laws, such as in Indiana, require local health departments to make sure that quarantined individuals have sufficient resources, including food. With incidents involving biological, chemical, or "dirty bomb" exposures, communities are likely to experience *triage inversion,* in which the least injured patients present first while the most severely injured are extricated at the scene. In this type of scenario, the contaminated victims may appear for care before hospitals have received information from the scene. Thus, preparations for surge capacity involve protecting hospitals from contamination and ensuring a mechanism for EMS to quickly communicate to hospitals so that they can set up the decontamination expeditiously.

Surge Capacity Planning

To estimate the potential requirements for increased personnel, assets, and other resources, a community has to inventory available sites of inpatient and ambulatory medical and mental health care; public health agencies; the volume, location, and services delivered; and the geographic area served. In addition, the community should survey organizations that serve vulnerable populations that might have functional needs. Once the capacity assessment is complete, coordination with community and regional resources is essential. As an example, when space is needed for any service, alternatives are schools, gymnasiums, military facilities (e.g., National Guard facilities), and conversion of existing space, such as hotels. The need for having this planning in place is highlighted by the problems following Hurricane Katrina when the organizations that had previously provided services to 45,000 people with functional needs could not agree on the nature of their clients' requirements.

Projections for increasing capacity can be determined by estimating the following:

- Potential types of casualties and care needed by the type of incident (e.g., highly infectious biological event versus single location blast event)

- Volume, intensity, and differing rates of morbidity and mortality among projected patients
- Impact of demographics
- Current services by location
- Knowledge and skill mix of current staffing
- Available treatment and triage on-site at the incident
- How much care can be delivered by primary care physicians, such as caring for the "worried well"
- Alternative sources for capacity (e.g., mutual aid agreements, Medical Reserve Corp)
- Expected time frame, length of the response, and work schedules
- Types of public health and health care services to be added or increased based on these estimates

Scheduling should allow for care or services to be provided over the entire projected length of a response so that staff is not "burnt out" within the first 6 hours. Capacity assessments might indicate that an agency needs to realign staffing assignments by shifting staff from one venue to another or from one location within an agency or facility to another. The same assessment is required for equipment and other resources. Once staffing projections are identified, plans should provide for training of surge staff in the following:

- Their role and responsibilities in the response
- The chain of command within the organization in which they will report
- Reporting protocols and any legal responsibility to report
- Clinical recognition of diseases (i.e., signs and symptoms) where indicated

Delivering Care Under Extreme Conditions

When planning for a disaster, health departments and health care facilities will initially prepare for the delivery of conventional medical care by sharing local, regional, and federal resources; developing strategies to conserve, reuse, adapt, and substitute supplies; and calling upon alternative care systems and facilities (e.g., home and community-based care).

However, the ability to provide conventional care could be hampered by the following:

- Loss of services, including power or water
- Inadequate supplies and pharmaceuticals
- Loss of infrastructure and medical records
- Shortage of personnel, including specialists and essential staff
- Surge in the number of patients seeking care, including those uninjured in the disaster but in need of care such as women giving birth
- Need for coordination among health care systems that are competing for scarce resources

- Communication barriers
- Need for enhanced security

Extreme weather events may further compound planning for vulnerabilities. First, the events may quickly affect uncommonly large, demographically diverse, and widespread populations. Second, the direct and indirect effects of disruption to the infrastructure can create a large and varied set of community burdens and needs. Extreme weather events pose direct threats to life and often present novel and unanticipated health concerns. In addition to increasing public health needs, when extreme weather knocks out the infrastructure required by disabled individuals (e.g., oxygen, power for electrical equipment), a community's health response is complicated and its capacity to respond reduced because of the additional need.

As these conditions deteriorate during a catastrophic disaster or incident, it is assumed that the provision of conventional health services will evolve into contingency care. When the growing demand for services cannot be met by the available resources, crisis standards for care may need to be initiated. When crisis standards are implemented, the needs of individual patients are set aside in order to distribute the greatest good for the greatest number of patients.

Crisis standards of care are formally declared by a state government and involve a substantial change in the organization of services and delivery of health care. A formal declaration to institute crisis standards of care legally protects health care providers as they allocate scarce medical resources and dramatically alter the operations at their facilities. Many states have executive orders that governors can sign when needed. Further, during a declared disaster, a waiver of requirements under Section 1135 of the Social Security Act suspends penalties for noncompliance with the Health Insurance Portability and Accountability Act of 1996 and Emergency Medical Treatment and Labor Act regulations (available at: http://www.idph.state.il.us/h1n1_flu/NEA_and_1135waivers.pdf). Planning for situations where crisis standards of care are needed will fortify a community's ability to respond in the most difficult circumstances.

Crisis standards of care should be formulated with strong ethical underpinnings and be fair and equitable, involve collaboration between the community and providers in a formalized process, and authorize providers to carry out necessary and appropriate actions and interventions in response to emergencies under laws that support the standards. Chapter 15 discusses ethical considerations in more depth. Crisis standards should:

- Be consistent across states with clear indicators, triggers, and lines of responsibility;
- Ensure attention to the requirements of populations with disabilities and access and functional needs;
- Adhere to ethical norms when making choices regarding the allocation of scarce health care resources;

- Legally protect providers and institutions by adjusting scopes of practice for licensed or certified health care practitioners; and
- Ensure consistency in the implementation of these standards through advisory committees which develop clinical guidance and protocols.

Exercises, Drills, and Training

The existence of a written emergency response plan does not ensure that it will be used or that the plan will be effective if needed. Exercises and drills are used to test the effectiveness of plans. Ideally, local public health and health care facilities are integrated into a community-wide plan that is exercised and evaluated at least once every 12 months. When all of the agencies that will be called upon to respond to a disaster, including public health, have participated in the plan's development, they are more likely to ensure that the full needs of the community are met and that individual organizations are not overburdened as a result of poor planning. In addition, health departments, hospitals, and other public health agencies should perform stand-alone exercises to ensure that their plans are effective.

Because disasters often cross political, geographic, functional, and jurisdictional boundaries, exercises and training are most effective when carried out on a multiorganizational, multidisciplinary, multijurisdictional basis. Coordination is also facilitated when participants are familiar with the skills, level of knowledge, and dependability of other responders upon whom they may one day need to rely. The full-scale exercise will often involve both prehospital and hospital response.

Exercises are used to improve planning. Exercises help officials and public health professionals test emergency preparedness and response capabilities and identify gaps in planning, conflicts with other plans, inadequate resources, and other opportunities for improvement. The *test-exercise cycle* begins with an assumption about how agencies will function in a response. Following training, an objective for an exercise is developed. The exercise is organized and conducted. An evaluation occurs and the plan is revised based on the evaluation. Responders are then retrained for the revised plan.

The National Preparedness Directorate of the Department of Homeland Security established a program with standardized methodology and terminology for preparedness exercises. The Homeland Security Exercise and Evaluation Program (HSEEP) provides tools and resources, such as the evaluation guides, to help jurisdictions and organizations test their plans and identify and remedy vulnerabilities prior to a real incident. To be considered HSEEP compliant, 4 performance requirements must be satisfied:

- Conduct a biannual training and exercise plan workshop and maintain a multiyear training and exercise plan.

- Plan and conduct exercises following HSEEP guidelines.
- Develop and submit the outcome of an exercise in an after-action report/improvement plan (AAR/IP). (An explanation of how to write an AAR/IP can be found at: https://www.cebma.org/wp-content/uploads/Guide-to-the-after_action_review.pdf.)
- Track and implement the corrective actions identified in the AAR/IP.

Table 4-2 identifies the types of activities that public health could practice in either agency-specific or communitywide exercises.

Types of Exercises

HSEEP has identified 2 types of exercises: (1) discussion-based exercises, such as seminars, workshops, and tabletop exercises; or (2) operations-based exercises, such as games, drills, functional exercises, and full-scale exercises (see Table 4-3).

Table 4-2. Public Health Activities for Disaster Plan Exercises

Category	Activities
Preparedness	Develop mutual aid networks for your community
Response	Escalate a response by activating federal resources and response
	Request, receive, and distribute medications, supplies, or equipment (such as ventilators) from the Strategic National Stockpile
	Distribute pharmaceuticals for treatment or prophylaxis
	Implement ring or mass vaccinations
	Activate social distancing, including isolation and quarantine
	Implement evacuation and sheltering in place
	Import health professionals from neighboring states
	Provide for requirements of functional needs populations
Delivery of health care	Care for mass casualties, including care for burns or other trauma
	Conduct decontamination
	Provide mental health support for responders, survivors, and other community members
	Coordinate among the various health care systems in the community or region
Communication	Activate the area Health Alert Network
	Operate a Joint Information Center
	Communicate with the public about health risks and protective behaviors
Operations into policy	Translate epidemiological investigations into policy, operational/management, and public communications actions
Dealing with remains	Set up a mass mortuary

Source: Adapted from U.S. Department of Health & Human Services (HHS). 2007. *Public Health Emergency Response: A Guide for Leaders and Responders.* Chapter 9. Washington, DC: HHS. Available at: https://www.hsdl.org/?view&did=481394. Accessed January 2, 2017.

Table 4-3. Homeland Security Exercise and Evaluation Program Exercises

Type	Use or Purpose	How Conducted
Discussion-Based Exercises		
	Used as starting point Usually emphasize existing plans, policies, agreements, and procedures Used to familiarize agencies and personnel with current and expected capabilities	Led by facilitators
Seminars	Orient participants or provide an overview Good start when developing or making changes to plans and procedures	Informal discussions led by a presenter
Workshops	Used to determine objectives, develop scenarios, and define evaluation criteria for exercise Produce new standard operating procedures, emergency operations plans, multiyear plans, or improvement plans	Focus on achieving or building a product (such as a draft plan or policy) Participant interaction is increased
Tabletop exercises: Basic	Evaluation of group's problem-solving abilities, handling of personnel contingencies, message interpretation, information sharing, interagency coordination, and achievement of specific objectives Key personnel discuss hypothetical scenarios in an informal setting	Situation established by the scenario; materials remains constant Players apply their knowledge and skills to a list of problems presented by the leader/moderator Problems are discussed as a group Leader summarizes the resolutions
Tabletop exercises: Advanced		Prescripted messages alter the original scenario Moderator introduces problems one at a time in various formats (e.g., message, simulated telephone call, videotape) Participants discuss issues raised by the simulated problem, applying appropriate plans and procedures
Games (simulations)	Simulation of operations involving teams; uses rules, data, and procedures in an actual or real-life situation Explore decision-making processes and the consequences of those decisions	Computer-generated scenarios and simulations Internet-based, multiplayer games

(*Continued*)

Table 4-3. (Continued)

Type	Use or Purpose	How Conducted
Operations-Based Exercises		
	Validate the effectiveness of plans, policies, agreements, and procedures	Actual reaction to simulated intelligence
	Clarify roles and responsibilities	Response to emergency conditions
	Identify gaps in resources needed to implement plans and procedures	Mobilization of apparatus, resources, and/or networks
	Improve individual and team performance	Commitment of personnel, usually over an extended period of time
Drills	Validate a single, specific operation or function in a single agency or organizational entity	Coordinated, supervised activity
	Provide training on new equipment	Narrow focus measured against established standards
	Develop or validate new policies or procedures	Immediate feedback
	Practice and maintain current skills	Realistic environment
Functional exercises	Validate and evaluate individual capabilities, multiple functions, activities within a function, or interdependent groups of functions	Activation and simulated activity of all sections of the ICS
	Simulates the reality of operations by presenting complex and realistic problems in a highly stressful, time-constrained environment	Test disaster plan in simulated field conditions
		Participants include players, simulators, controllers, and evaluators
Full-scale exercises	Validate many facets of preparedness	Scripted scenario with built-in flexibility to allow updates to drive activity
	Responders get to know each other and their roles, gain experience working with the community's plan, and understand what must be done—thus enhancing their ability to rely on each other's activities	Conducted in real time in stressful, time-constrained environment that closely mirrors actual events
	Implement and analyze plans, policies, procedures, and cooperative agreements	Personnel and resources are mobilized and deployed to the scene where they conduct activities as if a real incident had occurred
	Presents complex and realistic problems that require critical thinking, rapid problem-solving, and effective responses	Multiagency, multijurisdictional, multiorganizational
	Test the mobilization of all or as many as possible of the response components using principles of the National Incident Management System	Participants include responder, controller, evaluator, and victims

Source: Adapted from U.S. Department of Homeland Security (DHS). 2013. *Homeland Security Exercise and Evaluation Program (HSEEP).* Washington, DC: DHS. Available at: http://www.fema.gov/media-library-data/20130726-1914-25045-8890/hseep_apr13_.pdf. Accessed January 2, 2017.

Note: ICS=incident command system.

At-Risk Populations

A cadre of people with access and functional needs have been involved as developers, trainers, and participants in emergency management training. Public health professionals should partner with these individuals and the organizations that serve them when developing exercises and training for responders. These individuals can:

- assist in the development of plans that consider access and functional needs,
- identify weaknesses and gaps in plans,
- articulate emergency needs within their communities,
- build awareness about access and functional needs when a community prepares for emergencies, and
- facilitate collaboration, coordination, and communication between responding agencies and those with access and functional needs.

Those responsible for integrating the needs of vulnerable populations into exercises and exercise programs should fully understand what the various groups would require by including representatives from these groups as active participants in exercises. People with disabilities and different access and functional needs can help identify issues and provide ideas for effective solutions. To ensure their active participation, transportation to and from the exercise and facilities where the exercises are conducted should be fully accessible. In addition, communication about and instructions during the exercises should be varied so all understand. Communities should not include very young children as participants in exercises because they may not be able to distinguish between an exercise and an actual event.

When an AAR/IP is developed, the specific communities with access and functional needs should be asked to provide feedback on and potential solutions to gaps that were identified in the exercise. Additional guidance on support services for those with functional needs is provided by FEMA at: http://www.phe.gov/Preparedness/planning/abc/Pages/funcitonal-needs.aspx. Additional guidance on serving at-risk populations can be found in Chapter 11.

CHAPTER 5

DISASTER SURVEILLANCE AND INFORMATION SYSTEMS

Surveillance and the exchange of gathered information guides both emergency response and long-term planning for public health and medical issues related to a disaster. This chapter examines disaster epidemiology and information systems (IS) throughout the disaster event, public health surveillance, and geographic information systems (GIS) in preparing for and responding to disaster.

Public Health Role

Develop, apply, and evaluate tools, methods, guidance, and protocols to improve investigation of public health emergencies at the federal, state, and local levels:

- Describe and monitor medical, public health, and psychosocial effects of disaster.
- Identify at-risk groups or geographic areas.
- Identify changes in agents and host factors.
- Detect changes in health practices.
- Detect illness or injuries—including sudden changes in disease occurrence—and determine when, where, and how injuries, illnesses, and deaths occur.
- Detect, investigate, and analyze collected data to identify necessary interventions.
- Monitor long-term disease trends.
- Provide evidence for establishment of response protocols.
- Provide information about probable adverse health effects for decision making.
- Identify what is a rumor and what is not.
- Determine needs by estimating the magnitude of a public health issue and match resources to needs in affected communities.
- Evaluate how personnel and partners are conducting surveillance activities for effective practice and the improvement of surveillance activities.
- Inform evaluation of the effectiveness of response activities.

At times, especially early in response to a disaster, public health professionals may need to carry out some or all of these functions with little to no information. This concept is often referred to as the *information lifecycle*. At the beginning of a disaster, public health officials often rely on the reports of perceptive clinicians who recognize the significance of their patient's symptoms, information captured through syndromic surveillance data feeds, or personal relationships with the provider community. As time goes on, interviews may be conducted with those thought to be at risk, such as through exposure or potential exposure to a contagious disease. Federal, state, or local health departments are asked questions to better understand the sequence of events. The collected information helps public health officials develop case definitions (see below) or hypotheses that are important preparatory steps before moving forward in an investigation. Often a determination is made to keep monitoring or to take action, such as collecting specimens and testing for specific agents or infections. The final steps in the information lifecycle are confirming or denying theories about what may be happening, implementing interventions where indicated, and evaluating the process.

Disaster Epidemiology and Surveillance

Epidemiology can be used to investigate the public health and medical consequences of disasters. The aim of disaster epidemiology is to ascertain strategies for the prevention of both acute and chronic health events as a result of the occurrence of natural or man-made hazards. Primary prevention seeks to prevent disaster-related deaths, injuries, or illness before they occur, such as by evacuating residents prior to landfall of a hurricane. With secondary prevention, the goal is to mitigate the health consequences of a disaster, such as by providing education about injury control during the cleanup and recovery period. Tertiary prevention minimizes the effects of disease and disability among those already ill, such as by setting up evaluation units where the chronically ill can obtain access to short-term pharmaceuticals when their usual source of care has been disrupted.

Disaster epidemiology includes rapid needs assessment; disease control strategies; assessment of the availability and use of health services; surveillance systems for both descriptive and analytic investigations of disease and injury; research on risk factors contributing to disease, injury, or death; and communication of beneficial and harmful behaviors to the public. Although this chapter focuses on surveillance and the tools used to conduct it, some of the systems discussed are used in other epidemiology tasks.

In disasters, surveillance concentrates on the incidence, prevalence, and severity of illness or injury as a result of ecological changes, changes in endemic levels of disease, population displacement, loss of usual source of health care, overcrowding, breakdowns in sanitation, and disruption of public utilities. Surveillance also monitors increases in communicable diseases, including vector-borne, waterborne, and person-to-person transmission. Data for disaster surveillance are collected through IS, which complements traditional reporting mechanisms that may not be fully functional following a disaster.

Types of Surveillance

To understand surveillance during disasters, it is helpful to review the 4 types of epidemiological investigation and how they are used in emergencies. The determination of which type of surveillance to implement, such as active, passive, or a combination of both, is determined by the specific disaster and the available resources.

Passive Surveillance

Passive surveillance involves the routine reporting of disease data by health institutions to health authorities. As a result of this passive notification by health care facilities or practitioners, there is no need for the epidemiologist to actively search for cases. For example, hospitals, clinics, public health facilities, laboratories, and other sources are required by state law to report to state or county health departments on the occurrence of a predetermined list of notifiable diseases. The National Notifiable Diseases Surveillance System collects information on selected infectious and noninfectious diseases and conditions—such as salmonellosis, West Nile virus, and carbon monoxide (CO) poisoning—that can be used as a data source during disasters.

The labor needed for data requested from passive systems is minimal compared to the manpower efforts involved in more complex surveillance systems. If a large geographic area needs to be covered, passive surveillance can be a cost-efficient strategy for collecting data. For example, following a disaster that is widespread, passive surveillance may be used to monitor the occurrence of vaccine-preventable diseases, such as tetanus.

Passive surveillance systems have limitations and technical difficulties that can impact the utility of the data in meeting the original need. Slow and inconsistent reporting, which can happen with passive surveillance, are concerns in a disaster. The quality and timeliness of data are difficult to control because passive systems depend on data reporting by health officials in different institutions that may not have the same procedures for providing the information. Further, reporting can be slow, variable, or incomplete if the responsible health officials do not submit the data regularly. Advantages of passive surveillance systems include:

- Cost efficiency;
- A minimal requirement of labor; and
- Due to the ability to gather information for a wider geographic span, passive systems can provide information for the health of that population.

Active Surveillance

Active surveillance utilizes designated staff members to regularly contact health care providers, laboratories, hospitals, the affected population, and others to seek out information about health conditions. Active surveillance is often more sensitive and thus able to better differentiate between those who do and do not have the disease being investigated. Active surveillance may also collect information that is more detailed than passive systems since staff can search or request specific details about cases.

During disasters, epidemiologists may use active surveillance systems to monitor the incidence of certain diseases and health-related outcomes. After Hurricane Andrew, for example, the Louisiana Office of Public Health, in coordination with emergency departments, public utility personnel, and coroners, used active surveillance to facilitate the reporting of health impacts in the affected areas.

Active surveillance is commonly used to collect data when tents, temporary shelters, mobile clinics, or other venues are established for short-term medical care by response agencies such as the American Red Cross (Red Cross), Department of Health & Human Services portable hospitals, and Disaster Medical Assistance Teams (DMATs).

Although active surveillance provides the most accurate and timely information, it is also expensive and labor intensive. Resource scarcity in disaster settings and the cost of conducting active surveillance might result in a health department deciding to limit its use to short periods of time and the investigation of only specific health concerns, such as diarrhea in a shelter or communicable diseases in the community. Agencies conducting active surveillance that are able to use both standardized questionnaires and clear directions for collecting and recording the data can enhance the ability to aggregate the collected data since these mechanisms help avoid differences in the format of the methods of data collection and reporting across sources. Advantages of active surveillance systems include:

- Complements regular reporting functions interrupted by the disaster event
- Provides more flexibility than regular reporting mechanisms
- Can be targeted to focus on the needs of specific populations
- Provides more complete information than passive surveillance

Sentinel Surveillance

Sentinel surveillance is an active or passive surveillance system that collects data about specific health events from a limited number of recruited participants or providers. By selecting a sample of reporting sources, public health professionals can often estimate trends in the larger affected population. Providers of sentinel data often include clinics, hospitals, other health care facilities, laboratories, and physicians. Providers are asked to report all cases of the conditions of interest. Sentinel surveillance can be established to supplement an existing surveillance system. For example, in order to target relief efforts to areas of need after the 2010 earthquake in Haiti, national and international agencies collaborated to form the National Sentinel Site Surveillance System to monitor disease trends, detect outbreaks, and characterize the health problem of the affected population. Over 3 months, 51 selected hospital and clinic sites provided daily reports by telephone or e-mail for 25 specified conditions. During that time, the sentinel system did not pick up any increases in unexpected disease clusters or outbreaks during the reporting period and was used as evidence to dispel rumors about disease clusters and outbreaks.

Although sentinel surveillance can be useful for detecting large public health problems, it may not detect rare events, such as the emergence of a disease new to that area, if that case occurs in a location not included in the sentinel surveillance. The sentinel sites selected also might not be representative of the larger disaster-affected area, depending on how the sample is selected.

The advantages of sentinel surveillance systems are that such systems:

- effectively monitor trends for a specified condition,
- overcome issues of underreporting because only a select number of sites are required to report,
- track a greater range of morbidity since data are reported on all conditions of interest,
- are less costly compared to other systems, and
- provide flexibility in scaling and recruiting additional surveillance sites.

Syndromic Surveillance

Syndromic surveillance can be useful in identifying emerging infections and outbreaks. Syndromic surveillance systems collect data describing actions that precede diagnosis, such as laboratory test requests, emergency department chief complaints, ambulance run sheets, prescription and over-the-counter drug use, and school or work absenteeism. Clusters of medical signs and symptoms may signal a sufficient probability of an outbreak to warrant further public health response.

Syndromic surveillance data are usually collected at the point of medical care and from existing data streams that can monitor disease patterns. Syndromic surveillance has 5 characteristics that make it ideal for identifying outbreaks. The data are routinely collected and do not rely on physician reporting. The data are immediately computerized, are population-based, and are categorized by syndrome. This approach to data collection and organization is extremely helpful because it allows analysts to query the data with specific keywords related to a given event. With unique words used as filters, these queries can identify medical records most likely associated with a specific illness.

This system of investigation is further distinguished from surveillance of mandated notifiable disease in that standard case definitions may not have been established and detection thresholds are flexible.

Hospital-based syndromic surveillance systems often report data from emergency departments. Daily or twice daily transfer of electronic data about patients with fever or respiratory and gastrointestinal illness allows for analysis and identification of increases 7 days per week. Data can be analyzed by hospital and by zip code and should be examined as close to the time the data were collected as possible.

When an alarm is sounded, it is necessary to distinguish between natural variability in the data (e.g., seasonal events, true outbreaks of an expected illness, data quality anomalies) or an event involving an infectious disease or biological agent. In evaluating the data, public health officials are often concerned if there is a sustained or increasing visit rate, if multiple hospitals are involved, if there are dual syndromes in the same area, if other surveillance systems are sounding an alarm, and if there is a strong geographic clustering. Of less concern would be a 1-day increase, only a single hospital involved, no other evidence of an outbreak, or a diffuse increase across the city or region. These guidelines, however, are not all-inclusive. Analysts familiar with the situation also take into account other factors like signals—signs that something may be happening across hospitals and geographic regions—sustained increases in visit rates, clustering of unique symptoms at the same time or same location, and knowledge of other relevant information (i.e., information that may lower the index of suspicion). For example, increases in respiratory-related syndromes due to influenza-like illness are expected each winter and an increase may not require further evaluation. Similarly, seasonal increases in pollen may produce increases in respiratory-related illness, which may cause statistical alerts in surveillance systems even though these events are expected.

To analyze syndromic surveillance data, time series methods that include regression models account for effects that are seasonal or attributed to the day of the week. If the assumptions that are the basis of those models do not fit well, analysts can use other methods based in statistical control charts, which are graphs that are used to study how an event changes over time. Among the statistical control chart methods, there are many variations—C1, C2, and C3; exponentially weighted moving averages (EWMA); and for small numbers, EWMA methods based on Poisson models.[1] Spatial statistical methods are also available—the most common is the SatScan method developed by Martin Kuldorf. Many syndromic surveillance systems automatically deploy these methods and present results to the public health analysts.

Some syndromic surveillance systems, such as the Electronic Surveillance System for the Early Notification of Community-based Epidemics (ESSENCE), allow the user to

1. Additional information about statistical control chart methods can be found in the papers authored by Carnevale et al. and Zikos et al. included in the Surveillance section in the references for this book.

add their own custom syndrome to the analysis. This is helpful when there is an outbreak of an unidentified disease or when one would like to track a specific disease or event of interest. During flu season, tracking is often done using the case definition for *influenza-like illness* to define the syndrome of symptoms being observed.

Sources of data for syndromic surveillance include:

- Emergency departments
- Urgent care centers
- Inpatient data
- Outpatient data
- Emergency medical services (EMS)
- Nurse hotlines
- Labs
- Prescription drug sales
- Over-the-counter drug sales
- Poison control
- School absenteeism
- Workplace absenteeism
- Animal health

Advantages of syndromic surveillance systems include:

- Timeliness because as soon as the data is received by the hospital (for example) the agency conducting the syndromic surveillance also receives it, often in real time
- Ability to detect outbreaks early on
- Ability to identify illness in a community does not require diagnoses or laboratory confirmation

Disaster Information Systems

Disaster Information Systems (DIS) amass data about the effects of a disaster during the impact phase, response phase, and early stages of recovery. DIS consist of integrated sets of files, procedures, and equipment for the storage, manipulation, and retrieval of information. The data collected through DIS are used to make decisions about the services that are needed postimpact, such as emergency and short-term relief, as well as long-term planning for recovery and reconstruction. DIS personnel examine how the everyday relationship between people and their physical and social environments has been disrupted by disasters, such as by lost productivity, as well as emerging problems or problems under control.

Data must be collected rapidly, sometimes under adverse circumstances. Quick processing, analysis, and interpretation ensures a timely flow of information to inform an

Table 5-1. Definitions and Formulas for Surveillance Parameters Used in Disaster Information Systems

Measure of Frequency	Measure	Definition
Counts	Incident cases	The occurrence of new cases of death, disease, or injury in a population over a specified period
	Prevalent cases	The existing cases of death, disease, or injury in a population over a specified period
Morbidity and mortality rates	Incidence rate (new cases)	The number of new cases of a disease or injury that occur during a specified period per unit of person-time at risk (can be stratified by age and sex)
	Prevalence or prevalence rate (total existing cases)	The proportion of people in a population who have a particular health condition at a specified point in time or over a specified period
	Crude mortality rate	The rate of death in the entire population (includes all people, regardless of sex or age)
	Cause-specific mortality rate	The mortality rate from a specified cause for a population in a specified period
	Age-specific mortality/morbidity rate (<5 years, >5 years)	A mortality/morbidity rate limited to a particular age group (e.g., under-5 mortality rate [U5MR] is the rate of death among children younger than 5 years in a population)
	Incidence proportion (attack rate, generally used for infectious conditions)	The proportion of an initially disease-free population that develops disease, becomes injured, or dies during a specified (usually limited) period
	Proportional morbidity/mortality	The proportion of all deaths/new or existing cases in a specified population over a period attributable to a specific cause
	Case fatality rate	The proportion of people with a health condition in a specified period who die from it
Program process rates	Health facility utilization rate	The number of outpatient visits per person per year (if it is possible, distinguish between new and old visits and use new visits to calculate the rate)
	Number of consultations per clinician per day	The average number of total consultations (new and repeat cases) seen by each clinician per day

Source: Adapted from Centers for Disease Control and Prevention (CDC). 2016. *A Primer for Understanding the Principles and Practices of Disaster Surveillance in the United States.* Atlanta, GA: CDC. Available at: http://www.cdc.gov/nceh/hsb/disaster/Disaster_Surveillance_508.pdf. Accessed January 2, 2017.

appropriate response. To enhance the ability of public health professionals to analyze the information, surveillance activities must be based on standardized data with the procedures established and teams trained in advance. DIS and the personnel working with information systems must be flexible, adaptable, and able to work under adverse conditions when either established procedures and/or trained teams that are ready to go into the field are not available. Table 5-1 summarizes the definitions and formulas for the parameters used in surveillance through DIS. Table 5-2 summarizes the types and uses of data collected through DIS.

Table 5-2. Disaster Information Systems Data Collection

Type of Data	Uses of Data
Deaths	Assess the magnitude of disaster
	Evaluate effectiveness of disaster preparedness
	Evaluate adequacy of warning system
Casualties	Estimate needs for emergency care
	Evaluate preimpact planning and preparedness
	Evaluate adequacy of warning systems
Morbidity	Estimate type and volume of immediate medical relief needed
	Evaluate appropriateness of relief
	Identify populations at risk
	Assess needs for further planning
Health needs	Prioritize services delivered
	Prioritize groups most affected
	Evaluate adequacy of resources
Public health resources	Estimate the type and volume of needed supplies, equipment, and services
	Evaluate appropriateness of relief
	Assess needs for further planning
Donated goods	Estimate the type and volume of needed supplies, equipment, and services
	Evaluate appropriateness of relief
	Assess needs for further planning
Hazards	Monitor health events, disease, injuries, hazards, exposures, or risk factors
	Support early warning system to forecast occurrence of a disaster event by monitoring conditions that may signal the event

Disaster Surveillance

To determine actions important for a public health response, managers assess concerns about public health issues and the necessity of monitoring disaster-related morbidity and mortality before initiating DIS. Considerations include whether existing systems could be used, which is preferable due to the level of resources required for active surveillance, though often not possible because of lost infrastructure; sufficient personnel are available, including volunteers such as medical, nursing, or public health students; the data are needed to influence the public health response; and data collection can be funded, either by the participating institutions or externally, such as support through the Robert T. Stafford Disaster Relief and Emergency Assistance Act of 1988 (see Chapter 3 for more information on the Stafford Act).

DIS personnel must ensure that they have the capacity to provide information that is both adequate and timely when existing systems, such as those established to track reportable diseases, will not collect sufficient information. The information in existing systems is often based upon reports coming passively from both labs and doctors and may not provide all of the information about the disaster that is needed. Further, these data are vetted by DIS personnel to assess whether the symptoms meet the definition of a case before being disseminated to the public. It is possible that data, especially event-specific data, during a disaster may not be complete if there are not enough people to gather and/or input it, such as when lab and hospital personnel are diverted to carry out tasks in another part of the response. As such, public health professionals have advocated for the automated electronic reporting of data to public health agencies, including electronic lab reporting and more recently, electronic case reporting.

Existing hospital-based data may provide an accurate representation of morbidity attributable to the disaster. Data can be obtained from mobile care sites and clinics. All health care facilities may be asked to participate in a syndromic surveillance system, or, given finite resources, selected sites may be chosen to provide a reasonable representation of the health effects being monitored. At a minimum, hospitals should report on surge capacity (e.g., beds, staffing, supply needs, availability), event-related data (e.g., numbers of patients seen, waiting to be seen, unidentified, deceased), and patient locator information (e.g., name, sex, and date of service for patients seen as a result of the disaster). During an emergency, a hospital may not be able to devote resources to providing these data; this is where DIS staff who can gather the data or automated systems may be of use. When there are concerns about infectious disease, syndrome-specific morbidity data may be requested from all sites providing care. Box 5-1 describes the surveillance in New York City during the Ebola virus disease outbreak in 2014.

Community clinicians play a key role in identifying and reporting cases, educating patients about infectious risks, and preventing the spread of infections. Interventions to improve detection and to ensure that information is reported quickly and correctly

Box 5-1. Ebola Surveillance in New York City

When New York conducted surveillance for possible cases of Ebola Virus Disease (EVD) in 2014, there was a statewide active monitoring of travelers arriving from Liberia, Guinea, and Sierra Leone. Using CDC guidelines to determine an individual's epidemiological risk, local health departments conducted different levels of surveillance based on that risk. Twice a day, health department personnel communicated by telephone with the traveler at "low but not zero" risk to assess for the presence of symptoms and fever and directly observed (in person or by video) travelers with "some" or "high" risk to assess their health and record their temperature. This active surveillance was enhanced by notifying area hospitals and EMS providers that an unidentified high-risk individual was in the area. EMS and area hospitals created a plan for transporting a patient with EVD, identified which hospital would receive the traveler, and detailed how the patient would enter the facility.

include outreach to both hospital-based and community providers through educational forums for clinicians, laboratorians, and trainees; health department mailings; health alerts by broadcast fax and e-mail; a provider portal, the Health Alert Network; and a public Web site.

Although the ability to collect surveillance information has expanded tremendously in the past few years, if existing systems do not meet the adequate and timely standard, temporary sentinel surveillance systems can be organized for the duration of the emergency period or at any point before, during, or after the disaster. To expedite DIS, epidemiologists should have access to additional data reporting systems, such as existing electronic disease reporting or temporary sentinel efforts established by state or local systems. Data should be collected using the standardized protocols established by the Centers for Disease Control and Prevention (CDC), including veterinary inputs. This may not be possible for temporary sentinel systems established during an emergency, but is a good goal to work toward. The collected data are then pooled by epidemiologists to create a larger picture of an event. After collection, pooling, evaluation, and analysis, the information should be presented in a simple format, in a manner easily understood by both public and emergency management officials. Table 5-3 lists some of the numerous surveillance systems in operation.

Establishing a Postimpact Surveillance System

Outcomes anticipated from a specific disaster must be identified initially (e.g., crush injuries from earthquakes, diarrheal diseases from floods, fever from infectious disease). From a sample of the disaster-affected population, epidemiologists determine associations between exposure and outcome (e.g., disease variables) by identifying demographic, biological, chemical, physical, or behavioral factors associated with outcomes of death, illness, or injury. The incidence of diseases endemic to an area prior to the disaster event would be expected to rise as a result of population displacement, increased population density, the interruption of existing public health programs, and breakdown in sanitation and hygiene. Examples of such exposure-outcome relationships in disaster settings are included in Table 5-4.

Case Definitions

To ensure uniformity, case definitions must be established in advance of the outcomes that will be measured. Four case classifications are used: confirmed; probable; suspect; or not a case because it failed to fulfill the criteria for confirmed, probable, or suspect cases. Without data based on standard case definitions, unusual occurrences of diseases might

Table 5-3. Surveillance Systems

System	Sponsor	Function
BioSense	CDC	Monitors and rapidly identifies possible health emergencies through continuous scanning of medical information from hospital emergency rooms and pharmacies
Biowatch	Laboratory Response Network	Uses air samplers to test for threat agents
Electronic Surveillance System for Early Notification of Community-Based Epidemics (ESSENCE)	DOD	Early notification of epidemics by monitoring health data to identify and control epidemics
EMERGency IDNET	CDC	Multicenter emergency department based network for research of infectious diseases; a goal is to identify emerging infections in emergency department patients
Geosentinel	International Society of Travel Medicine and the CDC	Conduct syndromic surveillance in international travel medicine clinics
Global Emerging Infections Surveillance	DOD	Protects DOD health care beneficiaries through domestic and international surveillance of respiratory infections, gastrointestinal infections, febrile illness syndromes, antimicrobial resistance, and sexually transmitted infections
Global Public Health Intelligence Network	Public Health Agency of Canada	Monitors global media sources (e.g., news wires, Web sites) as web-based "early warning" system of public health events in 7 languages in real time around the clock
Global Outbreak Alert and Response Network	World Health Organization	Technical collaborative network where human and technical resources are pooled for rapid identification, confirmation, and response to international outbreaks
Infectious Diseases Society of America Epidemic Intelligence Network	Infectious Diseases Society of American	Provider-based emerging infections sentinel network
International Emerging Infections Program	CDC Global Disease Detection Program	Sites track global diseases to detect unusual changes in trends that may signal an outbreak

(*Continued*)

Table 5-3. (Continued)

System	Sponsor	Function
National Electronic Disease Surveillance System (NEDSS)	CDC	Integrated and interoperable surveillance systems for all levels of government to detect outbreaks rapidly
National Notifiable Infectious Conditions	CDC	Voluntary national collection and publication of data for notifiable diseases
National Outbreak Reporting System	CDC	Web-based system for reporting of waterborne, food-borne, enteric person-to-person, and enteric zoonotic (animal-to-person) disease outbreaks
Program for Monitoring Emerging Diseases (ProMED)	International Society of Infectious Diseases	Global electronic reporting system for outbreaks of emerging infectious diseases and toxins
PulseNet	CDC	Facilitates early identification of common source outbreaks
Real-Time Outbreak Disease Surveillance	University of Pittsburgh	Biosurveillance research laboratory
Syndromic Reporting Information System	Universities of New Mexico and Arizona	Real-time, web-based early warning system to prevent the spread of infectious disease and limit the effectiveness of bioterrorism attacks

Note: CDC=Centers for Disease Control and Prevention; DOD=Department of Defense.

Table 5-4. Exposure–Outcome Relationships in Disaster Settings

Timing	Disaster	Exposure	Outcome
Preimpact	Cyclone	High winds	Injury, death
		Presence of functioning warning system	Evacuation or not
	Tornado	High winds	Injury, death
		Presence of functioning warning system	Evacuation or not
Impact	Flash flood	Motor vehicle occupancy	Death by drowning
	Volcanic eruption	Ash particulate of respirable size	Silicosis
Postimpact	Earthquake	Building type, age, indoor cleanup	Injury, death
	Cyclone	Flood level	Death by electrocution
		Outdoor cleanup	Injury during cleanup

not be detected, trends cannot be accurately monitored, and the effectiveness of intervention activities cannot be easily evaluated.

Case definitions often evolve over time as the effect of a disaster on a community develops. Case definitions may be looser early on in the investigation following a disaster when the consequences of the events are not fully understood. Having a case definition that is not as well defined helps ensure the capture of information about the entire desired population. Over time, these definitions become more stringent as the event and its implications become clearer. Within the case definitions, detection thresholds must be flexible enough to respond to changing levels of risk and the priorities for detection. The CDC and the Agency for Toxic Substances and Disease Registry (ATSDR), collaborating with the Council of State and Territorial Epidemiologists, published and distributed standard case definitions to states and jurisdiction enabling the collection of uniform national data sets. However, standard definitions are not as useful in the early response to a disaster because information take times to get reported and vetted by state or local health departments and because new case definitions take time to create and disseminate.

Analysis

Appropriate methods for analysis must be considered and applied. Examples include descriptive (e.g., age, gender, ethnic group), geographic location, rates of disease or death, secular trends, and an analytic time series defining the total number of cases and trends over time.

Criteria for evaluating morbidity include clinical signs and symptoms, results from laboratory tests that confirm a diagnosis, and epidemiological limits on person, place, and time. In addition, sources of comparison data, such as local or regional incidence of a disease in the same month or time period during prior years, should be identified for use in the epidemiological analysis.

Data Collection Used for Decision Making

To enhance data collection during a disaster, it is important to identify the elements in advance. The public health and responder community will be interested in hospital capacity, such as bed, staffing, and supply needs and availability; event-related visits; and information from the patient locator system. Different emergencies require different levels of medical care and it will be essential to know the exact types of care that a hospital can provide and what outpatient services are still functioning.[2] A web-based collection system is best, but alternative collection through fax and phone should be established in case the web-based system fails. If a preexisting system is not in place when a disaster hits, an interim system should be developed. Finally, business rules need to be defined, such as who gets access to hospital-specific, aggregate information.

Since response activities and planning for relief and recovery are based on the data collected, the information should reflect as accurate and reliable a picture of the public health needs as possible. Hazard mapping and vulnerability assessments (discussed in Chapter 6) provide useful background information about the disaster event that can be used both for planning programs for disaster preparedness, and for determining response activities and evacuation plans. Although this information is usually available from the local emergency management office, geological institutions, or departments related to natural resources and the environment, public health professionals can work with these groups to create assessments that highlight public health concerns.

Information about the incident itself often includes the following:

- Demographic characteristics of affected areas
- Assessment of casualties, injuries, and selected illness
- Numbers and characteristics of displaced populations
- Type of volunteers needed (e.g., medical, mental health, search and rescue) for coordination of deployment
- Management of health care infrastructure
- Storage and distribution of relief materials, including food, water, and medical supplies
- Public information and rumor control

Possible reporting units for data collection include all the institutions that provide information for the surveillance system (e.g., hospitals, clinics, nongovernmental organizations, long-term care facilities, temporary shelters). Information can often be obtained

2. When entire hospitals needed to be evacuated during the response to Hurricane Sandy, administrators learned that hospitals defined their level of care differently. The capabilities of caring for a patient in an intensive care bed in the major teaching centers was not the same across the city. This complicated the ability of nursing personnel in finding a transfer bed where the necessary and appropriate level of care could be provided for patients in the hospitals providing quaternary care.

from existing data sets (e.g., census, state hospitalization data), hospitals and clinics (e.g., emergency departments, patient medical records, electronic health records, e-codes), health maintenance organizations and insurance companies, private providers, temporary shelters (e.g., daily shelter census, logs at medical facility in shelter), first responder or patient logs, and mobile health clinics, such as those run by the military and volunteer medical groups (e.g., patient logs, records of prescription medications dispensed). The patient logs are now collected electronically, easing the importation of the data into syndromic surveillance systems such as ESSENCE, discussed below.

Where hospitals are using radio-frequency identification (RFID) chips or scannable bar codes inside patient wristbands in lieu of traditional medical record retrieval and when legal agreements are established in advance, health departments can have instant access to hospital-uploaded databases through smartphones, personal data assistants, or notebook computers equipped with RFID or bar-code readers. Bar-coded scanning technology was deployed during the response to the bombing during the Boston Marathon in 2013 and used to inform Boston's mental health surveillance.

Due to time constraints and adverse environmental conditions, use of rigorous epidemiological methods may not be feasible in the postimpact phase. In disaster situations, assessment team members often use "quick and dirty" methods; "quick" in that they are simple, flexible, and can be used under difficult circumstances, and "dirty" in that numerator and denominator data may be rough estimates that, although they are subject to bias, serve to answer immediate questions whose answers are needed for the response.

Uniformity in Data Collection

Traditional public health surveillance is dependent on medical providers reporting unusual diseases or patterns of disease and laboratorians reporting unusual clinical isolates or patterns of routine isolates. The establishment of national standards for the interchange of electronic data can facilitate communication and integration with a breadth of information systems if the data definitions, coding conventions, and other specifications are identical. To ensure that data can be compared across jurisdictions by reducing incompatibilities across data, a number of efforts are being made to establish uniform definitions for data capture.

Examples of Disaster Information Systems

The availability of preexisting DIS expanded greatly as the need became better understood across the country. During the response to Hurricane Katrina, the CDC collaborated with many agencies, including DMATs, the U.S. Public Health Service (USPHS), and the Red Cross. DMATs provided triage and medical care and assisted with evacuation while providing information used for surveillance. Many epidemiology and surveillance team members were activated from within the USPHS. The Red Cross provided shelter, food, and health and mental health services while gathering information used for surveillance. Coordinating with these agencies, the CDC conducted ongoing surveillance in 12 states. Data sources included hospitals, emergency departments, clinics, DMATs, military treatment units, and evacuation centers. Table 5-5 identifies key steps in surveillance conducted in the Gulf Coast area following Hurricane Katina and the subsequent flooding. Box 5-2 describes disaster surveillance following Hurricane Sandy.

Although in the United States' multiple systems support the collection and reporting of information to public health labs, the clinical community, and state and local health departments, many of these systems operate in isolation without a mechanism to exchange consistent response, health, and disease-tracking data between systems. On the federal level, the CDC and ATSDR developed an ensemble of data collection systems that build on common technical standards and infrastructure. These initiatives include surveillance capacity, e-mail and message centers, and communication networks. On the state and local level, systems were built that function both in unique ways suitable for the locality and in ways that interface with the federal architecture.

Table 5-5. Sentinel Surveillance Post-Katrina

- Louisiana Health Department suffered loss of infrastructure
- Concern for outbreaks
- Sentinel (enhanced) surveillance implemented in New Orleans
- Captured data on every patient that accessed care in a New Orleans health care facility
  - 8 hospitals
  - 6 Disaster Medical Assistance Teams
  - 5 clinics
  - 10 military facilities
- Form captured
  - 30 disease syndromes
  - 4 mental health conditions
  - 15 trauma conditions
  - Medication refills
  - Severity
  - Disposition
- Clinical encounter forms collected every 24 hours
- Forms completed by facility or CDC staff through record review
- Data collection was labor intensive
- Paper form had to be transferred to electronic database
- Identified cases reported to the Louisiana Health Department and CDC
- Transitioned to automated syndromic surveillance after 6 weeks

Note: CDC=Centers for Disease Control and Prevention.

Box 5-2. Disaster Surveillance Following Hurricane Sandy

Disaster surveillance was a key component in the recovery from Hurricane Sandy that struck 24 states in 2012. Following the storm, the New Jersey Department of Health (NJDOH) developed indicators to enhance syndromic surveillance for extreme weather events. The NJDOH used EpiCenter, an online system that collects and analyzes real-time chief complaint data for emergency department (ED) visits and classifies each visit by indicator or syndrome. To determine which indicators they wanted to include during severe weather, the NJDOH included key words through a review of chief complaints from cases where diagnostic codes met selection criteria and excluded other key words by evaluating cases that lacked selected diagnostic codes.

Spikes in the number of ED visits were observed immediately after the hurricane for carbon monoxide (CO) poisoning. Using statistics that examined data by zip code, they found clusters of CO poisoning and an increase in the refilling of prescriptions during the 2 weeks after Hurricane Sandy. CO poisoning clusters were identified in areas that experienced power outages of 4 days or longer. The results yielded valuable information that can aid New Jersey in their preparedness plans to monitor the effects of future severe weather disasters.

Immediately after the hurricane, surveillance systems were also used to track potential outbreaks of infectious disease for 42 reportable diseases that could have been affected by hurricane-related exposures. Only legionellosis was found to have a statistically significantly increase in flooded/impacted areas following the hurricane. This finding facilitated public health action to promptly curtail the outbreak.

Data Mining to Develop Novel Systems

Data mining is the processing and analyzing of data from different sources and summarizing it into useful information. A variation of data mining has been applied to the early detection of infectious disease outbreaks. A robust field of biosurveillance modeling has emerged and has advanced our understanding of the dynamics of the transmission of infectious disease (e.g., risk factors, virulence, and spatiotemporal patterns of spread) at the population and individual levels. These biosurveillance models may be used to detect or forecast when an infectious disease becomes an emergency, to assess risk, or to understand the elements that can change the outcome of an event. As with a hypothesis where the investigator decides what the inputs will be before they collect data and do an analysis, these mathematical models are determined in advance and can integrate diverse data sources (e.g., demographics, remotely sensed measurements and imaging, environmental measurements) with surrogate data (e.g., news alerts and social media). In addition, early research is examining data at the omics level (i.e., the study of large biological data) to aid in forecasting future epidemics. Examples include phylogenetic techniques for predicting pathogen mutations, algorithms for identifying novel microbials, metagenomic analysis, and examination of multiscale systems of biology. At present, these models do not have the sensitivity and specificity needed to forecast or predict the occurrence of disease.

Several models are used to create and analyze biosurveillance systems. The categories are not mutually exclusive.[3]

- **Risk Assessment** models determine the risk of an outbreak occurring under specified conditions. Those calculating the risk of disease correlate factors that might affect that risk for a specific location based upon weather and other covariates. This type of model is commonly referred to as *disease risk mapping*.
- **Event Prediction** models are used to assign a probability for when (time period) and where (location) a disease event is likely to occur based upon data sources and variables.
- **Spatial** models, which can change in time, forecast the geographic spread of a disease after it occurs based upon the correlation between the outbreak and GIS factors.
- **Dynamical** models examine how a specific disease moves through a population or when the pathogenicity will change. These models may include parameters that could be used as interventions, such as the restriction of movement that could impact the severity of an epidemic.
- **Event Detection** models are used to identify outbreaks by detecting increases in signs, symptoms, or syndromes that are indicative of spreading infectious disease, either through sentinel groups or through the collection of real-time diagnostic, clinical, or syndromic data.

Disaster Surveillance Work Group

In 2006, the CDC established the Disaster Surveillance Work Group (DSWG) to coordinate surveillance activities following a natural disaster. DSWG partners with state and local health departments and the agencies with response authority for Emergency Support Functions #6 and #8. In the event of a disaster, DSWG provides technical resources to its partners and facilitates the methodology for capturing data used for surveillance. To standardize data collection, DSWG developed morbidity and mortality surveillance tools and training materials available at: https://www.cdc.gov/nceh/hsb/disaster/surveillance.htm.

---

3. Readers interested in learning more can refer to the work of Corley et al. listed in the Surveillance section of References for this book.

Council of State and Territorial Epidemiologists Disaster Subcommittee

The Disaster Epidemiology Subcommittee of the Council of State and Territorial Epidemiologists convenes colleagues to share best practices and collaborate on investigative approaches for improving the profession's capacities for all-hazard disaster preparedness and response. The contribution of epidemiologists in these areas is enhanced by using epidemiologic principles for describing the distribution of injuries, illnesses, and disabilities; rapidly detecting outbreaks or clusters; identifying and implementing timely interventions; evaluating the impacts of public health efforts; and improving public health preparedness planning. The activities of the subcommittee fall within the following categories:

- Defining disaster epidemiology
- Identifying training needs and developing training opportunities
- Developing a repository of tools and methods for responding to and evaluating the impacts of disasters
- Additional information can be found at: http://www.cste.org/group/disasterepi.

Public Health Information Network

In order to enhance early detection of public health emergencies and to facilitate the gathering, storage, and dissemination of electronic information, a framework called the Public Health Information Network (PHIN) was established by the CDC. This framework includes the following guidance and tools:

- **Public Health Directory (PHIN DIR):** The PHIN DIR is a repository of information about people, organizations, and jurisdictions that are important to public health programs and includes the roles that people play within organizations. PHIN DIR is not a single directory but is a distributed network of related directories. Every PHIN partner (e.g., state health departments, larger local health departments, and the CDC) is responsible for managing its own directory and maintaining and updating information about its own workforce and about the people and organizations within its jurisdiction that play a role in PHIN systems or in the partner's emergency response plan.
- **PHIN Messaging System (PHIN MS):** The PHIN MS is the CDC-provided software that enables public health information systems to reliably exchange critical and sensitive data, even among systems with different architecture. PHIN MS can securely send and receive any type of message over the Internet, facilitating interoperability among multiple public health information systems.

- **PHIN Message Quality Framework (PHIN MQF):** The PHIN MQF is an automated testing tool that ensures messages adhere to standards defined in the messaging guides by: validating the structure of the message, validating that the messages are following the business rules defined for the message, and verifying that the vocabulary defined for the message is utilized. This tool is hosted at the CDC and can be accessed via a public Web site available at: https://phinmqf.cdc.gov.
- **PHIN Vocabulary Access and Distribution System (VADS):** PHIN VADS uses standard terminology in a web-based system for accessing, searching, and distributing vocabularies used in public health and clinical care practice. By using a common vocabulary, PHIN VADS supports the exchange of consistent information among public health partners.

Public Health Surveillance System and Geographic Information Systems

When combined with GIS, public health surveillance systems can be a powerful tool for analysis. As data are loaded into the system, the information goes through geocoding, which provides the latitude and longitude of the information so that the user can see the mapping both visually and in a tabular report. Seeing the data visually is like viewing a series of transparencies overlaid on top of one another, each with a new set of information. The ability to visualize the data permits modeling of activity based on parameters set by the user. RiskMap and WebFOCUS are commercially available software programs that build a tunnel and provide an interface between the GIS and CDC's National Electronic Disease Surveillance System (NEDSS) databases. (RiskMap is available at: https://www.riskmap.com; WebFOCUS is available at: http://www.informationbuilders.com/products/webfocus.)

To understand the advantages that this technology offers, it is worthwhile to describe how GIS operate and the opportunities for public health response and preparedness in emergencies.

GIS can be a useful tool to support epidemiology and surveillance in preparation for and in response to disasters. GIS technology allows the user to digitally link data, spatial information, and geography and display the information in an easy-to-understand visual medium. GIS data combine information about *where* things are with information about *what* things are so that we can identify which groups with different features are located together. Using spatial database management, visualization, mapping, and spatial analyses, this technology allows us to see spatial and temporal relationships among data. These systems allow researchers, public health professionals, and policy makers to better understand geographic relationships that affect health outcomes, public health risks, disease transmission, access to health care, and other public health concerns as they relate to all emergencies. GIS data are precise to 15 centimeters and can show buildings shifting after a disaster. GIS maps allow departments to switch from an overview of sections of a city to the location of individual objects. For example, if a hospital needs to bring nurses from home following an emergency, using MapPoint software, GIS can provide information about transporting them to your hospital, department, and so forth by identifying safe

Table 5-6. Public Health Uses of Geographic Information Systems Data in Emergency Preparedness

Community Preparedness Efforts

- Assess community risks
- Identify high concentrations of vulnerable populations
- Estimate populations in hazard zones
- Map demographic factors (e.g., housing type, age, those needing special assistance) to target preventive activities for specific populations
- Develop treatment profiles of physicians so officials know how to target education (e.g., large number of physicians prescribed 3 pills of ciprofloxacin as prophylaxis for anthrax following the anthrax mailings in 2001)
- Predict location of disease-transmitting vectors (e.g., mosquitoes)
- Predict, by model, demand for a service for known emergencies (e.g., in regions with frequent flooding, earthquake, or hurricane) both before and after event
- Identify capacity of the health care system:
    - Identify the market/treatment area for health care systems
    - Locate specialty physicians and specialized services in a community
    - Conduct small-area analysis to see how services are used by defined population
- Better distribute services in future disasters or reallocate preventive services in advance of emergency by analyzing both residence and treatment zip codes to identify where victims sought services
- Develop training scenarios

Response Capabilities

- Conduct infection surveillance by identifying geographic spread of disease
- Monitor and track spread of infectious disease and predict path of disease by searching for spatial relationships
- Inform establishment of medical care sites (e.g., points of distribution) or shelters by locating injuries/illness by zip code in relation to existing health care services
- Produce accurate maps for urban search and rescue
- Monitor asset management
- Manage field data in real time
- Improve data-sharing capabilities
- Locate resources
- Notify and update residents on status of basic services, utilities, transportation
- Track location and real-time capacity of shelters
- Risk and vulnerability assessments
    - Estimate extent and location of potential damage
    - Identify where centers delivering services are to discover gaps
    - Map patterns of destruction, targeting recovery and reconstruction efforts
    - Track plumes of chemicals to see how they spread through air, soil, or water and who and what will be affected
    - Determine evacuation zone
- Evaluate response

passageways. Further, a process available through GIS, geographic allocation process analysis, helps determine where gaps in service exist. GIS can be supported in a network environment. Table 5-6 identifies the many public health uses of GIS data in emergencies.

How to Use Data in Geographic Information Systems

The purpose of a geospatial system is to combine data with the questions that are asked administratively. GIS provides spatial information in response to the query, *what should I look at next?* While analyses from relational databases present tabular data in tables and charts, GIS provides a more descriptive view of the information and expands what can be done beyond traditional aggregate reports. Built upon an underlying data model, GIS presents data about locations and attributes by looking spatially at layers of information.

The development of GIS as a management tool for public health as part of the larger community is best achieved through collaboration among several agencies. Establishing a team of GIS personnel often requires volunteers from many disciplines. A GIS volunteer list should include professionals or students who are vetted and credentialed in advance like other public health and mental health personnel. GIS volunteers need to be oriented in advance to the current GIS being used in the community, the configuration of the files, and so forth, so they can quickly help in the event of disaster.

Traditionally, communities collect and use their data in stovepipes, where each agency creates and analyzes its own databases, often without sharing information with sister agencies. The National Spatial Data Infrastructure[4] Executive Order encouraged geospatial data acquisition and access throughout all levels of government, the private and nonprofit sectors, and the academic community. Importantly, the order targeted data needed for emergency response efforts. An enterprise GIS solution, where all agencies have access to a centralized data set of geographic data layers, reduces redundancies of data collection, maintenance, and processing. GIS applications such as ESRI (available at: http://www.esri.com) and ArcPad (available at: http://www.esri.com/software/arcgis/arcpad/index.html) can be used in the field on smartphones and personal data assistants, allowing field-level assessments in real time and the transmission of information back to the Emergency Operations Center. Interactive mapping applications, such as GeoMAC (available at: http://www.geomac.gov/index.shtml) can be used to assess disaster conditions from anywhere in the United States.

Through GIS, we can map case distributions and variability in disease agents and analyze temporal and geographic trends in disease outbreaks, all of which can inform our decisions on targeting interventions and preventive activities. By matching addresses through geocoding we can convert each address to a point on a map. For example, by

4. Exec. Order No. 12,906, 59 Fed. Reg. 17671–17674 (April 13, 1994); amended by Exec. Order No. 13,286, 68 Fed. Reg. 10619–10633 (March 5, 2003).

creating a zip code map of high risk (e.g., areas of outbreaks and areas with large numbers of non-English-speaking residents) public health can identify where the development of educational materials in multiple languages is needed. By mapping the areas that lack accessible services, have high-density residential housing, and the historical sites where injuries occurred in a previous disaster, public health may be better able to plan the locations for temporary treatment centers or DMATs. By mapping data from syndromic surveillance systems with GIS, we can predict where infections or outbreaks will spread. We can use a GIS-based application coupled with an automated telephone dialing system to communicate an emergency message, such as warning citizens about impending or ongoing disasters. As an example, NEDSS data are collected and entered at the hospital and automatically shipped to the state, which customizes the data by setting the parameters for analysis. When analyses are run and maps created that identify a community at risk, the system can trigger an automatic telephone notification in which a series of phones ring or texts automatically and prerecorded messages tell people what to do depending on their address and its proximity to the emergency.

Using GIS, departments of health working with the state or local offices of emergency management have overlaid census data with information about power outages and roadmaps to see which major populations were being impacted. GIS has been used to map sites of dead crows and locate pockets of breeding mosquitoes, helping identify where West Nile virus and Zika virus were spreading. In the response to the World Trade Center attacks of 2001, officials used GIS to create a frame of reference for understanding where the buildings had been. They used GIS to see if buildings next to the site were shifting dangerously. Furthermore, thermal maps were overlaid on orthoimagery to identify where fire suppression was necessary and where to avoid sending workers. More recently, the National Capital Region Geospatial Data Exchange (NCR GDX) was created for the Washington, D.C., metropolitan area to facilitate the sharing of GIS data among local, regional, state, and federal partners. Through the NCR GDX, participating jurisdictions are improving decision making by sharing real-time data through regional mapping applications.

Where to Get Data

The potential sources for locating data are limitless and any data describing a characteristic of a community can better inform decision makers. Some data are available without cost, while some must be purchased. For example, ArcGIS (available at: http://www.esri.com/software/arcgis/index.html) has many links that permit the download of state level information (available at: http://www.esri.com/industries/stategov/index.html). The Web site GeoPlatform (available at: https://www.geoplatform.gov) hosts geographic maps for all levels of jurisdiction and serves as a GIS data clearinghouse. The site includes many data sets and services that were formerly published by ESRI. In addition, GIS departments have parcel maps available for sale.

When locating or purchasing GIS data, it is important to use managed (versus unmanaged) data if they are available. Managed data are a potentially more reliable source that will reduce error in notification of emergencies or other public service announcements, as well as in determining evacuation routes, issuing shelter-in-place instructions, or responding to the correct location.

Let us suppose that you, the reader, are interested in building a GIS database for public use during an emergency. When looking for data to create a database for your community, the local zoning and planning commission and local tax commission are the best sources of data. Since they make money from tracking activities of daily living, they can be depended on to track such activities accurately. Property tax databases contain the names and phone numbers of homeowners (i.e., information that can be imported into an emergency telephone notification application). Information is available from the Department of Transportation, federal railways, census bureau, schools, the White Pages phone book, and so forth. To obtain additional data, search the Internet by entering the search term "GIS data." Locating a GIS user network in your area is an important place to get started since these groups will know where data sets are "buried."

Furthermore, research and nonprofit institutions may have data sets that will be valuable to your community. Rich data sets are possible in locales where land is owned by state or federal governments, county governments, other public agencies, or public-interest organizations. To expand data and improve resource and facility management, electronic blueprints can be created by zooming in on individual hospitals and getting a detailed map of which facilities are operational by tying hospital floor plans to the community's disaster plans. Two publicly available software packages, CATS for emergency response (Consequences Assessment Tool Set, available at: http://www.esri.com/industries/public-safety/tools/cats) and HAZUS software (Hazards U.S., available at: http://www.fema.gov/hazus-software), use GIS (e.g., ArcView and ArcGIS) and include extensive national data sets of assets necessary in disaster response. The assets include hospitals, pharmacies, and nuclear plants that can be mapped by GIS. The following are types of data sets that are useful when public health professionals work with GIS:

- Airports
- Community-based organizations
- Community centers
- Demographics of the community
- Doctors' offices at which patients have signed Health Insurance Portability and Accountability Act (HIPAA) authorization
- Fire and other emergency services
- Government buildings

- Hospitals
- Hospital surveillance
- Law enforcement facilities
- Long-term care facilities
- Major highways and railways
- Pharmacies
- Phone lines
- Power-generating plants
- Schools and school surveillance
- Sentinel reporting systems
- Toxics Release Inventory
- Veterinary clinics
- Vital statistics

It is very important that complete and current data be obtained about both the assets available to the community and the potential hazards when planning a GIS-focused disaster management program. It is also useful to collate and regularly update the contact names, current mobile telephone numbers, and e-mail addresses of GIS personnel and current emergency management contacts. GIS data sets should be updated periodically because many communities build new roads and buildings and data should reflect that.

Because it is difficult to know what data will be needed post-disaster, the goal should be to create as rich a data set as possible, including as many types of information as available. Once the data sets have been located, it should be ensured that they will be immediately available following a disaster by negotiating data-sharing agreements before the data are needed. Sharing data facilitates a community's coordinated planning and response through public-private partnerships. The directory structure of your GIS data set should be logical because many people may use it after the disaster, which is a particularly stressful time. For naming conventions of the data files, use simple, descriptive labels that will be easily recognizable.

Planning With Geographic Information System Data

Once the data sets have been assembled, the analysis should begin with identification of vulnerable assets, including critically important facilities. Examples include the following:

- Structures used for communication
- Fire and rescue
- Hospital and nursing facilities
- Pharmacies

- Police
- Schools and day care facilities
- Shelter
- Transportation
- Utilities

Facilities whose destruction could result in severe public health problems for a community should also be examined, such as hazardous material storage sites, food and water sources, and sanitation centers.

Developing the Data Set

An initial step is to identify the historical events that have been hazardous to a community and prioritize those events according to frequency, magnitude, and area of impact. High-risk areas get assigned a risk level based on probability and historic occurrence. Because critical decisions will be made based on the data, it is important to keep a log of the pedigree of the data one is using, such as summaries of origin, update schedules, and contact numbers for data librarians. The pedigree of the data may influence some decision making about public health interventions. Some data, such as those collected through active short-term surveillance systems, may be incomplete and require follow-up data cleaning. For example, corrections to the record of reportable disease can be made by utilizing address data as geographic identifiers. Furthermore, when data are obtained from a variety of data sources, it is often necessary to convert the data to make them usable and compatible. Finally, although specific data sets can be established as shapefiles for each hazard, another robust format is the Spatial Data Transfer Standard, which was designed so that spatial data could be easily used on different computer platforms.

Social Vulnerability and Community Preparedness

GIS is useful to identify people or neighborhoods most at risk of suffering adverse outcomes as a result of their social vulnerability, enhancing a community's preparedness efforts and targeted response and recovery. Although vulnerability (or those at risk) is discussed at greater length in Chapter 11, it is sufficient here to define socially vulnerable individuals as those with access and functional needs and those without financial resources, women, children, and the elderly. Entire communities may also be vulnerable.

A tool called the Social Vulnerability Index (SoVI) measures the social vulnerability of U.S. counties to various hazards. The index combines 32 socioeconomic variables that predict a community's inability to prepare for, respond to, and recover from hazards.

SoVI highlights the geographic variation in social vulnerability and enables the planner to identify which communities might not have the capacity to prepare or respond and where resources might be used most effectively to reduce the preexisting vulnerability. SoVI can also be used to indicate different rates in the recovery of communities. (More information on SoVI is available at http://www.222.sovius.org.)

The process of determining who is vulnerable in a community can be straightforward. As an example, start with a single agency by gathering the addresses of the individuals of interest. After collecting the addresses of clients who are served, service providers, facilities, and staff, geocode each of these addresses. Overlay the addresses onto the potential hazardous area (e.g., a known flood zone). Finally, prepare the maps and discuss the results with the planners.

HIPAA compliance can be ensured by obtaining authorizations from the individuals involved or using registries of individuals who want to be notified about emergencies. In addition, guidelines should be established between emergency management and public health agencies about data-sharing for individuals with disabilities and others with access and functional needs. When using GIS data in syndromic surveillance, the analysis is limited to zip code or a larger spatial resolution to aggregate data sufficiently to protect patient privacy under HIPAA rules.

The University of North Carolina (UNC) Gillings School of Global Public Health's North Carolina Institute for Public Health recently developed Collect SMART, a suite of software designed to help agencies manage and implement community-based data collection efforts. With direct funding from the UNC Preparedness and Emergency Response Learning Center, Collect SMART was developed as a free mobile platform for obtaining high-quality, representative data to assist local health agencies with data collection projects, including community health needs assessments and pre- and post-disaster assessments. To date, Collect SMART has been implemented in 7 North Carolina communities with the assistance of more than 350 health agencies and community members who provided feedback to refine and improve Collect SMART tools.

Use of Geographic Information Systems in Mitigation

GIS products and spatial analysis allow the user to precisely map where hazards exist and to visualize that information so that decisions can be made about possible preventive activities. GIS can be used to combine areas of high risk with areas where many high-value assets or vulnerable populations are found. An example is wildfire-prone areas where brush could be cut back. Once a community determines the areas and populations at risk, public health can work with emergency management and community leaders to target areas where preventive or mitigation activities would be beneficial.

Since many communities use GIS to create assessment maps of economic damage, the foundation has been set to create assessment maps for public health. Public health planners can focus mitigation efforts where calculations show a probability that a hazard common to the community would cause an unacceptable level of morbidity and mortality.

If you are concerned about risks in your area, check the GIS assessment systems identified in Table 5-7.

Maps

Following an emergency, there will be a high demand for spatial information by many sectors involved in the response. Where a disaster has destroyed a neighborhood or a community's landmarks, a geographic visualization of the area can help with reorientation and stabilization of the site. Maps provide a common platform for everyone to visualize needed information about the location of events, resources, transportation, emergency networks, and so forth, facilitating communication and decision making. Further, through social networking sites on the Internet and interactive mapping programs, public health workers can inform a community about interventions and recovery progress, enabling real-time online changes.

GIS can create individualized maps, customized to the features needed in the user's tasks. As a start, it is necessary to create what are known as *basemaps,* basic generic maps used as a reference to the location of preexisting community data. The attributes of basemaps will vary according to the risks of the community. Because disasters are not confined to jurisdictional boundaries, basemaps often cross territorial lines. Multiple basemaps with differing attributes may be needed. As an example, for responders who travel from out of the area, to help them become oriented to their surroundings, the basemaps need to be very specific about any landmarks that may still be standing. Basic operational field maps are valuable for directing off-site support teams in the field, in identifying where supplies are needed, and so forth. One basemap may be needed that locates pet shelters, and others to show the preexisting locations of hospitals and schools.

Part of the implementation of GIS is the establishment of a system to create and distribute maps. The jurisdictional Office of Emergency Management is often the agency responsible for the distribution of the maps. Three types of maps should be distinguished: standard, templates, and at risk. Maps can be created by using desktop mapping products such as ArcGIS and a relational database such as SQL Server. By permitting online requests for maps, one can establish and track the parameters of map requests. This online site can also provide the complex array of Incident Command System forms that are so often requested by responders and agencies.

Table 5-7. Hazard-Specific Geographic Information Systems Tools

Hazard	Digital Mapping Projects/Tools	Web Resource
Earthquakes	California Geological Survey	http://www.conservation.ca.gov/cgs/information/geologic_mapping/Pages/Index.aspx
	U.S. Geological Survey Earthquake Hazards Program, national seismic hazard maps	http://earthquake.usgs.gov/hazards
Fires	U.S. Wildland Fire Assessment System, fire danger rating maps	http://www.wfas.net
	California Department of Forestry and Fire Prevention, Fire and Resource Assessment Program, maps of fire hazard severity zones	http://www.fire.ca.gov/fire_prevention/fire_prevention_wildland_zones_maps
Floods	Federal Emergency Management Agency National Flood Insurance Program, Flood Hazard Mapping, flood insurance rate maps	https://www.fema.gov/national-flood-insurance-program-flood-hazard-mapping
	Sea, Lake, and Overland Surges from Hurricanes, hurricane storm surge inundation area maps	http://www.fema.gov/plan/prevent/nhp/slosh_link.shtm
Hurricanes	Consequences Assessment Tool Set	http://www.esri.com/industries/publicsafety/tools/cats
	U.S. Geological Survey Center for Integration of Natural Disaster Information	https://pubs.er.usgs.gov/publication/fs00301
Landslides	Association of Bay Area Governments Resilience Program, Landslide Maps and Information	http://quake.abag.ca.gov/landslides
Toxic spills, explosions, and fires	HAZUS	https://www.fema.gov/hazus
Tsunamis	California Department of Conservation, Tsunami Inundation Map	http://www.conservation.ca.gov/cgs/geologic_hazards/Tsunami/Inundation_Maps
	University of Southern California Tsunami Research Center	http://www.tsunamiresearchcenter.com

As maps can undergo numerous changes, users of GIS should develop a log that tracks the history of each map and the data used to build each one. It is important to keep a record of earlier maps and the data used because, as was the case at the World Trade Center site, officials may not know the types of hazardous substances at the site until sometime later. Public health professionals will want to trace exposures over time, especially as new information is added or if stations for decontamination are moved.

The National Oceanic and Atmospheric Administration's Office of Response and Restoration provides comprehensive modeling programs and data sets (available at: http://response.restoration.noaa.gov/maps-and-spatial-data). Table 5-8 describes some of the modeling programs available.

Evaluating Disaster Surveillance

Finally, a DIS must be evaluated within the disaster setting to know when the system is no longer needed. This endpoint is often determined by assessing both the resources and personnel available to run the system and the ability to merge the emergency system into routine surveillance. In addition to describing the attributes, usefulness, and cost of DIS, evaluations can lead to recommendations on the initiation and conclusion of future surveillance related to disasters.

The CDC developed a guide to evaluate surveillance systems. Their evaluation focuses on the public health importance of the health-related event under surveillance, the purpose and operation of the system, and resources used to operate the system. Additional information can be found at: http://www.cdc.gov/mmwr/preview/mmwrhtml/rr5013a1.htm. See Chapter 14 for more information on evaluation methods.

Table 5-8. Representative Modeling Programs

Agency	Program	Tool	Function	Source
NOAA	Assessing Risk to Ecological Resources		Assessing hazardous waste sites	
		Environmental Sensitivity Index map	Summary of coastal resources that are at risk if an oil spill occurs nearby	Office of Response and Restoration, NOAA's National Ocean Service; Environmental Sensitivity Index Metadata, Emergency Response Software and Data Sets (http://www.response.restoration.noaa.gov)
		Risk and Vulnerability tool	Interactive online tool that assists in identification of individuals, property, and resources that are at risk during a hazardous event or natural disaster	Can be accessed for free (http://gcmd.gsfc.nasa.gov/KeywordSearch/Metadata.do?Portal=GCMD&MetadataType=1&MetadataView=Full&KeywordPath=&EntryId=NOAA_RVAT)
	Emergency Response Program		Build and sustain NOAA's ability to respond effectively to emergencies	
		Environmental Response Management Application	Assists in response planning Accessible to both the command post and to assets in the field during an actual response incident, such as an oil spill or hurricane	Office of Response and Restoration, NOAA's National Ocean Service; Environmental Response Management Application Web Portal page (http://www.response.restoration.noaa.gov)
		Mapping Application for Response, Planning, and Local Operational Tasks (MARPLOT)	Simple mapping application allowing download of maps of any area of the country	Emergency Management, U.S. EPA (https://www.epa.gov/cameo/marplot-software)

(Continued)

Table 5-8. (Continued)

Agency	Program	Tool	Function	Source
		Aerial Locations of Hazardous Atmospheres (ALOHA)	Gas-dispersion modeling software that uses information the user provides, along with physical property data from its extensive chemical library, to predict how a hazardous gas cloud might disperse in the atmosphere after an accidental chemical release	Emergency Management, U.S. EPA (http://www.epa.gov/osweroe1/content/cameo/aloha.htm)
	Responding to Oil Spills		Support effective and safe responses to oil spills in the coastal environment	
		ADIOS	Designed to help answer typical questions during oil spill response and cleanup Used to help assess where the oil was going from the Deepwater Horizon spill	Office of Response and Restoration, NOAA's National Ocean Service; ADOIS2, NOAA's Emergency Response Program page (http://www.response.restoration.noaa.gov)
		GNOME	Oil spill trajectory model	Office of Response and Restoration, NOAA's National Ocean Service; GNOME, Emergency Response Software and Data Sets page (http://www.response.restoration.noaa.gov)
FEMA		HAZUS	Loss-estimation modeling which allows users to forecast most probable physical and economic damage to a community Models earthquakes, floods, and hurricanes Bundled with federal data sets, but can be customized with local data FEMA offers a training course on HAZUS	HAZUS: FEMA's Methodology for Estimating Potential Losses from Disasters (http://www.fema.gov/plan/prevent/hazus)
National Hurricane Center		Sea, Lake, and Overland Surges from Hurricanes (SLOSH)	Evaluate storm surge threat from hurricanes and tropical cyclones Emergency managers use these data to determine which areas must be evacuated	National Weather Service Meteorological Development Laboratory page (http://www.nws.noaa.gov/mdl)

Note: ADIOS=Automated Data Inquiry for Oil Spills; EPA=Environmental Protection Agency; FEMA=Federal Emergency Management Agency; GNOME=General NOAA Operational Modeling Environment; HAZUS=Hazards U.S.; NOAA=National Oceanic and Atmospheric Administration.

CHAPTER 6

RISK AND RAPID HEALTH ASSESSMENTS

Assessments are foundational to public health practice in times of disaster. Of the types of assessments that are conducted in disaster preparedness and response, 2 merit an in-depth focus. Estimations of both risk and health needs must be tailored to the timing, size, and impact of a specific disaster. In the first, key steps to assessing risks are identifying the hazards or threats, determining who is at risk of being harmed, and assessing the probability of the hazard actually occurring. Once risk is determined, decisions can be made on preventive action and the capabilities needed to respond. In the second, rapid health assessments are used to collect information about the health status and needs of the population impacted by the disaster. This information is critical to understanding the magnitude of response required.

This chapter reviews a rationale for assessing risk, the Federal Emergency Management Agency's (FEMA) threat and hazard assessment process, hazard identification and analysis, determining the context of potential hazards and threats, and establishing targets for tasks needed in a response. This chapter also includes guidance for conducting rapid health assessments: specifics on assembling a team, the tools needed, what to look for and what can be accomplished within specific time frames, conducting an assessment for a disaster that develops over time, sources for data collection, and the use of Community Assessment for Public Health Emergency Response (CASPER).

Public Health Role

- Identify disaster-related hazards, threats, and associated vulnerability in a community.
- Determine risk of likely public health needs due to disaster.
- Prioritize necessary health and public health requirements following a disaster based on information from community needs assessment.
- Provide decision makers with objective information to guide prevention, mitigation, and response to disease.

Rationale for Assessing Risk

Different types of disasters are associated with distinct patterns of morbidity and mortality. To develop location-specific strategies for reducing negative health outcomes, public health officials and disaster managers must be aware of the types of hazards most likely to affect specific communities. Although all-hazards planning is efficient for the utilization of resources, preparedness often focuses on the events that are most likely to occur. For example, health planners in Florida might prepare primarily for hurricanes, whereas those in California would prepare more for earthquakes and wildfires.

Following an analysis of hazards and threats, vulnerability and risk, 6 categories of public health prevention measures can be implemented:

- Performing activities that prevent or remove a hazard (e.g., providing guidance on mold remediation due to flooding)
- Moving those at risk of being harmed away from the hazard (e.g., evacuating populations prior to the impact of a hurricane, including hospitalized patients or residents of long-term care facilities located in a flood zone)
- Providing public information and education (e.g., providing information concerning measures that the public can take to ensure that their food is safe to eat and drinking water safe to drink following a tornado)
- Establishing early warning systems (e.g., conducting syndromic surveillance to identify early trends of infectious disease)
- Reducing the impact of the disaster (e.g., providing influenza immunization before a pandemic reaches your region)
- Increasing local capacity to respond (e.g., coordinating a plan utilizing the resources of the entire health community, including health departments, hospitals, community clinics and home care agencies)

Federal Guidance—the Threat and Hazard Identification and Risk Assessment

The federal government designed a process for assessing a community's risks from natural, technological, and human-caused threats and hazards; for determining how capabilities (methods to accomplish a critical task) will be employed; and for estimating the resources needed to reduce the impacts of these threats. This guidance is found in the *Comprehensive Preparedness Guide (CPG) 201: Threat and Hazard Identification and Risk Assessment (THIRA) Guide* (Second Edition). The THIRA process helps communities understand what they need to prepare for, the resources required in order to be prepared, actions that can lessen or eliminate the threat or hazard, and potential impacts that need to be incorporated into the community's recovery preparedness planning. By understanding the potential threats and hazards, communities can make informed decisions about how to manage the identified risks and then develop needed capabilities.

The 4-step process for developing a THIRA includes:

1. Identify the Threats and Hazards of Concern—Based on the experience of the community and input from experts and other available resources, including forecasting, recognize and name threats and hazards.
2. Give the Threats and Hazards Context—Describe how the identified threats and hazards may affect the community.
3. Establish Capability Targets—Following a description of how the threats and hazards of concern may affect the community, develop a target that describes what the jurisdiction hopes to be able to accomplish for an entire capability or component of a capability.
4. Apply the Results—For each core capability, estimate the resources required to achieve the capability targets. These goals can be met through the use of community assets and mutual aid.

Public Health Role in THIRA

This 4-step risk assessment process is administered by FEMA and every state emergency management office is required to complete it. States submit a State Preparedness Report, which is a self-assessment of how their preparedness capabilities compare with the needs established in the state's THIRA. This report must include activities and input from public health departments and the health care sector who participate actively in its preparation. In addition, public health agencies receiving public health emergency preparedness funding are required to complete risk assessments to identify the potential hazards, vulnerabilities, and risks within their community that relate to the public health, medical, and behavioral health systems and the functional needs of at-risk individuals. These risk assessment activities must be coordinated with the state's emergency management and homeland security programs, support whole community planning, and inform the development of the THIRA of that jurisdiction. By partnering with emergency management as communities understand and plan for future disasters, public health agencies enhance the way their community will respond, potentially reducing morbidity and mortality. Most health departments adopt the risk assessment developed by the office of emergency management in their jurisdiction.

Hazard Identification and Analysis

The first step of the THIRA is to identify the hazard or threat. Hazard identification is used to determine which events are most likely to affect a community. This step is critical in determining actions that can be taken to mitigate the potential harm to a community and its residents. To identify threats and hazards of significant concern, public health professionals should consider (1) the likelihood, or chance, that something might happen and (2) how significant the effects might be to their community. Start by looking at what threats and hazards have historically affected them and what threats and hazards might exist in the future (e.g., earthquakes, industrial accidents, or potential terrorist attacks). After-action reports for previous disasters, scientists and appropriate subject-matter experts, and historical archives (e.g., newspapers or the local library) are all potential sources. The significance to a community will vary, depending on the magnitude of previous and potential incidents, the ability of the community to manage, and whether complex interagency or intergovernmental coordination would be required to respond.

Public health and mental health professionals determine risks to the medical and behavioral health of a community by assessing its infrastructure and systems, the probable human impact from the threats and hazards, and potential interruption of public health, medical, and mental/behavioral health services. For example, a public health assessment of the threat from a highly infectious disease might include:

- Identifying potential scenarios of highly infectious disease and their exposure pathways;
- Identifying populations that might be exposed, facilities that might be impacted, and environments that might exacerbate the spread or containment of the infectious disease; and
- Estimating the health impact of the potential spread of the highly infectious disease and the requirements for health care facilities and public health intervention.

Table 6-1 describes Centers for Disease Control and Prevention (CDC) guidance on identifying hazards and threats to public health, specific concerns, and potential sources of information.

Data Collection

Information from several sources, including data from previous disasters, is needed to predict future events and assist in the development of appropriate mitigation measures. Historical data include the nature of previous hazards, the direct causes or contributing factors of previous events (e.g., where the location of a health care facility in a flood zone led to evacuation in a hurricane), the frequency and intensity of past disasters, the magnitude or power of past hazards (as measured with established standards, such as the Richter scale for earthquakes or the Saffir-Simpson

Table 6-1. Conducting a Public Health Threat and Hazard Assessment

Guidance	Specific Concerns or Elements	Sources for Identification
Written plans should include policies and procedures to identify at-risk populations (e.g., disabled, elderly, pregnant women and infants, individuals with other acute medical conditions, individuals with chronic diseases, underinsured persons, persons without health insurance)	• Poor health status • Limited access to neighborhood health resources • Reduced ability to hear, speak, understand, or remember • Reduced ability to move or walk independently or respond quickly to directions during an emergency • Populations with health vulnerabilities that may be caused or exacerbated by chemical, biological, or radiological exposure	• Existing health department data sets • Existing chronic disease and maternal child health programs • Community profiles • Local or regional strategic advisory council • Service agencies in the community who are familiar with the populations served
Written plans should include a jurisdictional risk assessment, utilizing an all-hazards approach (e.g., potential hazards, vulnerabilities, and risks related to the public health, medical, and mental/behavioral health systems) • Probable human impact; interruption of public health, medical, and mental/behavioral health services • Impact of those risks on public health, medical, and mental/behavioral health infrastructure	• A definition of risk • Use of geospatial informational system or other mechanism to map locations of at-risk populations • Evidence of community involvement in determining areas for risk assessment or hazard mitigation • Assessment of potential loss or disruption of essential services such as clean water, sanitation, or the interruption of health care services or public health agency infrastructure	• Public health and nonpublic health subject matter experts • Emergency management risk assessment data • Health department programs, community engagements, and other applicable sources

Source: Adapted from Centers for Disease Control and Prevention (CDC). 2011. *Public Health Preparedness Capabilities: National Standards for State and Local Planning* 16–17. Washington, DC: CDC. Available at: https://www.cdc.gov/phpr/capabilities/dslr_capabilities_july.pdf. Accessed January 13, 2017.

Hurricane Wind Scale for hurricanes), and the reported effects of an event at a given location (e.g., number of homes destroyed by tornado, number of people displaced by flood).

The jurisdictional office of emergency management is likely to collect baseline data to assess the full range of potential hazards in a community, from the location of dams, levies, and other flood control mechanisms to facilities that store infectious waste. That assessment will provide valuable information for determining the types of events that could impact the public health of the community.

Scientific Resources

Data from meteorology, seismology, volcanology, and hydrology should be used to provide important predictive information concerning hazards. These data can be obtained from a variety of government agencies and private institutions, including the National Oceanic and Atmospheric Administration, the National Weather Service, the U.S. Geological Survey, and the Natural Hazards Center at the University of Colorado. In addition, decision-support systems can analyze data from several core databases, such as municipal or regional data on building inventories, infrastructure, demographics, and risk. These systems can simulate "what if" scenarios to aid in planning. Finally, mobile and Web apps, such as Temblor, estimate risk for a specific hazard. Temblor estimates the likelihood of seismic shaking by address in the United States (available at: http://temblor.net).

Hazardous Materials Documentation

In the United States, the Superfund Amendment and Reauthorization Act (42 U.S.C. § 9601 (1980), *amended by* Pub. L. No. 107-377 (Dec. 31, 2002)) requires that all hazardous materials manufactured, stored, or transported by local industry that could affect the surrounding community be identified and reported to health officials. In most communities, gasoline and liquid petroleum gas are the most common hazardous materials, but other potential hazards include chlorine, ammonia, and explosives. Material safety data sheets (MSDS) provide a standardized method of communicating relevant information about each material, including its toxicity, flammability, and known acute and chronic health effects. MSDS are provided by the manufacturers of individual chemicals and can be searched via databases available on the Internet, such as CHEMTREC (available at: http://www.chemtrec.com). Table 6-2 provides scientific and other sources of data to aid in the identification of threats and hazards.

Table 6-2. Data Sources on Threats and Hazards

Sources to Identify Threats and Hazards
Existing threat and hazard assessments
Records from previous incidents, including historical data and disaster declarations (http://www.fema.gov/disasters)
Analysis of critical infrastructure interdependencies, including disruptions and failures that may originate elsewhere but produce cascading effects experienced locally (e.g., an electrical power disruption that spreads both geographically and across sectors)
Local or regional National Weather Service offices
State radiation control programs, radiological subject matter experts (http://www.crcpd.org/Map/RCPmap.htm)
Local/state fire, police, emergency medical services, health departments, and hospital associations
Infrastructure owners and operators
NOAA Areal Locations of Hazardous Atmospheres (http://response.restoration.noaa.gov/aloha)
FEMA Hazus (http://www.fema.gov/hazus)
FEMA HURREVAC (http://www.hurrevac.com)
U.S. Department of Energy LandScan (http://web.ornl.gov/sci/landscan)
Current hazard zone maps:
• United States Geological Survey ShakeMaps (http://earthquake.usgs.gov/earthquakes/shakemap)
• National Weather Service Sea, Lake and Overland Surges from Hurricanes (SLOSH) models (http://www.nhc.noaa.gov/surge/slosh.php)
• FEMA Q3 Flood Data (https://www.fema.gov/media-library/assets/documents/3846)
NOAA and its agencies/programs:
• National Centers for Environmental Information (https://www.ncei.noaa.gov)
• National Weather Service (http://www.nws.noaa.gov/view/national.php?thumbs=on)
• NOAA Sea Level Rise and Coastal Flooding Viewer (https://coast.noaa.gov/digitalcoast/tools/slr)
U.S. Army Corps of Engineers Hurricane Debris Estimating Model (http://dps.sd.gov/emergency_services/emergency_management/images/dmgappa.pdf)
National Drought Mitigation Center, University of Nebraska Lincoln (http://un-lincoln.academia.edu/Departments/National_Drought_Mitigation_Center/Documents)
Temblor mobile app (http://temblor.net)

Source: Adapted from U.S. Department of Homeland Security (DHS). 2013. *Threat and Hazard Identification and Risk Assessment Guide: Comprehensive Preparedness Guide (CPG) 201*. 2nd ed. Washington, DC: DHS. Available at: https://www.fema.gov/media-library-data/8ca0a9e54dc8b037a55b402b2a269e94/CPG201_htirag_2nd_edition.pdf. Accessed January 13, 2017.

Note: FEMA = Federal Emergency Management Agency; NOAA = National Oceanic and Atmospheric Administration.

Hazard Analysis

Following compilation, the information is analyzed to determine which hazards are most likely to affect a given community and to make decisions about who or what to protect. Data analysis attempts to predict the nature, frequency, and intensity of future hazards; the area(s) most likely to be affected; and the onset time and duration of future events. This assessment should be conducted at a level appropriate to both the perceived risk and the availability of resources.

Hazard Mapping

With the wealth of gathered data, the location of both previous and potential hazards can be mapped. Aerial photography, satellite imagery, remote sensing, and geographic information systems (GIS) technology can all provide information through hazard mapping. Remote sensing can show changes to land-use maps over time. GIS models enable managers to develop plans with information consolidated from numerous disciplines, including engineering, natural sciences, and public health. Various types of maps are available for different hazards both macro and micro in scale, including inundation maps for floods and seismic zoning maps for earthquakes. Maps detailing the location of industrial sites and hazardous material storage facilities can also be used. Multihazard maps are available from the scientific community, industry, the media, and governmental jurisdictions.

Give the Threats and Hazards Context

The second step of the THIRA process is to describe how the identified threats and hazards may affect the community, known as *context descriptions*. The THIRA guidelines direct planners to develop more than one context description for a threat or hazard because these events can have different impacts depending on the time, place, and conditions in which they occur. For example, coastal communities may need multiple context descriptions for hurricanes to account for varying storm intensities (e.g., Category 1 where dangerous winds produce some damage versus Categories 4 or 5 where catastrophic damage occurs), landfall locations (e.g., urban areas with large residential populations versus rural areas that are mainly farmland), and landfall times (e.g., night when most people are at home versus day when people are not at home). Considerations when developing the context description include the time, place, and conditions in which the threats or hazards might occur. This context can be informed by consulting with experts who are knowledgeable or by the determinations of a vulnerability analysis.

Vulnerability Analysis

Part of the context description is a vulnerability analysis. A vulnerability analysis is used to develop appropriate prevention strategies by obtaining information about the susceptibility of individuals, property, and the environment to the adverse effects of a given hazard. The analysis of this information helps determine who is most likely to be affected, what is most likely to be destroyed or damaged, and what capacities exist to cope with the effects of the disaster. A separate vulnerability analysis should be conducted for each identified hazard or threat. Variables that might impact the public health preparedness and response include:

- The timing of an incident and if that affects the community's ability to manage it
- The time of day and/or seasons that potentially have the greatest impact
- Locations that affect the community's ability to manage it and which locations have the greatest impacts (e.g., populated areas in a tornado, coastal zones in a hurricane and flood, industrial or residential areas in a chemical release)
- Sections and individuals in a community that are vulnerable and most likely to be affected by a particular hazard (e.g., individuals living in or near flood plains, numbers of elderly and/or immobile people living in high rises who would be isolated during a blackout)
- A community's risk of adverse health effects caused by a specified disaster (e.g., traumatic deaths and injuries following an earthquake)
- Delivery systems or facilities that are vulnerable in this type of incident (e.g., health care, mental/behavioral health, long-term care)
- Existing measures and resources that reduce the impact of a given hazard (e.g., robust community of behavioral health professionals available after an incident of terrorism)
- Areas that require strengthening to prevent or mitigate the effects of the hazard (e.g., development of common electronic medical record so that patients can be transferred easily between medical institutions if one facility is inoperable during a disaster)

A focus on the populations at greatest risk will aid in identifying who may need the most help early on (the 5 categories of being at-risk are described in Table 6-3).

A community's capacity, or resilience, to withstand the effects of a disaster is determined by collecting data on numerous variables. (See Chapter 8 for information on resilience.) Information on the size, density, location, and socioeconomic status of the community at risk of being harmed can be obtained from local government officials. Public utility companies, health departments, hospital associations, and school authorities can provide data on the location and structural integrity of lifeline structures (i.e., electricity, gas, water, and sewer) as well as buildings with high occupancy. Information on the location and structural integrity of private dwellings is also useful. A structural engineer may be required to review these data. Additional community capacity elements to be assessed include the presence of early warning systems, the number of available emergency responders and medical personnel, the level of technical expertise among emergency responders, the availability of supplies, and the status of emergency transportation and communication systems.

Table 6-3. Categories of Being At-Risk

Category	Measures
Proximity and exposure	Identify population(s) vulnerable because they live or work near a given hazard
Physical	Assess vulnerability of buildings, infrastructure, agriculture, and other aspects of the physical environment as a result of factors such as site, materials used, construction technique, and maintenance
	Evaluate transportation systems, communication systems, public utilities (e.g., water, sewage, power), and critical facilities (e.g., hospitals) for weaknesses
	Estimate potential short- and long-term impact of hazard on crops, food, livestock, trees, and fisheries
Social	Identify population most vulnerable to the effects of disaster who require targeted planning (e.g., older adults, children, single-parent families, the economically disadvantaged, those with functional needs)
	Estimate the level of poverty, jobs that are at risk, and the availability of local institutions that may provide social support
Economic	Determine the community's potential for economic loss and recovery following a disaster
Capacity	Evaluate the availability of human resources, material resources, and the presence of mutual aid agreements with neighboring communities
	Review the existence and enforcement of government regulations that mitigate the effects of certain disasters (e.g., building codes)

Assessment of Risk

The likelihood that an event of a given magnitude will occur in a certain area over a specified time interval is determined through a risk assessment. This determination of risk, reflected in the THIRA process, is used as a diagnostic and planning tool to inform prevention and preparedness actions. The major components of a risk assessment include hazard identification and analysis and vulnerability analysis. The risk assessment also answers the questions: "What can happen?" "How likely are each of the possible outcomes?" and "When the possible outcomes happen, what are the likely consequences and losses?"

Risk is frequently presented as a probability estimate whereby this estimate is calculated to determine the possibility that a specified outcome will occur based on an analysis of vulnerability to a given hazard. As example, one might ask, how many excess cases of outcome A will occur in a population of size B, due to a hazard event C of severity D? Several statistical formulations can be used to determine the probabilities; however, risk is frequently depicted by the following useful formula (although the association is not strictly arithmetic): risk = hazard × vulnerability. More complicated formulations take into account not only the hazard and vulnerability estimates, but also mitigation efforts to reduce vulnerability and disaster management issues. Although these estimates cannot predict the exact timing of an event, they can be used to guide the allocation of resources in preparing for likely hazards or threats.

Modeling to Determine Potential Impact

To conduct a risk assessment, public health professionals identify a hazard or threat and calculate a potential impact on a community with known vulnerabilities and coping mechanisms (risk=hazard×vulnerability). The probability may be presented as a numeric range (e.g., 30% to 40% probability) or in relative terms (e.g., low, moderate, or high risk). A good example of how such models are used in daily life is the environmental and climate prediction services provided by the National Weather Service. The results of this modeling are broadcast by the media to warn communities of the risks of thunderstorms, blizzards, tornadoes, and hurricanes.

Models can also be used to guide appropriate responses to disasters. For example, plume dispersion modeling has shown that the most appropriate response to a major chemical release is evacuation of the surrounding community. Other strategies, such as "sheltering in place" (i.e., remaining indoors with windows and doors closed), provide less protection to the population. Similar dispersion models are also used to determine the risks of other technological hazards, including releases from nuclear installations. Further, mathematical and simulation models have been used to plan for the public health and health sector response to epidemic infectious disease, including the staffing and distribution requirements for vaccine and antibiotic distribution. Table 6-4 lists some resources for risk assessment modeling.

Capabilities and Context Descriptions

Those receiving funding through the 2016 Hospital Preparedness Program and Public Health Emergency Preparedness cooperative agreements are required to complete risk assessments of their jurisdictions in order to identify potential hazards, vulnerabilities, and risks within the public health, medical, and behavioral health systems of the community that would affect the functional needs of at-risk individuals. These risk assessment activities are to be coordinated with the community's emergency management programs in support of the jurisdictional THIRA. Coordinating preparedness activities with their emergency management and homeland security counterparts enhances operational partnerships that will facilitate an effective public health response when a disaster strikes a community. Such collaborative action also contributes to the federal requirement that states prepare a comprehensive state THIRA with input from public health agencies. Many health departments use their state's risk assessment to meet these criteria because they have been active partners in the state's THIRA process.

Since THIRA is a process with FEMA oversight, public health departments and health care sector professionals identify which of the FEMA Core Capabilities would be required to respond to a specific hazard or threat (see Appendix G for a list of FEMA Core

Table 6-4. Risk Assessment Modeling Resources

Tools	Function	Web Resource
EPA superfund and ecological risk assessment modeling	Modeling tools to evaluate potential risks from environmental contamination	https://www.epa.gov/risk/superfund-risk-assessment; another site provides detailed information about ecological risk assessments: https://www.epa.gov/risk/ecological-risk-assessment
EPA risk assessment tools and databases	Risk assessment resources used by EPA scientists to assess risks due to environmental hazards	https://www.epa.gov/risk/risk-tools-and-databases
Adaptive Risk Assessment Modeling System	Determine safe and cleanup target levels for military relevant compounds and evaluate remediation alternatives	http://www.erdc.usace.army.mil/Media/Fact-Sheets/Fact-Sheet-Article-View/Article/500113/adaptive-risk-assessment-modeling-system-arams
Hazus (Hazards U.S.)	Analyze potential losses from floods, hurricane winds, and earthquakes	http://www.fema.gov/hazus
Environmental Health Shelter Assessment Tool	Conduct rapid assessment of shelter conditions; assessment form covers 14 general areas of environmental health, documents immediate needs in shelters	https://emergency.cdc.gov/shelterassessment

Note: EPA = Environmental Protection Agency.

Capabilities). While the FEMA capabilities are broad objectives and the definitions are not exactly the same as the Public Health and Health Care System Preparedness Capabilities, 4 of the FEMA capabilities are focused on public health and health care, and 1, fatality management, includes the tasks of providing counseling to the bereaved.

By prioritizing the capabilities and functions that impact public health services and the delivery of health care, planners will be able to identify which public health resources may be needed in a disaster response. Public health professionals assess the role of departments of health, hospitals and other health care facilities, health care manpower, etc. and determine the responsibilities of each for a given hazard. Table 6-5 provides a sample context description for an earthquake and for terrorism and identifies the probable capabilities that would be required in a response.

THIRA: Capability Targets and Applying the Results

The THIRA process includes 2 additional sets of actions. In the next step, communities establish specific and measurable targets for each core capability, known as *capability targets*. These targets are goals for successfully responding to each hazard or threat and describe what the community wants to achieve in its response. The goals should contain quantifiable measures to help assess whether a jurisdiction can achieve or has accomplished its desired outcomes. In the final step, communities identify what resources are needed to prepare for, mitigate, or respond to each threat or hazard.

When establishing the capability targets, communities should consider what both the potential impacts might be and the desired outcomes for each threat and hazard. A description of impacts illustrates how a threat or hazard might affect a core capability, such as a tornado that interrupts a water system requiring public health to provide information and warning about safe water and to screen, search, and detect people in the community who might have gotten sick from drinking unsafe water. The size and complexity of response needed to a specific hazard or threat will shape the potential impact. Larger, more complicated threats and hazards might cause bigger impacts requiring a more involved, multifaceted response requiring numerous capabilities.

The description of impacts should be specific and include quantitative descriptions as much as possible to allow jurisdictions to gain an understanding of what is needed to manage risk.

Examples of potential impacts include:

- Size of geographic area affected (i.e., neighborhood or region)
- Number of displaced households (i.e., dozens, hundreds, thousands)
- Number of fatalities (i.e., a few, hundreds, thousands)
- Number of injuries or illnesses (i.e., sprains and broken bones, epidemic cases of gastrointestinal disease)

- Disruption to critical infrastructure, including health care and mental/behavioral health (i.e., loss of power triggering use of generators, need to evacuate)
- Effects of supply chain disruption (i.e., delayed for hours, days)

The THIRA guidance defines *desired outcomes* as the description of the time frame or level of effort needed to successfully deliver the core capabilities. To respond or meet the capability target, a community has to have the necessary resources in place. For example, the capability target might require a community to complete physical protective measures within a certain time frame (e.g., within 48 hours). The targets for other tasks may be defined as a percentage (e.g., ensure 100% screening, search, and detection). Different threats and hazards may require different elements of a core capability, resulting in a more complicated process of developing capability targets.

In the last step, communities list the actions required to successfully manage the identified threats and hazards and then estimate the community resources and mutual aid required to meet the capability targets. Communities can also use the list of resources needed (known as *resource requirements*), to support decisions of the allocation of resources, planning for operations, and activities aimed at mitigation. Because of the variability across a state in population density, geography, and topography; in available professionals and health care systems; and in resources, the THIRA process is most accurate at the local level.

The next section discusses assessments conducted after a disaster has struck when public health professionals are determining who and how many people need health assistance.

Rapid Health Assessment

Rapid health assessments are used in the early stages of disaster response, often simultaneously with emergency response, to characterize the health impact of the disaster on the affected community. Such assessments are common in international settings and the World Health Organization recommends that these rapid assessments be completed as soon as possible following a disaster. The primary task of the multidisciplinary assessment team is to collect, analyze, and disseminate timely and accurate health data. These data assist public health professionals in determining health needs, prioritizing response activities, initiating an appropriate emergency response, and evaluating the effectiveness of the response. Even if the rapid health assessment is only a basic estimate, it facilitates the rational allocation of available resources according to the true needs of the emergency.

Community plans for disaster response should include teams to provide medical care that are functionally separate from the team(s) conducting the rapid health assessment. Appropriate medical responses can be planned in advance since specific disasters are

Table 6-5. Core Capabilities and Context Descriptions With the Public Health Role

THIRA Process Step	Earthquake	Terrorism
Context Description	A magnitude 7.7 earthquake along the New Madrid Fault occurring at approximately 2:00 PM on a weekday with ground shaking and damage expected to affect millions of people, including those in the cities of St. Louis, Missouri, and Memphis, Tennessee	A potential threat exists from a domestic group with a history of using small improvised explosive devices as part of hate crimes. There are a number of large gatherings planned during the summer at open air venues sponsored by various ethnic and religious groups. Attendance at these events average 10,000 people daily
FEMA's Core Capability Where Public Health and Health Care Systems Have a Role	Environmental response/health and safety Health and social services Mass care Providing counseling to the bereaved (under fatality management) Public health/health care and emergency medical services	Environmental response/health and safety Health and social services Mass care Public health/health care and emergency medical services

Source: Based on U.S. Department of Homeland Security (DHS). 2013. *Threat and Hazard Identification and Risk Assessment Guide. Comprehensive Preparedness Guide (CPG) 201*. 2nd ed. Washington, DC: DHS. Available at: http://www.fema.gov/media-library-data/8ca0a9e54dc8b037a55b402b2a269e94/CPG201_htirag_2nd_edition.pdf. Accessed January 13, 2017; Federal Emergency Management Agency. Core capabilities. Available at: https://www.fema.gov/core-capabilities. Accessed January 13, 2017.
Note: FEMA = Federal Emergency Management Agency; THIRA = Threat and Hazard Identification and Risk Assessment.

associated with predictable patterns of morbidity and mortality. Although rapid health assessments provide for the early collection of health data, emergency response activities to save life and limb and to rescue trapped or isolated individuals may be initiated before the results of the rapid health assessment are available. Subsequent detailed needs assessments are often conducted during the recovery and rehabilitation phases of the disaster cycle to provide information over time.

Objectives and Methods

The primary objectives of rapid health assessments are to assess the following:

- Presence of ongoing hazards (e.g., a persistent toxic plume following a major chemical release)
- Nature and magnitude of the disaster (e.g., number of people affected or geographic area involved)
- Major medical and public health problems of the community (e.g., risk of further morbidity and mortality; observed patterns of injury, illness, and death; need for food, water, shelter, and sanitation)
- Availability of resources within the local community and the impact of the disaster on those resources
- Community need for external assistance
- Augmentation of existing public health surveillance to monitor the ongoing health impact of the disaster

Before field visits and preliminary data collection can begin, a team must be assembled. Members of this multidisciplinary team could include an epidemiologist, a clinician, an environmental engineer, and a logistician. If the area affected by the disaster is large and crosses jurisdictions, several assessment teams may be required, as might specialty teams to concentrate on transportation, communications, and infrastructure. It is important to coordinate with local agencies to ensure that each assessment will yield new information and that the information is shared with those who need it. If more than one assessment team is required, all teams should use the same standardized assessment form. Data forms can be developed in advance using existing protocols, such as the rapid health assessment protocols developed by the World Health Organization for various events, including sudden impact natural disasters, chemical emergencies, and sudden population displacements.

Baseline data gathered prior to the field assessment are essential. This information includes background on the population size and demographics, including the presence of vulnerable groups such as older adults, children, and people with functional needs. Census data can provide an accurate estimate of the number of people affected by the disaster, though estimating the actual number of individuals present in the disaster area at the time of impact (e.g., after evacuation following hurricane warnings) can be difficult.

Advanced information on the health care infrastructure is also critical. The location, bed capacity, and capabilities of local and regional health facilities must be documented. The status of local emergency medical services (EMS) must be assessed as well, including search and rescue capabilities. This determination of available EMS resources can serve as a surrogate measure of likely response in case of disaster. Similar information on the location and status of public utilities (i.e., provision of water, sanitation, and electricity) will also assist assessment efforts.

Detailed maps are essential for rapid health assessments. These maps should show high-risk areas, including at-risk populations; major transport routes; main utility lines; locations of health facilities and water sources; and concentrations of residential, office, shopping, and industrial areas. These maps are often available from government departments, academic institutions, and utility companies. (See Chapter 5 on GIS maps.)

All these data will be wasted if not supplied to decision makers with authority to shape the disaster plan. The rapid health assessment should be an integral component of emergency response planning.

Timeline

For acute onset disasters, such as transportation crashes and hazardous material incidents, the initial on-scene assessments should be conducted within minutes if possible, but might not occur for a few hours. When multiple casualties are suspected, such as following an earthquake or tornado, the initial assessment should be completed within several hours of impact. Any assessment should be completed as soon as possible as the majority of deaths will occur within the first 24 to 48 hours. This early information will be critical in identifying the need for EMS and urban search and rescue teams.

For slower-onset disasters, information can be collected during the first 2 to 4 days (e.g., floods, epidemics, population displacements). An even longer time frame may be used for assessments of droughts and famines. In these settings, it is often more appropriate for health officials and disaster managers to collect baseline data and then follow trends with ongoing public health surveillance.

Categories of Data and Priorities for Collection

Data collection priorities differ for sudden impact disasters (e.g., earthquake, tornado) and gradual onset disasters (e.g., famine, complex humanitarian emergency). Teams often have limited time in which to collect data for a rapid health assessment. In these situations, only the most relevant health-related information should be collected. The specific elements of data will vary according to the type of disaster and the stage of the response. A concise checklist, developed prior to the field visit, will ensure that the most critical health issues are assessed.

Sudden Impact Disaster

Days 1 to 2: Baseline information should be gathered as discussed previously. The sole objective is to collect information needed for immediate relief. The priority at this stage is the emergency medical response to save life and limb. Since obtaining accurate data can be difficult directly after impact, initial relief efforts are frequently guided by rough estimates. Key data include the following:

- Ongoing hazards, since persistent hazards that pose a risk to rescue personnel must be eliminated or controlled prior to initiating relief efforts
- Injuries, since the number, categories, and severity of injuries help characterize the impact of the disaster and prioritize relief activities
- Deaths, since the number and causes of death help characterize the impact of the disaster (however, information about deaths is not as important in guiding relief efforts as injury data)
- Environmental health and the status of community lifelines (e.g., water, sewer, power), since an early estimate of the population's needs for shelter, food, water, and sanitation may prevent secondary disaster-related health problems
- Health facilities, since the impact of the disaster on the physical integrity and functioning of the health infrastructure may indicate the need for temporary medical shelters and external medical assistance

Days 3 to 6: At this stage, information will be needed to guide secondary relief. Emergency medical interventions and search and rescue activities may be less important, as more than 96% of critically injured patients will already have received medical care in the event of an earthquake or building collapse. However, flood or hurricane disasters may destroy the health care infrastructure, and assessments should identify the need for care of chronic conditions and other problems, such as loss of medication or medical supplies. If disaster-related deaths are still occurring, any persistent hazards causing or contributing to these deaths must be identified. Injuries as a result of cleanup activities and secondary impact from the disaster (e.g., fire, electrocution, hazardous material release) must be monitored carefully to optimize recovery efforts. Ensuring the availability of and access to primary health care becomes more important at this point than emergency care since disaster-affected populations still require routine medical services.

Assessment of environmental health and utilities must clarify the longer-term needs related to food, water, sanitation, shelter, and energy.

Day 6+: During the recovery stage, disaster plans should be fully implemented and resources made available for all sectors. Surveillance should concentrate on both rates of illness and injuries determined from information available from all health facilities and the occurrence of infectious disease, since outbreaks are uncommon after sudden impact disasters unless major population displacement or disruptions of the public health system occur. The surveillance system should track diarrheal disease and acute respiratory infections if people are displaced into overcrowded shelters or if there is a disruption of environmental health services. The status of health facilities, the number of health personnel, and the availability of medical and pharmaceutical supplies should be accurately tracked. Environmental health (e.g., water quantity and quality, sanitation, shelter, solid waste disposal) and vector populations must be monitored carefully. Floods are often associated with swells in mosquito populations, increasing the risk of arboviral infections such as St. Louis encephalitis. Surveillance for arboviruses can assist in determining the need for vector control following flooding.

Gradual Onset Disaster

Baseline assessments are conducted and a surveillance system established. Background information must include population size and demographics, major causes of morbidity and mortality, sources of health care, and the status of preexisting public health programs, such as immunizations. Key health indicators address both morbidity and mortality. For mortality, the crude mortality rate (deaths/10,000/day) is the most sensitive indicator of the population's health. Age- and sex-specific rates should be collected. The under-6 mortality rate is used to assess the health status of one of the most vulnerable groups in the population. For morbidity, information must be collected on rates of disease with public health importance, including diarrheal disease, respiratory infection, measles, malaria, and hepatitis. Rate of malnutrition in children younger than 6 years of age is the second-most important indicator of the population's health. Data on environmental health should be collected and compared with the standards of 16 to 20 liters of water per person per day and 1 pit latrine per family.

The disaster impact on the health system can be assessed by measuring (1) the loss of staff since major population displacements and complex humanitarian emergencies are frequently associated with health professionals not being available to communities; (2) the status of health infrastructure since populations may no longer have ready access to health facilities, and hospitals and clinics are frequently damaged or destroyed; and (3) the status of public health programs since immunization programs, maternal and child health services, and vector control programs may all have been disrupted.

Sources and Methods of Data Collection

Data collection methods may be classified as primary (direct observation or surveys) or secondary (interviews with key informants or review of existing records).

Direct observation can be completed on the ground or from the air. Direct on-the-ground observations can provide team members with a firsthand view of the impact and extent of the disaster. Major health problems in the observed area may be identified but may not be generalizable to other sites. Where possible, team members should conduct informal interviews with victims and responders. Aerial observation allows team members to confirm the geographic extent of the disaster and to view the impact in inaccessible areas. In addition, by viewing the entire geographic region, the most severely affected areas may be identified so that relief efforts can be more appropriately targeted.

Four types of surveys can be conducted. First, focused surveys may be used to collect health data. These are relatively resource-intensive and should therefore be reserved for data that are necessary but are not available through other sources. Second, surveys based on convenience samples may be conducted relatively rapidly and provide a gross estimate of the health care needs of the affected community. However, convenience samples do not provide population-based information, so are likely to be sources of bias. Third, telephone surveys using randomly selected telephone numbers may be useful in determining the impact of the disaster and the health care needs of the community. Phone surveys require an intact communications system and may not provide a representative sample. People who are at home during the time of calling (e.g., elderly) may be overrepresented, introducing a potential source of bias. Fourth, surveys based on cluster-sampling methods are being used more frequently in disaster settings. Sampling methods such as simple random sampling, stratified random sampling, and systematic random sampling are time- and resource-intensive, making them impractical for the purposes of a rapid health assessment. Cluster-sampling methods for natural disasters are based on the World Health Organization's Expanded Programme on Immunization method for estimating immunization coverage.

Cluster-sampling techniques provide population-based information to both guide and evaluate relief operations. Modified cluster-sampling methods can be used to estimate the size of the population in the disaster-affected area, the number of people with specific health care needs, the number of damaged or destroyed buildings, and the availability of water, sanitation, food, and power in the community. Cluster surveys can usually be conducted rapidly, and the results made available within 24 hours. Follow-up surveys can be repeated in the same area over the following 3 to 14 days. Cluster surveys are particularly useful when the area of damage is generally uniform, such as after a hurricane. They have been less useful following earthquakes, where the distribution of damage may vary widely between locations. Among displaced and famine-affected populations, such as large refugee settlements, cluster surveys have been used to estimate the prevalence of acute malnutrition, disease rates, the major causes of mortality, and access to health care services.

For secondary data collection, interviews with key health and emergency personnel can be useful in obtaining qualitative data concerning the disaster. Gross estimates of the impact and population needs may also be available. Attempts should be made to corroborate these data with those collected through primary methods. Interviews may be conducted with hospital emergency room staff, medical personnel at temporary health facilities, community providers, public health officials, incident commanders, paramedics, police and fire department officials, Red Cross representatives, and coroners. To augment and confirm these interviews, an effort should be made to review documented medical records from health facilities. Health data may be available from hospital emergency rooms and inpatient units, temporary health facilities, community providers, public health officials, and coroners' offices.

Limitations of Data Assessment

Health officials and disaster managers should be aware of the limitations of data that are collected during the rapid health assessment. Assessment team members must balance their preferences for sound epidemiological methodology against the time constraints and other limitations of the data collection process. Inaccuracies may result from logistical, technical, and organizational problems. Potential limitations include incomplete data, poor internal or external validity, and reliance on secondary sources of information. Unless population-based methodologies are used, data collected may not be representative of the community being assessed, and data collected from one population may not be generalizable to those in other regions. Further, information may not be available from certain disaster-affected areas as a result of poor access and communications. Finally, underreporting of health events by rescue and medical personnel may occur because accurate documentation ranks as a low priority during the initial disaster response, particularly during sudden impact disasters.

Community Assessment for Public Health Emergency Response

The CDC's CASPER is used to conduct rapid need and rapid health assessments. Based on statistical methods, CASPER standardizes the assessment procedures and assists public health and emergency management officials in determining the health status and basic needs of a community following a disaster. This tool was designed to guide public health in prioritizing their response and to create a basis for distributing resources in a quick and low-cost manner.

A CASPER toolkit was developed to provide specific guidelines for developing an instrument for data collection; developing a methodology for conducting a rapid assessment; selecting a sample; setting steps for data collection; and training those carrying out the assessment, conducting the analysis, and writing the report. CASPER collects information at the housing-unit level to determine the population affected by a disaster. Any community considering the use of CASPER should evaluate both the available resources and recommended timeline to determine whether CASPER is the appropriate sampling methodology. (The CASPER toolkit can be found at: https://www.cdc.gov/nceh/hsb/disaster/casper/default.htm.)

Collect SMART

A suite of software that can be uploaded to mobile devices, known as Collect SMART, was developed by the North Carolina Institute for Public Health based on CASPER (available at: http://sph.unc.edu/nciph/collectsmart). This tool can be used for rapid health assessments. Through a 2-stage cluster sample conducted door to door, Collect SMART's data collection and analysis provide information to estimate an affected population's health status and access to care, determine health priorities, assess community preparedness, and identify services that need improvement. Data collection can be completed in 2 days with an additional 2 days of analysis. Collect SMART is integrated with the CDC's Epi Info app, a mobile application available through the Google Play Store and Apple App Store.

CHAPTER 7

DISASTER COMMUNICATIONS

Communications before, during, and after disaster strikes dictate the success of prevention and relief efforts. This chapter reviews both the strategies and methods of communicating with other responding agencies and the public during a disaster and the equipment and systems that public health officials and responders will rely on or use. Specific chapter units include the communication of risk, who is the audience, internal and external communications, communicating warnings and response needs, channels of communication, working with the media, communications systems, the use of social media in disasters and best practices, smartphones and other communication tools, radio operations, the specific communications systems used by public health officials, and disaster recovery and information technology (IT) continuity.

Public Health Role

- Communicate about health and public health matters with the following:
  - Health care providers (e.g., hospitals and their emergency departments, community providers, and other public health and social service agencies)
  - First responders (e.g., fire, police, emergency medical services) and other responders (e.g., national guard)
  - Local and regional laboratories
  - General public
  - Officials, mayors, governor(s)
  - Partners (e.g., emergency management, American Red Cross [Red Cross], public works)
- Set up communications networks with health-related agencies, the media, and the public by providing public health reports to the media on regular basis.
- Share information and conduct data analysis across agencies and organizations.

Communicating About Threats Related to Emergencies

Historically, communicating about threats or risks has been part of the responsibility of professionals working in environmental areas. Now, the evolution of practice requires all public health leaders to effectively communicate information about potential dangers.

Not only does our community look to us for information and guidance, but our colleagues, especially those in governmental agencies, seek our assistance in evaluating and informing them and the public about health risks.

When communicating in disasters, strategies used in environmental practice can be applied. These strategies incorporate principles that influence people's perception of risk. The principles established by Fischhoff et al. in 1981, are likely to have direct application to our communication practice during the threat of or following disasters. Individuals are less willing to accept risks that they perceive as imposed on them or controlled by others, having little or no benefit, unevenly distributed among different groups, created by humans, catastrophic or exotic in occurrence, generated by an untrusted source, and mostly affecting children. By contrast, individuals are more willing to accept risks perceived as voluntary and under an individual's control, having clear benefits, fairly distributed or of natural causation, generated by a trusted source, mostly affecting adults, and whose occurrence is a statistical probability.

Who Is the Audience?

Communication is a task carried out by every person involved in disaster response. The purposes of each communication will vary, depending on whether the person has primary responsibility for communicating (such as an agency official or communications director) or simply considers communications to be part of their job as an agency employee. The more you know about those with whom you are communicating—what their concerns are, how they perceive the emergent threat, and whom they trust—the greater the likelihood that you will successfully communicate with the people who make up your audience. The characteristics of audiences will vary, and this variance may affect how and what you communicate, such as the nature of their concerns, attitudes, level of involvement, level of knowledge, and experience. Depending on what the individuals experienced and what they were exposed to in the emergency, or their responsibility in responding to the emergency, the audience may be concerned about health and safety, impacts on the environment, economic implications, fairness as to exposure to the health risks, the process of responding, or the legalities of the process. In the response phase of an emergency, health and safety are likely to be the chief concerns. Finally, those responsible for communicating must be sure that the information gets out to the intended audience, a process referred to here as *transmission,* and that the intended audience has received and understood the information, here called *reception.*

Internal and External Disaster Communications

During the impact and postimpact phases of a disaster, communications occur both internally and externally. Public health agencies communicate internally to provide information to other responders and to solve problems. Internal communications also occur among an organization's staff and includes call-up and notification of the emergency, assignments to work, sharing of information, status reporting, monitoring and tracking of public health concerns, and so forth. Internally, a first step in preparing to communicate during an emergency is to compile a 24-hour contact directory so that supervisors can reach staff at any time. This directory—including full names, contact information, and credentials—should be updated regularly due to changes in personnel (e.g., new hires, changing positions, retirements, departures) and e-mail and phone numbers. External communication occurs among health departments, hospitals, community providers, ambulatory care facilities, emergency management and first responders, laboratories, pharmacies, veterinarians, community decision makers, community-based organizations, other responders, volunteers, the media, area residents, and the general public. External communication to the media and area residents must provide factual information that the public finds credible. Information being communicated is referred to as the *message*.

Initially, a spokesperson has 15 to 30 seconds to get an agency's message across to those responding to an emergency, who are likely to have an "adrenaline high." Thus, it is important to develop strategies in advance for communicating immediately after the event occurs and during the response phase. There will be more time to plan communications during recovery. Strategies may be different in each phase. Further, when communicating about preparedness and threats such as terrorism or releases of toxic agents, governmental spokespersons should deliver consistent messages that motivate protective actions by those who hear the message.

Three actions are critical to communicating during an emergency: advance planning, collaboration, and updating the message as needed. When planning for your agency's overall response, include communication as a section in the plan. This component should describe how you will communicate information about the emergency and who will deliver the message. Identify what information could be needed for different emergencies and establish ways to gather that information as quickly as possible. Prepare communication messages to have on file or locate how you will access them through federal agencies. Be sure that hard copies of the messages are readily available in case there is a loss of power and computer files cannot be accessed.

Collaborate with other agencies responsible for communicating in an emergency. Arrangements for release of public information should be worked out in advance, including how you will communicate with community leaders and build on their views that public health professionals are the "go-to" source for health information.

It is important to build vertical connections among the local, state, and federal levels and across response sectors. To create efficiencies in these networks, the channels of communication need to be *interoperable* (i.e., the parts of a system able to work with or use the parts or equipment of another system). As neither natural nor man-made or technological disasters respect borders and boundaries, regions should try in advance to agree on best strategies for handling information about hazards and threats across jurisdictions. The development of inter- and intra-agency procedures may involve cross-state cooperative agreements. A broad range of media can be used for communicating to both the press and the public. It is important to involve the stakeholders (e.g., public, responders, government officials) and incorporate their views into your message. Finally, during an event, you should track the public's perceptions and alter the message when needed.

Communicating Warnings and Response Needs

With improved forecast technology, such as the tracking of storms through satellite imagery from government and commercial sources, we can issue advance warnings to allow timely evacuation before hurricanes, taking shelter against tornadoes, and taking active steps toward vector control. Messages communicated to the public should be positive and reassuring yet factual. These bulletins must translate technical information into lay language that will result in the average person taking the desired action. The messages must be accurate, timely, and congruent for both the internal and external audiences so that consistency exists between the actions of the response agencies and the actions requested of the public. Messages should be clear, concise, and credible and include information about the nature of the expected hazards, specific step-by-step actions regarding safety precautions, where to go and what to bring if evacuating, and requirements for sheltering in place, when necessary. When possible, warnings should give sufficient time to enable everyone to take whatever preventive actions are required.

Public health leaders in the stricken community are often inundated with requests for information, and these requests interfere with the more urgent need to educate the public about injury prevention and food and water safety, request supplies, and share surveillance information with community officials. Knowing that this is likely to happen, part of the initial organizational response should be the establishment of and notification about a victim locator service. More information about victim locator services can be found in Chapter 8.

Communication can be a weak aspect of a disaster response without safeguards to ensure both the transmission and reception of information. Senders of all messages must request and receivers supply verification that the transmission was both received and understood. Validation that the intent of the message was understood is evident by observation of safety responses by citizens, use of shelters, and other appropriate actions.

Frequently, residents do not want to evacuate areas threatened by impending disasters. In disasters for which adequate warning is available, such as hurricanes, communities can prevent morbidity and mortality by making appropriate decisions, disseminating information, coordinating warnings, and posting messages that are easily understood and motivate evacuation. In disasters such as earthquakes and tornadoes, for which advance warning is rare, the risk of injury and death increases. However, even with tornadoes, morbidity and mortality can be lessened by warning through a variety of media as soon as conducive weather conditions are identified or the funnel cloud itself is spotted. Nocturnal tornadoes result in the most injuries because people do not hear the warnings.

Unfortunately, some officials withhold warnings until the last possible moment, sometimes until it is too late to take effective protective action. This has been attributed to the mistaken belief that panic is a likely response and that panic following a call for evacuation might cause more deaths and injuries than would the disaster itself.

Requests for aid following a disaster require the same clarity as warnings issued in advance. Otherwise, donations may be inappropriate (e.g., wool blankets shipped to hurricane victims in the Caribbean, shipment of outdated medications) and cause additional problems on the receiving end. The management of donations is one of the most time-consuming and difficult response activities in both large domestic and international disasters. The Pan American Health Organization developed a supply management system known as SUMA that facilitates the sorting, classifying, and inventorying of the supplies sent to a disaster-stricken area. However, the stricken locale has to sort and distribute what is sent, which takes manpower away from the disaster response. Monetary donations can be used more flexibly. Preventing the broadcast of broad appeals for help and volunteers often requires advance education of the media, local government officials, and even disaster relief organizations.

Channels for Communication

Effective communication depends on utilizing specific methods appropriate for both the message and the audience. Different messages are required for different audiences and media. Table 7-1 describes channels of communication that are mapped for delivery to different audiences.

Working With the Media

A strategically planned campaign, worked out well in advance, will most likely lead to success in working with the media. Designate either a spokesperson or public information officer who can guide the implementation of a comprehensive communications plan and through whom all information is provided to the media. A designated spokesperson coordinates messages so that the organization speaks with a single voice and provides a consistent point of contact for media representatives. It is also important to assign an alternate

Table 7-1. Audience and Communication Channels

Audience	Communication Channels
Colleagues	Blogs
	CCTV cameras
	Datacasting
	FirstNet Hotlines
	Intranet
	Internet forums
	Meetings to address questions and concerns
	Microblogs (e.g., Twitter)
	News releases and fact sheets
	Site tours
	Social networking sites
	Podcasts
	Reverse 911
	RSS feeds
	Text messaging
	Unit newspaper articles
Area residents	Community meetings
	Direct mailings
	Fliers
	Image/video sharing (e.g., Flickr, YouTube)
	Internet forums
	Films, videos, and other materials at libraries
	Newspaper articles and ads
	Microblogs (e.g., Twitter)
	Mobile Web sites
	Podcasts
	Radio and TV talk shows
	RSS feeds
	Social marketing
	Social networking sites
	Text messaging
	Widgets
Elected officials, agency leaders	Advance notices
	Fact sheets
	Frequent telephone calls
	Invitations to community meetings
	Microblogs (e.g., Twitter)
	Mobile Web sites
	News releases
	Personal visits
	RSS feeds
	Widgets
Media	Blogs
	Clear, informative fact sheets
	Microblogs (e.g., Twitter)

(*Continued*)

Table 7-1. (Continued)

Audience	Communication Channels
	Mobile Web sites News releases that focus on your message News conferences Podcasts RSS feeds Site visits Text messaging Widgets

Source: Based on Currie D. 2009. *Expert Round Table on Social Media and Risk Communication During Times of Crisis: Strategic Challenges and Opportunities. Special Report.* Washington, DC: Booz Allen Hamilton. Available at: https://www.boozallen.com/content/dam/boozallen/media/file/Risk_Communications_Times_of_Crisis.pdf. Accessed January 18, 2017.

or two because the designated spokesperson may not always be available. The spokesperson will establish relationships with media professionals in advance and prepare advance protocols for the release of information, including situation-specific messages. Part of a communications campaign will include media training for public health leaders.

The establishment of a Joint Information Center (JIC) as part of the community's response plan is critical to the success of communicating a uniform message and part of preparations under the National Incident Management System (see Chapter 3). The JIC should provide information consistent with information provided by the state JIC in a statewide emergency. The local JIC must have multiple-line phone banks for answering calls from the public and redundant communications systems in case the phone lines are down.

Preparing for an Interview

This section provides some specific tips about interviewing with the media. When the press calls, remember that reporters are usually working on a deadline. Call back right away. Since reporters' schedules may change if events create "breaking" news, interviews may get canceled or rescheduled for a more urgent story. However, in emergencies, your story is most likely the urgent one.

Ask for the reporter's name and the media organization for which he or she is reporting. Ask the subject, format, and duration of the interview; some sample questions; and who else will be interviewed. If you need time to prepare and the deadline allows, offer to call back at a specific time and follow up. If a reporter arrives in your office or calls at a time when you are unprepared, try to schedule the interview for later in the day so you can prepare. If you are not the best person to interview because you lack the necessary knowledge, let the reporter know that.

Prepare by thinking through the interview in advance. The media will be seeking information on who, what, when, where, why, and how. For broadcast media, prepare a 10- to 12-word "sound bite," and for print media prepare a 1- to 3-line quote for each of 2 or 3 main points about your subject. To support your ideas, gather facts and figures presented in printed material that can be given to the reporter to help minimize errors. If time allows, offer to fax or mail the reporter the printed information in advance of the interview. Anecdotes can also be useful in connecting your information to the experience of the reporter's audience. Prepare responses to other questions that the reporter might ask.

Choose a location where you can screen out extraneous noises such as background hums from air conditioning or heating units, phones, computers, or printers. Find out in advance whether the interview will be edited or will be live. In a live interview, be prepared to think on your feet and respond "off the cuff." In edited interviews, pause briefly before answering a question to give yourself time to think out your answer and to give the reporter a "clean" sound bite. In a TV interview, look at the reporter and not the camera. The only exception is for a satellite interview, for which the reporter or anchor may not be on location. If you are uncertain where to look, ask.

For television interviews, dress in a subtle manner. Wear solid-colored clothing and simple accessories. Stripes, plaids, or other designs can cause problems with the picture on color televisions. Before you go on the air, practice how you will deliver your key points. If possible, look in a mirror before going on camera. Television magnifies images, so be sensitive to nonverbal messages that you may communicate. Do not allow your body language, position in the room, or dress to be inconsistent with your message. Be aware of your nonverbal communication, particularly gestures or nervous habits. Assume you are on camera at all times, from all angles. Make an effort to appear to be a good listener when other people are speaking.

Sit or stand stationary in front of the radio or TV microphones and avoid moving from the microphone. Moving to and from the microphone can cause the recorded volume to rise and fall.

During the Interview

If you are being interviewed by phone, the reporter is required to tell you when you are being recorded. Ask whether the interview is being taped if you are uncertain. Be brief in your responses. Television and radio stories may use only a 10- to 30-second sound bite. The shorter your comments, the less likely they are to be edited.

State your conclusions first and then provide supporting data. Stick to your key message(s) and main points. Provide information on what your agency is doing to respond to the emergency or issue. Emphasize achievements made and ongoing efforts to respond. Don't talk too much and try not to raise other issues. Assume that everything you say and do is part of the public record. Repeat your points if necessary if you have wandered onto a tangential issue. Since you want your response to be understood on its own if the reporter's question is edited out, speak in complete thoughts.

Don't overestimate a reporter's knowledge of your subject and don't assume the facts speak for themselves. Offer background information where necessary. Explain the subject and content by beginning at a basic level using positive or neutral terms. Avoid academic or technical jargon and explain all terms and acronyms. Don't rely on words alone; visuals can be helpful to emphasize key points if the interview is in person. If you do not understand a question, ask for clarification rather than talking around it. Do not assume that you have been understood. Ask whether you have made yourself clear. It's acceptable to say, "*This is an important issue and I want to be sure I convey our position precisely. Would you mind reading back what you just heard me say?*" If you do not have the answer, say so. Offer to get the information or tell the reporter where to find the information.

Rather than say, "*No comment,*" tell the reporter if you cannot discuss a subject. For example, say, "*I can't answer that because I haven't seen the research you are referring to.*" Be honest and accurate. Don't try to conceal negative information. Let the reporter know what you are doing to solve a problem. If you make a mistake, correct yourself by stating that you would like an opportunity to clarify.

Finally, do not assume the interview is over or the recording equipment is turned off until you are sure that it is off.

After the Interview

Specify for the reporter how you would like to be identified. You will probably not be able to check the reporter's story before it appears. However, you can ask questions at the end of an interview. For example, you might inquire, "*What do you think is the main story?*"

Most reporters will be able to tell you when the story will appear. If you feel that you misspoke or gave incorrect information, call the reporter as soon as possible and let him or her know. Similarly, you can call with additional information if you forgot to make an important point. If an error appears, let the reporter know right away. Sometimes a correction can be printed or aired. You also will want to prevent the incorrect information from being used as background for future stories.

Watch for and read the resulting report. Thank the reporter if the story is even fairly good. If you are unhappy with a story, share your concerns with the reporter only if the story is factually wrong. For radio and TV stories, obtain a tape of the final broadcast if possible and critique your own performance, looking for ways you might improve in the future.

Communications Systems

Because multiple agencies must be able to share information and communicate without interruption during the impact and postimpact phases of a disaster, responding agencies should prepare to use interoperable information and communications systems. Communication lines must also be available between fixed and mobile locations. It is essential to build redundancy in communications systems as a result of technological limitations and the vulnerability of public networks.

Plans for communicating in emergencies need to ensure interoperability in 3 conditions: when technology is totally intact; when some technology is intact (e.g., wind or snowstorm); and in spartan conditions when no or little technology is intact (e.g., electrical blackout). The building of compatible systems that do not operate as silos requires careful interagency planning, partnering with the private sector, and implementation of integrated systems and policies based on industry standards. Public health officials must have alternative systems for communication and must be able to establish a link to the community's Emergency Alert System (EAS). Radio systems and radio frequencies must be established, with staff trained on the use of these systems. Protocols should be developed between the 911 system, hospitals, and health departments so that public health agencies are among the parties regularly notified as part of the community's emergency response. Users of cellular, analog, and radio communications must recognize that these networks are not secure and that anyone with a receiver can hear the conversations.

Following both natural disasters (e.g., earthquakes, hurricanes, and tornadoes) and man-made or technological disasters (e.g., power blackouts), telephone landline services and data systems are likely to be nonfunctional. Arrangements must be made to receive calls through an emergency telecommunications system if the landline circuits are overloaded or not operational. A redundant, robust phone and data network includes landlines with phone-only units that plug directly into a wall jack, cell or smartphones, Wi-Fi, or wireless Internet devices, beepers, and walkie-talkies (e.g., Nextel). Cell phones, one solution for telecommunications during disaster response, depend on the existence of relay stations or cells. Each cell has a limited capacity for simultaneous communications and covers only a defined radius. If too many people are using their cell phones, these systems will crash. Further, it may not be possible to guarantee security or privacy on cell phones. More importantly, cells are usually located in urban areas and along major traffic routes. Rural areas, where disasters are as likely to occur, may not be covered by such systems.

An alternative wireless model is available without a fixed infrastructure. The mobile ad hoc network (MANET) establishes high-speed communications among mobile devices, which double as routers. MANETs can carry all types of digital information, including text, voice, graphics, and video. To send information from one device to another, low-powered radio signals relay the data in short hops from one node to the next until the data reach their destination. MANETs can extend the range beyond that of traditional radios, and signals can penetrate tall buildings. If a mobile computing device can accept the required communications card, it can serve as a node on a MANET. Other models include using a fixed communications station, such as a computer in a vehicle, linked to the Internet via satellite. A vehicular ad hoc network is a form of MANET that provides communications between nearby vehicles and nearby fixed (usually described as *roadside*) equipment.

In all cases, the system must have off-site data backup. Some organizations will establish access to duplicate or triplicate networks. These might include separate access cables coming into a building with cable connections that are physically distant from each other. Further protection is provided by upgrading from basic straight-line links to more modern systems. Consider upgrading systems so they can route calls by firing signals through the air in light beams or radio signals. Such systems shoot invisible beams capable of transmitting volumes of data between building rooftops. Some high-speed Internet providers can support voice service, thus enabling multiple functions. Although some cable television systems offer redundancy, with cables run separately from phone lines, the downside is that transmission can slow down as the number of users increases, because cable lines are shared. Fixed facilities (e.g., hospitals and health departments) should also have standby sources of power to support communications equipment in addition to lighting, ventilation, heating, and air conditioning.

Health departments and hospitals should have several unlisted phone numbers so that they can more easily make outgoing phone calls. Telephone lines coming into communications centers should be buried, clearly marked, and protected from damage. Records of the location of telephone lines must be maintained and updated so they can be located quickly postimpact.

For office-based communication about disaster-related activities, public health officials need basic computer equipment. Computers must have continuous Internet e-mail capacity and sufficient security (e.g., firewall, password protection, virus scanning) to protect data and prevent intrusion. Backup power supplies are essential, as is off-site data backup and storage. A system for broadcasting health alerts 24 hours a day, 7 days a week (24/7) must also be maintained.

Alerting and Warning Systems

Communication during disasters involves the ability to notify authorities and for authorities to notify members of the community that there is an emergency. For citizens to notify authorities, 911 emergency calling and reverse 911 must be accessible to people with hearing, speech, and vision disabilities. The systems used to notify communities are varied.

Communities are alerted to impending hazards through the EAS and the National Oceanic and Atmospheric Administration's (NOAA) Weather Radio All-Hazards (NWR).

Initiated in 1997, EAS superseded the Emergency Broadcast System (and the Control of Electromagnetic Radiation System, commonly known as CONELRAD). Most emergency warnings in the United States are issued through EAS and are generated by the National Weather Service (NWS). EAS can be activated by authorities at all levels, including police, fire, weather, and other governmental authorities. Each state and several territories have their own EAS plans.

Working with the EAS, the NWR is a nationwide network of radio stations that broadcast comprehensive weather and emergency information for natural, environmental, and public safety hazards 24/7. NWR requires a special radio receiver or scanner capable of picking up its signal. Broadcasts are found in the VHF public service band at 7 megahertz (MHz) frequencies: 162.400, 162.425, 162.450, 162.475, 162.500, 162.525, and 162.550.

The national EAS broadcasts alerts over television, radio, cable, and satellite. With the growth of electronic media, Congress passed the Warning, Alert, and Response Network (WARN) Act in 2006 to establish a voluntary, national notification network that would modernize and expand EAS by providing geographically targeted alerts to wireless phones, Web browsers, and other electronic devices. To implement the WARN Act, in 2008 the Federal Communications Commission (FCC) adopted system requirements that guided commercial mobile service providers (CMSP) in transmitting emergency alerts to their subscribers, if they choose to do so.

Under the rules adopted by the FCC:

- The Wireless Emergency Alerts (WEA) consist of an end-to-end system by which an alert aggregator/gateway receives, authenticates, validates, and formats federal, state, tribal, and local alerts and then forwards them to the appropriate CMSP Gateway. The CMSP Gateway and associated infrastructure processes the alerts and transmits them to subscribers.
- Subscribers can receive up to 3 classes of text-based alerts, such as presidential, imminent threat (e.g., tornado), and Amber Alerts.
- Subscribers automatically receive these alerts if they have a WEA-compatible phone. There are no subscriber opt-in requirements.
- To ensure that people with disabilities have access to alerts, CMSPs must provide a unique audio attention signal and vibration cadence on WEA-compatible phones.
- CMSPs generally must transmit alerts to areas no larger than the targeted county. However, CMSPs may transmit to areas smaller than the county if they choose to do so.
- Subscribers receiving services will receive alert messages if: (1) the operator of the network is a participating CMSP; and (2) the subscriber's mobile device is configured for and technically capable of receiving alert messages from the network.
- WEA messages will not preempt calls in progress.

Enhancing the notification services that governments already operate to provide emergency alerts and information on mobile devices, cell phone subscribers will automatically receive information about disasters without having to subscribe. Emergency managers can develop alerts, send them to a national center where alerts are authenticated, and then the national center will aggregate the alerts and send them to WEA for distribution in the affected area.

FEMA created the Common Alerting Protocol *(CAP),* a standard for formatting messages so a single message can activate multiple warning systems over various media using numerous applications. The CAP allows a consistent digital message to be disseminated simultaneously over many different communications systems.

System of Systems

In order to provide life-saving information quickly, governmental authorities at all levels use the Integrated Public Alert and Warning System (IPAWS), which integrates the nation's alert and warning infrastructure. Local communications systems that use CAP standards can be integrated with the IPAWS infrastructure. IPAWS uses the EAS, WEA, NWR, and other public alerting systems from a single interface.

A system-of-systems approach facilitates the delivery of information quickly and efficiently to a diverse population that uses a variety of tools to communicate. Rather than depending on a single mode, this aggregated system of communication methodologies provides for redundancy. Where one communication system may fail to reach the intended audience, another may be successful. A system-of-systems structure is the foundation for creating statewide warning approaches. Local systems, regardless of the modes of communication, can tie into the statewide system.

Examples of the components of a system-of-systems include the following:

- Landline or cell phone calls based on geography or special groups
- Sirens or other mass notification for communities or buildings
- Messages on social media sites
- Pop-up or instant messages on desktop computers
- Push messages on smartphones
- E-mail with links to a multimedia system for the deaf
- Messages on digital signs (e.g., Amber Alerts)
- Messages to encoded receivers via FM radio
- Messages to Web media

Notification systems utilizing electronic media have been used for hurricane warnings. Communities can develop lists of phone numbers and e-mail addresses with priority messages sent to the entire list. These systems have been used to instruct residents to shelter in place after a chemical plant explosion spread a plume of black smoke across nearby communities.

An Example of a Regional Intranet

Jurisdictional agencies (i.e., office of emergency management, department of health, mayor or governor's office) and first responders need to be able to share information and data in a reliable and secure manner through communications systems available on demand during both emergencies and daily operations. Video surveillance is one technique used to communicate such information where interoperability is critical. Through closed-circuit television (CCTV), video cameras transmit a signal to a preestablished place, on a limited set of monitors. In the National Capital Region (NCR), comprising Washington, D.C., and surrounding counties in Maryland and Virginia, many government jurisdictions and agencies use different CCTV cameras and video management software. Through the use of video-sharing architecture, one agency can see another agency's video in their own viewing application without the need to purchase new CCTV software or systems. The jurisdictions of the NCR developed a smartphone application to enable them to share video via mobile devices even when they use different video management systems. Further, the NCR developed an interconnection network, known as NCRnet, to connect 24 regional jurisdictions and municipalities and the Metropolitan Washington Council of Governments. NCRnet is a high-speed network primarily comprising dedicated fiber optic strands. It implements regional interoperability and connects community leaders and first responders across the metropolitan area.

The Creation of FirstNet

Historically, communities used land mobile radio (LMR)—wireless communications systems that were independent or connected to other fixed systems or cellular networks, such as two-way radios in vehicles—to communicate in an emergency. These conventional radio systems have dedicated frequencies and channels assigned to a group of users. The use of LMRs has been problematic during disasters. When a user makes a call and selects a channel, other members of the group cannot use the channel until the call is over. Further, many radios purchased from different vendors are not interoperable, resulting in responders not being able to communicate with each other. An alternative—trunked systems—are computer-controlled and assign a pool of channels for use by multiple individuals. When a call is made by a user on a trunked system, an available channel is automatically selected by the system from the pool of available channels, leaving the remaining channels available for others.

Some states, regions, and large urban areas migrated from basic systems to computer-based or Internet Protocol-based systems, which allowed agencies to increase the number of users on a system, enhance capabilities, and improve interoperability. However, not all of these systems are compatible with each other, inhibiting the ability of public safety responders and officials to talk to each other during emergencies.

To overcome these challenges, in February 2012, Congress passed the Middle Class Tax Relief and Job Creation Act, which required the establishment of a national broadband network for public safety known as the National Public Safety Broadband Network. The act mandated that technical standards developed for the new network incorporate commercial standards for Long Term Evolution (LTE).[1] In response, the First Responder Network Authority (FirstNet) was created within the National Telecommunication and Information Administration of the Department of Commerce to provide a nationwide high-speed broadband network to be used for public safety. FirstNet can increase the safety of first responders by heightening situational awareness, improving communications, and enhancing productivity through extensive coverage with reliable high-speed data services. When completely developed, FirstNet will provide a single interoperable platform for communicating about emergencies on a dedicated 700 MHz spectrum, ensuring communications for first responders everywhere in the country. The development of a unified national network helps the United States achieve the long-sought goal of robust, interoperable communications for those responding to disasters.

Datacasting

When responders use communications systems that are not interoperable during a disaster, it is often difficult to get the same information to a wide group at the same time. In addition, cellular networks become congested with consumer use during a disaster. In order to send and receive information quickly, datacasting is used to disseminate data over a wide area via radio waves. Datacasting facilitates simultaneous secure communication in real time and allows for sending encrypted information (i.e., live videos, files, alerts, and other critical data) using the broadcast frequencies of public television stations. Through this technology, public television stations are a wireless data network that is invisible to traditional television viewers. With television networks switching to digital signals, unused bandwidth becomes available for programs like datacasting. This technology allows first responders to access important information without depending on cellular networks that may not be designed to handle large amounts of data.

Such was the case in April 2016, when severe storms caused serious flooding in Houston, Texas. First responders relied on KUHT and TV8 to share critical information. In addition, Houston fire and police used datacasting technology at Houston Public

1. LTE is the standard that increases the mobile bandwidth available to wireless networks, which dramatically increases the flow of information. Using LTE, users in the field can send real-time data, such as high-definition video, in seconds rather than minutes. The capability of smartphones (discussed later in this chapter) has been substantially enhanced with this wireless technology.

Media to deliver live video of the flooding from a mobile phone in a helicopter to the Emergency Operations Center (EOC). Through a mobile app, GoCoder, they sent live images from a mobile device to the encoder at Houston Public Media, which carried the video to city officials over the public television broadcast spectrum. Through this technology, first responders and emergency management agencies were able to communicate, assess the damage, and determine the best response.

SAFECOM

SAFECOM, operated by the U.S. Department of Homeland Security (DHS) Office of Emergency Communications, is a public safety-driven communications program working to improve emergency communications. More than 70 members represent both emergency responders at all levels of government and major intergovernmental and national public safety associations. The members of SAFECOM collaborate with policy makers to improve the interoperability and compatibility of multijurisdictional and intergovernmental communications. One product is the annual *SAFECOM Guidance on Emergency Communications Grants* available at: https://www.dhs.gov/publication/funding-documents.

Social Media in Emergency Preparedness and Response

Communication in disasters requires reaching all audiences, whether they use traditional or the latest communication modes, e-mail or text messaging, landline or cell phone, or are individuals who are disabled or are non-English speaking. Throughout history, societies have used available technology, such as the teletype during World War II, to broadcast information about emergencies. More recently, communication relied on traditional mediums: radio, telephone, television, handouts, and posters. Technological innovation has exponentially expanded the pathways and today emergency communication occurs through a wide variety of tools.

Web-based and other electronic technologies used for interaction are known as social media. Public health agencies can leverage the networks created by social media to convey alerts and create dialogues that result in speedy community response to disasters. Alerts can be sent and received in real time and anywhere there is a cell tower or satellite reception. Using social media brings the message directly to the user audience. Social media can reach groups who do not depend on or who may be hard to reach through traditional channels. Importantly, web-enabled technologies address the problem of interoperability that has plagued traditional communications systems.

Social media is useful in the breadth of emergencies—an expert can supply guidance about an emerging infectious disease or a governmental agency can direct communities

Table 7-2. Functions of Social Media in a Disaster

Disaster Social Media Use	Disaster Phase
Provide and receive disaster preparedness information	Pre-event
Provide and receive disaster warnings	Pre-event
Signal and detect disasters	Pre-event → Event
Send and receive requests for help or assistance	Event
Inform others about one's own condition and location and learn about an individual's condition in a disaster-affected area	Event
Document and learn about what is happening in a disaster	Event → Post-event
Deliver and consume news coverage of the disaster	Event → Post-event
Provide and receive disaster response information; identify ways to assist in the disaster response	Event → Post-event
Raise and develop awareness of a disaster; donate and receive donations; identify and list ways to volunteer or help	Event → Post-event
Provide and receive disaster mental health/behavioral health support	Event → Post-event
Express emotions, concerns, well-wishes; memorialize victims	Event → Post-event
Provide and receive information about and discuss disaster response recovery and rebuilding; recount and hear stories about the disaster	Event → Post-event
Discuss sociopolitical and scientific causes and implications of responsibility for events	Post-event
(Re)connect community partners	Post-event
Implement traditional crisis communication activities	Pre-event → Post-event

Source: Adapted with permission from Houston et al. 2015. Social media and disasters: a functional framework for social media use in disaster planning, response, and research. *Disasters.* 39(1):1–22.

to take preventive actions. Emergency broadcasts through social media can help governmental agencies deliver a unified message about an emergency, direct traffic in evacuations, or issue shelter-in-place or other advice to minimize injury and illness. Using networks as a pathway for notification, social media can educate the public and promote preparedness before a disaster strikes. Officials can monitor what is happening on the ground in real time so they have a better understanding of the situation. Through social media, the many people who want to help can form a *crisis crowd,* where the people in the community provide information about events. Collaboration in sharing information and best practices during an emergency is improved using social media. Communication plans that are activated during a disaster should include social media as one of the channels of communication. Table 7-2 describes the functions of social media in a disaster.

How Social Media Can Be Used

In a disaster, it is critical to notify the public and to reach a broad audience as soon as possible. A study that was conducted following a chemical spill in West Virginia found that timely communication of emergency information resulted in a greater perception of risk and, therefore, greater compliance with recommendations. To reach a broad audience quickly, people must be reached at work, at school, at home, at play, or in transit. People could be on their computers, surfing the Internet, watching television, listening to the radio, talking or texting on their cell phone, using a social networking site, receiving updates from a Web site such as Twitter, or not near a media outlet at all. Communication strategies need to be all encompassing. Using social media during and after disasters can be an effective tool for fast and economical distribution of public health information. Further, social media is now universally used for the rapid mobilization of equipment, supplies, and people and for fund-raising after a disaster. Following the 2013 Typhoon Haiyan in the Philippines, the World Health Organization established Facebook, Twitter, and Instagram accounts to disseminate public health information and found that utilizing social media during and after disasters was an effective method for quickly and inexpensively disseminating public health information.

The range of potential media that can be applied is vast and reshaping the dissemination of emergency information. Services such as Twitter or text messages are used to quickly broadcast alerts and announcements. Preparedness and response apps may push out notifications to users. Blogs and podcasts broadcast messages and encourage a conversation with the audience. Social networking sites, like Facebook, are connected to NWS feeds and are used to disseminate real-time weather alerts, warnings, and other preparedness information. Internet forums generate public participation or comment. Staying current with quickly changing events is effortlessly possible through a Web format known as Really Simple Syndication (RSS). By aggregating multiple data feeds into one location, RSS provides timely updates about a topic to users without their having to visit many sites individually or to join multiple newsletters. RSS can be used to notify users that a site has new information.

Our government and other public safety authorities are disseminating information through social media to help citizens understand what it means to be ready or prepared for responding to disasters. FEMA initiated a readiness campaign that provides practical advice on preparing for and surviving a disaster. The Centers for Disease Control and Prevention (CDC) has a Twitter account on which they post instant updates on the status of a variety of public health topics. The CDC provides information accessible from smartphones on Zika virus, public health emergencies, and more. State agencies are working with YouTube and Google to develop their own social networks. The NWS uses Skype to talk to the local media during a weather event. Medical Reserve Corps chapters use Facebook to improve recruitment. Finally, it is now possible to reach people around the world using social media and current technology. People trapped in rubble after the 2010 earthquake in Haiti used their cell phones to call relatives in the United States to ask them to send help.

One of the drawbacks of social media is that the deluge of posts and texts can overwhelm the system; thus, proper technical planning is critical. When a survivor tweeted about the need for water after tornadoes struck Alabama in April 2011, more than 20 voluntary agencies responded because there was no coordination and therefore no feedback that the request was fulfilled. In addition, where there is a limited amount of bandwidth, neighboring communities may need to provide the emergency information. With social media fully integrated into basic emergency preparedness and response, community groups, faith-based organizations, and local public health officials can effectively communicate with more people before, during, and after disasters. By being integrated into social media, public health agencies ensure that accurate information is available to the public as quickly as possible.

In 2014, Facebook launched the "I'm Safe" feature. The feature allows users to announce on their Facebook page that they are safe, check on others, and check notifications in the event of a disaster. Those involved in the 2014 earthquake in Nepal and the 2015 terrorist attacks in Paris used this feature, which can be launched across 80 languages simultaneously. In 2016, Facebook announced that it would start experimenting with community-activated Safety Checks. With the new system, Safety Check would be triggered when a certain number of people post about a particular event and Facebook receives an alert from one of its third-party sources. Users would also be able to share their status and spread the word once the Safety Check was activated.

Best Practices Using Social Media

Regular use of social media in disaster and emergency management has the potential to engage stakeholders and the public in better preparedness. A summary of best practices on the use of social media in the management of disasters is provided below:

- Implementation: Set up accounts as "public" to allow for maximum accessibility and use social media as an additional platform to communicate with the public.
- Education: Provide education and training to staff who will be managing the site on a regular basis about posts, Tweets, and interactions with followers.
- Collaboration: Have friend and follower lists capture as many stakeholders as possible so they in turn can follow your account. This can be done by proactively reposting or re-Tweeting information from other agencies. When possible, keep the message in its original format to decrease the chance of passing along incorrect official information.
- Communication: Engage with the public as much as possible. This is one of the more challenging tasks due to the number of staff and resources needed to maintain communication 24 hours a day.

The Mayo Clinic provides resources for health care and public health practitioners interested in learning more about navigating social media through the Mayo Clinic Social Media Network (available at: https://socialmedia.mayoclinic.org).

Examples of Social Media

Social media outlets have dramatically changed the way communities handle emergency response and have facilitated better decision making based on more accurate and timely information. Through these interactive channels, broader audiences can receive the critical information needed to take protective action during and after disasters.

The NWS, FEMA, and the National Hurricane Center all provide RSS feeds. Many news-related sites, Weblogs, and other online publishers syndicate their content as an RSS feed. When preparing or posting RSS feeds, it is advisable to include the full date and time in the heading or title of the updated post or press release. The viewer saves time by knowing when the event occurred and whether the report is an update without clicking on the feed. Feed readers or news aggregator software, available for different platforms, is needed to read an RSS feed. My Yahoo, Bloglines, and Feedly are popular web-based feed readers. Many sites display a small icon with the acronyms RSS, XML, or RDF to indicate that a feed is available. CrisisCommons (available at: http://crisiscommons.org) uses technology to share best practices and lessons learned in response to disasters. Through CrisisCamp, an international network supported by CrisisCommons, volunteer users solve problems through technology to help people and communities in crisis. Table 7-3 describes social media techniques being used by emergency management.

Twitter, Facebook, LinkedIn, Instagram, Flickr, YouTube, and Thunderclap

When landlines are not functioning but cell phone coverage is still intact, Twitter and Facebook are available. Twitter and Facebook are 2 of the most widely used social media platforms. Communities use Twitter, with its 140-character limit, to communicate the broadest range of short messages with immediate distribution with unlimited reach—traffic delays to bomb threats. Twitter has provided on-the-ground information used for rapid damage assessments, individual requests for help, anecdotal information about relief efforts, even messages of hope for those affected by a disaster. Twitter is used in Southern California to track a wildfire, assess the fire from multiple locations, and inform all about the progression of the fire. By creating graphs of the data streams of a given topic among tweets, it may be possible to use the information for decision making. As an example, graphing keywords in tweets, such as cough or diarrhea, may serve as a surveillance tool (see Chapter 5). Another use of Twitter is to analyze the number of tweets related to a particular disaster or epidemic. Tweets can be uploaded into a computer-assisted qualitative data analysis software research tool, such as NVivo, and perform a word search of key terms and concepts related to topic of interest. This computer-assisted qualitative data analysis software will not analyze the data, but it is useful to organize and

Table 7-3. Examples of Social Media Techniques for Emergency Management

Location or Agency	Tool	Use
San Francisco, CA	• Facebook, Twitter, YouTube	• Disseminate information about emergency preparedness • Issue public warnings
San Francisco, CA	• AlertSF	• Text-based notification system for emergencies
Manor, TX	• CiviGuard • Smartphones	• Location-specific emergency alerts • Send response data from field to emergency responders
U.S. Geological Survey	• Twitter Earthquake Detector • Twitter Associated Press International	• Monitor feeds to rapidly detect earthquakes • Conduct search for earthquake and aggregate information based on number of tweets
Virginia Department of Emergency Management	• Virginia Interoperability Picture for Emergency Response	• Geographic Information System platform that integrates feeds from 250 sources • Emergency response personnel can use single source of information to understand events
U.S. Department of Defense	• All Partners Access Network	• 380,000-user network • Community of communities Web site using wikis, blogs, forums, and file sharing • Exchange of information with authorized mission partners • In Haiti response, posted that fully functioning hospital had no patients and hospital reached capacity the next day
Department of Homeland Security	• First Responder Communities of Practice	• Online network of emergency response professionals • Share best practices

Source: Based on Yasin R. 2010. 5 ways to use social media for better emergency response. *Government Computer News.* Available at: https://gcn.com/articles/2010/09/06/social-media-emergency-management.aspx. Accessed January 18, 2017.

understand it. Practitioners and investigators can do a word search of key terms and concepts related to topics of interest, create word clouds, look up the references, and conduct text searches. Finally, Social Media for Emergency Management (#SMEMchat) is a community of emergency managers who share valuable information about using social media as part of preparedness. With the increase in the use of social media sites, individuals can follow disaster-related discussions or experts in the field. Table 7-4 describes how to use Twitter to disseminate information.

State and federal agencies, including FEMA, have Facebook pages. Those in the community who are signed up as friends have access to real-time updates and can post relevant information that will reach a broad audience. Through Facebook, nonprofits have organized relief efforts and facilitated a quick response of dollars and resources, such as the global disaster relief after the 2010 earthquake in Haiti.

Instagram and Flickr are social media sites where users can share real-time images of a disaster from which public health professionals can gain valuable information to enhance their response. Both government agencies and the public use the sites to post pictures from disasters as they occur. In addition, researchers have begun using social media platforms to derive information about the nature of specific events during a

Table 7-4. Use of Twitter During an Emergency

Set up a Twitter account so that you have followers before an emergency occurs
Messages must be 140 characters or less
Keep messages short and to the point
Monitor 24/7 to watch for and respond to rumors and misinformation
Use hashtags (#) for broader reach

disaster. Following Hurricane Sandy, the number of photographs showing varying degrees of damage, which were uploaded to Flickr, correlated with physical variables that characterize natural disasters, such as atmospheric pressure and its impact. The correlation suggests that digital traces of a disaster can help determine its strength or impact.

Disaster management is also found on the business-focused social networking site LinkedIn. Government agencies, nonprofits, and researchers use LinkedIn to feature updated disaster and emergency preparedness content and best practices. Among the numerous groups organized around interests related to disasters and emergency management, Disaster Researchers and Disaster Management Professionals and Emergency Managers Global Forum are active groups that share disaster-related information.

FEMA started a Thunderclap campaign in 2014 called "Resolve to Be Ready." Thunderclap is a crowd-speaking platform that helps people share their voices as a unit, rather than as individuals. Supporters of an idea sign up and agree to share a message, which amplifies the idea and its significance. In order to "support" the message, people have to connect with the Thunderclap platform and give it permission to access their social media accounts and send messages on their behalf. The messages are all sent simultaneously, only reaching people who are on social media when the message is sent.

Many governmental departments and nonprofits are utilizing YouTube. Government agencies take advantage of media advertising policies and expand their market by running informational videos before the entertainment on YouTube or other video hosting sites, like Hulu. FEMA's Ready Campaign (available at: http://www.ready.gov) is one example of the use of this strategy. WorkSafeBC, a Canadian organization committed to promoting health and safety for workers, has a dedicated channel on YouTube. WorkSafeBC posts public service announcements and provides training videos, including during a disaster or large-scale incident.

Smartphones and Other Communication Tools

Laptops and cell phones have limitations during disasters. Although laptops allow work to be done outside of the traditional on-site work environment by accessing information from any location, their bulk and weight make them impractical for emergency workers in the field. Laptops also have relatively short battery lives and require connectivity within the range of a Wi-Fi network. To send an e-mail from a laptop, it has to be turned on and connected to a virtual private network, which may take several minutes. Traditional cell phones allow communication from the field but don't have adequate storage to handle data-enabled applications.

Smartphones are small and lightweight, have increased reliability, and allow a user to send an e-mail or text instantaneously. Smartphones are also used to provide guidance to those directly impacted. Tsunami warnings via text messaging and e-mails are part of the plan to alert the deaf community in Australia.

Smartphones converge voice, database access, productivity applications, and multimedia on a single device. Smartphones have redundant communication options—voice, short message service (SMS) text messaging, e-mail over cellular, Wi-Fi, and satellite capability—which enable communication and information access when any one network is not working. Smartphone software, with easy access to the resources of the Internet, enables the user to access information, pictures, and maps and allows the download of health, safety, and preparedness applications before and during an emergency. Personnel can access information from the field as if they are at their desks. Door-to-door field assessments are made easier when assessment forms can be readily completed on the screen of a cell phone with the data automatically loading to a centralized database. Rapid health assessments can be completed in hours. Financial software can be preloaded to track all expenses as they occur, improving on-the-ground financial accounting. Rescue and medical care are also made easier. Phones with global positioning system (GPS) capability have been used to locate people who are trapped in rubble. In Haiti, responders placed cell phones on the chests of the injured and transferred electrocardiogram readings to medical units. Crisis Mappers (available at: http://www.crisismappers.net) facilitate a rapid response by combining GPS, mobile phones, statistical modeling, and visual analytics to map needs and requests following a disaster.

With a wireless connection on a smartphone, responders can do the following:

- Manage incidents and emergency alerts.
- Report on an incident.
- Disseminate emergency procedures within seconds on an incident report.
- Access preformatted messages, such as "shelter in place" or "evacuate immediately."
- Send message blasts without having to use multiple methods.
- Receive confirmation that the message was received.
- Send messages within and between agencies.
- Use streaming video to enhance situational awareness.
- Store documents.
- Carry out tasks even if roads are impassable.

Many emergencies require a multiagency response. Smartphones can be preprogrammed with contact information so that interagency communication is facilitated.

Smartphones can be used to exchange text messages so that information that might otherwise be communicated over a radio is not misunderstood. Since available dedicated channels on two-way radios can be quickly used up during a disaster, communication is quicker because text messages are not affected by heavy traffic in wireless networks.

Databases can be stored on smartphones using a removable SD ("secure digital") card. Wireless Information System for Emergency Responders (WISER), a free database that contains information from the National Library of Medicine's Hazardous Substances Data Bank, is available for download as a standalone application on smartphones, Microsoft Windows PCs, iPod Touch, Google Android, and Blackberry devices. Responders in the field can find out whether they need to take protective action against hazardous materials by checking WISER (available at: http://wiser.nlm.nih.gov).

Employees can access their organization's disaster response plan from their smartphones. They can look up directives, management and inventory records, and emergency medical procedures. Specialized calculators can be used to determine wind speed and direction, radioactive fallout zones, and so forth. Smartphones can even become tactical tools through the use of specialized mapping software. Maps of an incident area can show the location, identity, and status of other responders or the location of individuals needing rescue.

Examples of categories of smartphone applications available for improved disaster preparedness and better management of communications during a crisis include the following:

Maps and Weather: Google Maps, Waze, and iOS Maps all provide traffic information and maps. Weather information is also helpful for first responders and the public, especially if bad weather is predicted.

Flashlight: Flashlight (for iPhone, iPod Touch, and iPad) and Brightest Flashlight (for Android) are simple apps that use the phone's small LED flash to illuminate an area.

Note-Taking and Recording: Many productivity tools aimed at a general audience are useful for emergency managers including:

- Evernote for uploading files, photos, audio and notes into one place
- ColorNote to make quick lists of tasks
- AudioNote for taking notes and recording voice notes (available for Mac, iOs, Android, and Windows)
- Basecamp suite of tools for project management, contact management, and chat
- Incident Command Table (for Apple) to plot events on Google Maps
- Dropbox to store important documents

Alerts: These apps alert others to disasters that occur within their jurisdiction as well as those occurring around the world:

- **Disaster Alert, developed by the Pacific Disaster Center, has an interactive map with real-time alerts around the globe.** A similar app, Streetsmart, was developed by the Xora software company. Streetsmart is a location-based app that although originally designed to manage workforce, can also be used to track damage during a disaster. Streetsmart was used to track the 2010 British Petroleum oil spill. The app enabled responders to identify where the damage was and make real-time decisions on response as on-site teams took pictures of the damage, provided details, and captured the GPS coordinates.

Emergency Prep: These apps provide technical information about preparedness and response:

- The Red Cross's applications are listed at www.redcross.org/prepare/mobile-apps and include apps for finding shelters and instructions for performing first aid.
- FEMA's app is at www.fema.gov/smartphone-app.
- The National Library of Medicine has a Web page that lists additional apps (available at: https://disasterinfo.nlm.nih.gov/dimrc/disasterapps.html). The page includes apps like Mobile REMM for responding to radiation and WISER for responding to hazardous materials.
- Developed by the National Fire Protection Association (NFPA), the NFPA 1600 provides a foundation for disaster and emergency management planning. The entire text is fully searchable and contains active links and phone numbers for NFPA and other agencies involved with emergency management programs, risk mitigation, and response. The NFPA 1600 standard is available at www.nfpa.org/codes-and-standards/all-codes-and-standards/list-of-codes-and-standards?-mode=code&code=1600.

Disaster Community: These apps aim to bring the disaster community together:

- IGLOO is a software available for purchase that enables users to create and manage an online community directly from the user's tablet. IGLOO has been used to collaborate in disaster response. One example is the Crisis Kitchen, which enabled and supported humanitarian relief in response to the earthquake and recovery in Haiti.
- ubAlert is a global social network that shares the knowledge of the world's citizens with those in danger. The app provides the information one needs to know about disasters happening across the world. Alerts contain basic event details, impact statistics, maps, images, videos, and more. One can instantly share alerts with coworkers, family members and friends via e-mail, Facebook, and Twitter.

Personal Use: These apps provide the following:

- In case of emergency (ICE) contact information is programmed into cell phones so that emergency responders can locate next of kin if needed. Smart-ICE expands that data to include personal and medical information. Available for iOS devices, smart-ICE has an automatic emergency tone that rings every 2 minutes after calling 911 so that if a caller is incapacitated, responders can locate the iPhone and ICE information. Phones can also be programmed so that emergency information is displayed on the lock screen so a professional does not have to be able to unlock the phone to retrieve information.

- Life360 allows the user to keep track of his or her family in an emergency. It sets up a personal network so one can send messages and share locations privately. It also has the capability to upload photos and can track loved ones via a map.

As part of disaster preparations, agencies can ask staff to preprogram their phones and provide information for them to update the information regularly. Some of the most basic information to program includes the following:

- Nonemergency numbers for police and fire
- Emergency contact information
- Medicines, medical conditions, and medical practitioners
- Emergency phone numbers for other staff and volunteers
- Meeting location where you will reconvene after an emergency
- Phone number to call to check "report to work" status

Other Communication Tools

FEMA's Web site is accessible from any mobile device with a Web browser and provides information on what to do before, during, and after a disaster (available at: https://www.fema.gov). Being able to access FEMA's Web site from a mobile device makes it easier to know how to take preventive actions. FEMA's mobile app has the following features:

- Push Notifications: "reminder feature" allows users to receive pre-scheduled safety and preparedness tips, including testing smoking alarms, practicing a fire escape plan, updating emergency kits, and replacing smoke alarm batteries
- Weather Alerts: provides warning on severe weather occurring in specific areas that users select, even if the phone is not located in the area
- Safety Tips: pointers on how to stay safe before, during, and after over 20 different types of disasters
- Disaster Reporter: site for sharing disaster-related photos
- Maps of Disaster Resources: driving directions to open shelters and disaster recovery centers
- Apply for Assistance: access to apply for federal disaster assistance
- Information in Spanish: defaults to Spanish-language content for smartphones that have Spanish set as their default language

In the aftermath of the 2015 earthquake in Nepal, rescuers used an advanced heartbeat detection technology known as Finding Individuals for Disaster and Emergency Response (FINDER), developed by the DHS and the U.S. National Aeronautics and Space Administration. FINDER units are about the size of a carry-on bag and are powered by a lithium battery. The units send out low-power microwaves that can detect subtle movements under debris, such as the slight pulsing of skin from a heartbeat. Using radar, the waves can penetrate into mounds of rubble at about 30 feet or into solid concrete at 20 feet.

Radio Operations

The emergency management sector will have radio networks available, and public health agencies should be linked as part of a community's emergency communication network. Communities use a variety of radio frequencies to communicate during emergencies. These include low frequency, very high frequency (VHF), ultra high frequency (UHF), and 800 MHz (digital). Both professional and amateur radio operators facilitate communication during emergencies.

Ideally, your community will establish a multichannel, multisite trunked 800-MHz radio system to provide two-way radio communications. Such a system has dual use: it can provide day-to-day communications in support of public safety and intra/interagency communications in the event of an emergency. Manufacturers recommend that the batteries of these radios be changed every 2 years.

To avoid overload on radio frequencies, protocols should be established to limit the length of conversations and to establish several radio transmitter-receivers operating on multiple frequencies. Radio transmissions should not last more than 30 seconds. If, while using a portable radio, the listener is unable to hear a transmission, the user should relocate his or her position. If poor reception is not corrected by relocating, portable users may need to spell out their message using the phonetic alphabet (Table 7-5). All times should be

Table 7-5. Phonetic Alphabet

A=Adam	J=John	S=Sam
B=Boy	K=King	T=Thomas
C=Charlie	L=Lincoln	U=Union
D=David	M=Michael	V=Victor
E=Eddie	N=Nora	W=William
F=Frank	O=Oscar	X=X-Ray
G=George	P=Paul	Y=Young
H=Henry	Q=Queen	Z=Zebra
I=Ida	R=Robert	

denoted as military time (e.g., 1:00 p.m. is 13:00 hours). An institution should designate persons responsible for carrying the radio and ensure that they are trained in its use.

It is important to follow the rules of etiquette established in your community when using the radios. Often these rules include identifying yourself and using the full name of your institution so that other users are aware of who is on the system at all times. If one party is transmitting and another party attempts to transmit, the second party's communication will not be received and the second party will hear a tone.

In order to test that the system is transmitting, most communities conduct a daily roll call of radio users. The response to the daily roll call is a simple "10-4" or "5 by 5." Table 7-6 identifies communications systems available to agencies and facilities.

Radio Amateur Civil Emergency Service

The Radio Amateur Civil Emergency Service (RACES) was founded in 1952 as a public service to provide a reserve communications group within government agencies in times of extraordinary need. The FCC regulates RACES operations; the amateur radio regulations (47 C.F.R. § 97.407) were created by the FCC to describe RACES operations in detail.

Each RACES group of licensed amateurs is administrated by a local, county, or state agency responsible for disaster services, such as emergency management, police, or fire and rescue services. In some parts of the United States, RACES may be part of an agency's Auxiliary Communications Service. Some RACES groups refer to themselves by other names such as *Disaster Communications Service* or *Emergency Communications Service.* FEMA provides planning guidance, technical assistance, and funding for establishing RACES organizations at the state or local government level. Citizen band radio operators run the General Mobile Radio Service (GMRS). By sharing repeaters, GMRS users can communicate over a much wider area.

RACES provides a pool of emergency communications personnel prepared for immediate deployment in time of need. At the local level, ham radio operators may participate in local emergency organizations or organize local "traffic nets" using VHF and UHF. At the state level, hams are often involved with state emergency management operations. Local, county, or state government agencies activate their RACES group. Traditional RACES operations involve the handling of emergency messages on amateur radio frequencies. These operations typically involve messages between critical locations such as hospitals, emergency services, shelters, and other locations where communication is needed. RACES communicators may become involved in communications about public safety, EOC staffing, and emergency equipment repair. RACES groups develop and maintain their communications ability by training throughout the year with special exercises and public service events. (A comprehensive RACES manual, *Guidance for Radio Amateur Civil Emergency Service*, is available online at: http://www.

Table 7-6. Communications Systems

Phone Service	Radios	Internal Communication Methods	External Information Systems	Contact Directories	Social Media
PBX	Radio link to local emergency management agency (800-MHz radio)	Walkie-talkies	Stand-alone computer and Internet access through dial-up and cable modems	Updated directories for internal and external contacts	Blogs
Analog phone lines	Ham radio (RACES)	Overhead speaker and paging systems	Staff have access rights to the HAN	Alert facility operator when EOC activated	E-mail alerts and instant messages
Long-distance service provider trunks		Runner system		Vendor contact numbers	Podcasts
Cell phones					Online and streaming video
Satellite phones					Microblogs (e.g.,Twitter)
Smartphones					Social networking sites (e.g., Facebook)
Skype					Mobile Web sites
					Widgets
					RSS feeds

Note: EOC=Emergency Operations Center; HAN=Health Alert Network; PBX=Private Branch Exchange; RACES=Radio Amateur Civil Emergency Service.

seattleyachtclub.org/files/FEMA%20Amateur%20Radio%20Guidance%20for%20Civil%20Emergencies.pdf.)

Hams also operate on the same radio wavelength through the Amateur Radio Emergency Service (ARES), which is coordinated through the American Radio Relay League and its field volunteers. In addition, in areas that are prone to tornadoes and hurricanes, many hams are involved in SKYWARN, operating under the NWS. Many national organizations have other formal agreements with ARES and other amateur radio groups including the National Communications System, the Red Cross, the Salvation Army, and the Association of Public-Safety Communications Officials.

In July 2010, the FCC amended the amateur radio services rules to permit amateur radio operators to also transmit messages, under limited circumstances, during disaster drills.

Public Health Emergency Communications Systems

Emergency communications systems (ECS) are web-based systems that ensure rapid, effective, and consistent communication to the news media, the public, and key stakeholders during public health emergencies, including terrorism events. Federal ECS facilitate an ongoing two-way dialogue with state and local health officers, public health information officers, clinician associations, policy makers, and other key stakeholders in all 50 states. Federal ECS have been used to respond to public inquiries, media telebriefings, press releases and interviews, and daily web-based updates.

There are 2 major components to ECS: the portal and the content. The portal serves as a single gateway to an organization's web-based information. Portals create efficiencies, facilitate the categorization of groups of information, and integrate applications while ensuring security. Structured levels of access can be granted for employees, public health professionals and community providers, the emergency management community, and the general public as well. By establishing a portal and by setting individualized security levels, organizations are able to control access to their web-based systems with a single username and password. When a user logs onto a portal, the system looks at his or her credentials and allows the person to access those areas for which they have authorization. The Public Health Information Network (discussed in Chapter 5) is an example of a portal, as are many of the health information networks established at the state department of health level.

Epidemic Information Exchange

During an emergency, the Epidemic Information Exchange (*Epi-X*) links the U.S. Department of Health & Human Services (HHS) and the CDC/Agency for Toxic

Substances and Disease Registry command centers with state surveillance and response programs, provides 24/7 emergency alerts, and creates a secure forum to share important disease information nationwide. Participation in *Epi-X* is limited to designated public health officials who are engaged in identifying, investigating, and responding to health threats. This secured communications network has been used to communicate with colleagues and experts about urgent public health events; to track information and create reports about outbreaks; create online conferences; alert health officials of urgent events by pager, phone, and e-mail; post and discuss newly emerging information from the CDC; and to communicate simultaneously with command centers at HHS, CDC, and all state and large metropolitan bioterrorism response programs. Available to its users in the field, in the laboratory, at the office, or at home, *Epi-X* was used to notify state epidemiologists by pager and phone of the first anthrax case in New York City and to track and notify new West Nile Virus activity throughout the United States. Other *Epi-X* reports included foodborne outbreaks, SARS activity, influenza surveillance, and H1N1 pandemic preparation.

The success of *Epi-X* depends largely on 3 principles: building community, being prepared, and responding to user needs. *Epi-X* does this by:

- Securing reports of health events (*Epi-X* reports)
- Securing discussions (*Epi-X* forum, comments on *Epi-X* reports)
- Notifying and alerting
- Securing user contact information (*Epi-X* directory)

Epi-X has over 6,000 users, approximately 35% are from state government, 35% are from local government, and 20% are from the CDC.

Health Alert Network

The most prevalent content-based ECS is the Health Alert Network (HAN), a subscription service for providers that was established to strengthen the public health infrastructure nationwide. HAN is used to ensure communications capacity at all local and state health departments and to update on the presence of disease as often as needed. Locally, HAN has daily practicality, including online dialogues where clinicians can confer with each other about syndromes presenting in their offices, emergency departments, and hospitals.

The numerous HANs—one in each state, the 3 largest city departments of health, and others—provide an alerting mechanism to pass on alerts that the CDC issues. The CDC established 3 categories of alerts: alert (do something now), advisory (important, may not require immediate action), and update (no action, information only). The alerting function uses various communication modalities to notify its user base: e-mail, fax, cell phone, and pager. There are both general (routine) and specific (emergency) alerts.

There is variability among the HANs as to their functionality. The most extensive web-based systems allow access to general and personalized information to the broadest community of users and access to more secure information to a more selected group. HAN utilizes both a *pull* and a *push* method of disseminating information. These HANs are multifunctional. HANs send out e-mails to all subscribers to notify them that a new alert has been posted through a multichannel broadcast. HANs also post health alerts, archive all alerts, have a document library, a bulletin board for posting and threaded discussions, multiple levels of security, and can conduct online conferences supplemented with visuals, such as Microsoft PowerPoint presentations.

Each HAN administrator determines the list of authorized users and their security level. Most users require a one-factor authentication, where the user name and password are linked with a professional license number or other identifier and a third-party certifying authority. Key health care, public health, and emergency response personnel undergo a two-factor authentication (i.e., they are issued a username and password with a token or digital certificate that is stored on a user's computer). Their access is controlled by the system administrator. Communication between the user's browser and HAN application is encrypted.

Disaster Recovery and Information Technology Continuity

It is critical that public health agencies and facilities develop an IT component as part of their disaster plan to mitigate the risks that could affect their ability to deliver public health services. The disaster plan should include arrangements for both clinical and business applications and detail a plan for recovery in the event of a disaster. The plan should be tested every 6 months to ensure that it is functional and viable. The test of the plan should be documented and the documentation retained.

The IT disaster plan should address the basic needs of the organization in maintaining continuity of operations and at a minimum include the following:

Prevention: A plan for protecting agency assets and identifying and managing the risks to the core activities of the organization, which includes:

- Inventory of critical forms, magnetic media, hardware, software, equipment, and supplies
- Development and maintenance of a vendor contact list
- List of critical organization applications
- Written vendor agreements
- Description of emergency recovery team roles and responsibilities
- Agreements with off-site data processing facilities in the event of an emergency

Response: Protocols for managing the crisis and its short- or long-term interruptions in agency operations, including:

- Procedures to notify employees and partners and to escalate response activities
- Backup procedures and data recovery procedures

Recovery: Recovery of all operations

Restoration: Repair and restoration of facilities and organizational operations

CHAPTER 8

BEHAVIORAL HEALTH STRATEGIES

While the health and medical needs of a community will vary based on the type and nature of a disaster, all traumatic events will result in the need for behavioral health services. Although different type of threats (e.g., terrorism or human-caused mass casualty, natural disasters, or pandemics) may involve different psychosocial risks, behavioral health is an all-hazards concern.

Most victims and workers in disasters respond normally to an abnormal situation. However, disasters can affect both short-term and long-term mental health when they destroy people's homes, their livelihoods, and the lives of loved ones. The long-term psychosocial effects of disasters are mitigated by understanding what is likely to occur and preplanning the management strategy. Many people may need support services in the immediate aftermath of a disaster and some will need long-term services. By knowing who is at greater risk, behavioral health professionals can triage and more closely monitor those most liable to have a difficult time adjusting. Behavioral health interventions following disaster include services and activities intended to keep adverse reactions from progressing into more serious physical and behavioral health conditions. This chapter reviews the psychosocial effects of natural and man-made disasters, special considerations and interventions needed for vulnerable populations (e.g., children, older adults, emergency workers), the impact of cultural backgrounds, the considerations of post-traumatic stress disorder (PTSD) and acute stress disorder (ASD), differences and similarities between natural and man-made disasters and terrorism, and resilience and how communities and individuals can develop this protective ability to "bounce back" from difficult experiences. Building upon that foundation, the chapter lays out a plan for organizing services for mental and substance-use conditions, including assistance centers and patient locator systems, and describes public health interventions, including psychological first aid.

Public Health Role

- Help restore the psychological and social functioning of individuals and the community.

- Reduce the occurrence and severity of adverse behavioral health outcomes caused by exposure to natural and man-made disasters through prevention, assessment, and response.
- Help speed recovery and prevent long-term problems by providing information about normal reactions to disaster-related stress and how to handle these reactions.
- Design, implement, and evaluate behavioral health programs.
- Provide practical, concrete services that address shelter, food, and employment issues, often in atypical settings such as shelters.
- Conduct rapid triage with a short time to intervene and little background info.
- Coordinate with medical providers to assist in the identification and referral of those in their practices who could benefit from further behavioral health intervention.
- Assure that coordination occurs as part of community planning in communities where services for mental and substance-use conditions are organized separately from public health.

Psychosocial Impacts of Disaster

Living through the experience of a disaster can have profound psychosocial effects and can alter social structure. The type of disaster predicts the level of psychological injury. Natural disasters have the lowest level of impact on behavioral health, followed by events resulting from human error, whereas violence and terrorism have the biggest impact. When planning a response to or delivering services in the aftermath of a disaster, public health professionals must consider the wide range of responses among victims and responders.

Disasters are very stressful, disruptive experiences that affect the entire community and can be life-changing. However, two-thirds of those who experience a disaster do not suffer long-term effects. Human behavior in emergencies generally adapts to meet immediate needs, with people behaving within their usual patterns pre- and post-disaster. The challenge of dealing with a disaster can also result in positive responses by both individuals and communities. Residents typically work together and support one another as they rebuild their lives and their communities. Residents of disaster-stricken areas tend to exhibit prosocial behaviors, are proactive in remediating the effects of the event, and are willing to help one another in their recovery. People generally provide assistance to one another and support those managing the response to the emergency. Volunteer activity increases at the time of the impact and continues throughout the postimpact period. More disaster tasks are carried out spontaneously by civilian bystanders (e.g., family, friends, coworkers, neighbors) than by trained emergency or relief personnel. We know that resilient individuals and communities recover sooner. The abilities of adjusting to the circumstances and taking positive actions are examples of resilience, as discussed later in this chapter.

In terms of morbidity, the social and psychosocial impacts of a disaster can greatly add to and often outlast the physical injuries. The social and psychosocial effects of disasters can last months, years, or an entire lifetime. People who are involved in disasters, as either victim or responder, may experience a wide variety of stress symptoms. These symptoms can have the broadest range of emotional, physical, cognitive, and interpersonal effects. In some disaster situations, victims recover quickly without long-lasting effects. In others, victims and responders suffer major problems with mental and substance-use conditions both immediately and for years after the event. They may have lost loved ones, need to adjust to new role changes, need to clean and repair property, or move from their home and neighborhood. In addition, peer support may be lost or victims may find that their peers are drinking more in response to stress.

Individual factors can influence one's psychological response. In addition to genetic vulnerabilities, an individual's prior history (e.g., child abuse, previous traumatic experience, experience of multiple stressors, prior psychological disorder, or none of these) and the family's emotional health and ability to provide support can all make an individual more or less vulnerable to long-term psychological difficulties. This principle was exemplified in individuals with a history of depression or anxiety who experienced more stress following Hurricane Sandy in 2012.

The severity of one's exposure is a risk factor for adverse psychosocial outcomes. One's proximity to the events and specific stressors, such as losing a loved one, being injured or seeing a family member injured, having your life threatened, or losing your home or community can all have significant effects on behavioral health. Both children and adults show a dose-response reaction to disaster threats—the greater the exposure, the greater the difficulties. Further, residents who experience physical injury, household damage, and displacement may experience higher levels of serious psychological stress. For example, the degree of exposure to Hurricane Sandy was strongly related to an individual's reported levels of subjective stress. Finally, loss of social support, particularly for those who are displaced from their home or community, lose their usual routine, or experience the death of significant others, will also negatively influence an individual's ability to adapt.

Both victims and responders experience a disaster as a crisis. Unusual events exacerbate the trauma, since there may be deaths of family or friends, injuries, job difficulties, illness, loss of personal belongings, and disruption of the regular routine. Initially, people feel numbness rather than panic. Those who experience a disaster want to talk about it with everyone who will listen. Victims may exhibit anger toward "the system," such as a perceived slow response by responding agencies. In time, everyone attempts to return to a normal routine, but delays in achieving normalcy impede emotional recovery.

Some predictors of potential long-term dysfunction can be managed. Fortunately, the mobilization of support can offset the impact of the severity of exposure. People who receive high levels of support are helped in dealing with the serious impacts of the disaster experience. Further, behavioral health problems following a disaster may not be distributed equally across geographic areas. After Hurricane Sandy, researchers found that risk factors in one neighborhood were not necessarily found in another. Resources should be allocated based on risk.

Normal Reactions to Abnormal Situations

In general, the transient reactions that people experience after a disaster, such as grief and stress reactions, represent a normal response to a highly abnormal situation. The goal is to assist individuals and communities experiencing transient dysfunction to return to their pre-disaster levels of functioning.

Victims of a disaster should be viewed as normal people, capable of functioning effectively, who have been subjected to severe stress and may be showing signs of emotional strain. Mild-to-moderate stress reactions during the emergency and in the early postimpact phases of a disaster are highly prevalent among survivors, families, community members, and rescue workers. Although some individuals may exhibit symptoms of extreme stress, these reactions generally do not lead to chronic problems. However, public health professionals should not ignore common stress reactions. Counselors may find that the marital problems that families have previously been working on are heightened following a disaster. Mental health professionals can help speed recovery and prevent long-term problems by providing information about normal reactions and educating victims about ways to handle those reactions.

A portion of the population will suffer more serious, persistent symptoms. Although most individuals exposed to traumatic events and disasters recover and do not suffer prolonged psychiatric illness, some exhibit behavioral change or develop physical or psychiatric illness. Troublesome reactions can result from exposure to both natural and man-made disasters and can include depression, alcohol abuse, anxiety, somatization disorder, domestic violence, difficulties in daily functioning, insomnia, and PTSD.

The following are common to all who experience a disaster:

- Concern for basic survival
- Grief over loss of loved ones and loss of important possessions
- Fear and anxiety about one's physical safety and that of loved ones
- Sleep disturbances, including nightmares and flashbacks from the disaster
- Concerns about relocation, potentially crowded living conditions, and being separated from support system
- Need to talk about events and feelings associated with the disaster
- Need to feel part of the community and its disaster recovery efforts

Behavioral Health Morbidity and Mortality

Adults and children manifest symptoms of distress differently. Disasters can have emotional, cognitive, physical, and interpersonal effects. For adults, the initial emotional response is usually shock and disbelief. This lasts from a few minutes to a few hours. Behavior is dazed or stunned. For the next several days, victims are willing to follow directions and are grateful for assistance. They may feel guilty for surviving.

In the next several weeks, victims will likely seek out others who were affected and participate in group activities of recovery. This activity is often followed by despair and depression. Victims can experience flashbacks, anger, emotional numbing, or dissociation, perceiving their experience as "dreamlike." Cognitive effects can include impaired memory, concentration, and decision making ability. Interpersonal relationships can become strained. Some victims worry about their futures and blame themselves. Furthermore, victims may increase their use of alcohol and over-the-counter sleep aids.

In the long term, there is a risk of decreased self-esteem and self-sufficiency. Some victims experience intrusive thoughts and memories. Physical effects can include sleep disturbances leading to insomnia and fatigue. Some victims and responders experience hyperarousal or a "startle" response. There can be somatic complaints such as headaches, gastrointestinal problems, reduced appetite, and decreased libido. Finally, disasters can have profound and widespread interpersonal effects such as alienation, social withdrawal, increased conflict within relationships, and both vocational and school impairment.

Symptoms of Distress in Vulnerable Groups

Those most at risk for psychosocial impacts are children, older adults, people with serious mental illness, families of people who die in a disaster, and responders. Different age groups are vulnerable to stress in different ways. Most people do not see themselves as needing services for mental and substance-use conditions following disaster and will not voluntarily seek out such services.

Children

Although a disaster affects everyone in the community, children are a particularly vulnerable group and require special attention and programs to avoid a traumatic experience. Children look to caregivers for support—parents, peers, and teachers will be the first responders to children in the preimpact and impact phases of disaster. For children, a key protective factor is their family. When a mother is resilient and adapts to the events, a child also adapts. This is especially true for children younger than 6 years old. For teenagers, however, their peer group is more influential. Because a child has a strong initial reaction does not mean that he or she will not recover. As families and social support are the primary protective factors, it is best to provide post-disaster counseling with families together.

Helping children will likely involve working closely with teachers and schools. The goal for those intervening with children is to help them integrate the experience and to reestablish a sense of security and mastery. Children who are most at risk are those who have lost family members or friends, who had a previous experience with a disaster, or who have preexisting family or individual crises. Children may not be able to describe their fears, which is a normal reaction stimulated by real events. Fear can outlast the event and can persist even if no physical injury occurred. Exposure to repeated media coverage can increase and prolong symptoms.

Preschool children needing extra help may appear withdrawn or depressed, or they may not respond to directed attention or to attempts to draw them out. They may exhibit thumb-sucking, bed-wetting, fears of darkness or animals, clinging to parents, night terrors, incontinence or constipation, speech difficulties, or changes in appetite. Preschoolers are vulnerable to disruptions in their environment, are affected by the reactions of their family, and are disoriented by changes to their regular schedule. Quickly reestablishing their regular schedule for eating, playing, and going to bed is important. Other interventions to help preschoolers include reenactment of the events in play (i.e., with fire trucks, dump trucks, ambulances), nonverbal activities such as drawing, and games that involve touching (i.e., Ring Around the Rosie; London Bridge; Duck, Duck, Goose). Verbal reassurance, physical comforting, frequent attention, expressions regarding loss of pets or toys, and sleeping in the same room as their parents may be helpful as well, because it should be temporary.

Children aged 5 to 11 years may exhibit irritability, whining, clinging, aggressive behavior, competition for a parent's attention, night terrors or nightmares, fears of darkness, and withdrawal from peers, as well as avoidance, disinterest, or poor concentration in school. Interventions for this age group include patience and tolerance, play sessions with adults and peers, discussions with adults and peers, relaxed expectations, structured free time with activities, and rehearsal of safety measures for the future. Children in this age group who reenact the events over and over and who have ongoing intrusive thoughts should be referred for evaluation.

Children aged 11 to 14 years can experience sleep disturbances, changes in appetite, rebellion at home, physical complaints, and problems with or less interest in school activities. At this age, children may benefit from encouraging the resumption of normal routines, organizing groups with peers, engaging in group discussions about the disaster, relaxing expectations temporarily, taking on structured responsibilities, and receiving additional attention as needed.

Children aged 14 to 18 years may exhibit psychosomatic symptoms, disturbances of sleep and appetite, hypochondriasis, changes in energy level, apathy, decline in interest in the opposite sex (or same sex, if that is their norm), irresponsible or delinquent behavior, fewer struggles for emancipation from parents, and poor concentration. School-age children in junior and senior high may become disoriented (e.g., confused regarding their name, town, the date), despondent, agitated, restless, severely depressed and withdrawn, unable to make simple decisions, and unable to carry out daily activities. These children may also pace, appear pressured, hallucinate, become preoccupied with one idea or thought, engage in self-mutilation, abuse drugs or alcohol, experience significant memory gaps, and become delusional or suicidal.

Interventions for 14- to 18-year-olds include encouraging participation in community reclamation, resumption of social activities, discussion of experience with peers, reducing expectations temporarily, and discussion of experience with family. Adolescent activities should end on a positive note, such as talk of heroic acts, helping the community, and preparing for the next time. Small groups could develop a plan to help the community rehabilitate. Adolescents who begin or increase risk-taking activities (e.g., substance abuse) should be referred for evaluation.

Finally, disaster plans can help protect the welfare of children by ensuring that all buildings where children congregate have written plans for all-hazards evacuation, for the relocation and reunification of children with their families or caregivers, and for the care of children with functional needs.

Older Adults

Older adults are in the highest risk group following a disaster. Generally, older adults have fewer support networks, limited mobility, and preexisting illness. In addition, disasters can trigger memories of other traumas experienced earlier in life. Older people worry about their deteriorating health and needing to be institutionalized and, as a result, may conceal the full extent of their physical problems. Research has shown that this population experiences a higher proportion of personal injury or loss because they often live in places more vulnerable to damage. For example, a significant number of older adults who lived in high-rise buildings during the New York City blackout in 2003 were unable to evacuate and had no air conditioning in high heat, no power for electrically powered medical devices, and no safe food. Since they experience a greater loss of mobility, their independence and self-sufficiency are harmed because they are less able to rebuild their homes, businesses, and other losses following a disaster. Living in assisted living or long-term care facilities may involve built-in supports that protect older adults.

Responders

Those whose job is to respond to disasters have physically demanding work that is tiring, may interrupt sleep patterns, and may expose them to hazards that are life threatening or have potential long-term health risks. Response tasks, such as search and rescue, expose responders to mutilated bodies and mass destruction. Their role as a help provider is also stressful. Some responders experience feelings similar to those experienced by the victims. They can be irritable, finding fault with things that never bothered them before. They can be suspicious and resent authority. They can be concerned for their own safety and the safety of their children. Responders can be stressed by their working environment, particularly in the presence of understaffing of their units, overwork, and conflicts with other professionals. Responders may face anxiety about their competence, are more affected by the impact of sights and smells, and can also struggle to balance family responsibilities and work demands in the face of an emergency.

Some responders may develop a condition known as critical incident stress syndrome. This syndrome must be recognized and treated because critical incident stress lowers group morale, increases absenteeism, interferes with mutual support, and adversely affects home life. The symptoms include deterioration in sense of well-being, exhaustion, depression, hostility, lost tolerance for victims, dread of new encounters, guilt, helplessness, or isolation. Burnout is often recognized by looking for either detachment or overinvolvement.

Cultural Considerations

With the population of the United States becoming increasingly more diverse, public health professionals can develop more effective behavioral health programs by understanding how people's ethnicity and culture impact responses to disaster. People's reactions to disaster, their ability to adapt, and their receptivity to assistance and services for mental health and substance-use vary according to their cultural traditions. Reactions to and recovery from disasters is influenced by one's ethnocultural background and the inherent life exposure and values embedded in that experience. The role of the family and who makes decisions also varies. In some cultures, elders and extended family play a significant role, whereas in others, nuclear families make the decisions. Behavioral health services following disasters are most effective when victims receive assistance that is consistent with their cultural beliefs as well as their needs.

Community is especially important for racial/ethnic minority groups. As discussed in the section on resilience below, intact communities provide strong social support. A community that is disrupted and fragmented is less able to provide the needed assistance, and this loss of social support can dramatically affect one's ability to adapt and recover. Refugees to the United States may have experienced a previous loss of social support, making them more vulnerable following repeated losses. Further, racial/ethnic minority groups may be severely impacted in areas where socioeconomic conditions cause the community to live in housing that is vulnerable to many disasters.

American Indian and Alaska Native tribes are federally recognized sovereign nations; thus, disaster response involves working with multiple agencies within the tribes and with all levels of government. In addition, tribes may work together to receive assistance and services. The Stafford Act provides that a state government must request a presidential disaster declaration on behalf of a tribe. Before a disaster declaration, responding agencies can work directly with a tribe to meet their needs using existing resources. Table 8-1 describes different aspects of daily life in which cultural customs should be considered by those providing disaster services to diverse populations.

Trauma- and Stressor-Related Disorders

The *Diagnostic and Statistical Manual of Mental Disorders,* Fifth Edition (*DSM-5*) organized an entire section covering trauma- and stressor-related disorders. Included are conditions where exposure to a traumatic or stressful event is specifically identified as a criterion for diagnosis. These disorders have been grouped into a separate category because there is variability in people's reactions and their clinical distress following exposure to devastating events. The disorders included are reactive attachment disorder, disinhibited social engagement disorder, PTSD, ASD, adjustment disorders, other specified trauma- and stressor-related disorder, and unspecified trauma- and stressor-related disorder.

When exposed to a traumatic or stressful event, the distress that a person experiences can vary greatly. Many individuals experience symptoms of anxiety or fear. Others who have similar exposure present observable characteristics such as a loss of the capacity to

Table 8-1. Cultural Views That Can Impact Response and Recovery

Communication: Culture influences how people express their feelings and what feelings are appropriate to express. The inability of both verbal and nonverbal communication can make both parties feel alienated and helpless.

Personal Space: Spatial requirements can be similar among people in a given cultural group. One person might touch or move closer to another as a friendly gesture, whereas someone from a different culture might consider such behavior invasive. Disaster crisis counselors must look for clues to a survivor's need for space, such as moving their chair back or stepping closer.

Social Organization: Understanding the influences of beliefs, values, and attitudes will enable the disaster worker to more accurately assess a survivor's reaction to the events. A survivor's answers to questions about hobbies and social activities can lead to insight into his or her life before the disaster.

Time: Perceptions of time may be altered during a disaster. Diverse cultures may view time differently, including their interpretations of the overall concept of time. Social time may be measured in terms of "dinner time," "worship time," or "harvest time." It is important to set time frames that are meaningful or realistic.

Environmental Control: Some people believe that events occur because of some external factor (e.g., luck, chance, fate, will of a higher being, or the control of others). These views can affect a person's response to disaster and the types of assistance needed. Those who feel that events and recovery are out of their control may be pessimistic about recovery, whereas those who believe that they personally can affect events may be more willing to take action.

Source: Adapted from Athey J, Moody-Williams J. 2003. *Developing Cultural Competence in Disaster Mental Health Programs: Guiding Principles and Recommendations.* Table 2-2. Important considerations when interacting with people of other cultures. Washington, DC: U.S. Department of Health & Human Services, Substance Abuse and Mental Health Service Administration.

experience pleasure (i.e., anhedonic symptoms); feelings of general dissatisfaction, restlessness, depression, and anxiety (i.e., dysphoric symptoms); withdrawal (i.e., dissociative symptoms); or symptoms where the person externalizes anger and aggression. Further, it is not uncommon for an individual to present with a combination of the above symptoms (i.e., with or without anxiety- or fear-based symptoms).

Although PTSD has been the subject of considerable research in recent years, other serious problems that can develop after a disaster include acute stress, major depression, generalized anxiety, and substance abuse. Acute stress disorder is characterized by post-traumatic stress symptoms lasting at least 2 days but not longer than 1 month following the trauma. In the long term, individuals who experience a disaster suffer more from depression than they do from PTSD. Finally, alcohol abuse can increase by 5% to 7% following a disaster. Given that this chapter is not meant to be a comprehensive guide for psychiatric diagnosis, the discussion focuses on PTSD and ASD in more depth. Those interested in more detailed information about these and other stress related disorders should refer to *DSM-5* (available at: http://www.dsm5.org/Pages/Default.aspx).

Post-Traumatic Stress Disorder

Post-traumatic disorders are best understood as a failure to recover. PTSD, a prolonged stress response associated with impairment and dysfunction, is a process, not a singular reaction or experience. How an individual perceives and experiences the disaster is a more salient factor in developing PTSD than the events themselves. While the duration and nature of the disorder varies, PTSD usually appears within 3 months of the trauma but may surface months or years later. Some individuals may be symptomatic longer than 12 months. Sometimes the symptoms of PTSD disappear over time, and sometimes persists for many years. PTSD has a range of significant impacts on individuals and the community. Those with PTSD have high levels of medical utilization, poor social and family relationships, absenteeism from work, and lower educational and occupational success. In the elderly, PTSD can be exacerbated by declining health or cognitive functioning and social isolation. Importantly, not all traumas cause this disorder.

Criteria for Post-Traumatic Stress Disorder[1]

A diagnosis of PTSD, as listed in *DSM-5*, requires that several criteria be met. *DSM-5* requires that PTSD symptoms continue for more than a month, but there can be delayed

---

1. American Psychiatric Association. 2013. *Diagnostic and Statistical Manual of Mental Disorders*, 5th ed. Washington, DC: American Psychiatric Publishing.

expression. If delayed, some symptoms may manifest immediately but the full diagnostic criteria are not met until at least 6 months after the event.

There are 8 criteria that must be met for a diagnosis of PTSD in adults, adolescents, and children older than 6 years of age:

1. The event was traumatic and evokes a significant response.
2. The person is reexperiencing the traumatic event through the presence of intrusion symptoms associated with the traumatic event, beginning after the traumatic event occurred.
3. The person is avoiding things that remind him or her of the traumatic event.
4. The person is experiencing increased arousal after the traumatic event.
5. The person is experiencing marked alterations in arousal and reactivity associated with the traumatic event, beginning or worsening after the traumatic event occurred.
6. For a diagnosis of PTSD to be made, the duration of the symptoms in the second, third, and fourth criteria must exceed 1 month.
7. The disturbance causes clinically significant distress in social, occupational, or other important functioning.
8. The disturbance is not due to substance abuse or another medical condition.

Post-Traumatic Stress Disorder in Children Age 6 and Younger

In the diagnosis of PTSD, a preschool subtype has been developed for children 6 years and younger. In the past, while the literature documented the types of behavioral health problems that children experience following a disaster, many cases were probably undetected because of the lack of diagnostic criteria. Without detection, children are unlikely to receive appropriate treatment. When developing *DSM-5*, a decision was made to create reliable diagnostic criteria based on previously documented cases, with a focus on behaviors rather than subjective experiences.

The way that children express their experience of the trauma can vary. Young children may have frightening dreams or may express their symptoms through play. Parents may be concerned about behavioral changes or changes in mood. (See previous section for more information.)

For children under 6 years of age, there are 7 criteria:

1. The child was exposed to actual or threatened death, serious injury, or sexual violence.
2. The child experiences 1 or more items of intrusion.
3. The child avoids or experiences negative alterations in cognitions items.
4. The child experiences 2 or more alterations in arousal and reactivity.
5. The duration lasts for more than 1 month.

6. The disturbance causes clinically significant distress in relationships with parents, siblings, peers, caregivers, or in school.
7. The disturbance is not attributable to substance abuse or another medical condition.

The complete *DSM-5* criteria are in Appendix K.

Post-Traumatic Stress Disorder Risk Factors/Predictors

Several factors can help predict which individuals might be at risk for PTSD. As previously discussed, the nature or severity of the trauma the person has experienced plays a major role, with more traumatic events leading to a greater likelihood of developing PTSD. Higher-risk scenarios potentially leading to long-term adjustment problems include exposure to life-threatening situations; death of a loved one; loss of home and belongings; exposure to toxic contamination; and exposure to terror, horror, or grotesque sights such as multiple casualties. Additional risk factors relate to life events before the disaster (i.e., childhood adversity and emotional problems by age 6). Being female, having lower socioeconomic status, having a history of prior exposure to trauma, having a history of psychiatric disorder, withdrawing during the event and continuing that withdrawal after, exhibiting inappropriate coping strategies, and experiencing concurrent or subsequent stressful life events all predispose to PTSD. While lacking social supports places individuals at risk, having social supports is protective in the development of PTSD. Family members of trauma victims and family members of disaster workers may also develop PTSD and related symptoms. Spouses and domestic partners should be included in debriefing, education programs, and treatment programs as indicated.

Severe Mental Illness and Post-Traumatic Stress Disorder

People with severe mental illness are more likely than other people to have experienced trauma in their lifetime and many have experienced multiple traumatic events. Further, following extremely stressful events, such as disasters, people with severe mental illness are more likely to develop PTSD even in the months and years following a disaster. While it is not fully understood why this population is so vulnerable, many are homeless, living on the streets or in homeless shelters, and are unlikely to be able to make necessary preparations or have a strong social network for support—all of which reduces their ability to develop resilience.

Further, extremely stressful events can exacerbate preexisting PTSD symptoms. People with severe mental illness may experience an increase in their PTSD symptoms, including (1) disturbing memories and nightmares about stressful events; (2) increased fear and wanting to avoid thoughts, feelings, and reminders about the trauma; and (3) increased problems with sleep, concentration, and hyper-alertness regarding potential danger. As a result, dedicated behavioral health services are likely to be required for this vulnerable population following a disaster.

Ethnocultural Issues in Post-Traumatic Stress Disorder

Rates of PTSD or other disaster-related impairment can differ among different racial or ethnic groups as a result of culturally varying perceptions of what constitutes a traumatic experience, as well as individual and social responses to trauma. PTSD has been detected in traumatized cohorts from very different ethnocultural backgrounds, and victims from all groups who meet PTSD diagnostic criteria have shown a similar clinical course and response to treatment. Assessments of the stress reaction of all individuals who have experienced a disaster should be carried out in a culturally sensitive manner, accounting for factors that may be unknown. Major depression, generalized anxiety disorder, and substance abuse are well documented after exposure to trauma and disasters. When planning interventions and developing programs, including members of the group in the planning and delivery of services and incorporating cultural aspects from the group's background will help give a sense of empowerment and result in better outcomes.

Acute Stress Disorder

The diagnostic criteria for ASD are similar to the criteria for PTSD, but there is a greater emphasis on dissociative symptoms (e.g., numbing, reduced awareness, depersonalization, or amnesia) in the criteria for ASD. For an ASD diagnosis, a person must experience 3 symptoms of dissociation, unlike a PTSD diagnosis, which does not include a dissociative symptom cluster. In addition, the diagnosis can only be made within the first month after a traumatic event. When symptoms continue beyond a month, clinicians should assess for the presence of PTSD. In 2016, the National Center for PTSD reported an ASD rate of 7% among survivors of a typhoon, 6% among survivors of an industrial accident, and 33% among victims of a mass shooting.

Risk for ASD Resulting From Trauma

The factors that place individuals at risk for developing ASD have not been studied as thoroughly as those for PTSD. Currently identified risk factors include exposure to prior trauma, more psychiatric dysfunction and treatment, depression, history of PTSD, and being prone to experiencing dissociation when experiencing traumatic stressors. Being diagnosed with ASD and not having received treatment is a predictor of subsequent PTSD.

Natural Disasters and Man-Made Disasters

The similarities and differences between man-made and natural disasters are strongly connected to the degree in which the events are felt to be preventable and controllable. The 2 types of disasters have in common the immediate threat and the potential for ongoing disruption. However, they differ with regard to whether someone can be blamed for the event and whether it could have been prevented. People understand that humans have little control over nature and that some geographic locations are more prone to some natural disasters than are others. By contrast, they believe people can control technology and thus feel a greater sense of a loss of control with technological or man-made events, since these events could have presumably been prevented.

Residents who are victimized by man-made disasters may have their stress exacerbated by knowing that their tragedy was caused by other human beings. Technological or man-made disasters of the same magnitude as natural disasters generally cause more severe problems with mental and substance-use conditions because it is harder to achieve psychological resolution and to move on following a technological event. During the nuclear disaster that followed the earthquake and tsunami in Japan in March 2011, the Japanese people were upset because they had been led to believe that their nuclear reactors were designed to prevent damage from earthquakes. Although many people initially doubted the official version of events, they became angrier when they learned that the government had issued inaccurate information.

For several reasons, man-made disasters present complex challenges for public health professionals. First, unlike the community cohesiveness that occurs after natural disasters, communities are often in conflict after an environmental disaster. Where the disaster involves contaminants that are usually invisible, great uncertainty often exists as to the risks of exposure. Contaminants may not have dispersed evenly, resulting in very different perceptions of the events by people living in the same community. Victims of man-made disasters often feel unsure about the long-term risks. Because of this ambiguity and insecurity, neighbors can become bitterly divided, and their support networks may be irreversibly damaged. Worse, residents of affected communities can be stigmatized by society as a result of the unknown risks of their exposure.

Man-made disasters often cause chronic uncertainty and distress. Unlike natural disasters, which generally have a low point after which things can be expected to improve, in disasters involving chemicals and radiation, those affected often do not know when all of the recovery activities will resolve. Uncertainty continues about the chronic health effects of exposure to invisible contaminants. Furthermore, long-term consequences, such as cancer, may take years to develop. Events that have a beginning and an end, such as tornadoes or hurricanes, allow the process of recovery to begin. Man-made disasters do not have this defined timeline, and as a result, the psychological threat can be continual and chronic.

Following a man-made disaster, psychophysiological symptoms are prevalent, along with chronic stress and demoralization. Psychological effects may result from either direct exposure or reaction to mitigation activities. Exposure to chemicals often does not result in a large number of exposed seeking immediate medical treatments. Here, concerns are long term. Information about the level of exposure or contamination may not be available for some time. Loss of social support and status can cause stress, especially if evacuation is required. These symptoms can manifest as physical complaints, can lead to increased morbidity of chronic diseases, such as hypertension, and can lead to medical problems attributable to the earlier exposure but appearing later in life. Groups at high risk for psychological health effects from environmental exposures include older people living alone, mothers with young children, evacuees, responders, and people with previous mental disorders. The following causes of stress can follow major environmental exposures[2]:

- Acute stress reaction
- Worry about long-term health effects
- Uncertainty about long-term effects
- Housing and job security
- Media siege
- Somatic complaints
- Stigma and social rejection
- Cultural pressures
- Inadequate medical follow-up and compensation

Terrorism

The mechanism of anticipatory anxiety—worrying about a possible, totally random horrific event that is not currently happening but could occur and impact that person—is the central tenet that makes the threat of terrorism so frightening. Like many psychological reactions, the individual response to terrorism has phases of adjustment. Repeated exposures to terrorism also impact our biological systems. Initially there is a high-alert phase that involves both a psychological (fear) and biological (fast heart rate) response. Without repeated exposure, this high alert dissipates. If the event is more intense and more frightening, individuals might experience an even stronger response. If the exposure to terrorism continues and becomes the norm, a person might adapt psychologically and biologically, but at a level that does not return to their baseline. This stress on a person's psychological, neural, neuroendocrine, and neuroimmune systems makes a person

2. Adapted from Baxter PJ. 2002. Public Health Aspects of Chemical Catastrophes. In: Havenaar JM, Cwikel JG, Bromet EJ, eds. *Toxic Turmoil: Psychological and Societal Consequences of Ecological Disasters.* New York, NY: Kluwer Academic/Plenum.

less able to respond to future attacks. People who are repeatedly exposed to traumatic events, such as terrorism, may have a diminished response to subsequent events, which is known as *habituation*. However, if a person is in a heightened state of fear or anxiety and is then exposed to trauma, such as terrorism, they can have an even stronger response, known as *sensitization*.

People who have experienced terrorist events, either as a victim or a relative of a victim, can suffer some psychological impairment. Prevalence varies by the specific events, differences in population involved, and nature of the events. Those most likely to be affected are those who were injured, first responders exposed to trauma, and those who were already at risk to develop psychological symptoms. People who are resilient have fared better even with repeated exposures. Further, individuals who experience violence through terrorism tend to be angrier about what has happened than are those who have experienced other kinds of disasters. Those who have uncontrolled anger and rage that persists over time can predictably have the worst outcome psychologically.

Resilience

The mental health of a community following a disaster is dependent, in part, on the community's preparedness, which includes: their organizational response, ability to protect those who are impacted from harm, and ability to provide needed assistance. The impact of disasters on individuals and on the larger community is also influenced by their resilience. Good community mental health is a precondition for community resilience and resilience is important in a community's effective response to disasters.

What Is Resilience?

While initially used to describe a psychological trait, the concept of resilience has become one of the fundamentals of emergency preparedness at all levels. In their 2010 *DHS Risk Lexicon*, the U.S. Department of Homeland Security defined resilience as the "ability of systems, infrastructures, government, business, communities, and individuals to resist, tolerate, absorb, recover from, prepare for, or adapt to an adverse occurrence that causes harm, destruction, or loss." To be resilient, individuals, families, and communities should be "informed, trained, and materially and psychologically prepared to withstand disruption, absorb or tolerate disturbance, know their role in a crisis, adapt to changing conditions, and grow stronger over time."

Developing resilience, the capacity of individuals and community to adapt following devastating circumstances, has become a focus of preparedness and effective response. The capacity to adapt is affected by both the way that communities have prepared and by the types, timing, and levels of support received. Further, social support and resilience can strengthen one's ability to withstand stress following a disaster. Although disasters often bring numerous losses, there are also opportunities for individual growth and improvements in the community. For example, Greensburg, Kansas, established itself as a futuristic model "green" town by building a new school at LEED (Leadership in Energy and Environmental Design) platinum standards after a tornado devastated the entire town in 2007.

Individuals

Individuals who are resilient are more able to positively adjust following adversity or severe stress. While individuals may struggle for a period of time and may not sleep well or work optimally during the process of recovering from disaster, resilient people are generally able to function in a healthy manner within a few months after life is more normal. Resilience is not based on how things work out, but how individuals adapt and "bounce back" along the way. Those who are resilient do as well or better than expected, maintain competence in their functioning under adverse conditions, and regain normal functioning.

The path to recovery is not always straight. For some, severe distress comes and goes in a cyclical pattern. Others face a delayed dysfunction, such as those who experience PTSD. Finally, there are individuals who encounter chronic dysfunction, where they suffer a significant reaction to the stress that continues after others have recovered.

Resilience for individuals varies in each phase of a disaster. When the disaster first strikes, an individual's capacity to adapt is dependent on their level of individual preparedness, household preparedness, and the individual's ability to manage by themselves. Those with lower incomes are often less prepared; disabled individuals with low income are even less likely to be prepared.

Those who are better prepared (i.e., because they have an emergency plan, have stored food and water, and are capable of communicating even without power) are better able to adjust. Those with stronger psychosocial resources before the disaster are likely to have greater resilience.

An individual's pace of adapting is also shaped by both one's ability to cope and the breadth of their social interactions. Those who have a strong connection to their community are often more concerned about issues facing the community and helping others. Action taken as a group to help the community recover, known as *collective action*, is dependent on the awareness, motivation, and willingness of individuals to act as agents for change in their community. People engage in collective action during disasters when they (1) see a positive benefit associated with working with the responding group; (2) see social injustice and believe that collective action will remedy it; and (3) believe that by responding to a disaster, it will help a community recover faster.

Community

Homeland Security Presidential Directive 21 (see Chapter 3) identifies community resilience as one of the 4 most critical components of public health and medical preparedness. The Office of the Assistant Secretary for Preparedness and Response (ASPR) defines community health resilience as "the ability of a community to use its assets to strengthen public health and health care systems and to improve the community's physical, behavioral, and social health to withstand, adapt to, and recover from adversity." Community resilience also is a domain in the Centers for Disease Control and Prevention's Public Health Preparedness Capabilities described through 2 components—community preparedness and community recovery. Community preparedness, defined by the ability to prepare for, withstand, and recover from public health incidents, is key to being resilient.

A resilient community is one that has developed resources to protect its residents from the impact of major disruptions. Having these resources in place in advance of a disaster helps communities take effective collective action after an adverse event. The capacity of a community to adapt is dependent on having both the necessary volume and diversity of resources to cope with any disruption and the systems and skills to coordinate and utilize those resources. Communities, and people, with fewer resources are less resilient because they are less able to cope with the loss of scarcer resources. As example, people who live in less prepared communities and who don't have the financial resources to prepare for disaster by storing supplies or modifying their residences, have been hit harder when disaster strikes their community because the supplies the need may not be immediately available or they may not have the money to replace what they lost.

Resilient communities have the capacity to anticipate, prepare for emergencies, and plan for the future. Resilient communities involve their residents in the process of responding and recovering with members of the community working with each other to plan and carry out tasks. They believe that individual preparedness is a public responsibility and that residents are partners who multiply the community's capacity to respond. Emergency planners bring the members of resilient communities into the process and assimilate and coordinate their perspectives within the emergency plan.

Communities are more resilient when *social capital*, the network of social connections between people, holds a community together. Individuals with large social networks are more resilient than are those acting alone, because of their collective resources. For example, the larger one's social network, the more likely the person will receive information about protective actions to take during an emergency. Communities in which evacuation programs use public facilities or churches to shelter people can create social environments in those facilities to connect people who know each other. Social media is an excellent example of an avenue for sharing information. Furthermore, those who have networks and relationships before an emergency can more rapidly mobilize necessary resources and support. To increase resilience, people in a community must be engaged in preparedness activities for themselves, their households, and their communities. In addition, responders should work to advance the development of naturally occurring social supports postimpact and during recovery.

Resilience and Disaster Recovery

Developing community resilience is mutually beneficial to both disaster planners and community members. Whereas some people are more resilient than others, an individual's ability to resist and overcome the hardship associated with disasters is dependent upon the resilience of the communities in which they live and work and vice versa. Communities develop resilience by creating the capacity to respond, by encouraging both preparedness and strong community systems, and by tackling the important factors that impact health and public health. Building upon key preparedness activities, such as organizations maintaining plans for continuity of operations and families reviewing reunification arrangements, resilience can be enhanced by encouraging social connections and improving the health and community systems that are already in place.

Vulnerability and Resilience

When a community is able to increase the resilience of individuals, including socially vulnerable populations, it increases its overall resilience. Unfortunately "raising all boats" is a difficult task since socially vulnerable populations are disproportionately exposed to risk and less able to avoid or adapt to potential harm. People with psychosocial problems before an emergency disproportionately experience lack of access to services; property loss or damage leading to displacement from their homes; injury, illness, and death; domestic violence; and loss of employment after a disaster. Individuals who are unable to prepare for, respond to, or recover from emergencies are considered to have *social vulnerability* (for a more detailed discussion, see Chapter 11). People with social vulnerability are less likely to be resilient and more likely to suffer disproportionately because they are more often socially isolated, have fewer institutional connections, and are less engaged with their communities. Social isolation is a key factor in an individual's preparedness and resilience.

The Federal Emergency Management Agency's (FEMA) National Mitigation Framework encourages local governments to identify the most socially vulnerable in their communities and to engage community organizations in the emergency planning process which might provide services to identified vulnerable groups. Any plans should include a clear set of actions to take that would reduce their risk. While the identification of socially vulnerable individuals within a community might result in a long list that appears challenging, working across organizations will maximize the ability to build capacity and resilience within these vulnerable groups.

One strategy is to identify those who will most likely be the first responders for vulnerable populations. For example, parents or teachers will probably be the first to help children during and following a disaster. Helping them prepare to respond effectively will improve resilience for the children in their charge.

Resilience for Children and Families

Following Hurricane Katrina, many lessons were learned about helping children and families adapt to the tremendous losses that they experienced. To foster child and family resilience, community officials and others involved in the response to an event should do the following:

- Promote control, empowerment, and normalcy.
- Reunite families as quickly as possible.
- Help families recognize strengths and resources.
- Assist the integration of those who were evacuated into the community.
- Encourage proactive measures to cope with change and losses.
- Provide ready access to basic human needs.
- Treat individuals with dignity and respect.
- Be sure that those with functional needs are assisted in the most appropriate way possible.

Resilience and Recovery Intervention Model

Although disasters affect a whole community or region, individuals within the same community or region do not all react in the same manner. Many individuals might need assistance, but not everyone will benefit from the same type of aid. The challenge is identifying those who need more support and proactively delivering those services. So the first step in building resilience is identifying those in need. Despite being traumatized, many who survive find themselves having a life experience that makes them feel stronger.

Increasing an individual's and a community's capacity (i.e., the resources that can be deployed to address community problems) to adapt requires an identification and implementation of protective actions. Several strategies can be implemented by community officials to foster the development of psychological body armor. These include the following:

- Be ready to support the community in all sectors of society, including government, nonprofit, and business sectors.
- Develop perception of credible and competent leadership.
- Provide practical preparation by establishing realistic expectations.

- Develop stress management and coping skills through preparatory training.
- Train civilian volunteers in basic skills, capacities, and an understanding of their responsibilities.
- Build redundancy into support systems, preparedness plans, and community capacity.
- Ensure effective communication with accurate information, reassurance, direction, motivation, and a sense of connectedness.
- Promote the development of social support and solid group structures.
- Build the perception of an ability to organize, take action, and view stressful events as challenges that can be overcome.
- Foster positive awareness and insight, as well as positive memories of those who have died.

Interventions to help people return to normal functioning include the following:

- Get people to a safe place and help them understand that they are safe.
- Use media to inform the public about risks and provide calming assurance.
- Provide accurate information from a trusted source about danger and options for action.
- Furnish needed resources.
- Provide needed care for medical, mental, and substance-use conditions.

Strategies to Build Resilient Communities

A community's recovery is dependent on its ability to collaborate with all community partners to plan and advocate for the rebuilding of public health, medical, and behavioral health systems. Community engagement to create resilience is enhanced through public health techniques—health education and promotion (i.e., incorporating behavioral health promotion through the training of a community's residents in psychological first aid), evaluation (i.e., evaluating the planning for continuity of operations for behavioral health programs and facilities), and community-based participatory research (i.e., engaging behavioral health and social service systems and the people they serve in an active role in a community's preparedness efforts, and bringing civic organizations together to develop emergency preparedness and response functions that support the health of the community).

Developing resilience to restore the community to at least the same level of health and social functioning involves a community understanding its vulnerabilities and building capacity in advance by taking the following actions:

- Engage across organizations to plan a response that identifies threats, has mechanisms to mobilize residents and volunteers, and reduces vulnerabilities including socioeconomic conditions by working with manpower and resources external to the community to create strong networks. Robust networks include social services,

behavioral health, community organizations, businesses, academia, at-risk individuals, and faith-based stakeholders in addition to traditional public health, health care, and emergency management partners.
- Strengthen public health, health care, and social services so that these systems can support health resilience during disasters and emergencies.
- Local leadership maintains a focus on preparedness and responding rapidly, effectively, and fairly by anticipating problems, opportunities to improve, and the potential for surprise.
- Conduct diverse and culturally relevant education about risks to the community.
- Encourage community members to engage in individual preparedness that is self-sufficient.
- Use what is learned from each disaster to strengthen the community's ability to withstand the next.

Building this capacity might include activities such as ensuring that people understand the risks and what they can do to protect themselves, have access to needed health care, watch out for elderly neighbors and relatives, and share complementary resources. Communities across the United States are working to improve their ability to withstand disaster. In 2015 Los Angeles released "Resilience by Design," which made recommendations to protect her residents by improving the city's capacity to respond to earthquakes.

Organizing Disaster Behavioral Health Services

Section 416 of The Robert T. Stafford Disaster Relief and Emergency Assistance Act of 1988 (Public Law 100-707; available at: http://www.fema.gov/pdf/about/stafford_act.pdf) establishes legislative authority for the president to provide training and services to alleviate behavioral health problems caused or exacerbated by major disasters. The act reads as follows:

> Crisis Counseling Assistance and Training. The President is authorized to provide professional counseling services, including financial assistance to State or local agencies or private mental health organizations to provide such services or training of disaster workers, to survivors/victims of major disaster in order to relieve mental health problems caused or aggravated by such major disaster or its aftermath. (42 U.S.C. § 5183, at 47.)

Federally, the Crisis Counseling Assistance and Training Program is funded by FEMA and administered through an interagency federal partnership between FEMA and the Substance Abuse and Mental Health Services Administration (SAMHSA) Center for Mental Health Services. Their *Field Manual for Mental Health and Human Service*

Workers in Major Disasters should be used as a guide for establishing community programs (available at: http://store.samhsa.gov/product/Field-Manual-for-Mental-Health-and-Human-Service-Workers-in-Major-Disasters/ADM90-0537).

In February 2014, the U.S. Department of Health & Human Services (HHS) released the *HHS Disaster Behavioral Health Concept of Operations*, which details the Concept of Operations plan (CONOPS; available at: http://www.phe.gov/Preparedness/planning/abc/Documents/dbh-conops-2014.pdf) that describes how HHS coordinates their department's federal response and recovery activities to help a community recover from the behavioral health effects of a disaster. While the CONOPS focuses on federal-level operations, it is recognized that most disaster behavioral health assets (e.g., personnel, facilities, support systems) operate at state and local levels. This conceptual framework aims to improve the coordination of federal efforts in support of the behavioral health services provided by states, localities, and territories.

At the state and local levels, key community services come from a system of voluntary organizations, government, academia, and behavioral health care and professional organizations. The federal role is to collaborate with these entities to promote a behavioral health response that is integrated into the broader public health and medical response and recovery efforts. In this role, federal agencies supplement the local response based on the state's defined behavioral health needs.

What Services Are Needed

The organization for and delivery of behavioral health services should be part of a community's overall disaster plan to avoid the difficult task of recruiting and orienting masses of professional volunteers in the chaos immediately following a disaster. Before developing the community plan for behavioral services, it is useful to consider the range and types of services that might be required and to understand the needs of those impacted by a disaster, the environments in which one will be providing service, and the manner in which services are to be provided. For example, agencies coordinating the management of human remains are encouraged to develop programs that provide psychological and emotional support and behavioral health care for workers during and after recovery activities. Table 8-2 describes the types of behavioral services that are likely to be required in a major disaster. Although the services needed may vary with the nature of the event, such as type of disaster, severity, and time of year, in previous events a pattern of social and counseling services has been required.

The Disaster Behavioral Health Capacity Assessment Tool is used to help state and local agencies as well as provider organizations assess the capacity of their community to provide behavioral health services following a disaster and then integrate those services into all planning, preparedness, response and recovery efforts. This tool helps a

Table 8-2. Community Behavioral Services Needed Following a Disaster

- Adult, adolescent, and child services
- Assessments, crisis interventions, evaluations, and referrals
- Bereavement counseling
- Business counseling
- Crisis counseling
- Debriefing groups for health care and emergency workers
- Drop-in crisis counseling
- Early intervention services
- Emergency services in medical emergency departments
- Family support center
- Individual and group counseling
- Mobile mental and substance-use crisis teams
- Multidisciplinary services to designated community sites (e.g., police precincts, fire departments, temporary business locations)
- Multilingual services
- Psychological first aid
- Outpatient behavioral health services and counseling
- Ongoing support groups
- Outreach to schools for students, parents, and teachers
- Outpatient services
- Risk and crisis communication with stakeholders
- School presentations
- Short-term treatment
- Telephone triage
- 24-hour emergency psychiatric service
- 24-hour crisis hotline
- Use of pharmaceuticals
- Walk-in services
- Weekly support groups

community identify specific elements of planning and preparedness, the existence of partnerships and how well they are integrated, availability of training, and mechanisms to providing a behavioral health response following a disaster. The tool is available at: http://www.phe.gov/Preparedness/planning/abc/Documents/dbh-capacity-tool.pdf.

Survey of Existing Services

With potential post-disaster needs understood, a jurisdiction can map those against the resources available to determine whether a community has the resources to deliver these extra services or whether additional capacity is needed. The behavioral health community should gather a compendium of available professionals and/or programs, including experts in critical areas (e.g., post-traumatic stress disorder, children's behavioral health, death and dying), and identify where gaps exist. The list should include the credentials and emergency contact information for the professionals and programs, the location of specialized treatment and outreach services in the community (such as employee assistance programs, housing, restoration of utilities), and be updated regularly.

Staffing

With the increased interest and training that has been initiated in every behavioral health discipline since the 2001 attack on the World Trade Center buildings, it is likely that larger communities can bring together a sufficient cadre of local behavioral health responders. It is advantageous, where possible, to establish a core of trained and credentialed culturally competent professionals from the providers within a community. The advantage of using local providers is that they are knowledgeable about and work with the community's resources and customs, existing organizations, and support networks on a daily basis. In the initial stages, victims are interested in getting relief for practical, concrete problems, such as loss of shelter or business interruptions, and volunteers from outside the community may not have information to match the local resources with the need. Further, in a major disaster, it will be an additional strain to divert staff to train out-of-town volunteers about the community.

Where there are identified service gaps in a community and when the need exceeds the capacity, the behavioral health community should expand its capacity or reach out for federal support because of an anticipated surge in those needing both short- and long-term services. The number of behavioral health professionals needed will vary by existing resources. Federal Mental Health Teams (MHTs) can be deployed as part of a state's request for services. The function of MHTs is described in the HHS CONOPS.

When conducting the needs assessment to determine the number of behavioral health providers required, look at the demographics of the community, the magnitude and scope of the disaster, the potential number of subgroups affected within the community and the number of individuals within those groups, the cultural issues of those subgroups, and the potential behavioral health resources available. Further, in the weeks and months during recovery, when volunteers have gone, programs should be instituted with sufficient staffing for those individuals who need long-term behavioral health intervention. Deployment of behavioral health staff will depend on the number of people affected and the circumstances of the event, but as a guide communities have previously activated 40 behavioral health professionals per 250 victims.

When behavioral health resources from outside the community are likely to be required, advance planning should include memorandums of understanding (MOU) with the organizations to be called on for additional manpower and support. Such MOUs address the use of multiagency providers and community providers, roles and boundaries of each agency, plans for deployment and delivery of service by type of service, and establishment of a chain of command for services for both concrete and behavioral and substance-use conditions following a disaster. When developing these memorandums, coordination with the state or local office of emergency management is needed to ensure that the plan conforms to the community's broader emergency management plans. Finally, reimbursement for delivering behavioral health services will likely be funded through a federal contract with the state department of mental health, which will in turn contract with the local department, which will contract with local agencies.

Following the school shooting at Sandy Hook Elementary School in 2012, a U.S. Public Health Service MHT was deployed to Newtown, Connecticut, to provide mental health support as part of the overall request for support sent by officials to the ASPR. In addition to the MHT, other federal staff, including regional emergency coordinators who served as HHS liaison officers to the commissioners for the department of health and for mental health and addiction services for the state of Connecticut were involved during the disaster response.

Volunteers

Immediately after a disaster, there is often an infusion of volunteer professionals from outside the community offering their assistance. The registration and orientation of the behavioral health volunteers who arrive from outside the impacted region is a time-consuming task. A mechanism for incorporating and credentialing these volunteer providers should be worked out in advance as part of a community's planning with local behavioral health agencies and the various responding organizations.

Community emergency response plans provide for the American Red Cross (Red Cross) to deliver disaster services. If response to a significant disaster is projected to exceed resources, the local Red Cross chapter alerts the state chapter, which alerts the national system. The national Red Cross determines if the response will be regional or national. When the Red Cross gets activated, it issues a call to respond to all chapters in that area. Although the Red Cross views all disasters as local, with municipal or county governments initiating response, in large-scale disasters activation may start before any official call is made. When the Red Cross mental health unit is activated, the local department of mental health is responsible for coordinating services delivered, although there will be close coordination with the Red Cross.

Mental health volunteers through the Red Cross are all credentialed or licensed professionals in the states in which they practice. Each chapter of the Red Cross is responsible for verifying the background of behavioral health volunteers, including receiving a copy of their professional license. These volunteers are trained in a 2-day, 16-hour course to provide crisis intervention with clients and modified defusing and debriefing for response workers. Another national nonprofit organization that identifies psychiatrists and credentials them before they arrive is Disaster Psychiatry Outreach.

Organizing Culturally Sensitive Services

To include culture considerations in behavioral health plans following disasters, service providers need specialized knowledge, skills, and attitudes. The agency organizing the culturally sensitive services needs appropriate policies and structures to offer supportive care to diverse populations. SAMHSA's Center for Mental Health Services published guidelines stating that behavioral health workers need to have the following traits to be competent in carrying out services to diverse populations. The behavioral health worker must:

- value diversity,
- have the capacity for cultural assessment,
- be aware of cross-cultural dynamics,
- develop cultural knowledge, and
- adapt service delivery to reflect an understanding of cultural diversity.

Those who need assistance may distrust offers of help from people who are not part of their group, and may be more willing to accept help if they are working with those of similar backgrounds. The availability of trained bilingual and bicultural staff is key to success. If indigenous workers are not available, agencies should work to recruit staff from other agencies or jurisdictions with the same racial or ethnic background and language skills as those affected by the disaster. It is preferable to work with trained translators rather than family members, such as children, because of the importance of preserving a parent's role in the family and general privacy concerns regarding behavioral health issues.

In addition, because some groups may not be familiar with the mechanisms required to apply for assistance, those working directly with disaster victims should ensure that their description of facts, policies, and procedures are understood and properly interpreted. Disaster information and application procedures should be translated into the primary spoken languages of the communities in the catchment area and also be available in recordings that can be viewed.

To develop a culturally competent behavioral health plan, planners must perform the following:

- Assess and understand the makeup of the communities to be served.
- Identify the needs of the communities that are associated with a culture.
- Know about institutions (both formal and informal) within the communities that can provide diverse behavioral health services.
- Establish working relationships in advance with organizations, service providers, and cultural leaders and gatekeepers who are trusted by diverse communities.
- Anticipate and identify solutions to culturally related difficulties that may arise in delivering disaster services.

Delivery of Services

Cultural background can influence how and whether an individual seeks help, uses natural support networks, and relies on their customs and traditions to deal with trauma, loss, and healing. Individuals from cultures that believe traumatic events have spiritual causes may be less receptive to help. In many cultures, individuals reach out to family, friends, or cultural leaders before seeking help from government or nonprofit agencies. They prefer to receive services from familiar community groups. Places of worship also function as an important support in ethnic communities. Further, some refugee groups, fearing deportation, may be reluctant to seek services.

Different cultural groups experience the phases of a disaster differently. There are cultural variations in the expression of emotion, the manifestation and description of psychological symptoms, traditions about death and burial, and views about counseling. For example, Hispanics are more likely than are non-Hispanics to seek information about disasters from social networks and to believe the information received through these networks. In some cultures, age also can affect how an individual responds, with the old and young responding differently. The old and young may have different needs in identifying with and functioning in cross-cultural environments. Finally, different cultures handle grief in different ways. Helping a community carry out their usual burial rituals can facilitate the return to normal functioning.

If a community remains intact, their cultural norms, traditions, and values will provide support. However, if a community is devastated, the usual cultural mechanisms can be overwhelmed and unable to meet the extraordinary demands. Behavioral health programs should work to expedite the rebuilding of the cultural community. In Asian American and Pacific Islander cultures, the individual does not exist apart from the group, so it is crucial to strengthen family relationships and their connection to the community.

Death Notification

In preparing for catastrophic disasters with many deaths, it is important to establish protocols in advance to ensure smooth coordination. Legally, notification of death is the task of the medical examiner who may extend that duty to local law enforcement. The Red Cross prefers that behavioral health professionals from the community sit with law enforcement officials when they speak to families about the death of loved ones. Behavioral health coordination with local law enforcement should outline how the 2 disciplines will work together as survivors file reports for missing persons, review death lists, and engage in DNA collection.

Staff Training

As part of the management plan for assessment, referral, and treatment, social service agencies should provide general information (e.g., fact sheets, contact information for resources and consultants) to all staff members. Similar documents can also be distributed to the public at the reception desk, waiting rooms, and cafeteria. Agencies should provide facts about expected normal responses to media spokespersons so that they can educate the community about issues related to grief and loss and explain the role of the mental health and behavioral response within the emergency. They should establish a toll-free hotline for the community, including 24-hour, 7-day coverage. Coordination with other behavioral health providers in the community—including hospitals, community mental health centers, youth services organizations, and group homes should be part of the plan. The behavioral health services plan must ensure that culturally competent providers will be available to meet the needs of their community both in the crisis period immediately after the disaster and in the months and years that follow. Finally, provisions should include a transition period for the staff and agencies involved in delivering services since these individuals will personally need time to reenergize and recover from their experience before they can go back to business as usual.

A community may not have a plan for providing behavioral health services. When determining whether to establish behavioral health and psychosocial services, 7 criteria have been suggested[3] for evaluating the need to develop these services. These criteria include the following:

- The role of epidemiology and community concerns in determining the prevalence of health and mental and substance-use conditions
- Predictability, rapidity of onset, duration of the crisis, and severity of the problems
- Adequacy of resources
- Sustainability
- Political and ethical acceptability
- Cultural sensitivity
- Effectiveness

Table 8-3 summarizes the steps in establishing disaster services for mental and substance-use conditions.

Setting Up Family Assistance Centers

In large-scale disasters, one of the first activities is the establishment of a central place where victims and their families can go for relief. Communities might consider establishing

3. Speckhard A. 2002. Voices From the Inside: Psychological Response From Toxic Disasters. In: Havenaar JM, Cwikel JG, Bromet EJ, eds. *Toxic Turmoil: Psychological and Societal Consequences of Ecological Disasters.* New York, NY: Kluwer Academic/Plenum.

Table 8-3. Establishing Disaster Behavioral Health Services

1. Establish a Disaster Behavioral Health Preparedness Committee whose membership represents administrative, environmental, allied behavioral health, and community agency interests.
2. Establish an organization chart to manage emergencies.
3. Establish objectives of disaster behavioral health services, including definition of roles and responsibilities.
4. Establish procedures for emergency response.
5. Establish procedures for evaluation of mental status and distribution of psychiatric drugs and assisted treatment for substance abuse.
6. Incorporate procedures into community's disaster plan.
7. Develop memorandums of understanding between each organization and other key agencies within the community (e.g., Red Cross, community agencies, medical examiner, law enforcement).
8. Train behavioral health staff in disaster behavioral health plan, roles, and responsibilities.
9. Prepare education materials and preassemble for distribution.
10. Schedule regular mock exercises with outside review.
11. Regularly review and update emergency plan, including evaluation of resources and potential impediments to implementation.

Source: Adapted from Department of Veterans Affairs (VA). 1997. *Disaster Mental Health Services: A Guidebook for Clinicians and Administrators.* Washington, DC: VA.

2 distinct assistance centers: 1 for the victims, their families, and friends, and 1 for the responders and caregivers. These centers are multipurpose, established to meet the needs of a broad group of people, and are intended to bring all of the agencies or services that a family needs to deal with to a single location. As part of a community's disaster plan, 2 elements should be identified in advance: location with adequate space and personnel.

The first component is the identification of a location with adequate space so that these centers do not have to be relocated once they are open. Sufficient space is needed for all of the functions, and private space must be carefully thought out to minimize retraumatization. Table 8-4 describes the type of services that might be provided at a family assistance center.

The organization of the space must accommodate desks or areas where each of these activities can occur. It is possible that need evolves in catastrophic disasters and that more space and services are required than initially thought. Dedicated areas should be designated where private conversations can occur and where a drop-in center, much like a surgical waiting room, can be an environment for social support. The child care center should be located away from places where there might be strong emotional reactions. The assistance centers can provide ample food and drink to the families and staff who use them, since families needing multiple services may spend many hours at the center. Staffing decisions should consider how many shifts will be needed and the number of people simultaneously served at each agency table. At the family assistance center set up following the 2001 World Trade Center collapse, the assignment of behavioral health staff ranged from 8 to 30 per shift.

Following disasters where there has been a great loss of life, some family members may wish to visit the center repeatedly, whereas others may not. To help those who prefer less contact, when establishing the registration process, try to identify all of the things that

Table 8-4. Services Provided at Family Assistance Centers

- Child care
- Crisis counseling
- Death certificate processing
- Disaster Medicaid
- Distribution of gifts and donations received
- Emergency financial assistance
- Employment assistance
- Family reunification
- Food stamps
- Follow-up phone calls to recipients of crisis counseling
- Health and medical assistance, including pharmaceuticals and durable medical equipment
- Housing assistance
- Immigration services
- Legal assistance
- Meals for victims, families, responders, and caregivers
- Medication assessments
- Personal care items
- Phone banks
- Relief application assistance through FEMA
- Small Business Association loans
- Stress management for relief workers
- Training for FEMA interpreters
- Transportation
- Workers' compensation

families need to bring to register a missing family member. This registration list should include legal documentation (e.g., birth certificate, driver's license, Social Security card, marriage license) and sources of scientific information (e.g., hair samples, dental records) used for DNA testing and victim identification when necessary. Expect variability in family reactions, their behavior, and how much families hear of what is said to them.

Especially following disasters where a prolonged search and rescue operation is necessary, the assistance center for responders and caregivers will provide food and drink, showers, sleeping cots, changing rooms, and debriefing areas. These should be located in close proximity to where the disaster occurred, whereas the family assistance center should be located in a different, more distant part of the community.

The second component is the designation of personnel (by title and organization) who will serve as the administrators of this center once it is opened. An advance agreement on leadership is essential to avoid spending time establishing the management scheme while trying to set up the assistance centers.

In planning for the establishment of assistance centers, it is useful to consider who the users will be. In planning for the delivery of services, it is important to have preestablished protocols for the delivery of basic crisis intervention, medical intervention (e.g.,

Table 8-5. Types of Individuals Using Family Assistance Centers

- Family members of the deceased
- Those displaced from or who lost housing
- Workers who lost jobs
- Those whose business was interrupted
- Those who experienced prior trauma or have preexisting mental health or substance- abuse conditions
- Those who lost financial and social supports
- Responders and other caregivers

prescriptions), psychiatric referrals for prescriptions, and services to those needing immediate attention. Table 8-5 lists the types of individuals who may use these centers.

Patient Locator System

After a disaster resulting in many injuries and deaths, the most pressing behavioral health needs are those of family and friends wanting to know what happened to their loved ones, employers wanting to track their employees, and authorities wanting to account for people who are missing. When telephones do not function, the ability to contact hospitals may be impeded. Even if loved ones can connect, hospital operators only have the names of those admitted to their facility. In incidents such as these, the need for a patient locator system is paramount. Although people want to know the information immediately, it may take several days to get the system running if it is not in place in advance. If no preexisting system is in place, hospitals will likely fax emergency department logs to a central collection point and volunteers will need to sort through the logs and organize a database. Importantly, there will be numerous legal hurdles to overcome because of privacy concerns.

To establish a patient locator system in advance, several steps are necessary. A Web site or placeholder on a Web site of a central authority, such as the state department of health should be created. Every hospital should be able to log in and use Public Health Information Network messaging standards to securely upload patient information to create a database searchable by match. Reportable information should include patients who present at each emergency department, including unidentified patients and those who come into a unit (e.g., a burn unit) and cannot speak. Data may not be precise, so it is better to include the name and age of all patients and sort the list later. Each list should identify the hospital and provide contact information. In time, the list will get cleaned as names of patients whose visits were unrelated to the disaster are removed. To ensure patient privacy, the lists should be constructed so that users search by typing in a name and seeking a match rather than scrolling through names. The plan for the patient locator system should include daily printing and posting of the identified list at the family assistance center(s). Plans for the system should include hospital switchboard training so those answering the phone can explain how the system is set up and how to provide information about patients who were treated and released, within the guidelines of the Health Insurance Portability and Accountability Act of 1996.

Public Health Intervention

Natural Disasters

The delivery of psychosocial services following a disaster strongly emphasizes the principle of prevention using a multifaceted, multilevel approach aimed at helping individuals, groups, and the community as a whole. Most of the early work will be the provision of concrete services to psychologically normal people who are under stress, such as information about available services, how to get insurance benefits or loans, assistance with applications at government agencies, health care, child care, transportation, and other routine needs. Public health workers should initiate counseling as a preventive measure and encourage open communication. Some of the most important ways of helping may be simply listening and indicating interest or concern.

If evacuation is required, responders should keep families together and try to keep support systems intact. Workers can also help in rebuilding support networks as quickly as possible. During the short- and long-term recovery phases, public health and human service professionals will visit community sites where survivors are involved in the activities of their daily lives. Such places include neighborhoods, schools, shelters, disaster application centers, meal sites, hospitals, churches, community centers, and other central locations. Among the services typically provided after disaster are telephone help lines, information and referral services, literature on the emotional effects of disaster, facilitation of self-help, support groups, crisis counseling, public education through the media, information sessions for community groups, grief support services, and advocacy services. Behavioral health workers are important members of the teams who help workers cope with the recovery and identification of dead bodies, and communicate positive identification to families, significant others and domestic partners.

Encouraging parents to reduce their children's exposure to the media is important, as is encouraging them to talk about their experiences. This includes reduction in exposure to graphic images on television, newspapers, and computers. In addition, it is important to reach out not only to those directly involved, but also to those with indirect exposure (e.g., having a friend who knew someone who was killed or injured). Further, it is important to ensure that trauma and grief counseling interventions are included in a community's disaster plan.

Psychological First Aid

While there are many approaches to providing behavioral services following a disaster (see Appendix M), psychological first aid (PFA) is commonly used to reduce initial distress and to nurture short- and long-term adaptive functioning. PFA is an evidence-informed approach for helping people in the immediate aftermath of disaster and terrorism. A brief outline of the PFA model is described in Appendix L.

The program can be used by first responders, incident command systems, primary and emergency health care providers, school crisis response teams, faith-based organizations, disaster relief organizations, Community Emergency Response Teams, Medical Reserve Corps, and the Citizens Corps in diverse settings.

A PFA mobile app is available at http://www.ptsd.va.gov/professional/materials/apps/pfa_mobile_app.asp. The Mobile App materials were adapted from the *Psychological First Aid Field Operations Guide* (Second Edition) available at: http://www.ptsd.va.gov/professional/manuals/manual-pdf/pfa/PFA_2ndEditionwithappendices.pdf.

Man-Made Disasters

There is evidence to suggest that the most advantageous intervention with communities exposed to a man-made disaster is to establish open communication between officials and the community. Because of the potential spread of toxic agents in environmental disasters, planning should be regional. It is important to establish cooperation among public health, medical, media, and advocacy groups as part of everyday practice around environmental issues, so that if a man-made disaster strikes a community, good working relationships are already in place. Part of the plan should include training service workers to have a basic understanding of the technical aspects of environmental contamination, as well as the needs of the community in these complex situations.

Interdisciplinary cooperation is needed among psychologists, social workers, and educators. As in natural disaster, initial programs should offer practical assistance with concrete services—advice, shelter, clothing, and referral to medical care and evaluation. Care should be coordinated among the breadth of health, mental health, and social service agencies and educational institutions. The community will need a broad range of social needs—family counseling, support groups, day care, play therapy, information services, and health education. Immediately after the incident or release, it is important to provide accurate health information, assure the availability of physical exams, provide supportive counseling, and prepare specialized materials to help the entire community understand and deal with the situation.

Throughout the disaster relief effort, several general management strategies should be followed:

- Show clear decision making in actions so victims feel that the designated leaders are active in the response.
- Issue warnings with instructions of specific actions to take.

- Plan ahead for necessary resources, with call-up procedures in place.
- Tailor activities and services provided in the aftermath of disaster to the community being served and involve them in the development and delivery of services.
- Target psychosocial services toward psychologically normal people responding normally to an abnormal situation.
- Identify people at risk for severe psychological or social impairment caused by their experience of the disaster.

Early Intervention With Mass Violence

The National Institute of Mental Health (NIMH) convened an expert panel to develop recommendations regarding early intervention following events involving mass violence. In addition, the U.S. Department of Justice and the Federal Bureau of Investigation developed a toolkit to help communities prepare for and respond to victims of mass violence and terrorism. The toolkit is available at: http://ovc.gov/pubs/mvt-toolkit/about-toolkit.html. The NIMH panel recommended that:

- Components of early intervention should include preparation, planning, education, training, service provision, and evaluation.
- In the immediate post-incident phase, expect a normal recovery.
- Do not presume a clinically significant disorder in the early post-incident phase, except when there is a preexisting condition.
- Participation of survivors of mass violence in early intervention sessions, whether administered to a group or individually, should be voluntary.
- Integrate mental health personnel into emergency management teams.
- People's "hierarchy of needs" should be recognized within the early intervention (e.g., survival, safety, security, food, shelter, health, triage, orientation, communication with family and friends).
- Follow-up should be offered to those:
  - who have ASD or other clinically significant symptoms stemming from the trauma,
  - who are bereaved,
  - who have a preexisting psychiatric disorder,
  - who require medical or surgical attention, and
  - whose exposure to the incident is particularly intense and of long duration.

Table 8-6 describes the components of an early intervention with those exposed to mass violence.

Table 8-6. Early Interventions Following Mass Violence

Activity	Actions
Psychological First Aid	• Protect survivors from further harm. • Reduce physiological arousal. • Mobilize support. • Keep families together and facilitate reunions with loved ones. • Provide information and encourage communication and education. • Communicate risk effectively.
Needs Assessment	• Assess current status of individuals, groups, populations, and institutions/systems. • Ask how well needs are being addressed, what the recovery environment offers, and what additional interventions are needed.
Monitoring Recovery Environment	• Observe and listen to those most affected. • Monitor the environment for toxins and stressors. • Monitor past and ongoing threats. • Monitor services that are being provided. • Monitor media coverage and rumors.
Outreach and Information Dissemination	• Offer information/education. • Use established community structures. • Distribute flyers. • Host Web sites. • Conduct media interviews and programs and distribute media releases.
Technical Assistance, Consultation, and Training	• Improve capacity of organizations and caregivers to provide what is needed to: ○ reestablish community structure, ○ foster family recovery and resilience, and ○ safeguard the community. • Provide assistance, consultation, and training to relevant organizations, other caregivers and responders, and leaders.

(Continued)

Table 8-6. (Continued)

Activity	Actions
Fostering Resilience, coping, and Recovery	• Encourage but do not force social interactions. • Provide coping skills training. • Provide risk assessment skills training. • Provide education on stress responses, traumatic reminders, coping, normal versus abnormal functioning, risk factors, and services. • Offer group and family interventions. • Facilitate natural support networks. • Look after the bereaved. • Repair the organizational fabric.
Triage	• Conduct clinical assessments, using valid and reliable methods. • Refer when indicated. • Identify vulnerable, high-risk individuals and groups. • Provide for emergency hospitalization.

Treatment	• Reduce or ameliorate symptoms or improve functioning via:
	  ○ individual, family, and group psychotherapy,
	  ○ pharmacotherapy, and
	  ○ short- or long-term hospitalization.

Source: Based on National Institute of Mental Health. 2002. *Mental Health and Mass Violence: Evidence-Based Early Psychological Intervention for Victims/Survivors of Mass Violence. A Workshop to Reach Consensus on Best Practices.* NIH Publication No. 02-5138. Washington, DC: US Government Printing Office. Available at: https://www.hsdl.org/?view&did=441844. Accessed January 20, 2017.

CHAPTER 9

ENVIRONMENTAL HEALTH ISSUES

Maintaining environmental health is essential to preventing disease following disasters. Because of the complexity of environmental issues, there is seldom a single environmental health specialist responsible for all of the environmental problems that follow a disaster. In complex large-scale disasters and disasters in urban areas, it is common for numerous governmental agencies and consultants at all levels to be pulled together to coordinate an environmental response. This chapter addresses common environmental problems that require intervention by public health professionals including ensuring proper sanitation and waste disposal, maintaining safety of water and food supplies, feeding and ensuring adequate heating and shelter for large numbers of people, controlling diarrheal diseases, safe use of generators, conducting mold remediation, and controlling vector populations.

Public Health Role

- Provide technical assistance in addressing environmental threats and hazards.
- Contain or remove sources of environmental contamination, or evacuate people to ensure that they are no longer exposed to the hazard.
- Conduct quantitative monitoring of environmental services, including environmental sampling.
- Ensure the replacement or repair of existing sanitary barriers and waste management.
- Provide guidance, education, and assurance of safe water, safe food, safe air, and safe shelter to compensate for disrupted clean environments.
- Ensure that people impacted by the disaster have sufficient cooking utensils, equipment, and fuel to cook and store food safely.
- Inspect temporary housing, mass feeding centers, drinking water distribution, and areas where waste disposal is handled.
- Provide commercial toilets and hand washing stations.
- Supervise construction of latrines, if toilets are not available.
- Provide regular advisories to the public and the medical community.

Reducing Exposure to Environmental Hazards

Disrupted environments have variable effects on health depending on the presence of endemic disease, the susceptibility and habits of the population, and the availability of protective measures. The types of illnesses most often spread, such as respiratory infections and gastrointestinal disease causing diarrhea, are those that have a short transmission cycle and incubation period and are widespread. Public health professionals can use 3 major approaches to reduce exposure to environmental hazards: instituting measures of control, establishing multiple barriers, and providing distance between hazards and populations at risk.

Instituting Measures of Control: Certain hazards move through the environment and cause harm to humans. Public health professionals can control disease by preventing the hazard from being released or occurring, by preventing the transport of the hazard, or by preventing people from being exposed to the hazard. For example, when trains carrying drums of toxic chemicals derail, responders first try to keep the chemicals from being released into the air, and if containment is not possible, potentially affected residents are asked to evacuate or advised to shelter-in-place with protective coverings over windows, doors, and vents to reduce their exposure to the chemical.

Establishing Multiple Barriers: Since no single environmental measure is fail-safe, redundant barriers must be set up between hazards and populations. Multiple sanitary barriers provide redundant protection where, for example, public health professionals protect surface water used for drinking. For drinking water, the redundant processes are physical (e.g., filtration, sedimentation, and distillation), biological (e.g., slow sand filters or biologically active carbon), and chemical (e.g., flocculation and chlorination and the use of electromagnetic radiation such as ultraviolet light). If on a given day, any of the redundant measures are not functioning, the others will reduce the hazard. Most waterborne outbreaks in the United States occur when multiple barriers fail simultaneously. Protection from environmental hazards depends on awareness of risk, diligence in surveillance, and investment in multiple barriers to keep the risk to populations low.

Providing Distance Between Hazards and Populations At Risk: In general, the distance needed to protect a population from exposure to a hazardous substance varies according to the volume and nature of the hazardous substance. The greater the distance existing between a hazard and a population, the greater the amount of time before an inadvertent release of the hazardous material reaches the populated area. With a longer time delay, the release is more likely to be detected in time for the population to take protective measures. Since most pollutants degrade or disperse over distance, providing space between hazardous materials and populations may by itself reduce human exposure.

Environmental Surveillance

Four conditions should be monitored to estimate the number of individuals whose environment is affected by a natural disaster: access to excreta disposal facilities, water consumption, the percentage of people consuming safe water, and air contaminants.

Access to Excreta Disposal Facilities: Public health officials must assess the number of people per latrine to determine the relative availability of latrines (or toilets) and the amount of sharing required. To estimate people per latrine, conduct a walk-through survey or interview people. For those who indicate that they have a family latrine, ask how many people are in their family and if they share it with anyone else. If families are using communal latrines, calculate sanitation coverage as the number of latrines divided by the number of people using them. Where people continue to live in dwellings in which not all toilets are functional, monitor the fraction of households with a functioning toilet or latrine as a proxy for sanitation coverage.

Water Consumption: Water consumption depends both on water availability and the population's ability to obtain the water. Shortages of water containers, security concerns, and long lines can all prevent plentiful sources from being fully utilized. If water companies do not have the tools for estimating demand, it is helpful for public health officials to survey the population and estimate water consumption by asking for a 24-hour recall of water use, or by monitoring how much water is collected at the various sources and dividing this by the number of people being served. Water consumption is defined in terms of gallons or liters per person per day.

Percentage of People Consuming Safe Water: In settings where groundwater supplies at wells or springs are determined to be safe to drink, monitor the fraction of people obtaining water from the safe sources versus unsafe sources. Public health workers should monitor the percentage of people who are getting safe water when it is being collected; remembering that collecting water from a safe source does not ensure that the water is safe at the time of ingestion. With piped systems, workers must collect samples at household taps throughout the system, with a collection scheme such that each sample represents a similar number of people (e.g., 1 sample per 10,000 people). The fraction of water samples that are safe corresponds to the fraction of people whose water arrives safely at the point where the water is collected.

Air Contaminants: Many disasters result in potential exposure to airborne substances, such as smoke, dust, or other contaminants. Departments of health (DOH) are responsible for monitoring the air immediately after an event occurs when there is a public health concern. DOH reviews the numerous air quality, debris sample, and personal air monitoring tests that other agencies may perform. Sometimes federal agencies, such as the Agency for Toxic Substances and Disease Registry or the U.S. Environmental Protection Agency (EPA), or the local department of environmental protection will be involved in the study of air and dust samples. These samples will be compared with standards, such as indoor air quality standards, to determine potential health effects. Exposures following disasters can also be measured by outdoor air monitors. One example, BioWatch, the system to monitor biological releases, is discussed in Chapter 12.

Sanitation During Disaster Situations

Sewage systems are a network of pipes that carry wastes away from a population. Sewers often become flooded or clogged during hurricanes, earthquakes, and floods. Hurricanes or other storms may cause untreated sewage to be washed into waterways. Clogged sewer lines may also cause waste to spill into the environment at locations where it is likely to expose large numbers of people to biological or chemical hazards. Typically, problems within sewage networks are mitigated by pumping or rerouting the sewage, which may not be possible following a disaster. Public health officials should document the location of bypass valves, confirm that they are functional and that auxiliary pumping capacity exists, and have an operational plan for storm events as part of a disaster preparedness program.

Where sanitation systems are destroyed, one of the first activities should be the reestablishment of a system of latrines since containing human excreta is the most protective environmental measure that can be taken following a disaster, depending on the type of disaster. When defecation fields are required in areas of temporary housing, their location must be thoughtfully planned. Proper spaces for defecation fields must be set aside and located away from water sources and downhill from living quarters. Latrines should be built before the population arrives at a relocation site. Importantly, to ensure personal hygiene, paper, water, and soap must be made readily available in or near the latrine, especially where diarrheal diseases and dysentery are likely to occur. Where extended recovery work is expected, set up porta-potties or workers.

The World Health Organization recommends the provision of 1 pit latrine per family. Where that is not possible, both the United Nations High Commission for Refugees and United Nations International Children's Education Fund have set a maximum target of 20 people per latrine (see Table 9-1). To the extent possible, households should not share latrines or toilets with others outside their household. Efforts should be made to build separate latrines for men and women or separate latrines for children. Privacy screens should be constructed. Establishing 1 latrine per household, rather than sharing latrines, increases the likelihood that the facilities will be kept clean. With mortality and morbidity rates among displaced populations often higher in the first days and weeks following an event, it is essential to persuade everyone to use the latrines that have been set up.

To increase use of latrines by young children, 2 approaches may be useful. First, educate child care providers about proper handling of children's feces and the importance of washing their hands after cleaning the child or handling the child's feces. Second, establish excreta disposal facilities that are child friendly (e.g., well lit, have an opening smaller than that used in adult latrines).

Public health information officers should promote hand washing, particularly after defecating and before preparing food to protect against fecal-oral illnesses. Educational messages should be short, relate to the route by which disease may be transmitted, and focus on behaviors that are key to the prevention of fecal-oral illness. Public health

Table 9-1. Minimum Water, Food, and Sanitation Requirements per Person Each Day

Essential Need	Category	Requirement
Water	Minimum maintenance	15 liters/person/day
	Feeding centers	30 liters/inpatient/day
	Health centers and hospitals	40–60 liters/inpatient/day
	1 tap stand/250 people, not >100 m from users	
Food	Maintenance	2,100 Kcals/person/day
	Shelter space	3.5 m^2/person
	Total site area	45 m^2/person for temporary planned or self-settled camps
Sanitation	Toilets	At least 1 for every 20 people
	Maximum of 1 minute walk from dwelling to toilet (≥19.7 feet and ≤164 feet)	

Source: Based on U.S. Agency for International Development (USAID). 2005. *Field Operations Guide for Disaster Assessment and Response.* Washington, DC: USAID. Available at: https://scms.usaid.gov/sites/default/files/documents/1866/fog_v4_0.pdf. Accessed January 20, 2017.

workers should likewise establish a simple monitoring component to ensure that increased hand washing (or other preventive behavior) is actually occurring.

Ensuring Water Safety

Providing people with a greater amount of reasonably safe water is more protective against fecal-oral pathogens than is providing people with a small amount of pure water. Public health officials should work closely with the agencies that are monitoring the availability of water. Estimate water consumption at least weekly during the postimpact phase. Measure water consumption by what people receive, not what the water operators produce. Water consumption can be measured through sampling, such as household interviews, or by the actual collection of water at watering points.

Attempts should be made to provide each family with their own water bucket to reduce the risk of illness. The average water consumption should be 3.9 gallons (15 liters) per person per day, with no one consuming less than 5 liters or 1 gallon per person per day. This recommendation includes 2.5 to 3 liters per day for basic survival (i.e., drinking and food), depending on the climate and individual physiology; 2 to 6 liters per day for basic hygiene, depending on social and cultural norms; and 3 to 6 liters per day for basic cooking needs, depending on the types of food prepared and social and cultural norms. Table 9-1 lists the basic water, food, and sanitation requirements following disasters.

A 3- to 5-day supply of water (5 gallons per person) should be stored for food preparation, bathing, brushing teeth, and dishwashing. Where residents are preparing supplies in advance of a disaster, such as earthquake-prone California, they should store water in sturdy plastic bottles with tight fitting lids. Stored water should be located away from the storage of toxic substances and should be changed every 6 months.

Water for Drinking and Cooking

Safe drinking water includes bottled, boiled, or treated water. Residents should drink only bottled, boiled, or treated water until the supply is tested and found safe. They must be instructed not to use contaminated water to wash dishes, brush teeth, wash and prepare food, or make ice. All bottled water from an unknown source must be boiled or treated before use. To kill harmful bacteria and parasites, residents should bring water to a rolling boil for 1 minute. To maintain water quality while in storage, add 2 drops of household bleach per gallon. Water may also be treated with 2 iodine tablets for 1 quart of water. Each 20 milligram tablet of tetraglycine hydroperiodide releases 8 parts per million of titratable iodine per tablet. Use 4 tables or 16 parts per million for water with heavy sediment. Chlorine can also be used by mixing 1/8 teaspoon of unscented household chlorine bleach (5.25% sodium hypochlorite) per gallon of water. Mix the solution thoroughly, and let stand for about 30 minutes. This treatment will not, however, kill parasitic organisms or remove chemical pollutants. Further, check expiration dates since household bleach degrades over time.

The United Nations High Commission for Refugees considers water with less than 10 fecal coliforms per 100 milliliters to be reasonably safe, whereas water with more than 100 fecal coliforms is considered unsafe. Because bacterial contamination cannot be detected by sight, smell, or taste, the only way to know if a water supply contains bacteria is to have it tested. Contaminated water sources should not be closed until equally convenient facilities become available.

It may be necessary to transport safe drinking water to the disaster site by truck. Trucks that normally carry gasoline, chemicals, or sewage should not be used to transport water. Trucks should be inspected and cleaned and disinfected before being used for water transportation because they may be contaminated with microbes or chemicals. Containers, such as bottles or cans, should be rinsed with a bleach solution before reusing them. Do not rely on untested devices for decontaminating water.

Water Supply

There are 3 sources of water outside the home: groundwater, surface water, and rainwater. Groundwater, although generally of higher quality microbiologically, is relatively difficult to access because it is located within the earth's crust. Surface waters, found in lakes, ponds, streams, and rivers, have predictable reliability and volume and are relatively easy to gather but are generally microbiologically unsafe and require treatment. Rainwater is seldom used because collection is unreliable. Water can also come from inside the home, including from the tank that heats water, from melted ice cubes made with water that was not contaminated, and from liquid in unopened, noncontaminated canned fruit and vegetables.

Collecting and Treating Surface Water

Those collecting water should seek a source that is free of chemicals. After removal of any sediment or particles, the water has to be treated to make it safe for consumption. The handling and storing of water is a key determinant in water safety. Once collected, water quality deteriorates over time. When water is collected from natural sources or nonpiped systems, it should be chlorinated either in the home or by health workers at the point of collection. People should be encouraged to wait for 30 minutes after chlorination before consuming water to allow for adequate disinfection to occur. When people use glasses or similar items to dip into household storage containers to get water, rather than pour from the container, it causes considerable contamination. To maintain clean stored water, water should be stored in sanitized containers. Table 9-2 provides guidance on adding chlorine bleach to purify water.

With a piped system, typically chlorine levels are adjusted to ensure that 0.2 to 0.5 milligrams per liter of free chlorine is in the water at the tap level where it is collected. During times of outbreaks or in systems where there are broken distribution pipes, water system workers should aim to have 0.5 to 1.0 milligrams per liter of free chlorine.

To prevent cross-contamination, water utilities in consultation with health officials should increase the pressure in the water pipes and increase the level of residual chlorine. Pressure can be augmented by increasing the rate of pumping into the system, by cutting down on water wastage, or by closing off sections of the distribution system. Because cross-contamination usually occurs in unknown locations in a distribution system, the chlorine residual must be kept high throughout the network. Monitoring of chlorine should be done throughout the system, and the dose put into the system should be set so that there is free chlorine in at least 95% of locations.

Table 9-2. Treating Water With Household Bleach

Volume of Water	Amount of Bleach to Add
1 quart	5 drops
1/2 gallon (2 quarts)	10 drops
1 gallon	1/4 teaspoon
5 gallons	1 teaspoon
10 gallons	2 teaspoons

Source: Adapted from Washington State Department of Health. 2013. Purifying water during an emergency. Available at: http://www.doh.wa.gov/Emergencies/EmergencyPreparednessandResponse/Factsheets/WaterPurification. Accessed January 20, 2017.

Accessing and Treating Groundwater

To collect spring water without contamination, workers should build a collection basin that has an outflow pipe constructed at or just below the point where the water comes to the surface. To prevent contamination in wells, they can build a skirt around the opening of the well or a plate sealing off the surface at the top of the well.

Water should be disinfected when household water contamination is high, when there is a high risk of a waterborne outbreak, or when the groundwater is of poor quality. Chlorine can be used in buckets when the water is collected or stored at people's homes. To chlorinate wells, use a chlorination pot or the method of shock chlorination described next.

A chlorination pot includes a small container, such as a 1-liter soda bottle, with a few holes punched in it. This container is filled with a chlorine powder and gravel mixture and placed inside a larger vessel (such as a 4-liter milk jug or a clay pot) that also has holes punched in it. The chlorine disperses from the double layered pot slowly. The number and size of holes in the vessels control the disinfectant dose and must be tailored to match a specific well volume and withdrawal rate. Invariably, the first water drawn in the morning will have an offensively high level of chlorine, and if a well has hours of very high use, the dose may become too low. Thus, pot chlorination schemes are not widely used and should not be started during the acute phase of a crisis when a lack of time and attention will prevent proper monitoring and adjustment of the chlorine levels.

Shock chlorination is conducted by adding 5 to 10 milligrams per liter to the water in a well and allowing it to sit unused for a period of hours. The first water drawn from the well after the disinfection period is discarded, and normal use is subsequently resumed. When a well is drawing from safe groundwater but has been contaminated by people or an unusual event, such as a major rainstorm, shock chlorination can eliminate a transient threat to water quality. Shock chlorination does not provide chlorinated water to the people in their homes because after the first few hours of use after treatment, little or no residual chlorine will remain in the drawn water.

Disinfecting Wells

The Centers for Disease Control and Prevention (CDC) recommends procedures for disinfecting wells following an emergency. Before any chlorine is added:

- All power sources should be turned off.
- Those in the field should wear protective gear, including shoes or boots with thick rubber soles, rubber gloves, waterproof apron, and protective face gear (e.g., goggles and a face shield).

- The area around the well should be cleared of any hazards, including debris and downed electrical wires that must be de-energized by the utility provider before work is commenced.
- The well should be checked for gases and vapors.

To disinfect bored or dug wells, use Table 9-3 to calculate how much liquid bleach to use. To determine the exact amount of bleach required, multiply the amount of disinfectant needed according to the diameter of the well and by the depth of the well. For example, a well 5 feet in diameter requires approximately 4.5 cups of bleach per foot of water. If the well is 30 feet deep, multiply 4.5 by 30 to determine the total cups of bleach required (135 cups). Using a 5-gallon bucket, mix the bleach (see Table 9-3) with 3 to 5 gallons of water. Splash the mixture around the wall or lining of the well. Be certain that the disinfectant solution contacts all parts of the well. Seal the well top. Open all faucets, and pump out water until a strong odor of bleach is noticeable at each faucet. Then stop the pump and allow the solution to remain in the well for at least 12 hours. The next day, operate the pump by turning on all faucets and continuing until the chlorine odor disappears. Adjust the flow of water faucets or fixtures that discharge to septic systems to a low flow to avoid overloading the disposal system.

It is important to boil water from the well (rolling boil for 1 minute) until the well water is tested and found to be safe with no presence of total coliforms or fecal coliforms. Before drinking or household use, wait 7 to 10 days after the chlorine has been added and then test after all traces of chlorine have been washed from the system. Additional samples should be tested, one in the next 2 to 4 weeks and another in 3 to 4 months.

Table 9-3. Bleach Required to Disinfect a Bored or Dug Well

	Diameter of Well					
Depth of Water	**0.5 foot**	**1 foot**	**2 feet**	**3 feet**	**4 feet**	**5 feet**
10 feet	.5 cup	1.75 cups	7 cups	1 gal	1.75 gal	2.75 gal
20 feet	1 cup	3.5 cups	14 cups	2 gal	3.5 gal	5.5 gal
30 feet	1.5 cups	5.25 cups	1.25 gal	3 gal	5.25 gal	8.25 gal
40 feet	2 cups	7 cups	1.75 gal	4 gal	7 gal	11 gal
50 feet	2.5 cups	8. 75 cups	2.25 gal	5 gal	8.75 gal	13.75 gal

Source: Adapted from Centers for Disease Control and Prevention. 2014. Disinfecting wells after a disaster. Table 1. Approximate amount of bleach for disinfection of a bored or dug well. Available at https://www.cdc.gov/disasters/wellsdisinfect.html. Accessed January 20, 2017.

Note: gal = gallon; 1 cup = 8 fluid ounces; 1 gallon = 16 cups. Use only unscented household liquid chlorine bleach; amounts are approximate; the goal is to achieve chlorine concentration of 100 milligrams per liter.

Emergency Basic Services

During catastrophic events, all basic services may need to be reestablished. Where the infrastructure to provide safe water and food is not intact, interim measures must be established to provide services until systems are fully operational. In catastrophic circumstances, public health officials may issue orders to boil water, warn about foods that may have spoiled during electrical outages, or announce where potable water will be provided.

Boil Water Order

Through the Safe Drinking Water Act, Congress requires the EPA to regulate contaminants that may be health risks and that may be present in public drinking water supplies. The EPA sets legal limits on the levels of certain contaminants in drinking water and establishes the water-testing schedules and methods that water systems must follow. The rules also list acceptable techniques for treating contaminated water. The Safe Drinking Water Act gives individual states the opportunity to set and enforce their own drinking water standards so long as the standards are at least as strong as the EPA's national standards. Most states and territories directly oversee the water systems within their borders.

The Total Coliform Rule sets legal limits for total coliform levels in drinking water and specifies the type and frequency of testing to determine if legal limits are exceeded. Coliforms are a broad class of bacteria that live in the digestive tracts of humans and many animals. The presence of coliform bacteria in tap water is an indicator that the treatment system is not working properly or that a problem exists in the pipes. Of particular concern is exposure to the bacteria called *Escherichia coli (E. coli)*. *E. coli*, expelled into the environment within fecal matter, can cause gastroenteritis, urinary tract infections, and neonatal meningitis. Virulent strains have caused bowel necrosis, peritonitis, mastitis, septicemia, and Gram-negative pneumonia.

This Total Coliform Rule was modified in the Revised Total Coliform Rule (RTCR). Unless a state determines an earlier effective date, all public water systems (PWS) (e.g., community water systems, nontransient noncommunity water systems, and transient noncommunity water systems) must comply with the RTCR requirements starting April 1, 2016.

The RTCR increases public health protection by reducing the potential pathways for fecal material to enter and contaminate water distribution systems. When water samples are tested, each sample found positive for total coliforms (TC+) must be tested for the presence of *E. coli*, and, if the laboratory doing the analysis finds the sample positive (EC+), the sample result must be reported to the state by the end of the day that the PWS is notified. If any routine sample is TC+, repeat samples are required. In general, 3 repeat samples must be taken for each routine TC+. If any of these repeats are TC+, then they must be tested for *E. coli* as well, with the same reporting requirements to the state. An additional set of samples must be repeated unless an assessment has been triggered. There are 2 levels of triggered assessments. A Level 1 assessment can be conducted by the water system operator. If a Level 2 assessment is required, it incorporates a wider scope of review and analysis, and is performed by a party approved by the individual state. Following a disaster that may compromise a community's water supply, those responsible for monitoring water safety may use the regular water-sampling plan or make modifications, depending on the severity and geographic location of concern. When a decision has been made that water sampled from one or more sites exceeds the Maximum Contaminant Level (MCL) and poses a threat to the public's health, a decision may be made to issue a boiled water order or advisory.

The EPA issued a revised set of Drinking Water Standards and Health Advisories in 2012, so that the targets are consistent with the agency's most current assessments of risk and safety. With few exceptions, the health advisory values were rounded to one significant figure. The Surface Water Treatment Rule requires systems using surface water or groundwater under the direct influence of surface water to disinfect and filter their water or meet criteria for avoiding filtration so that these contaminants are controlled at the levels summarized in Table 9-4. The MCL goal, which is not enforceable, refers to the maximum level of a contaminant in drinking water at which no known or anticipated adverse effects occur and that allows for an adequate margin of safety. The MCL standard, which is enforceable, identifies the maximum permissible level of a contaminant in water that is delivered to any user of a public water system. Treatment technique is an enforceable procedure or level of technical performance that public water systems must follow to ensure control of a contaminant. Table 9-4 describes possible health effects, sources of contamination and treatment techniques for contaminated water and Table 9-5 identifies methods for removing contaminants in drinking water.

Public Notice Templates

The EPA has developed templates that can be used by water suppliers to ensure that the notice that they provide is complete. These public notice templates can be downloaded from the EPA Web site (available at: http://www.epa.gov/region8-waterops/reporting-forms-and-instructions-public-notification). Other information about the public notification rule is available at: http://www.epa.gov/dwreginfo/public-notification-rule. Because some states have different requirements for identifying violations or for the wording of any notice, check with your state office handling environmental affairs.

Air Contaminants

The EPA established standards about particulate exposures that direct public health actions. Those at increased risk from exposures to contaminants include pregnant women

Table 9-4. Health Effects, Sources of Contaminants, and Treatment Techniques

Microorganisms	Maximum Contaminant Level Goal (mg/L)	Maximum Contaminant Level or Treatment Technique	Potential Health Effects From Ingestion of Water	Source of Contaminant in Drinking Water
Cryptosporidium	-	Filter to remove 99%	Gastrointestinal disease	Human and animal fecal waste
Giardia lamblia	0	99.99% killed or inactivated	Giardiasis, a gastroenteric disease	Human and animal fecal waste
HPC	N/A	≤500 bacterial colonies per milliliter	HPC has no health effects but can indicate how effective treatment is at controlling microorganisms	N/A
Legionella	0	No limit; EPA believes that if *Giardia* and viruses are inactivated, ***Legionella*** will also be controlled	Legionnaire's disease (pneumonia)	Found naturally in water, multiplies in heating systems
Total coliforms	0	≤5.0% samples total coliform positive in a month. Every sample with total coliforms must be analyzed for fecal coliforms. No fecal coliforms are permitted	Used as an indicator that other potentially harmful bacteria may be present	Human and animal fecal waste
Turbidity	N/A	Turbidity (cloudiness) must be ≤5 NTU	Turbidity has no health effect but can interfere with disinfection and provide a medium for microbial growth. It may indicate the presence of microbes.	Soil runoff
Viruses	0	99.99% killed/inactivated	Gastrointestinal disease	Human and animal fecal waste

Source: Based on Environmental Protection Agency (EPA). 2012. *Drinking Water Standards and Health Advisories.* Microbiology table. Page 11. Washington, DC: EPA. Available at: https://www.epa.gov/sites/production/files/2015-09/documents/dwstandards2012.pdf. Accessed January 20, 2017; Centers for Disease Control and Prevention (CDC). 2009. Fact sheet for healthy drinking water: drinking water treatment methods for backcountry and travel use. Atlanta, GA: CDC. Available at http://www.cdc.gov/healthywater/pdf/drinking/Backcountry_Water_Treatment.pdf. Accessed January 20, 2017.

Note: EPA=Environmental Protection Agency; HPC=heterotrophic plate count; NTU=nephelometric turbidity units.

Table 9-5. Methods to Remove Contaminants in Drinking Water

Microorganism	Boiling (rolling boil for 1 minute minimum)[a]	Filtration	Disinfection: Iodine or Chlorine[b]	Disinfection: Chlorine Dioxide	Combination Filter and Disinfection
Protozoa–Cryptosporidium	++++	+++ Absolute ≤ 1 micron filter (NSF 53 or 58 rated "cyst reduction/removal" filter)	–	+ to ++	++++ Absolute ≤1 micron filter (NSF 53 or 58 rated "cyst reduction/removal" filter)
Protozoa–Giardia lamblia	++++	+++ Absolute ≤1 micron filter (NSF 53 or 58 rated "cyst reduction/removal" filter)	+ to ++	+++	++++ Absolute <1 micron filter (NSF 53 or 58 rated "cyst reduction/removal" filter)
Bacteria–*Campylobacter, Salmonella, Shigella*	++++	++ Absolute ≤.3 micron filter	+++	+++	++++ Absolute <.3 micron filter
Viruses–enterovirus, hepatitis A, norovirus, rotavirus	++++	–	+++	+++	+++

Source: Adapted from Centers for Disease Control and Prevention (CDC). 2009. Fact sheet for healthy drinking water: drinking water treatment methods for backcountry and travel use. Atlanta, GA: CDC. Available at http://www.cdc.gov/healthywater/pdf/drinking/Backcountry_Water_Treatment.pdf. Accessed January 20, 2017.

Note: –=not effective; +=low effectiveness; ++=moderate effectiveness; +++=high effectiveness; ++++=very high effectiveness.

[a]At altitudes greater than 6562 feet, boil for 3 minutes.

[b]Water that has been disinfected with iodine is NOT recommended for pregnant women, those with thyroid problems, those with known hypersensitivity to iodine, or continuous use for more than a few weeks at a time.

and their unborn children, children, the elderly, those with chronic conditions such as heart disease and asthma, and workers. Table 9-6 shows the EPA particulate standards.

The response of public health agencies should include monitoring the air with test equipment that permits a direct reading for conditions immediately dangerous to life or health and other conditions that may cause death or serious harm (e.g., combustible or explosive atmospheres, oxygen deficiency, toxic substances). Depending on the disaster, the community may need instruments that provide instantaneous readings for the review of the air quality tests because of the length of time it takes to get a laboratory analysis. The National Institute for Occupational Safety and Health (NIOSH) and the CDC developed guidance on the installation of filtration and air cleaning systems that can protect building environments from airborne agents. The Hazardous Waste Operations and Emergency Response (HAZWOPER) data should inform both the use of personal

Table 9-6. U.S. Environmental Protection Agency Particulate Standards

Primary[a]/Secondary[b]	Average Exposure Time	Level of Concern	Form
Primary	$PM_{2.5}$	12.0 μg/m³	Annual arithmetic mean, averaged over 3 years[c,d]
Secondary		15.0 μg/m³	Annual arithmetic mean, averaged over 3 years[c,d]
Primary and Secondary		35 μg/m³	98th percentile, averaged over 3 years[e]
Primary and Secondary	PM_{10}	150 μg/m³	Not to be exceeded more than once per year on average over a 3-year period

Source: Adapted from U.S. Environmental Protection Agency. 2012. Particulate matter (PM) standards-table of historical PM NAAQS. Available at http://www3.epa.gov/ttn/naaqs/standards/pm/s_pm_history.html. Accessed January 20, 2017.

Note: $PM_{2.5}$=fine particles 2.5 micrometers in diameter and smaller; PM_{10}= inhalable coarse particles smaller than 10 micrometers; μg/m³=micrograms per cubic meter of air.

[a]Primary standards provide public health protection, including protecting the health of "sensitive" populations such as asthmatics, children, and the elderly.

[b]Secondary standards provide public welfare protection, including protection against decreased visibility and damage to animals, crops, vegetation, and buildings.

[c]The level of the annual standard is defined to one decimal place (i.e., 15.0 μg/m³) as determined by rounding. For example, a 3-year average annual mean of 15.04 μg/m³ would round to 15.0 μg/m³ and, thus, meet the annual standard, while a 3-year average of 15.05 μg/m³ would round to 15.1 μg/m³ and, hence, violate the annual standard (40 C.F.R. § 50, app. N).

[d]The EPA tightened the constraints on the spatial averaging criteria by further limiting the conditions under which some areas may average measurements from multiple community-oriented monitors to determine compliance (see 71 Fed. Reg. 61165–61167).

[e]The level of the 24-hour standard is defined as an integer (zero decimal places) as determined by rounding. For example, a 3-year average 98th percentile concentration of 35.49 μg/m³ would round to 35 μg/m³ and thus meet the 24-hour standard and a 3-year average of 35.50 μg/m³ would round to 36 and, hence, violate the 24-hour standard (40 C.F.R. § 50, app. N).

protective equipment and actions public health officials can take such as advising a community that it is safe to reenter homes and businesses. HAZWOPER guides public health actions by requiring an ongoing air monitoring program for workers in the types of emergencies covered under the standard (see Chapter 10 for more information on HAZWOPER). A full description is beyond the scope of this book, but more information is available through the publications included in the reference section.

Careful thought should go into communicating information about the risks from potential air contaminants to the public (discussed more fully in Chapter 6). DOHs should develop advisories that can be communicated both to the public and to rescue personnel on air quality issues and on practical information about the particular hazards posed by the disaster. Examples include the advisories that the New York City Health Departments posted about using wet methods, such as wet mopping or high-efficiency particulate vacuum, after the collapse of the towers at the World Trade Center in 2001.

Food Defense and Safety

Governments are concerned about food contamination as a terrorist act because it does not require much technical skill or an extensive organization to cause widespread public health consequences. Protecting food from intentional contamination is known as *food defense*. Risk of contamination can occur at any point, including growing, manufacturing, transportation, and distribution. Contamination of the food supply is a risk to supermarkets, restaurants, and other food establishments, as well as food distribution centers and warehouses. Threats to food can occur as follows:

- Unintentional contamination (e.g., food-borne illness, outbreaks)
- Deliberate contamination (e.g., explosive or spray devices, food tampering)
- Transportation accidents (e.g., train, truck)
- Natural disasters (e.g., fires, floods, hurricanes, tornadoes)
- Building events (e.g., explosions, ammonia leaks)
- Hoaxes

Five federal agencies are responsible for ensuring food safety and defense:

Food and Drug Administration (FDA): Oversees domestic and imported food, animal drugs, feeds, and veterinary devices. Working closely with state and local food safety officers, the FDA conducts scientific evaluations to analyze potential hazards, identifies points of potential hazard, and establishes preventive measures.

United States Department of Agriculture (USDA): Oversees ongoing inspection of foods to ensure they are safe and accurately labeled, enforces sanitary requirements through monitoring and surveillance, and samples for harmful zoonotic diseases.

CDC: Reports and tracks food outbreaks and works with state and local health officers to investigate and control disease.

EPA: Evaluates levels of pesticides and herbicides.

United States Customs and Border Protection: Monitors imported food.

The key public health task is to distinguish between intentional and unintentional outbreaks. Communities should have food defense plans as part of their emergency response action plan. The food defense plan should include procedures for identifying food-borne illness, food recalls, and food safety following natural disasters or pandemics. Several tools have been developed to help bolster the country's food defense strategies. The Food Defense Plan Builder is a software program designed to help operators involved in food production, manufacturing, transportation, and sale minimize the risk of intentional contamination at their individual food facilities. The Food Defense Plan Builder is available at: http://www.fda.gov/Food/FoodDefense/ToolsEducationalMaterials/ucm349888.htm. The Food Related Emergency Exercise Bundle (FREE-B) is a collection of food safety scenarios designed to help public health and other regulatory agencies assess the efficacy of food emergency response plans, protocols, and procedures. The FREE-B can be used by multiple jurisdictions and organizations (e.g., medical community, private sector, law enforcement, first responder communities) or by a single agency. The FREE-B is available at: http://www.fda.gov/Food/FoodDefense/ToolsEducationalMaterials/ucm295902.htm.

Food Safety

Improper food storage is associated with *Bacillus cereus*, *Clostridium perfringens*, *Salmonella spp.*, *Staphylococcus aureus*, and group A *Streptococcus*. Lack of hand washing and personal hygiene are associated with shigellosis, hepatitis A, gastroenteritis, and giardiasis. Three food-handling techniques are a major source of food-borne illness following disaster: improper storage, inadequate cooking, and poor personal hygiene. In addition to careful hand washing, cooking utensils must be washed in boiled or treated water before being used, if contaminated due to the disaster.

Stored Food

When preparing for disasters, residents should store at least a 3-day supply of food. Canned foods and dry mixes will remain fresh for about 2 years when stored in a cool, dry, dark place away from ovens or refrigerator exhausts at a temperature of 40°F to 60°F. Residents should date all food items and use or replace food before it loses freshness. Food items should be heavily wrapped or stored in airtight containers above the ground to both prolong shelf life and to protect it from insects and rodents. Cans that bulge at the ends or that leak should be discarded.

Refrigerated Food

Ideally, meat, poultry, fish, and eggs should be refrigerated at or below 40°F. Refrigerators, without power, will keep foods cool for about 4 hours if left unopened. Block or dry ice can be added to refrigerators if the electricity is off longer than 4 hours. Perishable food in the refrigerator or freezer should be used before stored food. Unrefrigerated cooked foods should be discarded after 2 hours at room temperature regardless of appearance. Only foods that have a normal color, texture, and odor should be eaten.

Frozen Food

Frozen food is safe when stored at or below 0°F. Generally, when a freezer is full, food will be safe for 2 days. When a freezer is half full, food may be safe up to 24 hours. Twenty-five pounds of dry ice will keep a 10-cubic-foot freezer below freezing for 3 to 4 days. Dry ice freezes everything it touches and must be handled with dry, heavyweight gloves to avoid injury. Thawed food can usually be eaten or refrozen if it is still refrigerator cold or if it still contains ice crystals. Any food that has been at room temperature for 2 hours or more or that has an unusual odor, color, or texture should be discarded.

Flooded Food Supplies

Discard all food not stored in a waterproof container. Undamaged, commercially canned foods can be saved by removing the can labels, thoroughly washing the cans, and then disinfecting them with a solution consisting of 1 cup of bleach in 5 gallons of water. Relabel the cans with a nonerasable marker and include the expiration date. Food containers with screw caps, snap lids, crimped caps (e.g., soda pop bottles), twist caps, flip tops, and home canned foods cannot be disinfected. Only pre-prepared canned baby formula that requires no added water should be used for infants.

Table 9-7 provides tips for safe food handling; Table 9-8 lists foods that cannot be salvaged following loss of power or exposure to contaminated water.

Feeding Large Numbers of Displaced People

Food requirements can be estimated by assessing the effect of the disaster on food supplies and the number of people who are without food. Seasonal variations may affect the availability of food. Estimates of food requirements should be calculated for 1 week and 1 month: 16 metric tons (35,273.6 pounds) of food is needed for 1,000 people for 1 month,

Table 9-7. Measures for Ensuring Food Safety

Potential Exposure	Preventive Action
Contamination of raw food	Buy from reliable source Stipulate requirements for production and transport Purchase from reliable source
Contamination of prepared food	Control temperature during storage and when being transported Cover and/or store foods in closed container Control and protect from pests
Contamination by growth of bacteria	Maintain correct temperature, only store safe duration, and rotate so older foods used first Ensure food is cooked thoroughly throughout (i.e., to temperature of 165°F minimum) Ensure food is kept hot (above 140°F) and limit exposure to room temperature Ensure food is quickly reheated Quickly cool food to temperatures below 40°F (i.e., store food in shallow trays so it can chill quickly)
Contamination from various sources	Wash hands before handling food Cover food properly, ensure no contact with raw foods and nonpotable water Separate cooked foods to prevent contact with raw foods Use only clean utensils to handle cooked food Prevent contact with nonpotable water Prevent cross-contamination via surfaces, cooking utensils Use boiled water for cooking Limit exposure of food to room temperature Serve food when it is still hot
Survival of pathogens	Ensure food is cooked thoroughly throughout (i.e., to temperature of 165°F minimum)
Growth of surviving bacteria, their spores, or production of toxins	Ensure that food is kept hot (i.e., above 140°F) Ensure that leftovers, or foods prepared in advance, are thoroughly reheated Cool food as quickly as possible to temperatures below 40°F Ensure enough space for cold air to circulate in the refrigerator or cold storage room During long periods of cold storage, periodically monitor temperature fluctuations

Source: Based on Wisner B, Adams J, eds. 2002. *Environmental Health in Emergencies and Disasters: A Practical Guide.* Table 9.1. Geneva, Switzerland: World Health Organization.

and 2 cubic meters (70.6 cubic feet) of space is needed to store 1 metric ton of food. The USDA produced a booklet, *Cooking for Groups: A Volunteer's Guide to Food Safety,* which guides volunteers preparing food for large groups. The publication is available at: http://www.fsis.usda.gov/wps/portal/fsis/topics/food-safety-education/get-answers/food-safety-fact-sheets/safe-food-handling/cooking-for-groups-a-volunteers-guide-to-food-safety/CT_Index1.

Table 9-8. Food Products That Should Be Destroyed

Food Type	Incident Type	Examples
Produce	Flood, loss of electricity	Lettuce, celery, cabbage
Packaged foods	Flood	In bags: coffee, tea, flour, cereals, beans, grains, sugars, nuts
		Paper- or cellophane-wrapped candles, cereals, breads, cakes, chewing gum, etc.
		Ice cream and dairy products
		Spices
		Salt, sugar, dried milk, powdered eggs, etc.
	Fire, extreme heat	Look for charred labeling or other package damage
Screw-top or crimped-cap containers with drinks	Flood	Canned soft drinks, beer, wine, and other liquor products
Frozen foods	Flood, loss of electricity	Partially or completely thawed; if properly stored in adequate refrigeration, can be sold as "freshly thawed"
Refrigerated foods	Loss of electricity	Should be discarded if temperature above 40°F for 4 hours or more
		Eggs whether frozen or in shell
		Fish and seafood products
Open barrels	Flood	Sauerkraut or pickles
Glass or plastic containers with cork stoppers	Flood	Catsup, vinegar, condiments, syrup, molasses, honey
Glass containers with anchor-type vacuum-packed tops	Flood	Must be completely cleaned and sanitized
		Home canned goods must be destroyed
Various	Fire, smoke damage, exposure to chemicals used in fire prevention, aerosols, insecticides	Meats, oil products (including butter), produce

Source: Adapted from Houston Department of Health and Human Services. 2005. Food Surveillance and salvage following disasters. Available at http://www.houstontx.gov/health/Food/food-surv.htm. Accessed January 20, 2017.

Food Safety Monitoring

At the CDC, the Foodborne Diseases Active Surveillance Network, known as FoodNet, is a web-based system that identifies the sources and monitors the burden of new and emerging food-borne diseases. As a collaborative project of the CDC's Emerging Infections Program (EIP), 10 EIP sites, the USDA, and the FDA, FoodNet uses active surveillance to strengthen the ability of state and local health departments to detect and respond to food-borne outbreaks. Public health officials contact laboratory directors to find new cases of food-borne diseases and report these cases electronically to the CDC. Because most food-borne infections cause diarrheal illness, FoodNet focuses on people who have a diarrheal illness. FoodNet could be used to detect and monitor the emergence of food-borne disease secondary to disaster or related to intentional poisoning.

Control Strategies for Epidemic Diarrheal Diseases

Diarrheal diseases are a common problem following natural disasters. Environmental measures and education campaigns should be specific to the fecal-oral disease public health officials seek to protect against.

Cholera

Public health bulletins must instruct residents to consume only chlorinated or boiled fluids and to eat only hot, cooked foods or peeled fruits and vegetables. Emphasize hand washing in food preparation and before eating. During a cholera outbreak, ensure that the water being consumed is chlorinated. Where chlorination is not possible, order the boiling of water or the addition of a lemon per liter (1 quart). Acidic sauces, such as tomato sauce, added to foods can provide some protection against food-borne cholera.

Typhoid Fever

As with cholera, residents must be told to consume only chlorinated or boiled fluids and to eat only hot, cooked foods or peeled fruits and vegetables. Public health officials must ensure that the water supply is chlorinated and emphasize hand washing in food preparation and before eating. Workers must also ensure that infected residents do not prepare food for others for 3 months after the onset of their symptoms.

Shigella

Public health campaigns must educate residents about a comprehensive personal hygiene program. Public health workers must provide soap and lots of water and promote hand washing, the chlorination of water, and the proper handling and heating of food. Educational efforts should be focused in households where cases have occurred because secondary cases within households are common.

Hepatitis A

Water is the main route of transmission during major outbreaks. The most common form of fecal-oral hepatitis, hepatitis A, is transmitted by food and other routes. Control measures should therefore concentrate on the chlorination of water. Since pregnant women are particularly vulnerable, special efforts should be made to educate them and help them carry out personal and food hygiene.

Heating and Shelter

Provision of sufficient shelter following disaster prevents, depending on weather conditions, hypothermia, frostbite, malaise, heatstroke, and dehydration.

In cold climates, higher caloric intake is required to maintain the same activity level. For each degree below 68°F, about 1% more calories are required. If a house is 50°F, residents will require 10% more food intake to sustain their activity level. Public health interventions following cold weather disasters include making high-energy foods available; providing blankets and sleeping bags; distributing plastic sheeting to cover windows and unused doorways; encouraging the sharing of a heated place by several people or households; and instructing residents of multistory buildings to heat the same room on each floor, allowing heat lost from one floor to augment heat in the room above. Educational messages should warn people about the signs of carbon monoxide poisoning and provide instructions to check for gas leaks.

In warmer climates, sheeting should be provided to keep people dry during rainstorms and to provide shade in the daylight.

Safe Use of Generators

The incorrect use of generators results in human deaths every year. Deaths from generator usage have been caused by poisoning from the toxic engine exhaust, by electrocution, and by fire. To avoid these outcomes, operators should consult the directions provided by manufacturers with each generator before installing or using.

Generators must never be used inside a building, garage, or near the air intake of a building, even if doors and windows are open, because of the risk of carbon monoxide poisoning. Further, generators are best installed more than 20 feet away from a building to keep carbon monoxide from entering the building. Carbon monoxide cannot be seen or smelled and the people inside nearby buildings can be exposed even if they cannot smell exhaust fumes. A safety precaution is the installation of battery-operated or plug-in carbon dioxide alarms and checking the detectors regularly to be sure that they are functioning properly. Anyone using a generator who starts to feel sick, dizzy, or weak should get to fresh air immediately, without delay.

Appliances attached to the generator need to be plugged in using individual heavy-duty, outdoor-rated cords. To avoid electric shock or electrocution, generators cannot be used in any conditions where there is moisture, including wet hands, and it is preferable to operate them on a dry surface where they are protected from precipitation. If water has been present anywhere near the electrical circuits and electrical equipment, the power should be turned off at the main breaker or fuse on the service panel.

If gasoline is used, it should not be stored indoors where the fumes could ignite. When using gasoline- and diesel-powered portable generators to supply power to a building, the main breaker or fuse on the service panel should be switched to the "off" position before starting the generator in order to prevent power lines from being inadvertently energized by backfeed electrical energy from the generators. Before refueling, generators must be turned off and allowed to cool down because gasoline spilled on hot engine parts could ignite.

Mold Remediation

Following hurricanes and floods, mold commonly grows on drywall, ceiling tiles, wood products, paint, wallpaper, carpeting, books, papers, and fabrics due to the exposure to water. In addition, molds can also grow on moist, dirty surfaces such as concrete, fiberglass insulation, and ceramic tiles. Exposure to molds can cause severe health symptoms such as nasal, eye and skin irritation and wheezing in susceptible people. Most molds reproduce by forming spores. When these spores are released into the air and land on a moist surface, they grow and release more spores and/or mycotoxins. Mycotoxins, produced by microfungi, are capable of causing disease and death in humans and other animals. People are exposed when they inhale microscopic mold spores and/or mycotoxins from the air, which are usually more concentrated in the air of contaminated homes than outdoors. Mold growth can be prevented by eliminating the source of the water, followed by thoroughly cleaning or removing and drying the affected building materials.

The National Institute of Environmental Health Science (NIEHS) recommends that all involved in cleaning objects with mold take the following protective actions:

- Avoid breathing dust and fungal spores generated by wet building materials.
- Use an N95 NIOSH-approved disposable respirator as a minimum when working with small areas of moldy or damp materials. More protection may be needed for extended work.
- Wear long gloves that reach the middle of your forearm. If you are using a disinfectant, a biocide such as chlorine bleach, or a strong cleaning solution, you should select gloves made from natural rubber, neoprene, nitrile, polyurethane, or PVC. Avoid touching mold or moldy items with your bare hands.
- Wear goggles that do not have ventilation holes. Avoid getting mold or mold spores in your eyes. Avoid the splashing of cleaning solutions in eyes.
- Consider discarding all water-damaged materials. Articles that have visible mold should be thrown away. (When in doubt, throw it out.)
- After working with mold-contaminated materials, wash thoroughly, including your hair, scalp, and nails.

Mold remediation is a multistep process that may require outside assistance, depending on the size of the contaminated space. While many homeowners and volunteers undertake the task of mold cleanup and treatment themselves, when the contaminated portion of a home is larger than 10 square feet, a qualified mold assessment and remediation specialist is recommended by the EPA, United States Department of Housing and Urban Development, and CDC. The New York City Department of Health & Mental Hygiene recommends professional specialists for extensive contamination larger than 100 square feet. Table 9-9 provides a checklist, developed by the EPA, of key steps in ensuring a safe mold remediation process.

A full description of mold remediation is beyond the scope of this chapter. Information on (1) the steps in conducting mold cleanup and treatment, (2) conducting a mold assessment, (3) selecting a qualified mold remediation contractor or mold inspector, (4) personal protective equipment and respiratory protection, (5) decontamination and cleanup procedures, and (6) the work sequence is detailed in *NIEHS Disaster Recovery Mold Remediation Guidance: Health and Safety Essentials for Workers, Volunteers, and Homeowners* (available at: https://tools.niehs.nih.gov/wetp/public/hasl_get_blob.cfm?ID=9795).

Integrated Pest Management

Vector control is always important for the prevention of communicable disease, but becomes even more important when there is the potential for increased spread of disease

Table 9-9. Checklist for Mold Remediation

Investigate and evaluate moisture and mold problems

- Assess size of moldy area (square feet)
- Consider the possibility of hidden mold
- Clean up small mold problems and fix moisture problems before they become large problems
- Select remediation manager for medium- or large-size mold problem
- Investigate areas associated with occupant complaints
- Identify source(s) or cause of water or moisture problem(s)
- Note type of water-damaged materials (e.g., wallboard, carpet, etc.)
- Check inside air ducts and air handling unit
- Throughout process, consult qualified professional if necessary or desired

Communicate with building occupants at all stages of process, as appropriate

- Designate contact person for questions and comments about medium or large-scale remediation as needed

Plan remediation

- Adapt or modify remediation guidelines to fit your situation; use professional judgment
- Plan to dry wet, nonmoldy materials within 48 hours to prevent mold growth[a]
- Select cleanup methods for moldy items[b]
- Select personal protective equipment—protect remediators[b]
- Select containment equipment—protect building, occupants[b]
- Select remediation personnel who have the experience and training needed to implement the remediation plan and use personal protective equipment and containment as appropriate

Remediate moisture and mold problems

- Fix moisture problem, implement repair plan and/or maintenance plan
- Dry wet, nonmoldy materials within 48 hours to prevent mold growth
- Clean and dry mold materials[b]
- Discard moldy porous items that can't be cleaned[b]
- Avoid exposure to and contact with mold
- Use personal protective equipment

(Continued)

Table 9-9. (Continued)

Questions to consider before remediating

- Are there existing moisture problems in the building?
- Have building materials been wet more than 48 hours?[b]
- Are there hidden sources of water or is the humidity too high (i.e., high enough to cause condensation)?
- Are building occupants reporting musty or moldy odors?
- Are building occupants reporting health problems?
- Are building materials or furnishings visibly damaged?
- Has maintenance been delayed or the maintenance plan been altered?
- Has the building been recently remodeled or has building use changed?
- Is consultation with medical or health professionals indicated?

Source: Adapted from Environmental Protection Agency (EPA). 2014. *Mold Remediation in Schools and Commercial Buildings*. Checklist for mold remediation. Washington, DC: EPA. Available at https://www.epa.gov/sites/production/files/2014-08/documents/moldremediation.pdf. Accessed January, 20 2017.

Note: This checklist was designed to highlight key parts of a school or commercial building remediation and does not list all potential steps or problems. For comprehensive guidance, please review *Mold Remediation in Schools and Commercial Buildings* in full or see: National Institute of Environmental Health Sciences. 2013. *Disaster Recovery, Mold Remediation Guidance: Health and Safety Essentials for Workers, Volunteers, and Homeowners*. Available at http://www.elcosh.org/document/3671/d001213/NIEHS%2BDisaster%2BRecovery%252C%2BMold%2BRemediation%2BGuidance.html?show_text=1. Accessed January, 20 2017.

[a]See Environmental Protection Agency (EPA). 2014. *Mold Remediation in Schools and Commercial Buildings*. Table 1: Water damage–cleanup and mold prevention. Washington, DC: EPA. Available at https://www.epa.gov/sites/production/files/2014-08/documents/moldremediation.pdf. Accessed January, 20 2017.

[b]See Environmental Protection Agency (EPA). 2014. *Mold Remediation in Schools and Commercial Buildings*. Table 2: Guidelines for remediating building materials with mold growth caused by clean water. Washington, DC: EPA. Available at https://www.epa.gov/sites/production/files/2014-08/documents/moldremediation.pdf. Accessed January, 20 2017.

Table 9-10. Potential Vectors in Disaster

Type of Vector	Examples
Arthropods	Insects and arachnids: • Ants • Cockroaches • Flies • Lice • Mites • Mosquitoes • Spiders • Ticks • Wasps • Yellow Jackets • Bees
Vertebrates	• Bats • Feral cats, dogs • Opossums • Rodents (e.g., roof rats, Norway rats, mice) • Snakes • Skunks • Squirrels

Source: Based on California Conference of Directors of Environmental Health (CCDEH). 2012. *Disaster Field Manual for Environmental Health Specialists.* Cameron Park, CA: CCDEH.

caused by the breakdown in environmental controls following disaster. The most effective way to control vector-borne disease is to establish sanitary disposal of waste as soon as possible. Where vector-borne disease is known to be endemic, control programs should be accelerated in the postimpact phase of a disaster. The principles of integrated pest management are to eliminate breeding sites, to eliminate food, and to control harborage (i.e., where pests can live). The California Conference of Directors of Environmental Health produced a comprehensive field manual with provides detailed information about vector control and the other topics in this chapter. Table 9-10 lists the types of vectors that could be problematic, depending on location and type of disaster. A community vector control program includes several components:

- Remove food sources, water, and items that provide shelter for rodents. Collect and dispose of garbage as soon as possible.
- Educate the public about rat and mosquito control.
- Eliminate mosquito breeding sites by overturning receptacles, covering swimming pools, and draining or covering other stagnant water sources.
- Reduce rat population and spread by closing up cracks in walls and using cats to chase the rats. Seal gaps and holes that are greater than a ¼-inch diameter with any

of the following: cement, light-gauge metal mesh, wire screening, hardware cloth, steel wool, caulk, expanding foam, or other patching materials.
- Store food in enclosed, protected areas.

In flooded areas, rats will search for dry places to hide. Rats and other vectors can feed off dead animals and other organic waste. Therefore, animal carcasses should be sprinkled with kerosene to protect them from predatory animals.

CHAPTER 10

OCCUPATIONAL HEALTH IN DISASTERS

Protecting the health and safety of everyone involved in responding to a disaster is the essence of public health prevention. A large number of people are potentially at risk from hazardous exposures during disaster response, including emergency responders, recovery workers, volunteers, providers of health care, community residents, and others. While this chapter focuses on occupational exposures, many of the strategies can be adopted by anyone for whom protective actions can be safeguarding. Specific topics in this chapter include federal regulations to ensure worker safety, protecting workers with disabilities, the use of personal protective equipment (PPE) including when caring for patients with highly infectious diseases such as Ebola and those exposed to hazardous materials, and handling human remains.

Public Health Role

- Provide technical assistance in addressing occupational health and safety concerns.
- Provide for commercial toilets and hand washing stations.
- Protect worker safety by:
  - training incident commanders and their team on hazard assessment, the risks to workers, monitoring illness and injury to inform modifications in the use of protective measures, and providing specialized medical care; and
  - training workers on the proper techniques for responding to and cleaning up after a disaster and ensuring the use of protective measures.

Worker Health and Safety

During the cleanup after a disaster, workers are exposed to numerous hazards (see Table 10-1), such as the release of contaminants or construction safety issues. Other occupational hazards at disaster sites include excessive noise, contaminated dust, heat stress from working in a hot climate or wearing PPE, cold stress from working in a cold environment for an extended period, working in confined spaces, injuries from dust or flying debris, and exposure to blood and body fluids. Workers may come in contact with plants that cause contact dermatitis or be potentially exposed to infectious disease when responding to disasters that occur in regions where such disease is endemic. Workers treating patients with Ebola must be vigilant about the proper use of PPE to avoid contracting the potentially deadly disease. In addition, workers are potentially exposed to chemicals and other toxic agents when a disaster involves their release.

Morbidity and Mortality

Depending upon the hazard, workers may experience bites from insects, mammals, or reptiles; carbon-monoxide poisoning; electrical shock; food-borne illness; entrapment or death by asphyxiation, constriction, or crushing; heat exhaustion and cramps to heatstroke; hypothermia or frostbite; infections from exposure to blood-borne pathogens; irritation or injury of eyes, nose, throat, or lungs; lacerations, abrasions, or puncture wounds; symptoms related to toxic agent exposures including death; temporary hearing loss or difficulty communicating with coworkers; traumatic injuries from falls; traumatic stress, and trench foot from extended exposure to water. A comprehensive list of potential safety hazards and protective actions that can be taken is described in Table 10-1.

Protection Through Immunization

In advance of traveling both domestically and internationally to respond to disasters, all personnel should take precautions to ensure their health and safety. The CDC provides guidance on necessary preventive measures for specific travel destinations (available at: http://wwwnc.cdc.gov/travel/content/relief-workers.aspx). In addition to the general guidelines provided, all routine immunizations should be up to date:

- Tetanus/diphtheria/pertussis or tetanus/diphtheria vaccine or booster (if already have had adult pertussis vaccine)
- Polio booster if traveling to a polio-endemic or epidemic area (see http://www.polioeradication.org)
- Measles for those who do not have documented immunity
- Influenza vaccine
- Hepatitis B
- Hepatitis A

Table 10-1. Safety Hazards and Protective Actions in Disaster Response and Recovery

Specific Hazards	Examples	Protective Action	First Aid
Potential response and recovery-related hazards that will vary depending on type and extent of disaster	• Animals and animal-borne diseases • Blood-borne disease • Carbon monoxide • Chainsaws • Confined spaces • Cuts and burns • Debris and unstable work surfaces • Driving and traffic issues • Electrical hazards • Exposure to infectious disease • Extreme heat and cold • Fire • Food-borne disease • Handling bodies • Hazardous materials • Heavy equipment • Insects and insect-borne diseases • Mold • Motor vehicles • Musculoskeletal hazards • Poisonous plants • Potential chemical exposures • Respiratory hazards • Slick and unstable surfaces • Traumatic stress	• The selection of protective equipment will be dependent on site specific conditions, hazards, and tasks, but general safety equipment includes hard hats, goggles, heavy work gloves, safety glasses with side shields, earplugs or other hearing protection devices, watertight boots with steel toe and insole, NIOSH-approved respirators for exposures to mold-contaminated materials/environments, or other recognized chemical, physical, or biological hazards. • PPE and infection control procedure will vary by the biological organism that workers are potentially exposed to. • Stay hydrated. • Take frequent rests. • For specific advice, see *Protecting Yourself by Helping Others* (http://www.asse.org/assets/1/7/NIEHS-ProtectingYourselfWhileHelpingOthers.pdf).	• Immediately clean all wounds and cuts with soap and clean water. • Seek medical help.

(Continued)

Table 10-1. (Continued)

Specific Hazards	Examples	Protective Action	First Aid
	• Sharp jagged debris • Snakes and other reptiles • Spills/tripping/falls • Standing water • Struck by/against • Structural integrity • Sunburn • Trench foot • Water-borne disease • Working from heights		
Vision	• Dust, concrete, and metal particles • Falling or shifting debris, building materials, and glass • Smoke and noxious or poisonous gases • Chemicals (e.g., acids, bases, fuels, solvents, lime, and wet or dry cement powder) • Cutting or welding light and electrical arcing • Thermal hazards and fires • Blood-borne pathogens from blood, body fluids, and human remains	• Based on assessment of conditions and hazards, at a minimum wear: ○ safety glasses with side protection ○ goggles when more protection is needed ○ hybrid eye safety products, like glasses with goggle-like enclosure ○ faceshield over glasses or goggles for greater protection ○ ull-facepiece respirator for the best overall protection • When cutting or welding, use a welding helmet, goggles, or welding respirator with the appropriate lens shade. • All involved, including bystanders should be protected from the light and sparks coming from torch cutting or welding.	***Specks in the Eye*** • Do not rub eye. • Flush eye with large amounts of water. • See a doctor if the speck does not wash out or if pain or redness continues. ***Cuts, Punctures, and Foreign Objects in the Eye*** • Do not wash out eye. • Do not try to remove a foreign object stuck in the eye. • Seek immediate medical attention. ***Chemical Burns*** • Immediately flush eye with water or any drinkable liquid. Open the eye as wide as possible. Continue flushing for at least 15 minutes. For caustic or basic solutions, continue flushing on the way to medical care. • If a contact lens is in the eye, begin flushing over the lens immediately. Flushing may dislodge the lens. • Seek immediate medical attention.

(*Continued*)

Table 10-1. (Continued)

Specific Hazards	Examples	Protective Action	First Aid
			Blows to the Eye • Apply a cold compress without pressure, or tape crushed ice in a plastic bag to the forehead and allow it to rest gently on the injured eye. • Seek immediate medical attention if pain continues, if vision is reduced, or if blood or discoloration appears in the eye.
Skin	• Chemical agents (i.e., direct contact with contaminated surfaces, deposition of aerosols, immersion, or splashes) • Mechanical trauma (i.e., friction, pressure, abrasions, lacerations and contusions, scrapes, cuts, and bruises) • Physical agents (i.e., extreme temperatures and radiation) • Biological agents (e.g., parasites, microorganisms, plants and other animal materials)		Options include: • Molten flush: immediately flush the skin with large amounts of water. • Soap flush: flush the skin with soap and water. • Soap wash: wash the skin with soap and water. • Water flush: flush the contaminated skin with water. • Water wash: flush the contaminated skin with water. For specific conditions, see *NIOSH Pocket Guide to Chemical Hazards* (http://www.cdc.gov/niosh/npg/firstaid.html).
Hearing	• Exposures to noise above a level equivalent to 85 dBa for 8 hours (i.e., noise from equipment such as chainsaws, backhoes, tractors, pavement breakers, blowers, and dryers)	• Earplugs or other hearing protection devices	

(*Continued*)

Table 10-1. (Continued)

Specific Hazards	Examples	Protective Action	First Aid
Respiratory		• Use proper engineering controls to exhaust and replenish enough fresh air when working indoors. • Use a HEPA-type vacuum when cleaning dust. When exposure to dust cannot be controlled or avoided, use a well-fitted, NIOSH-certified air-purifying respirator (such as an N95 or more protective respirator) to reduce the effects of dust.	• Respiratory support: If a person breathes large amounts of hazardous chemical, move the exposed person to fresh air at once. If breathing has stopped, perform artificial respiration. • Fresh air: if a person breathes large amounts of a hazardous chemical, immediately move exposed person to fresh air. • Fresh air, 100% O_2: If a person breathes large amounts of a hazardous chemical, immediately move the exposed person to fresh air at once. If breathing has stopped, perform artificial respiration. When breathing is difficult, properly trained personnel may assist the affected person by administering 100% O_2. Keep the affected person warm and at rest. Get medical attention as soon as possible.

Source: Based on National Institute of Environmental Health Sciences. 2007. *Hurricane Response Orientation, Safety Awareness for Responders to Hurricanes: Protecting Yourself by Helping Others*. Available at: http://www.asse.org/assets/1/7/NIEHS-ProtectingYourselfWhileHelpingOthers.pdf. Accessed January 20, 2017; Centers for Disease Control and Prevention. 2007. *Workplace Safety and Health Topics, Emergency Response Resources*. Available at: http://www.cdc.gov/niosh/topics/emres/ppe.html. Accessed January 20, 2017; Centers for Disease Control and Prevention. 2013. *Skin Exposures and Effects*. Available at: http://www.cdc.gov/niosh/topics/skin. Accessed January 20, 2017; Centers for Disease Control and Prevention. 2013. *Eye Safety: Emergency Response and Disaster Recovery*. Available at: http://www.cdc.gov/niosh/topics/eye/eyesafe.html. Accessed January 20, 2017; Centers for Disease Control and Prevention. 2016. *Noise and Hearing Loss Prevention*. Available at: http://www.cdc.gov/niosh/topics/noise. Accessed January 20, 2017; Centers for Disease Control and Prevention. 2012. *Worker Safety During Fire Cleanup*. Available at: https://www.cdc.gov/disasters/wildfires/cleanupworkers.html. Accessed January 20, 2017; Centers for Disease Control and Prevention. 2016. *NIOSH Pocket Guide to Chemical Hazards*. Available at: http://www.cdc.gov/niosh/npg. Accessed January 20, 2017.

Note: HEPA=high efficiency particulate air filter; NIOSH=National Institute for Occupational Safety and Health; O_2=oxygen; PPE=personal protective equipment.

Specific vaccinations or protective actions are required when traveling to areas where the following are endemic:

- Japanese encephalitis (vaccination with the full course of immunization completed at least 10 days before departure and access to medical care during this 10-day period)
- Rabies
- Yellow fever
- Typhoid
- Cholera
- Malaria prophylaxis

Federal Guidance on Worker Safety

To minimize worker injury in disaster response and recovery, planning is essential. Numerous standards have been developed to guide the protection of workers who are responding during disasters.

The National Response Framework (NRF) includes a support annex (see Chapter 3) entitled "Worker Safety and Health," which outlines the national and regional assistance that will be provided to safeguard the health and safety of workers during disasters requiring a coordinated Federal response. These services vary, based upon the scope, complexity, and hazards associated with the disaster and can include the following:

- Identify and assess the health and safety hazards at the disaster site and in the environment.
- Assess resources needed to protect workers and identify available sources.
- Provide technical expertise in industrial hygiene, occupational safety and health, structural collapse and safety engineering, radiation safety, biological and chemical agent response, and occupational medicine.
- Create and implement a site-specific health and safety plan.
- Monitor and manage through on-site identification, evaluation, analysis, and mitigation of personal exposure to hazards.
- Assist in development, implementation, and monitoring of the PPE program.
- Coordinate collection and management of exposure and accident/injury data.
- Coordinate and provide worker training related to specific incidents.
- Assist with development and distribution of educational materials on preventing and mitigating hazards.

The Occupational Safety and Health Administration (OSHA) is the primary federal agency for the coordination of technical assistance and consultation for worker health and safety during emergency response and recovery. In their role as federal lead, OSHA developed a National Emergency Management Plan (NEMP) that clarifies procedures and policy regarding employee roles during responses to nationally significant incidents (e.g., a presidential declaration, the activation of the NRF, or a request for assistance from the Department of Homeland Security). The NEMP requires that each OSHA region develop a Regional Emergency Management Plan that coordinates federal and state plans for protecting workers. Further, it outlines logistical and operational procedures to ensure the health and safety of emergency responders and recovery workers. Where response activities are provided by contractors, communities should review their contracts to ensure that full health and safety protection is provided by both the contractors and any subcontractors who would be involved in search and rescue and/or recovery activities.

OSHA published the *Principal Emergency Response and Preparedness: Requirements and Guidance*, which summarizes the requirements to protect workers in emergencies. This guidance includes general requirements for workplaces (e.g., design of exit routes and medical services, first aid), additional requirements for specialized types of operations (e.g., process for safety management of highly hazardous materials and hazardous waste operations), requirements that support emergency response and preparedness (e.g., PPE, hazard communication, and respiratory protection), the requirements of the Hazardous Waste Operations and Emergency Response (HAZWOPER), a fire prevention plan, and also references the emergency planning and response requirements in many other OSHA standards. Key to these protective actions is the development and implementation of an emergency action plan (EAP; available at: https://www.osha.gov/pls/oshaweb/owadisp.show_document?p_table=STANDARDS&p_id=9726#1910.38(a)). The *Guidance* is available at: https://www.osha.gov/Publications/osha3122.html. HAZWOPER and EAPs are discussed below.

HAZWOPER

HAZWOPER (29 C.F.R. 1910.120) is a useful framework for organizing the protection of those responding to a disaster involving hazardous substances and certain biologic agents.[1] Among the requirements relevant to disaster response and recovery, HAZWOPER requires (1) extensive safety and health training, including instruction in: (a) decontamination for personnel, equipment, and hardware, (b) response required by levels A, B,

1. Hazardous substances covered by HAZWOPER include those defined under § 103(14) of the Comprehensive Environmental Response Compensation and Liability Act (42 U.S.C. 9601), which states: biologic and other agents can "cause death, disease, behavioral abnormalities, cancer, genetic mutation, physiological malfunctions (including malfunctions in reproduction) or physical deformations in such people or their offspring…." Hazardous materials are covered under 49 C.F.R. 172.101 and its appendices, and other hazardous waste defined in 40 C.F.R. 261.3 and 49 C.F.R. 171.8.

and C, (c) establishing appropriate decontamination lines with the proper donning and doffing of protective equipment; (2) the development of and implementation of a written safety and health program; (3) a medical surveillance program; (4) an effective site safety and health plan; (5) an emergency response plan and procedures; (6) provision of recommended sanitation equipment; (7) development of work practices to minimize employee risk from site hazards; (8) safe use of engineering controls, equipment, and relevant new safety technology or procedures; (9) establishing methods of communication, including those used while wearing respiratory protection; and (10) provision of PPE.

Emergency Action Plan

OSHA standard 29 C.F.R. 1910.38 requires that an employer have an EAP that provides for worker safety when required by the agency. An employer must review their organization's EAP with each employee when the plan is developed, an employee is initially assigned to a job, the employee's responsibilities under the plan change, or the plan is changed. An EAP must have the following minimum elements:

- Be in writing, kept in the workplace, and available to employees for review (an employer with 10 or fewer employees may communicate the plan orally)
- Procedures for reporting a fire or other emergency
- Procedures for emergency evacuation, including exit route and assignments
- Procedures to be followed by employees who remain to operate critical plant operations before they evacuate
- Procedures to account for all employees after evacuation
- Procedures to be followed by employees performing rescue or medical duties
- The name or job title of every employee who is responsible for providing more information about the plan, including an explanation of employee duties under the plan
- A working employee alarm system that uses a distinctive signal for each purpose and complies with the requirements in 29 C.F.R. 1910.165
- Designated and trained employees who assist in the safe and orderly evacuation of other employees

OSHA's Employee Emergency Plans and Fire Protection Plans (29 C.F.R. 1910.38) include EAP requirements that are also applicable to the protection of rescue workers. These additional requirements include (1) use of various types of fire extinguishers; (2) first aid, including cardiopulmonary resuscitation; (3) the requirements of the OSHA blood-borne pathogens standard; (4) chemical spill control procedures; (5) use of self-contained breathing apparatus; (6) use of other PPE; (7) search and emergency rescue procedures; (8) emergency communication; and (9) hazardous materials emergency response in accordance with 29 C.F.R. 1910.120. In addition to employers' providing these measures, workers must be trained in their use. Finally, it is important to ensure that subcontracts, where used, provide the same protections for their workers.

Protecting Workers With Disabilities

At the federal level, both executive actions and legislation have established requirements for protecting workers with disabilities in times of emergency and disaster. The Americans with Disabilities Act of 1990 requires employers who have an emergency evacuation plan to include actions that protect people with disabilities. Employers must also implement OSHA standards that require consideration of employees with disabilities in the development of their EAP. In 2004, President George W. Bush issued Executive Order 13347, Individuals with Disabilities in Emergency Preparedness, which directs all levels of government to work together with private organizations to address the safety and security needs of people with disabilities. The Office of Disability Employment Policy, at the U.S. Department of Labor, provides the following recommendations for implementing workplace emergency preparedness procedures for people with disabilities:

- When developing a plan, employees should be involved in all aspects of emergency preparedness.
- Workers with disabilities should take responsibility for their safety by offering their ideas and input.
- Develop the plan in consultation with local fire, police, and emergency departments, and community-based organizations.
- The plan should be periodically revised and updated to reflect changes in technology, personnel, and procedures.
- The plan should address:
  - evacuation after the day shift ends;
  - a method to identify visitors with special needs;
  - a detailed method for communicating with hearing-impaired workers when they are away from their work areas;
  - equipment needs to ensure the safety of all, including those with special needs;
  - service animals; and
  - a redundant buddy system for people with disabilities, including cross training for all buddies.
- The plan should be easy to read and understandable.
- The plan should be distributed in a format accessible to all employees and be incorporated into standard operating procedures.
- Drills should be performed regularly and encompass the needs of workers with disabilities.

Alerting Hearing-Impaired Employees

Although employees typically receive notification of an emergency through auditory devices, hearing-impaired workers may have difficulty understanding what is communicated over a public address (PA) system. A PA system is ineffective in communicating emergencies if the alarm interferes with or drowns out voice announcements. OSHA's Employee Alarm Systems standard (29 C.F.R. 1910.165) requires that an alarm system be able to alert all employees and be heard above ambient noise. Strobe lights or similar lighting and tactile devices meet the standard for hearing-impaired employees. Visual alarms must be installed so that hearing-impaired people can see them. The Underwriters Laboratories Standard for Emergency Signaling Devices for the Hearing-Impaired (UL 1971) establishes criteria for systems used for emergency notification.

A range of alerting device options is available to alert those with severe to profound hearing loss or mild hearing impairment. The hearing-impaired employees or an occupational audiologist can help determine the device or combination of devices that work best for their particular situation. Some alerting device options include the following:

- Exit signs set to flash when an emergency alarm sounds
- Strobe lights or vibrating alarm signals
- Visual or vibrating alarm signals at the employee's workstation
- Vibrating pagers worn by hearing-impaired workers
- Vibrating watches or other type of body alarm worn by hearing-impaired workers
- Sound amplifiers carried in a pocket
- Two-way vibrating pagers for text messages
- Hearing dogs trained to alert the hearing-impaired worker
- Buddy systems in which a coworker alerts a hearing-impaired worker
- Amplified telephone ring signaler to alert the worker to a phone ringing
- A captioned telephone that displays the words said by the caller during the conversation or a modem that converts a personal computer into a telecommunications device for the deaf (i.e., text telephone or TTY)
- Instant messaging or e-mail pop-up
- A flashlight provided to hearing-impaired individuals for signaling their location in the event they are separated from the rescue team or buddy

Personal Protective Equipment

Safety equipment, such as PPE, must meet the criteria contained in the OSHA standards (29 C.F.R. 1910.132 to 1910.138) or described by a nationally recognized standards producing organization. A determination of the nature and breadth of the hazard, through hazard assessment, is key to knowing which PPE is indicated to protect those responding to a disaster. Employers are responsible for surveying the area on foot to identify potential sources of hazards to workers and coworkers. The hazard categories to consider in determining the appropriate PPE include:

- Impact (i.e., potential for falling or flying objects)
- Penetration (i.e., sharp objects piercing foot or hand)
- Compression (i.e., roll-over or pinching objects)
- Chemical exposure (i.e., through inhalation, ingestion, skin contact, eye contact or injection)
- Temperature extremes (i.e., high heat or sub-zero cold)
- Dust/flying debris (i.e., is there grinding, chipping, sanding, etc.)
- Fall (i.e., is there a risk of slip/trip, scaffolds, or work at elevated heights)
- Light radiation (i.e., presence of nonionizing ultraviolet or infrared light, welding, brazing, cutting, furnaces, etc.)
- Noise (i.e., presence of mechanical rooms, machines, cage washing, jackhammers, etc.)
- Electrical (i.e., is there a potential for shock, short circuit, arcing, static)

Employers are responsible for assessing if hazards are present in the workplace and which hazards necessitate the use of PPE. If PPE is indicated, employers must select and have each affected employee use properly fitting and appropriate PPE for each type of hazard. There are both employer and responder (i.e., employee) responsibilities in ensuring the proper use of PPE. Employers are responsible for:

- Performing a "hazard assessment" of the workplace to identify and control physical and health hazards
- Identifying and providing appropriate PPE for employees
- Training employees in the use and care of the PPE
- Maintaining PPE, including replacing worn or damaged PPE
- Periodically reviewing, updating, and evaluating the effectiveness of the PPE program

Responders (i.e., employees) are responsible for:

- Properly wearing PPE
- Attending training sessions on PPE
- Caring for, cleaning, and maintaining PPE
- Informing a supervisor of the need to repair or replace PPE

The National Institute of Occupational Safety and Health (NIOSH) published additional guidance, *Recommendations for the Selection and Use of Respirators and Protective Clothing for Protection Against Biological Agents,* in the event of a terrorist attack involving biologicals (available at: http://www.cdc.gov/niosh/docs/2009-132). Table 10-2 lists the 4 types of PPE and their uses.

Table 10-2. Levels of Personal Protective Equipment

Level	Use	Apparatus
Level A	Greatest level of skin, respiratory, and eye protection is required	Fully encapsulated SCBA Disposable protective suit, gloves, and boots (depending on suit construction, may be worn over totally encapsulating suit)
Level B	Highest level of respiratory protection is necessary, but with a lesser level of skin protection	Encapsulated SCBA Hooded chemical-resistant clothing (e.g., overalls and long-sleeved jacket, coveralls, 1- or 2-piece chemical-splash suit, disposable chemical-resistant overalls)
Level C	The concentration(s) and type(s) of airborne substance(s) are known and criteria for using air purifying respirators are met	Full-face or half-mask, air purifying respirators (NIOSH approved) Hooded chemical-resistant clothing (e.g., overalls; 2-piece chemical-splash suit; disposable chemical-resistant overalls)
Level D	The atmosphere contains no known hazard Work functions preclude splashes, immersion, or the potential for unexpected inhalation of or contact with hazardous levels of any chemicals	Work uniform with standard precautions (e.g., gloves, mask)

Source: Adapted from Occupational Safety and Health Administration (OSHA). 1994. *OSHA Regulation Standard 29 C.F.R. 1926.65*. Appendix B. General description and discussion of the levels of protection and protective gear. Washington, DC: OSHA. Available at http://www.osha.gov/pls/oshaweb/owadisp.show_document?p_table=STANDARDS&p_id=10653. Accessed January 20, 2017.
Note: NIOSH=National Institute of Occupational Safety and Health; SCBA=self-contained breathing apparatus.

Although OSHA requires that employers are responsible for ensuring that their employees have adequate respiratory protection, depending on the size and location of the disaster, state and local departments of health (DOHs) may assess initial safety and health practices at the site of the disaster and provide the initial distribution of PPE. An appropriate respirator program involves medical screening, fit testing, and training. Training includes instructing the workers on how to wear, clean, and maintain the respirators.

Employees exposed to accidental chemical splashes, falling objects, flying particles, unknown atmospheres within adequate oxygen or toxic gases, fires, live electrical wiring, or similar emergencies need PPE, including the following:

- Safety glasses, goggles, or face shields for eye protection
- Properly selected and fitted respirators
- Hard hats and safety shoes for head and foot protection

- Whole body coverings (e.g., chemical suits, gloves, hoods, and boots for protection from chemicals)
- Body protection for abnormal environmental conditions such as extreme temperatures

Finally, a mechanism is needed to monitor environmental exposures of the community and of response workers. The establishment of a worker injury and illness surveillance system will permit the generation of daily injury reports that can guide the modification of prevention measures and the types of PPE needed. More specific information is available in the Occupational Safety and Health Standards (29 C.F.R. 1910), which are the OSHA general industry standards (available at: http://www.osha.gov/pls/oshaweb/owastand.display_standard_group?p_toc_level=1&p_part_number=1910).

Emergency Communication

Effective emergency communication is vital, especially when using PPE with highly contagious infections or dangerous materials. A system should be established to account for personnel once workers have been deployed or evacuated, with a person in the control center responsible for notifying police or emergency response team members of people believed missing. Management should provide emergency alarms and ensure that workers know how to report emergencies within the response activities. Handout materials need to be developed that are simple to read. Key ideas can be listed on a card, such as site safety rules or the use of PPE. The card can be laminated so that it can be posted on equipment used in the rescue or recovery.

PPE and Ebola

While a variety of clinical situations necessitate that providers of medical care to wear PPE to protect themselves and their environment from contamination, caring for patients with highly infectious and potentially deadly diseases requires an additional level of diligence. When health care workers developed Ebola after caring for the first infected patient in the United States in 2014, CDC and OSHA updated detailed guidance on the use of PPE when caring for a suspected or definite Ebola patient.

Key to the guidance is that everyone caring for patients must be properly protected. Protection includes training employees in proper donning and doffing techniques for the PPE they will be using. In addition, a trained observer should observe the donning and doffing procedure. The doffing procedure requires that the PPE be removed slowly and carefully to reduce the risk of contamination. An observer also watches providers who are working at the patient's bedside for potential contamination. The observer provides directions on personal decontamination, where needed. Table 10-3 describes

Table 10-3. Recommended Administrative and Environmental Controls for Health Care Facilities Caring for Ebola Patients

Who Takes Action	Action	Specific Step
Facility's infection control team, in collaboration with occupational health and other clinical departments	Establish and implement triage protocols to promptly identify patients who could have Ebola.	
	Designate site managers responsible for (1) implementation of routine and additional precautions for health care worker and patient safety, and (2) ensuring the safe delivery of clinical care to patients with Ebola.	Site managers should have experience in implementing protocols for employee safety, infection control, and patient safety.
	Site managers responsible for all aspects of Ebola infection control: (1) access to supplies; (2) ongoing evaluation of safe practices; and (3) direct observation of care before, during, and after staff enter an isolation and treatment area.	At least 1 site manager should be on-site at all times in the location where a patient with Ebola is receiving care.
	In advance: • identify critical patient care functions and essential health care workers needed to care for patients with Ebola, • collect laboratory specimens, and • manage the environment and waste.	Consider engaging the hospital incident command structure to further facilitate implementing Ebola-specific precautions.
	Ensure health care workers have been trained and evaluated in all recommended protocols to safely care for patients with Ebola before they enter the patient care area.	
	Ensure that workplace safety programs are in place and have been followed for OSHA's blood-borne pathogens, PPE, and respiratory protection standards.	
	Coordinate with safety program administrators to ensure that (1) all PPE has been selected to meet needs from a written risk assessment and (2) requirements for medical surveillance and clearance, fit testing, training, maintenance, storage, reporting, etc. are in place for all workers with potential exposure to Ebola.	

(Continued)

Table 10-3. (Continued)

Who Takes Action	Action	Specific Step
	Train health care workers on all PPE recommended in the facility's protocols.	
	Health care workers should practice donning and doffing procedures and must demonstrate competency through testing and assessment **before** caring for patients with Ebola.	
	Health care workers should practice simulated patient care activities while wearing the PPE to (1) understand the types of physical stress that might be involved and (2) determine tolerable shift lengths.	Use trained observers to ensure that PPE is being used correctly and that donning and doffing PPE protocols are being adhered to Use a checklist to verify compliance with each step of the donning and doffing procedure. Personnel who are unable to correctly use PPE and adhere to protocols should not provide care for patients with Ebola.
	Document training of observers and health care workers	
	Document proficiency and competency in donning and doffing PPE and in performing all necessary care-related duties while wearing PPE.	
	Designate distinct spaces so that PPE can be donned and doffed in unconnected areas to prevent any cross-contamination.	
Use key safe work practices	Identify and promptly isolate the patient with Ebola in a single patient room with a closed door and a private bathroom or covered bedside commode.	
	Limit room entry to only those health care workers essential to the patient's care and restrict nonessential personnel and visitors from the patient care area.	

(Continued)

Table 10-3. (Continued)

Who Takes Action	Action	Specific Step
	Monitor the patient care area at all times, and, at a minimum, log entry and exit of all health care workers who enter the room of a patient with Ebola.	
	Establish procedures to ensure that staff can safely conduct routine patient care activities (e.g., obtaining vital signs and conducting clinically appropriate examinations, collecting and appropriately packaging laboratory specimens).	
	Dedicate a trained observer to watch closely and provide coaching for each donning and each doffing procedure to ensure adherence to the protocols for each.	
	Ensure that health care workers take sufficient time to don and doff PPE slowly and correctly without distraction.	
	Reinforce the need to keep hands away from the face during any patient care and to limit touching surfaces and body fluids.	
	Frequently disinfect gloved hands by using an alcohol-based hand rub, particularly after contact with body fluids.	
	Prevent needlestick and sharps injuries by adhering to correct sharps handling practices.	Avoid unnecessary procedures involving sharps. Use needleless IV systems whenever possible.
	Immediately clean and disinfect any visibly contaminated PPE surfaces, equipment, or patient care area surfaces using an EPA-registered disinfectant wipe. (See http://www.epa.gov/oppad001/list-l-ebola-virus.html.)	
	Regularly clean and disinfect surfaces in the patient care area, even in the absence of visible contamination.	Only nurses or physicians should clean and disinfect surfaces in the patient care areas to limit the number of additional health care workers who enter the room.

(Continued)

Table 10-3. (Continued)

Who Takes Action	Action	Specific Step
	Site manager, or his/her designee, observes health care workers in the patient room if possible (e.g., through a glass-walled intensive care unit room, video link) to identify any unrecognized lapses or near misses in safe care.	Establish a management plan for unexpected exposures that addresses decontamination and follow-up of health care workers and training and review.

Source: Adapted from Centers for Disease Control and Prevention. 2015. *Guidance on Personal Protective Equipment (PPE) to Be Used by Healthcare Workers During Management of Patients With Confirmed Ebola or Persons Under Investigation (PUIs) for Ebola Who Are Clinically Unstable or Have Bleeding, Vomiting, or Diarrhea in U.S. Hospitals, Including Procedures for Donning and Doffing PPE.* Section 1. Recommended administrative and environmental controls for healthcare facilities. Available at: http://www.cdc.gov/vhf/ebola/healthcare-us/ppe/guidance.html. Accessed January 20, 2017.

Note: EPA=U.S. Environmental Protection Agency; OSHA=Occupational Safety and Health Administration; PPE=personal protective equipment.

recommended administrative and environmental controls for health care facilities caring for Ebola patients.

Selecting PPE With the Proper Protection

PPE recommendations are based on the patient's clinical status and activities being performed (e.g., interview of patient, blood draw, hands-on care with patient who is vomiting and/or has diarrhea). The risk of exposure is low for health care workers caring for a patient being evaluated for Ebola who does not have bleeding, vomiting, or diarrhea, and there is specific PPE guidance for these instances. The risk of exposure is higher when patients are known to have Ebola or when patients under evaluation have bleeding, vomiting, or diarrhea, and workers should follow the guidance for PPE that provides protection for that higher risk.

Some literature suggests that the Ebola virus can be transmitted via infectious aerosol particles both near and at a distance from infected patients, although this has not been universally accepted or reflected in federal guidance. Brosseau and Jones posit that body fluids (e.g., vomit, diarrhea, blood, and saliva) can produce inhalable aerosol particles in the area near an infected person. Some of these are small enough to be inhaled. Using the precautionary principle (i.e., if a serious threat exists, lack of scientific knowledge should not stop people from taking protective measures), the highest level of PPE should be used to protect those caring for patients with Ebola. If Ebola can be transmitted via aerosolized particles, or aerosol transmissible, then health care workers should wear respirators with an assigned protection factor greater than 10, not facemasks because facemasks do not offer protection against inhalation of small infectious aerosols since they have no or limited filters and allow air in between the mask and the face. Therefore, a higher level of protection may be necessary. Using the Canadian control-banding approach, while caring for a patient in the early stages of disease (e.g., no bleeding, vomiting, diarrhea, coughing, sneezing), Brosseau and Jones recommend the use of a negative pressure air-purifying half-facepiece respirator such as an N95 filtering facepiece respirator, with fit testing. When caring for a patient in the later stages of disease (e.g., bleeding, vomiting, diarrhea), they recommend a negative pressure air-purifying full-facepiece respirator or a positive pressure half-facepiece powered air-purifying respirator (PAPR), with fit testing. Where patients are in rooms with negative-pressure airborne infection isolation, they recommend a PAPR with a loose-fitting facepiece or with a helmet or hood that does not need fit testing. In addition, clinical laboratories and health care facilities may decide to include additional PPE.

When choosing PPE, the focus should be on the performance characteristics of the gear and suitability for use during the specific tasks rather than on the specific type of equipment. Critical features include impermeability or fluid resistance to protect from body fluids and viruses; FDA clearance on isolation gowns and coveralls; protection rating appropriate for the intended use; and the ability to safely put on and remove the equipment. A garment that is labeled as "fluid-resistant" may not provide resistance to blood, body fluids, or viruses. Manufacturers of PPE suitable for Ebola-level protection should meet the specifications outlined in the guidance document (available at: http://www.cdc.gov/vhf/ebola/hcp/procedures-for-ppe.html). Product information on gowns and coveralls should state the standards to which the garments conform, including those for impermeability or fluid resistance. Since altering PPE may affect the ability of the garment to protect the user, before making a change to any garment, consult the manufacturer to determine if changes to the garment will maintain the provided protection. Health care administrators should be aware of the cost of procuring the necessary PPE. A PAPR, depending on the brand and type, can cost $600 to $1,200. Outfitting a single provider in the most protective PPE can cost hundreds to thousands of dollars. Table 10-4 describes the principles of PPE when caring for patients with Ebola.

Coveralls that meet NFPA 1999 (amended April 2015) will protect health care workers treating confirmed Ebola patients because its standard for viral penetration resistance of both fabric and seams meets the specification in the updated PPE guidance (available at: http://www.cdc.gov/vhf/ebola/hcp/procedures-for-ppe.html). NPFA 1999 also provides performance requirements beyond those in the updated PPE guidance as discussed in the CDC's *Considerations for Selecting Protective Clothing Used in Healthcare for Protection Against Microorganisms in Blood and Body Fluids.* This guidance provides an in-depth explanation of the scientific evidence and national and international standards, test methods, and specifications for impermeable protective clothing used in health care (it is available at http://www.cdc.gov/niosh/npptl/topics/protectiveclothing/default.html). More detailed information on OSHA's *PPE Selection Matrix for Occupational Exposure to Ebola Virus* is available at: https://www.osha.gov/Publications/OSHA3761.pdf. Specific recommendations for PPE for some non-health care workers were issued by NIOSH and, while they are not being updated at this time, they have been archived online (available at: http://www.cdc.gov/niosh/topics/ebola/nonhealthcare.html).

Finally, protective garments must be used correctly in order to ensure intended protection.[2] The CDC recommends that a health care worker wear an apron over their gown

---

2. Additional guidance is available at Centers for Disease Control and Prevention. 2015. *Guidance on Personal Protective Equipment (PPE) to Be Used by Healthcare Workers During Management of Patients With Confirmed Ebola or Persons Under Investigation (PUIs) for Ebola Who Are Clinically Unstable or Have Bleeding, Vomiting, or Diarrhea in U.S. Hospitals, Including Procedures for Donning and Doffing PPE.* Section 9. Recommended sequences for donning PPE. Available at: http://www.cdc.gov/vhf/ebola/healthcare-us/ppe/guidance.html. Accessed January 20, 2017; Centers for Disease Control and Prevention. 2015. *Guidance on Personal Protective Equipment (PPE) to Be Used by Healthcare Workers During Management of Patients With Confirmed Ebola or Persons Under Investigation (PUIs) for Ebola Who Are Clinically Unstable or Have Bleeding, Vomiting, or Diarrhea in U.S. Hospitals, Including Procedures for Donning and Doffing PPE.* Section 1. Recommended administrative and environmental controls for healthcare facilities. Available at: http://www.cdc.gov/vhf/ebola/healthcare-us/ppe/guidance.html. Accessed January 20, 2017.

Table 10-4. Principles of Personal Protective Equipment When Caring for Patients With Ebola

Procedure	Guidance
Donning	• PPE must be donned correctly, in proper order, before entry into the patient care area, with no modifications while in the patient care area. • The donning activities must be directly observed by a trained observer.
During Patient Care	• PPE must remain in place and be worn correctly for the duration of work in potentially contaminated areas. • PPE should not be adjusted during patient care. • In the event of a significant splash, the health care worker should immediately move to the doffing area to remove PPE. • One exception—visibly contaminated outer gloves can be changed while in the patient room and patient care can continue. • Contaminated outer gloves can be disposed of in the patient room with other Ebola-associated waste. (See http://www.cdc.gov/vhf/ebola/healthcare-us/cleaning/waste-management.html.) Health care workers should perform frequent disinfection of gloved hands using an alcohol-based hand rub, particularly after contact with body fluids. • If during patient care any breach in PPE occurs (e.g., a tear develops in an outer glove, a needlestick occurs, a glove separates from the sleeve), the health care worker must move immediately to the doffing area to assess the exposure. • The facility exposure management plan should be implemented; including correct supervised doffing and appropriate occupational health follow-up, if indicated by assessment. • In the event of a potential exposure, blood-borne pathogen exposure procedures must be followed in accordance with the OSHA Bloodborne Pathogens Standard (see https://www.osha.gov/SLTC/healthcarefacilities/standards.html)
Doffing	Removing used PPE is a high-risk process that requires a structured procedure, a trained observer, a doffing assistant in some situations, and a designated area for removal to ensure protection. PPE must be removed slowly and deliberately in the correct sequence to reduce the possibility of self-contamination or other exposure to Ebola. A stepwise process should be developed and used during training and patient care.

Source: Adapted from Centers for Disease Control and Prevention. 2015. *Guidance on Personal Protective Equipment (PPE) to Be Used by Healthcare Workers During Management of Patients With Confirmed Ebola or Persons Under Investigation (PUIs) for Ebola Who Are Clinically Unstable or Have Bleeding, Vomiting, or Diarrhea in U.S. Hospitals, Including Procedures for Donning and Doffing PPE.* Section 2. Principles of PPE. Available at: http://www.cdc.gov/vhf/ebola/healthcare-us/ppe/guidance.html. Accessed January 20, 2017.

Note: OSHA = Occupational Safety and Health Administration; PPE = personal protective equipment. Double-gloving provides an easy way to remove gross contamination by changing an outer glove during patient care and when removing PPE. Beyond this, more layers of PPE may make it more difficult to perform patient care duties and put health care workers at greater risk for percutaneous injury (e.g., needlesticks), self-contamination during care or doffing, or other exposures to Ebola. If health care facilities decide to add additional PPE or modify this PPE guidance, they must consider the risk/benefit of any modification and train health care workers on how to correctly don and doff for the modified procedure. Donning and doffing steps may need to be adapted on the basis of the specific PPE that is purchased by the hospital. If adaptations are made, facilities must select PPE that offers a similar or higher level of protection than what is recommended here, train health care workers in its use, and ensure they demonstrate competence in its use before caring for a patient with Ebola.

or coveralls any time a patient is vomiting or has diarrhea to minimize exposure to the PPE and provide an easily discarded layer if the apron becomes soiled. If there is significant soiling of the PPE, the health care worker should leave the patient care area and take off the PPE in the doffing area under the observation of a trained observer. Continuing to work in equipment that is soiled creates additional risks for contamination. Health care workers preparing to remove PPE should ask the trained observer to visually inspect their PPE. The health care worker should then use disinfectant wipes to remove as much of the soil as possible in order to decrease the risk of contamination before beginning the doffing process. PPE must be removed slowly and deliberately in the correct sequence to reduce the possibility of self-contamination or other exposure to Ebola virus.

PPE and Hazardous Materials

In addition to protection against highly infectious disease, health care workers need protection when caring for patients endangered by hazardous materials or biological or radiological exposures. OSHA has issued a best practices document to guide hospitals who are receiving victims of incidents involving hazardous materials. It is assumed that hospitals will have little or no warning before patients who have been exposed to toxic materials will arrive in emergency departments. OSHA requires Level B protection or self-contained breathing apparatus when patients may be exposed to unknown substances. (This detailed program is available at: https://www.osha.gov/dts/osta/bestpractices/html/hospital_firstreceivers.html.)

When patients go directly to hospitals, rather than being evaluated by first providers in the field, hospitals have to consider decontamination of patients (gross or secondary) in the event that the incident involves hazardous materials or biological or radiological exposures. Preparedness requires the purchase and stocking of PPE so that providers can perform patient care. PPE items typically include an impervious gown or suit to protect the skin; gloves to protect hands; boots/shoe covers to protect feet; and a surgical mask, N95 respirator, or PAPR for respiratory protection. PPE must be appropriate to the level of risk and be accepted by the users, and hospitals have to provide training on the use of PPE so that providers are familiar with it in advance. It is critical that hospitals have to establish a mechanism for medical surveillance and fit testing so that all personnel are ready to use PPE quickly in an emergency.

Blood-Borne Pathogens

The OSHA Bloodborne Pathogens Standard (29 C.F.R. 1910.1030) was developed to reduce the potential exposure of health care personnel to blood-borne pathogens.

All U.S. laboratories handling patient specimens are required to continuously comply with this standard, with strict adherence being an initial step in providing protection to personnel. To minimize risk to personnel, a site-specific assessment of potential risk must be performed by the laboratory director, safety officer, and other responsible individuals prior to receiving blood-borne specimens in order to determine the potential for exposure from sprays, splashes, or aerosols generated during work in the laboratory. To mitigate risks, laboratories should implement engineering controls, administrative and work practice controls, employee training, and require the use of the appropriate level of PPE. Additional guidance is available at: https://www.osha.gov/Publications/osha3187.pdf.

Recovery and Handling of Human Remains

When establishing a temporary mortuary, look for a secure building that has the capacity for a reception room, a viewing room, a place for storing bodies at 39°F, and rooms for records and personal effects. Mortuary personnel should wear gloves and protective clothing and wash thoroughly with a disinfectant soap. Mortuary supplies include stretchers, leather gloves, rubber gloves, overalls, boots, caps, soap, cotton cloths and disinfectants, property bags, body bags and labels, wheeled trolleys to transport bodies, and plastic sheeting for the floor. In the United States it is common to use ice skating rinks, where available, to store remains and refrigerator trucks to transport the bodies. When setting up a facility for the identification of bodies, the World Health Organization recommends 2,187 square yards (1,828.6 square meters) for 1,000 unidentified bodies.

When a disaster involves the recovery of human body parts, there is no threat of a general outbreak of infectious disease. Workers are at risk of viral or bacterial infection if they cut themselves with an object contaminated with blood, body fluids, or tissue, or if these materials touch the rescuers' eyes, nose, mouth, or areas of broken skin. Bad odors coming from decomposing bodies are not harmful.

Rescue workers who expect that they might have direct contact with human remains should be advised to do the following:

- Take universal precautions for blood and body fluids.
- Be sure that their hepatitis B vaccination is current.
- Wear heavy-duty waterproof gloves to protect against injury from sharp environmental debris or bone fragments; a combination of gloves with an inner layer that cannot be cut and an outer layer of latex or something similar is preferable.
- Protect your face from splashes of body fluids and fecal material. Use eye protection and respirators equipped with organic vapor/acid gas (OVAG) cartridges to protect eyes, nose, and mouth from splash exposures and noxious odors; where

OVAG protection is not available, workers can use a plastic face shield or a combination of eye protection (indirectly vented safety goggles if available) and a surgical mask. If nothing else is available, use a cloth tied over the nose and mouth to block splashes.

- Wear protective garments to protect skin and clothes, including gloves. Footwear should similarly protect against sharp debris.
- Protect hands from direct contact with body fluids, and from cuts, puncture wounds, or other injuries that break the skin because of sharp environmental debris or bone fragments.
- Immediately wash hands with soap and water or with an alcohol-based hand cleaner after removing gloves.
- Use alcohol-based hand sanitizers only when hands are not visibly soiled.
- Promptly care for any wounds received while handling remains, including immediate cleansing with soap and clean water and getting a tetanus booster.
- Avoid cross-contamination of personal items.
- Thoroughly disinfect vehicles and equipment.
- Participate in available programs to provide psychological and emotional support for workers handling human remains. (See Chapter 8 for more information.)

CHAPTER 11

PEOPLE WITH DISABILITIES AND OTHERS WITH ACCESS AND FUNCTIONAL NEEDS

Individuals who may be disproportionately impacted during emergencies and may require specific resources to ensure that their needs are included in planning, response and recovery include those with disabilities or access and functional needs. This chapter defines who is at risk for significant adverse outcomes following a disaster, provides an overview of federal guidance on emergency preparedness for these populations, and describes disaster planning councils, community planning, and the training of response personnel to effectively help these at-risk populations. This chapter also discusses the pros and cons of the use of registries, specific strategies for protecting selected populations, steps to ensure individual preparedness, preparedness in shelters, ensuring accessible communications and transportation, preparedness in buildings, and the gathering and maintenance of emergency health information.

Public Health Role

- Ensure that the planning process includes the whole community and the organizations that serve them.
- Ensure that community preparedness plans accommodate the needs of populations with disabilities and others with access and functional needs.
- Educate the community about actions that can be taken to protect those with disabilities and others with access and functional needs in times of emergency.
- Coordinate preparedness in health care delivery sites, shelters, and distribution centers for those with disabilities and others with access and functional needs.
- Ensure that resources are accessible to all individuals, including those with access-based needs.

Who Is At-Risk?

Section 2814 of the Pandemic and All-Hazards Preparedness Act requires that emergency planning include the needs of at-risk populations who may require additional assistance during a response. In their definition, the Office of the Assistant Secretary for Preparedness and Response (ASPR) and the U.S. Department of Health & Human Services (HHS) followed the description of at-risk populations found in the National Response Framework (NRF).

The populations of individuals who are likely to need additional assistance in a disaster is quite broad and includes people with access and functional needs that may interfere with their ability to receive health care, take care of themselves, get to shelter, take preparatory actions, or understand the implications of what may be happening before, during, or after a disaster. The term "access and functional needs" is not tied to a specific diagnosis, status, or label and is used to describe a broad set of common and overlapping necessities before, during, and after a disaster.

- *Access-based needs* refers to ensuring that resources, such as human services, housing, information, transportation, and medications to maintain health, are available to all individuals.
- *Function-based needs* refers to restrictions or functional limitations that interfere with an individual's ability to perform fundamental physical and mental tasks or activities of daily living, such as eating, toileting, or bathing. This definition reflects the capabilities of the individual, not the condition, label, or medical diagnosis.

Examples of these populations include children, older adults, and individuals with disabilities who live in institutional settings, are from diverse cultures, have limited English proficiency or are non-English speaking, lack access or the ability to use transportation, are homeless, have chronic medical disorders, rely on electricity to power life-sustaining medical and assistive equipment, or have pharmacological dependency.

Individuals who have disabilities and others with access and functional needs often need additional support and/or specific equipment or services before, during, and after a disaster in one or more of the following areas, commonly known as C-MIST:

Communication: No or limited ability to receive or respond to emergency information. Includes ability to hear announcements, see directional signage, and understand how to get assistance.

Maintaining Health: During an emergency, people may be separated from family or caregivers. These individuals may require assistance in personal care and/or in maintaining their activities of daily living.

Medical Care: Individuals with chronic medical illness need continued access to medical care following a disaster to avoid a worsening of these conditions.

Independence: Individuals with access and functional needs often require help to be independent in daily activities when their usual support is lost in a disaster, including replacement of lost durable medical equipment and essential supplies.

Support and Safety: During a disaster or emergency, some people with behavioral health conditions (i.e., addiction problems, Alzheimer's disease, dementia, schizophrenia, or severe mental illness) or traumatic brain injury may become anxious. While some individuals are able to function well, others require services and support.

Self-Determination: Individuals with access and functional needs want to be able to make choices and decisions based on their own preferences and interests. People with disabilities are the most knowledgeable about their own needs.

Transportation: Often these individuals cannot drive because of their disability or they do not have transportation. Their transportation needs may include accessible vehicles equipped with lifts or oxygen.

Several national groups provide leadership in this area. The ASPR supports the Advisory Committee on At-Risk Individuals and Public Health Emergencies, which focuses on public health emergencies as they relate to at-risk individuals. The Federal Emergency Management Agency (FEMA) appoints a disability coordinator to provide guidance on planning requirements and direct emergency management activities for individuals with disabilities. FEMA has established the Office of Disability Integration and Coordination (ODIC), which advises FEMA, serves as liaison to the Department of Homeland Security (DHS) and other federal partners, and implements the requirements of the Post-Katrina Emergency Management Reform Act of 2006 (PKEMRA; see below). The ODIC ensures that the federal government provides needed services to individuals with disabilities during disasters. ODIC lists extensive resources on its Web site (available at: https://www.fema.gov/office-disability-integration-and-coordination).

People With Disabilities

The National Organization on Disability defines individuals with disabilities as those who have a physical or mental impairment that limits their major life activities, who have an ongoing or chronic physical or mental condition, or who are regarded by the community as disabled even without a condition.

According to the data collected in 2010 from the survey of income and program participation by the U.S. Census Bureau, 56 million Americans (almost 20% of the population) have a disability, with 12.6% or 38.3 million people having a severe disability. This group includes 1.8 million unable to see words in print; 4 million who require assistance with dressing, eating, or bathing; 28 million with hearing loss, of which 1 million are unable to hear conversations; 3.3 million older than age 14 years who use a wheelchair; and 10 million who require the use of canes, crutches, or walkers. Furthermore, there are over 4,000 adult daycare centers in the United States and about 800,000 people living in assisted care facilities. These statistics may not account for the additional segment of the population with chronic illnesses that would inhibit their ability to function in a disaster situation. There are many more people who experience disabilities and functional needs than the commonly referred to "1 in 5 individuals." This segment of people is estimated to be up to 50% of the population. In disasters, functional needs can increase significantly when people do not have access to their devices, equipment, supplies, or aids due to changes in their everyday environments. This lack of access can contribute to decreased independence and increases the potential number of those needing assistance.

National Guidance

Key federal documents provide direction that is helpful in planning for at-risk populations. The NRF defines the term *functional needs populations* and addresses specific issues regarding these individuals in the appropriate operational protocols. The National Incident Management System stresses the importance of the accessibility of emergency communications, effective outreach to populations with functional needs, and the addition of a special-needs advisor within the incident command structure. FEMA and the DHS Office for Civil Rights and Civil Liberties developed a guidance document, *Accommodating Individuals with Disabilities in the Provision of Disaster Mass Care, Housing, and Human Services: Reference Guide* (available at: https://www.fema.gov/media-library-data/20130726-1617-20490-6430/section689referenceguide.pdf). The DHS Grants Program includes planning for functional needs populations (available at: https://www.fema.gov/grants). In addition, 8 federal laws prohibit discrimination in emergency preparedness and response on the basis of disability:

- Americans with Disabilities Act of 1990 (ADA)
- Robert T. Stafford Disaster Relief and Emergency Assistance Act of 1988
- PKEMRA
- Rehabilitation Act of 1973 (including Section 508)
- Fair Housing Act of 1968
- Architectural Barriers Act of 1968
- Individuals with Disabilities Education Act of 1975
- Telecommunications Act of 1996

These statutes apply in activities of preparation, notification, evacuation and transportation, sheltering, first aid and medical services, temporary lodging and housing, transition back to community, and cleanup. Two key regulations are discussed next.

American With Disabilities Act Guidance

Preparedness for disasters should include specific safeguards to ensure the safety of those with disabilities both in the workplace and in the community. The ADA (Public Law 101-336, July 26, 1990) mandates "reasonable accommodation" or ensuring the same level of safety and utility for people with disabilities and other limitations as that provided to the entire population. The ADA provides a process to determine if individuals with disabilities have been discriminated against or denied services because of their disability, including the emergency preparedness activities of a community. The process involves a complaint filed with the U.S. Department of Justice, followed by an investigation, mediation, litigation, or suit.

The ADA Accessibility Guidelines (ADAAG), which primarily cover new construction and alterations, include specifications for accessible means of egress (ADAAG 4.1.3[9], 4.3.10), emergency alarms (ADAAG 4.1.3[14], 4.28), and signage (ADAAG 4.1.3[16], 4.30). State and local governments have additional ADA requirements, including the provision of auxiliary aids and services, the acquisition or modification of equipment or devices, appropriate adjustment or modification of training materials or policies, the provision of qualified readers or interpreters, and other similar accommodations. In addition, 47 C.F.R. § 79.2 obliges distributors of video programming to make emergency information accessible to people with hearing disabilities or vision loss.

Post-Katrina Emergency Management Reform Act

On October 4, 2006, Congress passed the PKEMRA in response to the deficiencies in the federal government's response to Hurricane Katrina. Although PKEMRA revamped the federal government's overall approach to managing preparedness, key sections required improving preparedness and response for individuals with disabilities. In PKEMRA, the term *individual with a disability* is defined by reference to Section 3(2) of ADA. Key sections include the following:

- **Section 689(a)** requires FEMA to "develop guidelines to accommodate individuals with disabilities" including accessibility of shelters, recovery centers, first aid stations, mass feeding areas, portable pay phone stations, portable toilets, and temporary housing.
- **Section 689(c)** amends the Stafford Act and provides temporary housing assistance to individuals with disabilities whose residence is rendered "inaccessible" as a result of a major disaster.
- **Section 689(e)** amends the Stafford Act to require FEMA to coordinate with state and local governments in the planning for population groups with limited English proficiency, to ensure that information is made available in formats that can be understood, and to develop and maintain an informational clearinghouse of model language assistance programs and best practices.
- **Section 689(a)** amends Section 308(a) of the Stafford Act to prohibit discrimination on the basis of "disability and English proficiency."

In addition, PKEMRA required that services be provided so that individuals with disabilities can maintain their health, safety, and independence in a shelter whose residents are from the general population. The *Functional Needs Support Services* (FNSS) regulations call for the provision of accessible supplies and services, including the following:

- Reasonable modification to policies, procedures, and practices
- Durable medical equipment
- Consumable medical supplies
- Personal assistance services
- Other goods and services as needed

Table 11-1 identifies some national standards that provide guidance in preparedness and response activities for at-risk populations.

Guidance for Children

In 2008, Congress authorized the formation of the National Commission on Children and Disasters to ensure that children's needs are considered in disaster plans at all levels of government. Before being terminated in April 2011, the Commission issued a report that recommended more than 30 improvements in emergency preparedness and response for children (available at: http://archive.ahrq.gov/prep/nccdreport/nccdreport.pdf). The report also included standards for the care of children in shelters, reflected in Appendix S. At shelters, children need safety, nutrition, waste disposal, protection against infectious disease, and stress management. Those setting up shelters should protect children from hazardous materials, trip hazards, and adult predators. All medication should be secured so they are not accessible to children. Finally, the frail elderly should be protected from unruly children.

FEMA established the Children's Working Group in 2009 to guarantee that federal planning in emergency management includes the needs of children. The Lessons Learned Information Sharing service working with the Commission and the FEMA Children's Working Group, created the Children and Disasters resource page to consolidate guidance documents, training programs, and lessons learned from exercises and real-world incidents involving children (available at: https://www.fema.gov/children-and-disasters).

The Pandemic and All-Hazards Preparedness Reauthorization Act of 2013 (Public Law 113-5) authorized the establishment of the National Advisory Committee on Children and Disasters (NACCD). This Committee was established under the oversight of the ASPR to provide advice and consultation to the secretary of HHS on issues related to the medical and public health needs of children during times of disaster. The NACCD established 2 working groups: surge capacity and health preparedness. The full report is

Table 11-1. National Standards in Preparedness and Response for At-Risk Populations

Organization	Guidance Name	What It Does	Source
FEMA	Comprehensive Preparedness Guide (CPG) 301: Interim Emergency Management Planning Guide for Special Needs Populations	Helps governments develop emergency plans for people with functional needs	http://www2.ku.edu/~rrtcpbs/resources/pdf/FEMA_CPG301.pdf
		Addresses planning considerations for range of hazards, security, and emergency functions	
		Provides general guidelines for developing a governmental household pet and service animal plan	
ADA and ADA Amendments Act (2008)	ADA Amendments Act	Requires equal access to all government programs	http://www.ada.gov
		Broadened scope of the definition of *disability*	
		Allows people with functional needs to seek protection under the ADA, including all disaster plans developed for a community under Title II	
ADA guide	Making Community Emergency Preparedness and Response Programs Accessible to People with Disabilities	Provides guidance for making local emergency preparedness and response programs accessible to people with disabilities	http://www.usdoj.gov/crt/ada/emergencyprep.htm

(Continued)

Table 11-1. (Continued)

Organization	Guidance Name	What It Does	Source
1986 Superfund Amendment and Reauthorization Act, Title III	LEPCs	Directs the creation and membership of LEPCs	https://www.epa.gov/laws-regulations/summary-emergency-planning-community-right-know-act
The Joint Commission	Emergency Management Standards of The Joint Commission	Oversees standard setting for health care facilities and accredits health care facilities	http://www.jointcommission.org
NFPA	NFPA 99, 1600	Recommends safety codes and standards for the prevention of fires and other hazards	http://www.nfpa.org
Federal Communications Commission	EAS Rules (47 C.F.R. Part 11)	Regulations regarding both EAS and closed-captioning	http://www.fcc.gov
	Closed-Captioning Rules (47 C.F.R. § 79)		
FEMA	Guidance on Planning for Integration of Functional Needs Support Services in General Population Shelters	Provides guidance for the implementation of practices so that individuals with disabilities can maintain their health, safety, and independence in a shelter whose residents are from the general population	http://www.fema.gov/pdf/about/odic/fnss_guidance.pdf

Source: Based on National Organization on Disability. 2009. *Functional Needs of People With Disabilities: A Guide for Emergency Managers, Planners and Responders.* Washington, DC: National Organization on Disability Emergency Preparedness Initiative; BCFS Health and Human Services. 2010. *Guidance on Planning for Integration of Functional Needs Support Services in General Population Shelters.* Washington, DC: Federal Emergency Management Agency. Available at: http://www.fema.gov/pdf/about/odic/fnss_guidance.pdf. Accessed January 21, 2017.

Note: ADA=American With Disabilities Act; EAS=Emergency Alert System; FEMA=Federal Emergency Management Agency; NFPA=National Fire Protection Association; LEPC=local emergency planning committee.

available at: http://www.phe.gov/preparedness/legal/boards/naccd/pages/recommendations.aspx.

In 2010, the Children's HHS Interagency Leadership on Disasters Working Group was established to integrate children's needs across the disaster policy, planning, and operations activities conducted by HHS. The working group's 2014 report made recommendations for 2 groups:

- Children at heightened risk (e.g., special health care needs)
  - Design messaging about disaster preparedness for low-income families with children.
  - Develop education and outreach to promote influenza preparedness for children with neurologic and neurodevelopmental disabilities.
- Neonates, pregnant/breastfeeding women
  - Disseminate a toolkit to assist public health departments in assessing the needs and outcomes of women of reproductive age after disasters.
  - Use prenatal care records and mobile-phone messaging as a communication tool to support disaster preparedness, resilience, and access to services for women.
  - Conduct research on the perinatal effects of recent natural disasters.

The report is available at: http://www.phe.gov/preparedness/planning/abc/documents/child-wg-report2012-2013.pdf.

Disaster Planning Councils for Populations With Disability and Others With Access and Functional Needs

Ideally, planning for people with disabilities and others with access and functional needs occurs at both the whole community and the individual levels. As part of community planning, one strategy is to organize a disaster planning council, which includes planning for at-risk populations. A disaster planning council is a network of representatives from neighborhoods, businesses, local organization and community groups who work together before and after a disaster to meet the needs of their community. In coordination with emergency management, public health professionals can reach out to the organizations that represent the breadth of individuals who have disabilities or access and functional needs. The planning group should identify what is needed during a disaster, what strategies can be used to address those needs, and which agency or group will be responsible for providing which services. Planning councils should always include people with disabilities or others with access and functional needs to ensure that the proposed solutions will work and also provide confidence to those who need them. Effective planning requires the utilization of multiple methods because the needs of at-risk groups are both broad and varied. Furthermore, it is crucial to inform the various groups of at-risk individuals how a community's specific disaster plans apply to them.

Disaster planning councils should include governmental agencies, community providers, community-based organizations (CBOs), advocacy groups, congregate living centers, and the local affiliate of national advocacy and disability organizations, where available. Because the definition of the individuals at-risk is so broad, communities might develop sections, such as school-based councils, to address the specific needs of a particular group. Disaster planning councils should be an essential part of a community's emergency response network, ensuring that the segment of the at-risk population that the CBOs serve is prepared. When forming the council, leaders from various segments of the at-risk population in the community should be located who will know the issues and agencies that need to be addressed. These leaders, often known as *advocates,* can help to identify both the groups that represent only their community and the organizations that represent the interests of more than one at-risk group. Table 11-2 lists examples of the potential groups who could participate in a planning council, though the names of these groups may vary by locale and region of the country. Because the official names of different types of organizations may not be the same in every community, public health professionals can work with an umbrella organization such as the United Way to identify which groups are present and active in a locale.

The disaster planning council can determine the specific plans, equipment, resources, and response activities required to ensure the safety of at-risk individuals during and in response to a disaster. Disaster plans for at-risk populations should specify the assignment of personnel, identify specialized equipment needed, and include information on the location of and availability of necessary assets. As part of preparedness activities, disaster planning councils can submit proposals to foundations to

Table 11-2. Potential Members of a Planning Council for At-Risk Populations

Government Agencies	Community Providers	Advocacy Groups
Mayor's office or county executive committee on people with disabilities	Visiting Nurse Service	National Association of the Deaf
Department of health and/or mental health	Meals on Wheels	Hearing Loss Association of America
Board of education	Residential and assisted-living facilities	Telecommunications for the Deaf, Inc.
Departments of rehabilitation and aging	Home health agencies	National Organization on Disability
Department of social services and regional centers	Ambulette and paratransit businesses	Local chapters of the American Foundation for the Blind and Council for the Blind
	After-school programs	Alliance for Technology Access
	Easterseals	Parent Teacher Association
	United Cerebral Palsy	Center for Independent Living

establish pre-disaster agreements so that, in an emergency, need for replacement equipment, medications, assistive devices, and the numerous other needs of at-risk populations can be quickly met.

Communities should designate a coordinator for populations with disabilities and others with access and functional needs who can work as part of the council and serve as liaisons with CBOs. The council can identify specific responsibilities that would be carried out by community and institutional providers in cooperation with advocacy-specific groups as part of a community's emergency response. Most importantly, members of the planning council have to be trained in developing a disaster plan for their organizations, their role and responsibilities as part of the overall community plan, and how to communicate and serve clients during an emergency.

Community Plans for Populations With Disabilities and Others With Access and Functional Needs

A community's plan should provide for guidance to its constituent organizations on improving preparedness for individuals with disabilities and others with access and functional needs in their homes and where they work, attend school, conduct activities of daily living, and receive services. A broad range of organizations provide service to these groups. Because the abilities and needs vary depending on the nature and severity of a disability and/or the type of access or functional need, it is important to develop emergency procedures that are specific to each group. For example, the range of disabilities that would impact one's ability to respond in a disaster is broad and whereas some disabilities are permanent, others are temporary. Both permanent conditions (e.g., arthritis) and temporary conditions (e.g., sprained ankle, broken leg) can limit one's ability to respond in a disaster. Planning is complicated because a person without disabilities may have what is called a *situational disability* because of the environment in which an emergency occurs. For example, many people would not be able to walk down a stairway of hundreds of steps in a high-rise building.

As some individuals with disabilities and others with access and functional needs may be connected through CBOs, home health care organizations, and health care providers, it is important to educate these groups to communicate and provide direct services to their clients in times of emergency. CBOs, community centers, and programs at which individuals with disabilities and others with access and functional needs spend time or receive services can distribute information about preparedness in their newsletters. Liaison relationships should be established with local social service departments to work out procedures for contacting clients in an affected disaster area. CBOs should encourage those with disabilities and/or access and functional needs to assess their own needs during a disaster and develop contingency plans.

Training

Training is necessary for response personnel so they are knowledgeable and skilled in using assistive equipment to aid individuals with disabilities and others with access and functional needs during emergencies. In addition, these individuals and/or their caregivers, need to know what to do in a disaster. Building on the materials developed by the American Red Cross (Red Cross) on sheltering and evacuation and emergency planning for people with disabilities and others with access and functional needs, the council can establish educational tools and work with the community to conduct "train-the-trainer" sessions about the creation of accessible facilities and services; transportation, lifting, or carrying; accessible communications and assistance; developing personal support networks (PSN); home preparation; preparation of Go Packs (discussed later in this chapter); and assistance animals.

Registries

The topic of registries is complex with many different layers and nuances. As an integral piece of community planning in the past, public health agencies were encouraged to work with CBOs to help create internal registries of the individuals they serve who have disabilities and others with access and functional needs. The rational was that these registries may help emergency management organizations understand how many individuals in the community have disabilities and access and functional needs and the range of problems that these individuals may encounter in a disaster. Once the registries are developed, public health can work with the local Office of Emergency Management to determine what services may be needed during a disaster.

Registries enable communities to develop specific disaster plans that include the necessary resources and response for at-risk individuals. Experience in previous disasters has demonstrated the need for preestablished procedures that facilitate the approval of and payment for medication and the replacement of durable medical equipment, such as wheelchairs, respirators, hearing aids, and other adaptive devices. This includes preestablished arrangements with designated pharmacies for the provision of pharmaceuticals on an emergency basis. Disaster plans could oblige utility companies to provide immediate notification to people who are dependent on life-sustaining electrical equipment, and listed on a registry, if they are aware that power is going to be reduced.

For communities that maintain these registries and distribute them to appropriate government departments and local emergency management teams, it is difficult to keep them current. Individuals should be asked to register annually, with periodic contact to determine whether they still need the registry's services. Information should be collected about alternative contacts for the registrant during the day since many individuals provide their home address to the registry but could be at school, work, or elsewhere when a disaster occurs. Registries should not be used as the definitive list for first responders since participation in registries is voluntary, and not everyone who potentially requires assistance during a disaster will enroll.

As developing comprehensive registries for at-risk populations may be labor intensive, several strategies can be used to minimize effort. A jurisdiction can target a registry to a segment or segments of the population. For example, a jurisdiction might choose to register individuals who will require evacuation or transportation assistance during a disaster. Communities may limit registries to individuals living in their own homes since the needs of individuals living in congregate settings, including group homes and other residential facilities, are known. The organization that manages these facilities should be encouraged to participate in community planning and to develop preparedness arrangements for their specific population.

Downside of Registries

The experience of past disasters has highlighted the complexities of maintaining such a registry. Privacy is a chief concern. The Health Insurance Portability and Accountability Act's (HIPAA) privacy rule permits covered entities, such as health care organizations and providers, to disclose information for public health purposes. Registry databases should be stored on a secure server with steps taken to protect the information, and this safeguard of privacy should be shared with registrants. However, it is becoming increasingly difficult to guarantee the privacy and security of registries from hackers.

There are also administrative issues with a registry. The maintenance of registries is a costly expense to the agency where it is housed. The need to both ensure that the information is current and continually validate the quality of the collected data results in substantial financial and manpower costs. In addition to potential modifications to where the registered person may be located at the time of a disaster, the condition for which they originally registered may have changed and a different level of assistance may be necessary when a disaster occurs. Further, many people with disabilities and others with access and functional needs lead full lives and may not be at the registered home address at the time of the disaster.

Registries may also give people a false sense of security about their safety during an emergency. If an individual knows that they are included in a registry for preparedness purposes, they may be less likely to prepare for an emergency since they may perceive that being included in a registry is a guarantee that they will receive assistance and evacuation services. This places unrealistic expectations on transportation providers and first responders.

More research is necessary on the utility of registries in disasters. There is little evidence demonstrating that the activation of registries for individuals with disabilities and other access and functional needs has resulted in lives being saved. Communities need to identify their disaster planning needs and decisions about registries should be made collaboratively with people with disabilities and others with access and functional needs, including their support systems.

HHS emPOWER Map

An example of a federal tool that incorporates elements of a registry is the emPOWER Map. The emPOWER Map was developed by the ASPR, in collaboration with the Centers for Medicare & Medicaid Services, to enhance the ability of jurisdictions at all levels to provide emergency services to Medicare recipients who live independently at home and rely upon medical and assistive equipment that is powered by electricity. These populations may be adversely affected during a disaster or extended power outage.

Using de-identified Medicare data that are updated monthly, the emPOWER Map applies a Geographic Information System to locate the total number of Medicare claims at a national, state, territory, county, and zip code level and couples these data with real-time tracking of severe weather provided through the National Oceanic and Atmospheric Administration (NOAA). Such maps can aid community agencies in identifying areas that may be impacted by severe weather and are at risk for prolonged power outages. Examples of electricity-dependent medical and assistive equipment that Medicare beneficiaries use include: ventilators, oxygen concentrators, enteral feeding machines, intravenous infusion pumps, suction pumps, at-home dialysis machines, wheelchairs, scooters, and beds.

These interactive maps can assist hospitals, first responders (e.g., fire, emergency medical services, law enforcement), shelters, community organizations, and electric companies to better anticipate, plan for, and rapidly identify areas and Medicare populations that may need assistance during a disaster. While the information in the emPOWER Map is presented in a way that protects patient privacy, in a disaster, additional information can be made available to a health department to facilitate a life-saving emergency response in a manner consistent with HIPAA.

Specific Strategies

Individuals with disabilities and others with access and functional needs should know where to go if they need shelter, transportation, and support services; keep needed assistive devices and equipment nearby; know their evacuation options; and repeatedly

Table 11-3. Descriptions of Access and Functional Needs

Planning for FNSS in general population shelters includes the development of mechanisms that address the needs of children and adults in areas such as:

- Communications assistance and services when completing the shelter registration process and other forms or processes involved in applying for emergency-related benefits and services including federal, state, tribal, and local benefits and services
- DME, CMS, and/or PAS that assist with activities of daily living
- Access to medications to maintain health, mental health, and function
- Available sleeping accommodations (e.g., the provision of universal/accessible cots or beds and cribs; the placement, modification, or stabilization of cots or beds and cribs; the provision and installation of privacy curtains)
- Access to orientation and way-finding for people who are blind or have low vision

Assistance for individuals with cognitive and intellectual disabilities:

- Auxiliary aids and services necessary to ensure effective communication for people with communication disabilities
- Access to an air-conditioned and/or heated environment (e.g., for those who cannot regulate body temperature)
- Refrigeration for medications
- Availability of food and beverages appropriate for individuals with dietary restrictions (e.g., people with diabetes or severe allergies to foods such as peanuts, dairy products, and gluten)
- Providing food and supplies for service animals (e.g., dishes for food and water, arrangements for the hygienic disposal of waste; and, if requested, portable kennels for containment)
- Access to transportation for individuals who may require a wheelchair-accessible vehicle, individualized assistance, and the transportation of equipment required in a shelter because of a disability
- Assistance locating, securing, and moving to post-disaster alternative housing, which includes housing that is accommodating to the individual's functional support needs (e.g., accessible housing; housing with adequate space to accommodate DME; or housing located in close proximity to public transportation, medical providers, job or educational facility, and/or retail stores)

Assistance with activities of daily living such as:

- Eating
- Taking medication
- Dressing and undressing
- Transferring to and from a wheelchair or other mobility aid
- Walking
- Stabilization
- Bathing
- Toileting
- Communicating

Source: Based on Federal Emergency Management Agency (FEMA). 2010. *Guidance on Planning for Integration of Functional Needs Support Services in General Population Shelters*. Pages 8–9. Washington, DC: FEMA. Available at: https://www.fema.gov/pdf/about/odic/fnss_guidance.pdf. Accessed January 21, 2017.

Note: CMS = consumable medical supplies; DME = durable medical equipment; FNSS = functional needs support services; PAS = personal assistance services.

practice their plan. This section highlights personal preparedness tips and examples of strategies specific to the needs of selected groups with access and functional needs. Table 11-3 describes the access and functional needs that may require additional assistance. Table 11-4 summarizes basic preparedness steps for individuals with disabilities and others with access and functional needs.

Table 11-4. Basic Preparedness Steps for Individuals With Disabilities and/or Access and Functional Needs

Disability/Need	Steps for Preparedness
Alzheimer's	Be listed in the emergency registry
	Wear an identification bracelet or necklace
	Carry papers with information about behaviors
	Carry contact information for family, friends, physician
Bedbound	Have an emergency transportation plan
	Stock supplies of daily care items (e.g., bedpans, adult diapers, linens)
Diabetes	Store special dietary foods
	Stock testing supplies
	Stock insulin supplies that do not require refrigeration
	Wear medical emblem on bracelet or necklace
Dialysis	Ensure dialysis facility knows where to find patient
	Start emergency diet as soon as aware of emergency situation
	Ensure that no one uses dialysis access for fluid or medication
	Make arrangements for dialysis at the evacuation destination
	Do not use disinfected water for dialysis
	Wear medical emblem on bracelet or necklace
Hearing impaired	Verify that the necessary equipment is available, or make special arrangements to receive warnings and communicate needs
Mobility impaired	Arrange for special assistance to get to a shelter
	Keep information readily available that details the proper way to transfer or move someone in a wheelchair and the best exit routes
Non-English speaking	May need assistance planning for and responding to emergencies
	Include community and cultural groups in preparedness efforts
Oxygen dependent	Stock oxygen supplies (including power source)
	Stock extra water for oxygen condensers
No vehicle(s)	Make arrangements for transportation
Special dietary needs	Stockpile an adequate emergency food supply

Source: Adapted from Federal Emergency Management Agency (FEMA). 2010. *Are You Ready?* Washington, DC: FEMA. Available at: https://www.fema.gov/pdf/areyouready/areyouready_full.pdf. Accessed April 4, 2017.

Overview

Despite any specific need, all individuals must follow 4 basics steps of preparedness:

1. **Get informed**: Know what hazards are most likely to affect your community and how you will need to prepare. Be aware of personal abilities and any limitations that may affect one's personal response to a disaster. Become familiar with the community disaster plan and communication systems. Connect with neighbors and let them know what might be needed in a disaster.
2. **Make a plan**: Develop a plan based on identified community hazards and personal needs. Share the information with family, friends, and caregivers. Set up an out-of-town

contact. Carry all useful information within one's wallet or purse. Information on a contact card and other elements of a plan can be found at http://elderaffairs.state.fl.us/doea/pubs/EU/DisasterPreparednessandtheDeafCommunity.pdf.

3. **Build a Go Pack and home kit:** Organize a Go Pack (i.e., pre-prepared kits with medication and other supplies that may be needed in the event of a disaster) based on the specific need.
4. **Maintain your plan, Go Pack, and home kit**: Review your plan every 6 months with family and friends. Regularly rotate all perishable items and change batteries in all essential devices.

When public health agencies are involved in preparing for and responding to a disaster, it is important that all plans and supplementary materials be developed in partnership with people with disabilities and others with access and functional needs. Preparedness information for the general population may not apply for people with disabilities. Materials that contain information about general emergency preparedness can be more inclusive when they contain information that focuses on specific functional needs, particularly in the areas where additional support is needed. Both plans and the response should include information that is useful and specific to people with hearing, vision, mobility, speech, and cognitive disabilities. Such information should be available in accessible formats and provide direction for retrieving these materials in alternative formats (i.e., large print, audio, disks, Braille, or primary language where English is a second language). All materials should use neutral terms to describe disability and be accurate and respectful.

When identifying mitigation strategies that individuals can carry out, it is helpful to focus on no-cost and low-cost preparedness in addition to costly activities since some populations with disabilities and others with access and functional needs cannot afford to buy emergency supplies and equipment.

Blind

Both people who are blind or partially sighted (and their service animal, defined below) are likely to need to be led to safety during a disaster. Some people who are blind or visually impaired may be reluctant to evacuate when the request comes from a stranger, and responders should be prepared to provide assurance of safety. Further, service animals could become confused or disoriented in a disaster and responders should receive training on handling these animals.

Service animals must be permitted to stay in emergency shelters with their owners. Section 36.104 of Title III of the ADA specifies that a service animal is "any guide dog, signal dog, or other animal individually trained to do work or perform tasks for the benefit of an individual with a disability." Section 36.302(c) requires public accommodations to modify policies, practices, and procedures to accommodate the use of service animals. In addition to guide dogs, this can include hearing dogs, seizure alert dogs, mobility dogs, and others. A service animal is not required to have any special certification or identification. The local emergency management office will have more information.

Children

Of the U.S. population, almost 25% are children who have functional needs during disasters. Children who are injured require pediatric-specific equipment, drug preparations, and delivery systems. Children who do not have parents or guardians present medicolegal challenges. A meta-analysis of 160 samples of disaster victims revealed that over the long term, only middle-aged women who are caregivers fare worse than children who have experienced a disaster. Disaster planning for children must be family centered and meet the needs of families who may have health care challenges. Since children spend much of their day in school, public and private schools need to be included in a community's emergency preparedness activities so that schools integrate with local response systems. Hospitals should include pediatric issues in their facility disaster plans and drills and information for pediatric discharge planning.

Emergency Information Form

Children with chronic medical conditions rely on complex management plans for problems that cause them to be at increased risk for poor outcomes in disasters. The emergency information form (EIF) was proposed as a means to provide rapid access to a health summary for children with special health care needs in a 1999 joint policy statement (reaffirmed in 2002) by the American Academy of Pediatrics and the American College of Emergency Physicians. It is a concise, single-sheet medical summary that describes a child's medical condition(s), medications, and health care needs, and informs those providing health care during disasters so that optimal emergency medical care can be provided.

An example of an EIF is available at: https://www.aap.org/en-us/about-the-aap/Committees-Councils-Sections/section-hematology-oncology/Documents/emergency_info_form.pdf.

Reunification

Following Hurricanes Katrina and Rita in 2005, the National Center for Missing & Exploited Children (NCMEC) received over 34,000 calls. On any given weekday, an estimated 67 million of children are in school and/or child care, and may be particularly at-risk because they are away from their families. The reunification[1] of unaccompanied minors and separated or missing children with their parents or legal guardians is a priority following a disaster.

Collaborative efforts between HHS, FEMA, the Red Cross, and the NCMEC generated guidance on reunifying children with their families following a disaster. The guide identifies existing state and national systems that function as a resource network for those involved in reunification and provides local and state jurisdictions with specific suggestions that enhance reunification through the establishment of shelters and other types of reception centers. The guide can be found at: http://www.phe.gov/preparedness/planning/abc/documents/children-reunification.pdf.

Another resource for reunification is RapidFTR (Family Tracing and Reunification), a volunteer-driven project developed by the Child Protection in Emergencies Team at UNICEF. RapidFTR is a mobile phone application and data storage system that facilitates the reunification process by assisting humanitarian workers collect, sort, and share information about unaccompanied and separated minors so that they can be registered for services and reunited with their families following disasters. RapidFTR is designed to expedite family tracing and reunification efforts immediately after a disaster and during the recovery phase. Additional information is available at: http://www.rapidftr.com.

Deaf and Hard of Hearing

The most underserved group during Hurricane Katrina were those who were deaf or hard of hearing. Less than 30% of shelters had access to American Sign Language (ASL) interpreters, 80% did not have text telephones (TTYs), and 60% did not have TVs with caption capability. Only 56% of shelters had areas where oral announcements were posted so people who are deaf, hard of hearing, or out of hearing range could go to a specified area to get or read the content of announcements. This meant that the deaf or hard of hearing had no access to the vital flow of information. This experience taught us that it is vitally important to be prepared to provide services to this population during a disaster. (See "Communication" below for more guidance.)

People who are deaf or hard of hearing should:

- Stockpile and maintain extra batteries for hearing aids, TTY devices when used, and light phone signalers.

1. Reunification is the process of assisting displaced disaster survivors, including children, and reestablishing contact with family and friends after a period of separation.

- Consider storing hearing aids in a container by the bedside that is attached to a nightstand using Velcro®. Some disasters, such as earthquakes, may cause personal items to shift location, if they are not secured, making them difficult to find.
- Install both audible and visual smoke alarms with at least one alarm that is battery operated.
- Determine how to communicate with emergency personnel by interpreter (if available) or by paper and pen (which should be stored).
- Carry preprinted messages such as "I speak American Sign Language and need an ASL interpreter."
- Determine which broadcasting systems will have continuous news that is captioned or signed. Captioned radio, known as HD radio, is available in many areas of the United States. HD radio transmits text, pictures, and graphics.

Life Support Systems

People who depend on life support systems (e.g., dialysis, ventilators, oxygen, suction, intravenous pump, or infusion therapy, enteral feeding machines, intravenous pumps, suction pumps) can enhance their preparedness by doing the following:

- Secure life support equipment so that it is not damaged by falling.
- Determine alternative facilities and providers who could help if the home system becomes inoperable or their provider cannot provide service.
- Identify and arrange for alternative power sources that could provide electrical service for 5 to 7 days if needed.
- Consider purchasing a generator.
- Determine whether manually operated equipment can be used.
- Determine whether the equipment can be powered from a vehicle battery and obtain necessary equipment for the hookup.
- Regularly test and charge stored batteries.
- Be aware of battery life and be sure to have enough charged batteries to provide power for 5 to 7 days.
- Those using breathing machines should have a 7-day supply of oxygen, tubing, solutions, and medications.
- Oxygen users should determine whether a reduced flow rate can be used. If possible, record the revised flow numbers on the equipment for easy reference.
- If necessary, post "Oxygen in Use" signs in the home so that responders are immediately aware of this.
- Keep the shutoff switch for oxygen equipment close by to enable a quick turnoff in case of emergency.

Older Adults

Older adults are at increased risk during a disaster because they may:

- Be dependent on wheelchairs, canes, or walkers to get around and unable to climb stairs as a result of impaired physical mobility
- Have chronic health conditions that:
  - can be exacerbated by exposure to conditions associated with many disasters, such as a lack of safe food and water, extreme heat or cold, stress, or exposure to infection;
  - require an emergency plan that accommodates medical devices and medications;
  - could make them prone to adverse medical events if essential medications and/or an individualized medication regime (e.g., insulin, blood thinners, psychotropic drugs) or special diets are not available during an emergency; and
  - could make them experience additional confusion and fear (e.g., people with dementia who are unable to take their medications)
- Be prone to heat stress and require adequate hydration
- Be dependent on caretakers and may not have a support system
- Lose their place to live and retirement security if the disaster destroys their home
- Lack sufficient income or other resources to enable preparations for disasters and to respond and adapt when they occur
- Be sensory impaired (hearing or sight) or cognitively impaired with difficulty understanding information or following directions
- Feel overwhelmed by a disaster because they have difficulty moving around, standing in line, or sleeping on a low cot in a noisy shelter
- Have difficulties evacuating if they no longer drive or do not own a vehicle
- Be reluctant to evacuate and leave behind lifelong possessions
- Be worried about their pets
- Be reluctant to accept assistance
- Fear institutionalization or loss of independence
- Perceive the task of rebuilding their lives as too much, leading to depression
- Be physically less able to go through the steps needed to meet basic needs following a disaster

Locally, organizations providing aging services should help older adults develop personal preparedness plans. Further, all sectors of the aging services network should participate in their community or state's preparedness and response planning. Potential partners in addressing the public health emergency preparedness, response, and recovery needs of older adults include a state's office on aging and municipal or county agencies on aging.

Where a community needs additional federal resources following a disaster, money is available for services to older adults. The Older Americans Act of 1965, last reauthorized for 3 years through the Older Americans Act Reauthorization Act of 2016 (S. 192), enables HHS's Administration on Aging to reimburse state agencies on aging for additional expenses incurred following a presidentially declared disaster. These funds can be used for outreach, counseling, food, cleaning of homes, emergency transportation, and medications for the elderly.

Specific Medical Needs

Where applicable, people with specific medical needs should:

- Have a 7-day supply of all medications.[2]
- Store medications in one location in their original containers.
- Have a list of all medications, including: name of medication, dose, frequency, and the name of the doctor who prescribed it.
- Have a 7-day supply of bandages, ostomy bags, or syringes.
- Determine whether an infusion pump has a battery backup and how long it would last without power.
- Learn about manual infusion techniques in case of a power outage.
- Attach written operating instructions to all equipment.
- Have a "Go Pack" ready at all times.
- Have copies of vital medical papers such as insurance cards, advance directive, and power of attorney.
- Discuss disaster plans with their home health care provider.
- Keep a contact list of providers and vendors for all equipment and supplies.

Ensuring Individual Preparedness

Individual can prepare for a disaster through their networks, which include family, coworkers and friends and by having a Go Pack ready.

Personal Support Networks

Community plans should encourage all at-risk individuals to develop a network of relatives, friends, or coworkers who can check on and assist them in an emergency. Often

2. After the tragic events in Japan in March 2011, U.S. emergency planners suggest that to prepare for catastrophic disasters, people should plan to be self-sufficient for at least 7 days.

referred to as PSNs, these networks help at-risk individuals evaluate their homes, prepare for a disaster by identifying and gathering the resources they'll need, and provide emergency assistance through a redundant set of people who know the individual's needs. At-risk individuals may need to organize more than one PSN (e.g., for home, school, and workplace), depending on where their time is spent. For example, if there are at least 3 people at each location where an at-risk individual regularly spends time, these individuals may be assured that there is redundancy in the plan. The members of each PSN should have a written list of what the individual needs as well as copies of medical information, medical or disability-related supplies and equipment list, evacuation plans, relevant emergency documents, and a personal disaster plan. Prearranged plans detailing the circumstances for when and how the members of the network will contact the person with a medical vulnerability or disability are essential. Members of a PSN should be provided with written instructions and trained in the location of the person's keys, the operation and movement of any adaptive or durable equipment used, locating their medical supplies, familiarity with any service animal, and needed personal care. Table 11-5 identifies basic elements of a personal assessment that will guide the plans worked out with the PSN. The personal assessment is best based on the environment after the disaster, individual capabilities, the individual's limitations, and the lowest anticipated level of functioning.

Go Packs

Everyone should prepare a "Go Pack." A Go Pack is an individualized portable kit (preferably housed in a waterproof plastic box) that is prepared in advance. For those on

Table 11-5. Elements of a Personal Assessment

- List personal needs and resources
- Evaluate activities of daily living
  - Assistance needed with personal care
  - Use of adaptive equipment to get dressed
- Assess needs if water service or hot water cut off for several days
- Identify equipment needed for personal care (e.g., shower chair, tub-transfer bench)
- Identify adaptive feeding devices and need for special utensils to prepare or eat food independently
- Arrange for continuation of electricity-dependent equipment (e.g., dialysis, electrical lifts)
- Plan for getting around if the disaster causes debris in home
- Plan for specially equipped vehicle or accessible transportation
- Practice evacuating a building in the community or at home
- Locate and plan for finding mobility aids and equipment necessary for service animal
- Evaluate ramp access
- Plan for care of service animal (e.g., provide food, shelter, veterinary attention) during and after a disaster
- Arrange for another caregiver for the service animal if unable to care for it

medications, it should include at least 7 days of medication stored at the recommended temperature, rotated every week to ensure that it has not exceeded its expiration date. For others, the Go Pack may include an extra cane, hearing aid batteries, a walker, a ventilator, lightweight emergency evacuation chair, augmentative communication equipment, insulin supplies, and food and water for a guide dog. This procedure was very effective in New York City after September 11, 2001, because it ensured that life-saving medication was available even when pharmacies were not. Note that some states will not permit patients on Medicaid to receive more than a 30-day supply of medication; it is important to check local state rules and determine what is allowed. Finally, if the individual receives Social Security benefits, the Go Pack should include a copy of the most recent award letter.

Shelters and Distribution Centers

In working with the community, public health can do a great deal to help at-risk populations prepare for evacuating from home during emergencies. At-risk individuals should be encouraged to plan how to get out of their home, work, or any building where they receive services, in the event of an emergency. Since some roads may be closed or blocked in a disaster, they should plan for 2 evacuation routes. These individuals should be encouraged to assemble a Go Pack as discussed above and store extra food, water, and supplies for any service animals.

State and local governments and other agencies, such as the Red Cross, may set up and run emergency shelters. Regardless of who operates the shelter, the ADA requires facilities to provide equal access to the assistance that they provide, such as food, showers, protection, and the support of family, friends, and neighbors. In general, the ADA does not require any action that would result in a fundamental alteration in the nature of a service, program, or activity or that would impose excessive financial and administrative burdens. Key issues in operating a shelter can be found at: https://www.ada.gov/pcatoolkit/chap7shelterprog.htm. The U.S. Department of Justice developed an ADA Checklist for Emergency Shelters that details the accommodations that must be made at facilities used to provide shelter during emergencies. These guidelines can be found online at: http://www.ada.gov/pcatoolkit/chap7shelterchk.htm.

The level of medical oversight that will be provided at each shelter must be determined as part of community planning. Planners must determine whether there will be different classes of shelters (i.e., medical management, mixed populations). With advance planning, it will be possible to ensure that the highly specialized medical needs of those using the shelter will be properly identified and addressed. Plans for shelters and distribution centers should provide for accessible and adequate electrical outlets so that adaptive equipment, such as battery-powered wheelchairs, light phone signalers, computers, and respirators, can be operated. Emergency running lights should be installed along floors. Preestablished procedures for shelters should include prior arrangements with providers of durable medical equipment that can loan, repair, or replace adaptive equipment (e.g., battery chargers, wheelchairs) following a disaster. Hotlines should include and publish TTY numbers.

Distribution centers for forms, food stamps, and hotel vouchers must meet the ADA standard of accessibility. Physical access must be ensured at the facility, in waiting lines, in restrooms, and to telephones. Educational and informational materials prepared for distribution in these shelters should be prepared in Braille, large print, languages other than English, and audiotape formats because the ADA requires that written materials used in disaster response be available in multiple formats upon request.

Phone communication following a disaster must be accessible for those who are deaf or hard of hearing, as required by the ADA. In all circumstances, the individual will need access to a device that has electrical power or is portable with working power. The use of TTY is waning as more people are using a video phone and video relay service (VRS), Internet Protocol Relay (IP Relay), or a captioned telephone (i.e., CapTel). Video relay service, a type of Telecommunication Relay Service (TRS), enables people who use ASL to communicate with voice telephone users through video equipment. The TRS phone plug is provided by telephone companies at no cost to the user; the costs of providing TRS are reimbursed from either a state or a federal fund. CapTel works like any other telephone for people with hearing loss. Using CapTel technology, users can listen to the caller and the system translates the voice into text so that the user can read the written captions in a display window. Where those who need service make a video phone call directly to a community organization or governmental agency providing assistance, the worker at the hotline would need to be able to speak ASL. Alternatively, the individual calling could use a VRS interpreter or captioned telephone that are both similar to a voice phone call.

Some community plans may incorporate alternative procedures to those who cannot access a shelter, such as the direct delivery of food and water. If this is the case, the method for making the contact to request assistance needs to be accessible. Another solution is to establish a process where community residents can access information and complete applications on the Internet, by phone, TTY, or e-mail. Finally, text messaging is being adopted by 911 systems and is likely to be used more widely in future disasters.

Communication

Emergency communication should be accessible for people with disabilities, limited English proficiency, and to members of diverse cultures. Although regulatory requirements specify the ways that emergency communications are to occur, public health should include targeted strategies to reach out to different populations. People who are deaf or hard of hearing cannot hear audible alerts sent via radio, television, or sirens.

Individuals who are blind or have low vision may not be aware of visual cues, such as flashing lights or emergency information scrolling on television screens.

Emergency alerts and warnings should be provided in languages other than English on public access channels and in cooperation with non-English radio and television stations. Some communities with high rates of limited English proficiency use bilingual staff or interpreters at radio and television stations to communicate information.

At-risk populations may need targeted education about the meaning of alerts and warnings. For example, some individuals who are blind may not be aware that an audible beep from a television signals that an emergency alert message is streaming as text across the bottom of the television screen, or that the listener should turn on a radio for more information.

Technology used to communicate with at-risk populations should be exercised regularly, and emergency plans should include redundant methods to provide a general notification for the community. Deaf, hard-of-hearing, and blind populations can be reached via closed-captioning, qualified sign language interpreters, Braille, text messaging, TTY, large print, and audiotape.

For the benefit of individuals with cognitive disabilities, the most pertinent information should be repeated frequently using a simple vocabulary. Pictorial representations can provide quick and easily understood instruction to many individuals including children, individuals with limited English proficiency, and some with cognitive disabilities.

Title II of the ADA provides that residents of a community must be able to contact emergency management agencies (including 911) directly via a TTY or through more current capabilities such as CapTel or VRS. Personnel answering emergency phones need to be trained to answer TTY calls, Voice Carry Over calls (a type of TTY/voice call where the hearing person can listen to the deaf or hard-of-hearing person talk and can then type back), and calls from the available Relay Services (a person who is deaf, hard of hearing, deaf-blind, or speech-disabled uses a TTY to type his/her conversation to the relay operator who then reads the typed conversation to a hearing person). The relay operator conveys the hearing person's spoken words by typing them back to the TTY user. For example, when calls are made to 911 from captioned telephones, the home phone number is visible through caller ID. Providers of VRS and IP Relay need to provide 10-digit telephone numbers to subscribers so that their Internet-based emergency calls automatically route to the call center responsible for answering calls to a community's emergency telephone number (known as the 911 Public Safety Answering Point dispatcher). A TTY allows an individual with hearing loss to send and receive text messages via a landline telephone connection and, in some instances, a mobile phone connection. Technology improvements now allow consumers to make digital wireless calls with TTY-compatible handsets, though as of this writing this is not the best solution due to the limits of the current technology. Some locations across the country are allowing receipt of text messages via instant messaging from wireless products.

Compliance With the Emergency Captioning Rules

The Federal Communications Commission (FCC) rules require broadcasters and cable operators to make local emergency information accessible to people who are deaf or hard of hearing and to those who are blind or have visual disabilities as part of a community's emergency plan. For public health, this means that emergency information must be provided both aurally and in a visual format. All information being communicated through video programming distributors (e.g., broadcasters, cable operators, satellite television services, and other multichannel video programming distributors) must meet this standard. Television stations can be helpful in broadcasting both text and audible emergency information to all their viewers.

Accessibility of Emergency Information Required

The FCC requires that for people who are deaf or hard of hearing, emergency information provided in the audio portion of programming must include either closed-captioning or other methods of visual presentation, such as open captioning or crawling or scrolling text that appears on the screen. No emergency information should block the closed-captioning, and closed-captioning should not block any emergency information provided in any other manner. For people whose vision is impaired, emergency information must be made accessible when provided in both the video portion of a regularly scheduled newscast or in a special newscast that interrupts regular programming. The oral description of emergency information must be included in the main audio portion of the broadcast. Emergency information provided in the video portion of any newscast through *crawling* or *scrolling* text must also be accompanied by an aural tone. This tone alerts people with any vision impairment that the broadcaster is providing emergency information, and that the viewer should turn on another source, such as a radio, for more information.

The delivery of emergency information must meet this standard for weather warnings and watches, community emergencies (e.g., discharge of toxic gases, widespread power failures, industrial explosions, civil disorders, school closings), and scheduling changes for school buses caused by any of these conditions. Information must be communicated about the specifics of the emergency, how to respond, if the community will be evacuated, the location of shelters, and how to shelter in place. Educational announcements made during and immediately after disasters such as earthquakes or tornadoes should encourage those with disabilities to check for hazards at home since items that have moved can cause injury or block an escape path for someone with limited mobility. Finally, announcements should inform those with chronic medical conditions to bring their medication(s) and medical supplies when they evacuate.

Some local news stations provide captions when broadcasting information on weather emergencies, such as tornadoes. An alternative source of notification is a NOAA-certified weather radio, which displays a short text message describing the nature of any emergency declared in the area. Weather radios can be indefinitely left on in standby mode. These radios are silent until an emergency is declared, at which time they sound an alarm and broadcast a spoken message concerning the emergency. Strobe lights and bed vibrators are available as attachments for people who cannot hear the alarm, and most models display text messages.

The CDC developed a series of video clips using ASL for public service announcements. Closed-captioned video clips using ASL are available on the CDC Public Service Announcements for Disasters Web page (at http://www.cdc.gov/disasters/psa/index.html). These clips cover broad topics, including preparing for a storm, cleanup, coping, safe food and water, and prescription drugs.

Specific Tools

A receiver system for NOAA Weather Radio All Hazards (NWR) is specifically available to provide an alert for the deaf and hard of hearing. NWR embeds nonverbal information in its broadcasts to provide warnings of life-threatening events. The warnings are delivered via connected vibrators, bed shakers, pillow vibrators, or strobe lights.

With specific area message encoding (SAME) technology, NWR receivers can be programmed to set off an alarm for specific events (e.g., tornado, flash flood) and specific jurisdictions. Basic NWR receiver systems are available with SAME technology and external alarm devices. These NWR receivers can be connected to existing home security alerting systems, similar to a doorbell or smoke detector. In more complex installations where wireless or wired remote modules are used, installation requires a connection to a device that allows the remote placement of alarms. Such alarms may require external power from batteries or modular power supplies. Ready-to-use systems are marketed by Silent Call Communications (available at: http://www.silentcall.com) and Harris Communications (available at: http://www.harriscomm.com).

Other devices that can be connected to external alarms require the skills of an electronics technician and are manufactured or sold by several companies, including Radio Shack, Midland, Uniden, and First Alert.

Transportation

Accessible transportation must be available for evacuation before, during, and after a disaster. As part of both community and facility planning, managers should ensure the availability of vehicles with wheelchair lifts or ramps. Although a community's emergency fleet can be assumed to be available to respond, redundant arrangements to use nonemergency vehicles should also be included in disaster plans, since it is likely that the number of specially equipped vehicles will be limited and thus not available or in service elsewhere. The National Fire Protection Agency released the *Emergency Evacuation Planning Guide for People with Disabilities* in 2016, which provides best practices and tools for evacuating at-risk populations. The report also includes a personal planning for evacuation checklist (available at: http://www.nfpa.org/disabilities).

Building Preparedness for Individuals With Disabilities

To develop an evacuation plan that accounts for both staff and visitors with disabilities, organizations and buildings should develop an emergency committee whose first task is to understand general evacuation issues. The evacuation committee might meet with the building management; local fire department, police, and HAZMAT personnel; a manufacturer of evacuation equipment; and other agencies and groups with evacuation interests involving people with disabilities and other at-risk users. In addition to identifying the individuals who regularly work in a building, preparations should be made for visitors who may require assistance. Furthermore, the committee should identify and train personnel who can properly lead individuals to safety who need assistance. Conducting regular drills and assessing performance are as essential to the evacuation plan as they are to the larger community preparedness plan.

It is useful to assess the number of employees and their types of needs and to meet with disabled individuals to discuss their preferences for evacuation as part of the committee process. The U.S. Equal Employment Opportunity Commission has stated that federal disability discrimination laws do not prevent employers from obtaining and appropriately using information necessary for a comprehensive emergency evacuation plan. Employers may ask employees to self-identify if they will require assistance in the event of an evacuation due to a disability or medical condition. This list, which will be essential if emergency evacuation is necessary, should be updated at least annually. Employers may obtain this information at 3 different times: after making a job offer, but before employment begins; during periodic surveys of all employees, when the employer indicates that self-identification is voluntary; and by asking employees with known disabilities if they will require assistance in the event of an emergency. An employer should inform and ensure individuals that the information is confidential and shared only with those who have responsibilities under the emergency evacuation plan. An employer may ask individuals who indicate a need for assistance because of a medical condition to describe the type of assistance needed. An employer can distribute a memo that includes a form requesting information from employees. The employer may also have individual follow-up conversations when necessary to obtain more detailed information. The ADA has provisions requiring employers to maintain confidentiality about employee medical information. In the event of an evacuation, employers can share medical information, including the type of assistance an individual needs, with safety personnel, medical professionals, emergency coordinators, floor captains, colleagues who are part of the employee's PSN, building security officers who need to confirm that everyone has been evacuated, and other nonmedical personnel who are responsible for ensuring safe evacuation under the employer's emergency evacuation plan.

Detection

The detection of some hazards (such as fires) often occurs through systems that function automatically. Automatic systems (e.g., with strobes, horns) must be compliant with the ADA regulations updated in 2014 (https://www.ada.gov/effective-comm.htm) and the Underwriters Laboratories Standard for Emergency Signaling Devices for the Hearing Impaired (UL Standard 1971). This standard requires that signaling devices alert those with hearing loss through the use of light, vibrations, and air movement. Where facilities use manual devices that require pulling, codes require that these pull stations be mounted at a height of 48 to 54 inches so that an individual seated in a wheelchair could reach the alarm.

Notification

Plans need to include a process of informing all building occupants that emergency action is needed. Because emergencies often disrupt technology, it is important to have low-tech solutions with built-in redundancy. Although specific considerations might be needed for those with disabilities, plans should consider the community in general because everyone benefits from improved notification systems.

The ADAAG provides specifications for emergency alarms so that they are accessible to people with disabilities, including those with sensory impairments (ADAAG 4.1.3[14], 4.28). Where emergency alarm systems are provided, they must meet criteria that address audible and visual features. It is important to install multiple systems because events may cause one or another system to fail. For example, audible signs may not be distinguishable above the sound of alarms, the signs may not be heard or distinguishable from siren alarms, or without electricity, the systems may not be operable. Further, interpreters must be provided where indicated.

Since audible instructions delivered via emergency paging systems are not effective for the hard of hearing or deaf, visual strobes with high-intensity flashing lights should be used to notify these individuals that the alarm has sounded. The ADAAG specifications for visual appliances address intensity, flash rate, mounting location, and other characteristics. Audible alarms installed in corridors and lobbies can be heard in adjacent rooms, but a visual signal can be observed only within the space it is located. Visual alarms are required in hallways, lobbies, restrooms, and any other areas for general and common use, such as meeting and conference rooms, classrooms, cafeterias, employee break rooms, dressing rooms, examination rooms, and similar spaces. Alternatively, visual instructions can be provided through television monitors, scrolling text, or pagers that vibrate. Finally, low-level signage should be placed 6 to 8 inches above the floor as a supplement to required exit signs placed higher on the wall because exit signs are usually located over exits or near the ceiling and can become obscured by smoke.

Tactile and Audible Signage

The ADAAG 4.1.3(16), 4.30 requires that certain types of building signs be tactile and use both raised and Braille characters. This is intended to include signs typically placed at doorways, such as room and exit labels because doorways provide a tactile cue to locating signs. Tactile specifications also apply to signs used to label the function of rooms and to the floor level designations provided in stairwells. Examples include signs labeling restrooms, exits, and rooms and floors designated by numbers or letters. The ADAAG also addresses informational and directional signs. These types of signs are not required to be tactile but must meet criteria for legibility, such as character size and proportion, contrast, and sign finish.

Braille signs, commonly found as raised patterns of dots on elevator control panels, have been installed in many buildings to assist people who are visually impaired. The usefulness of these panels is limited because the person must be at the location of the Braille signs to feel them. Plans should include an alternative way to provide directional guidance to exits, such as audible directional signage.

Audible directional, or remote, signage, is a device used to inform those with visual impairments about their environments. Audible instructions are transmitted by low-power radio waves or infrared beams. Small receivers, carried by the individuals, pick up these signals and are equipped with a voice that announces directions (e.g., "the exit is 10 steps from the front desk") or a word identifying where they are (e.g., "stairway," "elevator"). One example of audible signs is Talking Signs, which provide those who are blind with the information that helps them navigate in the environment. These signs "speak" by sending information from installed infrared transmitters. Handheld receivers pick up information from the transmitters and give verbal directions to those carrying them. Alternatively, some devices include a two-part, battery-operated smoke detector and transmitter that are attached to a wall and a companion vibrator device that is either placed on a desk or held in the hand. The vibrator is activated when a smoke detector transmits a signal to the receiver.

Preparedness at the Building Level: Evacuation

Moving people to safe areas is an important part of any disaster response, especially in tall buildings. Although contingency plans should be developed for providing evacuation assistance for all building occupants, there will always be someone in such buildings who will need assistance in any emergency in which evacuation is required. Further, unique evacuation problems are created where the elderly or disabled live or work on higher floors in high-rise buildings.

The methods of accommodation and the choice of assistive devices should be discussed with those needing them. When assisting individuals with vision impairments, a building's emergency plans should provide for announcing one's presence when entering the area, grasping the elbow of the person requiring assistance for guidance, and describing what he or she will be doing, including the mention of stairs, doorways, narrow passages, and ramps. Someone should remain with such an individual until he or she is safe.

There may be different procedures or preferences among local fire departments regarding evacuation procedures for people with disabilities, but many evacuation plans will include the use of evacuation chairs for those needing assistance. These devices are designed with rollers, treads, and braking mechanisms that enable a person to be transported down stairs with the assistance of another individual. For additional information, planners should check with the local fire, police, or HAZMAT department.

Following an inventory of the number of employees requiring assistance and estimating the number of visitors to the building, it will be possible to determine how many evacuation chairs are needed. Decisions may be made to also stock heavy gloves to protect individuals' hands from debris when pushing their manual wheelchairs, a patch kit to repair flat tires, and extra batteries for those who use motorized wheelchairs or scooters. It is also the individuals' responsibility to ensure that required emergency supplies are stocked appropriately. Staff should be trained on the use of evacuation chairs, through viewing the training videotape provided by the manufacturer as well as receiving on-site training from the manufacturer. When buildings conduct mandated fire drills, part of their exercise should test the ability to evacuate those with disabilities. Drills should focus on the use of evacuation and other assistive devices and occur on all shifts so that evening and night staff are familiar with the procedures and their responsibilities. Drills also provide an opportunity for individuals requiring assistance to practice transferring into and out of the evacuation chairs. It is important to practice evacuation procedures with blocked exits and service animals such as guide dogs, who accompany their owners during the evacuation. Drills can include the use of protective gear, such as booties made of Velcro for service animals to wear when evacuating from fire or walking over glass. (See Chapter 4 for more on drills and exercises.)

In planning for people with limited mobility, such as in residential institutions, there may be scenarios where sheltering in place is the best plan, even temporarily. Disaster plans should include the designation of several offices as waiting areas where individuals using wheelchairs or mobility devices and others can report and await assistance from the fire department, as is required in new construction (ADAAG 4.1.3[9], 4.3.11). Known as *areas of rescue assistance* or *areas of refuge*, in new construction these spaces must meet specifications for fire resistance and ventilation and are often incorporated into the design of fire stair landings, but can be provided in other recognized locations meeting the design specifications, including those for fire and smoke protection. An exception is provided for buildings equipped with sprinkler systems that have built-in signals used to monitor the system's features. In older buildings, offices designated as areas of refuge can be located at different parts of the building (e.g., front, back). Each designated area of refuge should have a preprinted sign requesting rescue assistance, a window, supplies that enable individuals to block smoke from entering the room from under the door, respirator masks, and a telephone and two-way radio (areas of rescue assistance must include two-way communication devices so that users can communicate about evacuation assistance). Employees should be instructed to post rescue signs in the window to alert the fire department of their location. The location of these waiting areas should be communicated to the local fire department.

Evacuation Equipment

The ability to evacuate during an emergency is highly dependent on one's mobility. The types of equipment discussed here are not meant to be all inclusive since experimental equipment is continuously being developed and improved. Wheelchair users are one group with mobility limitations. Because wheelchairs are frequently fitted to the specific physical needs of the user, those evacuated will need to have their own chairs returned to them if they are separated during the evacuation.

Several types of evacuation or fold-up chairs allow for people to be moved up or down stairs, and can be permanently installed within stairways to accommodate wheelchair users or stored near emergency exits. In one type, the person transfers or is transferred from the wheelchair to a portable chair. These chairs are designed to move down stairs on special tracks equipped with friction braking systems, rollers, or other devices that control the speed of descent. With another device, the wheelchair user rolls onto the transporter and the wheelchair is secured to the device as it descends. In addition, there are chairs that can be rolled down stairs. Table 11-6 describes examples of devices that can be used to evacuate individuals who need assistance. Contact information for the manufacturers of these devices is found in Appendix T.

Table 11-6. Assistive Devices for Evacuation

Evac+Chair	Weighs 18 pounds and has a 300-pound carrying capacity
Evacu–Trac	Designed so passenger's weight propels it down the stairs, and has a 360-pound carrying capacity
Ferno Rescue Seat, Evacuation Chairs	Adjustable and portable devices enable easy maneuvering through confined spaces with a 350-pound carrying capacity
LifeSlider	Flat-bottomed, toboggan-like device that slides down stairs, around landings, through small doorways, around inside corners, and across pavement
Rescue Chairs	Designed to go up and down stairs with a 300-pound carrying capacity
Scalamobil	Battery-operated portable stair climber, attaches to most manual folding wheelchairs, and has a 264-pound carrying capacity

Carrying Techniques

Wheelchair users are trained in special techniques to transfer from one chair to another. There are 2 techniques for carrying people in an emergency: the cradle lift and the swing or chair carry. If possible, always check with the individual first before starting to lift. The cradle lift is preferred when the person to be carried has little or no arm strength. It is also safer if the person being carried weighs less than the carrier. In the cradle lift, the person needing assistance is sitting and the carrier bends his knees and places one arm under the person's legs and the other arm around the person's back. The person being carried puts an arm over the shoulder of the carrier. The carrier lifts up with the person in front of him or her.

For the swing or chair carry, a two-person technique, the carriers stand on opposite sides of the individual. They take the arm of the person and wrap it around each of their shoulders. Each carrier grasps their partner's forearm at the small of the back of the person being carried. They reach under the person's knees and grasp the wrist of the carry partner's other hand. Both partners lean in close to the person and lift on the count of 3. The carriers should continue pressing into the person being carried for additional support.

Service Animals

In preparation for any emergency, those who have service animals should ensure that the animal's identification tags, licenses, and vaccinations are current, and that the tags display the owner's contact information and an out-of-town contact. The ADA requires state and local government agencies, businesses, and nonprofit organizations that provide goods or services to make "reasonable modifications" in their policies or procedures when necessary to accommodate people with disabilities. Service animals are included under this principle. Accordingly, entities that have a "no pets" policy generally must modify the policy to allow service animals into their facilities. Owners should prepare an emergency supply kit for the animal, which includes bowls for water and food, food, plastic bags, a toy, a collar, an extra leash or harness, and medications.

Plan Implementation and Maintenance

After the final evacuation plan is written, a copy should be distributed to all company employees and key personnel. In addition, evacuation drills should be regularly performed to make sure all employees are familiar with the plan. To ensure that accommodations continue to be effective, the plan should be integrated into the standard operating procedures, practiced, and accommodations updated periodically. In addition, a system for reporting new hazards and accommodation needs should be developed; a relationship with local fire, police, and HAZMAT departments should be maintained; and new employees should be made aware of the plan. Finally, all accommodation equipment used in emergency evacuation should be inspected and maintained in proper working order.

Emergency Health Information

Everyone who has a diagnosis that may impact emergency treatment should always carry information about their health needs and emergency contacts, updated twice a year, with a copy given to a family member and a friend or neighbor. This emergency health information lets others know about their medical condition or disability if they are unable to provide information. For those with disabilities, this information should detail special equipment and supplies that they use, such as hearing aid batteries; information about the specifications of their medication regime, including current prescription names and dosages, shelf life, and temperature at which it should be stored; and the names, addresses, and telephone numbers of doctors and pharmacists.

Emergency health information should be kept in emergency supply kits, wallets (i.e., behind driver's license or official identification card), and wheelchair packs. A MedicAlert tag or bracelet identifies the type of disability or medical condition and includes a toll-free number for an office at which the wearer's current medication and diagnosis are on file. MedicAlert bracelets are available at pharmacies. Figure 11-1 provides a template for collecting a person's emergency health information.

The Vial of Life is another tool that can be used in the event of a disaster. The Vial of Life form contains important medical information and emergency contacts that can assist emergency personnel in administering the proper medical treatment. Individuals complete the Vial of Life form, either by hand or online, and then place the completed form in a plastic bag with the Vial of Life decal. They secure the plastic bag to the

Emergency Health Information	Date:		Updated:
Name			
Address	City	State	Zip
CONTACT METHOD	HOME	WORK	
Phone:			
Cell:			
E-mail:			
Fax/Pager:	Fax: Pager:	Fax: Pager:	
Birth Date	Blood Type	Social Security No.	
Health Plan	Individual #:	Group #:	
Emergency Contact:			
Address	City	State	Zip
CONTACT METHOD	HOME	WORK	
Phone:			
Cell:			
E-mail:			
Fax/Pager:	Fax: Pager:	Fax: Pager:	
Primary Care Provider:			
Address			
City	State	Zip	
Phone:	Fax:	E-mail	
Disability/Conditions:			
Medication:			
Allergies:			
Immunizations	Dates	Immunizations	Dates
Communication / Devices / Equipment / Other:			

Source: Reprinted with permission from Kailes JI. 2011. *Emergency Health Information.* Pomona, CA: Center for Disability and Health Policy. Available at: http://webhost.westernu.edu/hfcdhp/wp-content/uploads/Emergency-v1.pdf. Accessed February 1, 2017.

Figure 11-1. Emergency Health Information

refrigerator door and place another decal on the front door so it can be easily visible to anyone responding to an emergency.

Finally, a copy of the checklist in Figure 11-2 should be distributed to personnel who are responsible for creating, reviewing, maintaining, practicing, and revising emergency plans.

DISABILITY-RELATED ISSUES FOR EMERGENCY PLAN COORDINATORS	
Date Completed	**Activity**
	Make sure a relationship is established with your local fire department that includes: ◆ Fire Department reviewing the plan at least once a year, ◆ Fire Department receiving a copy of a current log containing names and location of all people needing assistance, ◆ The plan being coordinated and practiced with fire department.
	Practice plans through regular drills.
	Know how to get to all the exits and practice this as part of regular drills.
	Practice using evacuation devices.
	Practice dealing with different circumstances and unforeseen situations, such as blocked paths or exits.
	Ensure that shift workers and others who are at the site after typical hours, (cleaning crews, evening meeting coordinators, etc.) are included in drills.
	Plans should include: ◆ People who are at the site on a regular basis; ◆ People who are at the site outside of the typical working hours; ◆ How visitors, guests and customers with small children who require extra time to evacuate will be assisted; ◆ Specific dates for revisions and updates.
	Orient all people to the plan.
	Plan Dissemination ◆ Have people read the plan? ◆ Have people been oriented to the plan? Placing plans in a drawer or even a prominent place on a bookshelf is as good as burying them. ◆ Is the plan distributed and reviewed with all people at the site? ◆ Do people get a copy of the plan in a usable format (Braille, large print, text file, and cassette tape, or in appropriate formats for non-English speakers and people who have poor reading skills)? ◆ Are these formats always updated when the plan is revised?
	Make sure that people know how to report safety hazards (i.e. fire extinguishers that need servicing, exits which are not kept clear, furniture and other items that block barrier-free passages).

Source: Reprinted with permission from Kailes JI. 2002. *Emergency Evacuation Preparedness*. Pomona, CA: Center for Disability Issues and the Health Professions. Available at: http://webhost.westernu.edu/hfcdhp/wp-content/uploads/Emergency_Evacuation.pdf. Accessed February 28, 2017.

Figure 11-2. Disability-Related Issues for Emergency Plan Coordinators

CHAPTER 12

PUBLIC HEALTH RESPONSE TO EMERGING INFECTIONS AND BIOLOGICAL INCIDENTS

Natural disasters visibly impact environments, leaving behind visceral images of destruction. Infectious disease and super-lethal microorganisms, or biological agents, can spread through the air without being visible. These invisible threats pose special concerns and response requirements for health departments and health care systems. Although fighting the spread of infectious disease is a core competency of public health professionals, the timely availability of health care teams and resources in an emergency may be inadequate if the public health infrastructure is not maintained at a sufficient level. Responding to a biological attack or event requires careful coordination between governmental departments and agencies that do not necessarily work together in the daily practice of their professions (e.g., law enforcement and health care providers). Both scenarios require a carefully planned response utilizing many of the principles discussed in this and other chapters in the book.

This chapter reviews the response to unknown disease, pandemic influenza, Ebola virus disease (EVD), Zika virus, chemical or biological warfare, the role of hospitals in responding to pandemic influenza and release of biological agents, point of distribution plans, the Laboratory Response Network (LRN), and legal issues. In recent years, there has been an increased emergence of novel infectious disease or strains globally. As discussion of the full range of emerging infections is beyond the scope of this book, this chapter focuses on a few known diseases where key principles, such as the use of quarantine and isolation, personal protective equipment (PPE), and surveillance can be adapted in novel circumstances until specifics are determined about how to handle each.

Public Health Role

- Develop and use multidisciplinary protocols for collaboration among state and local public health agencies, community hospitals, academic health centers, community health care providers, laboratories, professional societies, medical examiners, emergency response units, manufacturers of safety and medical equipment, the media, government officials, regional airports, and federal agencies such as the U.S. Office of the Assistant Secretary for Preparedness and Response, the Centers for Disease Control and Prevention (CDC), and the Agency for Toxic Substances and Disease Registry.

- Establish specific criteria for monitoring emerging infections and activate surveillance systems that can quickly identify emerging or reemerging diseases, closely monitor unexplained morbidity and mortality caused by infectious disease, and improve surveillance for influenza-like illness.
- Increase lab capacity, educate microbiologists about reporting, and establish communication linkages with the LRN for the rapid evaluation and identification of biological agents.
- Develop and activate diagnostic clinical and treatment protocols that are communicated to the medical community and that improve rapid reporting of suspect cases, unusual clusters of disease, and unusual manifestations of disease.
- Plan for and respond, when necessary, to reduce the morbidity and mortality from pandemic influenza, an emerging novel disease, or a biological incident by stockpiling antibiotics, developing vaccines, preparing multilingual patient information, developing contingency plans for the full range of social distancing techniques, and developing community plans for the delivery of medical care to large numbers of patients, as well as to those who are not ill but seek medical treatment for reassurance (these patients are known as the *worried well*).
- Utilize and expand access to the Health Alert Network (HAN) during epidemics.
- Develop contingency plans with the local medical examiner for mass mortuary services, including plans for the utilization of federal Disaster Medical Assistance Teams and Disaster Mortuary Operational Response Teams.
- Train all health organizations required to deliver care.
- Communicate emergency instructions, prevention, control, and treatment information to the provider community.
- Communicate with the public about risks, preventive actions, and actions being taken by the government and public health agencies.
- Build and leverage relationships with communities that can help control the disease that is circulating (i.e., local residents from Liberia, Guinea, Sierra Leone, and Mali during the Ebola outbreak).
- Resolve legal issues related to public health authority in emergencies.

Response to Unknown Disease

With climate change; globalization of commerce, recreation, and humanitarian work; inadvertent transport of vectors; zoonotic disease; and antigenic shift, it is inevitable that the U.S. public health system will continue to confront serious diseases that are not common today. Furthermore, although pandemic influenza may overwhelm our health care delivery systems and incidents involving CBRNE[1] (chemical, biological, radiological, nuclear, and high-yield explosives) may involve many victims and damage to buildings and other property, these emerging infections and incidents are dissimilar to typical disasters in several ways. A major difference between natural disasters and an event involving an infectious disease is the widespread health impact. Officials may not recognize that an incident is underway until several casualties, outbreaks of infection, or multiple releases have occurred. The scope of the incident may expand geometrically and affect multiple jurisdictions since victims unknowingly spread infection or carry the agent to health care facilities and across geographic areas. The fear of the unknown may generate concern from the public, resulting in larger numbers of worried well than of actual victims. The workings of the typical response team could be disrupted as the scope of events requires expansion of the emergency response personnel who normally work together.

Depending on the infectiousness of the emerging infection or type of agent used, there may be a shortage of any of a number of medical resources including intensive care unit (ICU) beds, ventilators and other critical care needs, appropriate PPE, and antibiotics and antiviral agents. If a release of a contagious disease, such as smallpox, occurs, several patients will likely appear in emergency rooms with rash illness that hopefully will be reported to authorities as suspected smallpox. Nontraditional treatment centers may need to be established on short notice. There is potentially a high demand for mortuary or funeral services and social and counseling services. Unlike morbidity and mortality associated with natural disasters, demands on medical care in each community are likely to be prolonged as the illness spreads among the population. The need for home care may increase if the elderly and other high-risk and vulnerable populations cannot or will not leave their homes to receive care for chronic medical conditions because of the threat of exposure to infectious disease. In addition to surveillance and activating the participation of other agencies, public health officials may initiate actions to protect the community, including social distancing, quarantine, and immunization. Further, the fire and safety workforce may be reduced in number and overwhelmed if first responders, who normally are the main core of personnel on the scene of an incident, become ill from early or repeated exposure to communicable disease. Finally, communities will need to be self-sufficient for potentially prolonged periods if resources cannot be diverted from other geographic areas because of regional spread.

Unlike the response to an overt chemical event for which fire, police, or hazardous material units are the first responders, the public health department is charged with

1. CBRNE include chemical (cyanide, incapacitating agents, pulmonary agents, vesicants), biological (bacteria, virus, toxins), radiological, nuclear (detonation or "dirty" explosives), and high-yield explosives (rapid release of gas and heat) agents. This chapter focuses primarily on the public health preparedness and response to biological agents, although many of the principles discussed in this book will apply to preparedness for other agents.

identifying infectious disease in a community. This response to emerging infections and bioterrorism requires an interdependent working relationship among local, state, and federal agencies and among community clinicians, emergency responders, and local public health personnel. Once a plan is in place, the public health response to outbreaks of unknown disease has 5 components: detection of unusual events, investigation and containment of potential threats, organization of care, laboratory capacity, and coordination and communication.

Pandemic Influenza

Preparing for the uncommon, but potentially devastating, occurrence of pandemic influenza is a national strategy for the United States. Before discussing pandemic influenza, it is important to understand seasonal influenza. Seasonal influenza, which occurs annually between late fall and early spring, is a common but frequently serious disease known as *flu*. Because flu can be transmitted by those who are infected but asymptomatic, the virus spreads from person to person rapidly, and public health agencies may notice simultaneous outbreaks across a region. Most people have some immunity to the circulating virus, either from previous infections or from vaccination, and recover relatively quickly. However, for groups at higher risk for complications from flu, including the very young, the very old, pregnant women, the immunocompromised, and those with chronic illnesses, even seasonal influenza can cause serious complications (e.g., pneumonia or death). The number of seasonal influenza-associated deaths fluctuates from year to year because the impact of flu each season varies in duration and severity. As a result, a range of estimated deaths is often used. In a 2010 *Morbidity and Mortality Weekly Report*, the CDC estimated that over the 40-year span from 1976–1977 to 2006–2007, annual flu-associated deaths ranged from a low of about 3,000 to a high of about 49,000 people.

Pandemic flu occurs on average every 3 to 4 decades when a new strain of the flu emerges. Pandemic influenza can be thought of as the flu on steroids, because in previous pandemics, influenza caused significantly more morbidity and mortality. When pandemics occur, they are followed by multiple waves after the initial outbreak, overwhelming public health and health care systems that have not prepared adequately.

Three groups of influenza viruses (A, B, and C) can cause illness in humans, but only group A viruses cause major epidemics or pandemics. The 2 major antigenic components of influenza A viruses (hemagglutinin [H] and neuraminidase [N]) are continually undergoing changes, known as *drift*. When drift occurs, these changes in antigenic structure cause illness in individuals because immunity from prior infections does not protect them from getting sick when exposed to the changed virus. Drift can result in annual epidemics. Pandemics of influenza arise when a reassortment, or *antigenic shift*, of the H and N components occurs. In this antigenic shift, humans, birds, or swine are simultaneously infected with 2 different influenza A viruses, resulting in a new or *novel* strain against which no one has immunity.

Most people have some immunity to seasonal influenza strains because they have circulated in previous years. By contrast, during pandemics, there is little natural immunity to the circulating novel strain. As a result, the virus can spread easily from person to person increasing the number of unexpected deaths.

Four major pandemics have occurred in the last century. The 1918 influenza pandemic caused more than 600,000 deaths in the United States and up to 50 million deaths worldwide. Although subsequent pandemics in 1957 and 1969 were less deadly, the number of excess U.S. deaths was in the tens of thousands. In 2009, a new flu strain (H1N1 or "swine flu") spread across the United States and the rest of the world. The CDC estimates that between 43 million–89 million people were infected with H1N1, resulting in 8,870–18,300 flu-related deaths. In addition to high morbidity and excess mortality, influenza pandemics have also been accompanied by social and economic disruption. Thus, the challenge of reducing the severity of pandemics is a critically important responsibility for public health professionals.

Twenty-First Century Influenza Strains

Starting in 2003, a highly pathogenic avian influenza strain (H5N1) caused widespread disease among birds. Although H5N1 did not spread extensively among humans, and illness in humans can be mild, it has been and continues to be associated with high case-fatality rates. On January 8, 2014, the first case of a human infection with H5N1 in the Americas was reported in Canada in a traveler returning from China. Other strains (H7N9) have caused illness in humans when there has been direct contact with infected poultry. There was concern that the avian virus could become more easily transmissible among humans. Before that could happen, H1N1, a novel influenza strain found in swine, spread worldwide.

Swine flu is a common respiratory disease caused by the type A influenza virus that typically infects pigs. In 2009, a novel swine flu virus spread worldwide and is now a seasonal flu virus affecting both humans and pigs. Before the spring of 2009, swine flu had only occurred periodically in the United States. The 1976 outbreak, first noticed in Fort Dix, New Jersey, prompted more than 40 million people to be vaccinated. In September 1988, a previously healthy 32-year-old pregnant woman died from pneumonia after being infected with swine flu. Between December 2005 and February 2009, 12 people were diagnosed with swine flu in 10 U.S. states.

The virus that circulated in 2009 was a new subtype of A/H1N1 not previously detected in swine or humans to which many people had no preexisting immunity. This contagious virus spread worldwide, killing nearly 13,000 and sickening more than

60 million just in the United States. In this pandemic, the H1N1 virus dominated other seasonal influenza viruses. Most strikingly, the severest cases occurred more often in younger age groups, reversing the usual seasonal influenza pattern. As part of the response, health departments around the country implemented their pandemic influenza plans, the CDC provided national guidance, and the Strategic National Stockpile (SNS) released antiviral drugs, PPE, and respiratory protection devices.

In the post-pandemic phase, as H1N1 spread around the globe, all age groups in many countries developed some immunity to the new virus, no large or unusual outbreaks occurred in the following year, and seasonal influenza was again the flu virus most likely causing illness. The H1N1 virus has continued to circulate since the 2009 pandemic and has caused and will likely continue to cause variable illness during each subsequent influenza season.

Stages of a Pandemic

In 2005, the World Health Organization (WHO) distributed a preparedness plan for global influenza that defines the stages of a pandemic, outlines the role of the WHO, and makes recommendations for national measures before and during a pandemic. In 2013, the WHO released an updated version that applies the principles of an all-hazards approach for the management of pandemic influenza risk (available at: http://www.who.int/influenza/preparedness/pandemic/influenza_risk_management/en). The updated guidance:

- underscores the need for appropriate and timely risk assessment that can guide evidence-based decision making at national, state, and local levels;
- enhances the content on the application of assessments of risk and severity to support implementation by individual countries;
- revises the approach to the classification of global phases in response to lessons learned from the 2009 pandemic of influenza A/H1N1 (i.e., virological, epidemiological, and clinical data now informs the identification of phases in describing the spread of a novel influenza subtype around the world);
- uncouples national actions from global phases, providing flexibility to regions of the world and encouraging the development of adaptable response plans based on a nation's assessment of their own risk with an understanding of the global risk assessment of WHO;
- includes the principles of emergency risk management for health and public health; and
- provides new and updated annexes based on assumptions for planning, ethical considerations, whole-of-society approach, parameters for determining severity, and measures for containment.

United States Pandemic Planning

The United States prepares and initiates a national response based on the pandemic phases tracked by the WHO and its own assessment. The CDC is involved in the global preparedness effort by supporting WHO activities and maintaining cooperative agreements for surveillance in other countries. The U.S. Department of Health & Human Services (HHS) pandemic flu Web site provides comprehensive information and planning tools as reference for public health agencies and providers across the United States (available at: https://www.cdc.gov/flu).

An *Updated Preparedness and Response Framework for Influenza Pandemic* was released by HHS in 2014, incorporating lessons from the 2009 H1N1 pandemic and the spread of swine-origin variant H2N2 virus. The updated guidance provides additional detail about the timing of key decisions and actions aimed at controlling the spread and mitigating the impact of an emerging pandemic through 6 phases for public health action. The 6 phases, also known as intervals, are (1) investigation of cases of novel influenza in humans or animals, (2) recognition of increased potential for ongoing transmission, (3) initiation of a pandemic wave with efficient and sustained transmission, (4) acceleration of a pandemic wave with consistently increasing cases in the United States, (5) deceleration of a pandemic wave (consistently declining cases), and (6) preparation for future pandemic waves (low pandemic activity). Response efforts will be organized in each phase in 8 areas: (1) incident management, (2) surveillance and epidemiology, (3) laboratory, (4) community mitigation, (5) medical care and countermeasures, (6) vaccine, (7) risk communications, and (8) state/local coordination. The updated guidance is available at: https://www.cdc.gov/mmwr/preview/mmwrhtml/rr6306a1.htm. A list of the WHO phases and actions to be taken are provided in Table 12-1. A framework for response to influenza A pandemic is found in Table 12-2. Table 12-3 describes intervention and mitigation strategies by setting.

Tools for Pandemic Risk Assessment

Although data needed to make decisions in the United States might be limited during the earliest intervals of an influenza pandemic, delaying action might weaken the effectiveness of the response. Therefore, estimating the likelihood of risks as early as possible, particularly the risks of transmissibility, severity, and antiviral resistance, is crucial to ensure a timely and effective management of pandemic influenza. To support the decision making process for pandemic influenza, several tools have been developed. These tools, combined with an application of transmission-defined intervals, provide information to guide decision making and inform appropriate risk communication strategies across different jurisdictions and levels of government.

Table 12-1. World Health Organization Pandemic Phases

Phase	Characteristics
Interpandemic period	Period between influenza pandemics.
Alert phase	Phase when influenza caused by a new subtype has been identified in humans. Increased vigilance and careful risk assessment, at local, national and global levels are characteristic of this phase. If the risk assessments indicate that the new virus is not developing into a pandemic strain, a decrease of activities toward those in the interpandemic phase may occur.
Pandemic period	Period of global spread of human influenza caused by a new subtype. Movement between the interpandemic, alert and pandemic phases may occur quickly or gradually as indicated by the global risk assessment, chiefly based on virological, epidemiological and clinical data.
Transition phase	As the global risk decreases, de-escalation of global actions may occur and reduction in response activities or movement toward recovery actions by countries may be appropriate, based on their own risk assessments.

Source: Based on World Health Organization (WHO). 2013. *Pandemic Influenza Risk Management: WHO Interim Guidance.* Geneva, Switzerland: WHO. Available at: http://www.who.int/influenza/preparedness/pandemic/GIP_PandemicInfluenzaRiskManagementInterimGuidance_Jun2013.pdf?ua=. Accessed January 23, 2017.

The Influenza Risk Assessment Tool (IRAT) is used by the U.S. government and the WHO Global Influenza Surveillance and Response System to gather data and then foster discussion and consensus-building among subject-matter experts to enable them to assign a score that reflects the risk of the virus spreading across communities and regions. Ten predefined elements are given a risk score. These 10 elements fall into 3 categories: (1) characteristics of the biologic properties of the virus (4 items), (2) characteristics of the population (3 items), and (3) characteristics of the ecology and epidemiology of the virus (3 items).

In 2007, as part of the interim guidance for community mitigation strategies, the Pandemic Severity Assessment Framework (PSAF) was introduced by CDC as a tool to define the severity of an emerging influenza pandemic. The PSAF is used to characterize the potential impact of a spreading illness relative to the impact of previous influenza epidemics and pandemics. To facilitate communication about assessed risk, the index had 5 categories similar to the hurricane severity scale, ranging from Category 1 (moderate severity) to Category 5 (most severe). The PSAF can be used early in a pandemic and assessments can be repeated as information changes. The PSAF was revised following the 2009 H1N1 pandemic in order to characterize the potential impact of a pandemic relative to previous experience with influenza epidemics and pandemics.

Comparing IRAT and PSAF

Each tool has a different function. While IRAT focuses on the risk of a novel virus emerging and the potential for significant impact if that occurs, PSAF focuses on the

Table 12-2. Preparedness and Response Framework for Novel Influenza A Virus Pandemics: WHO Phases and CDC Intervals, With Federal and State/Local Indicators

WHO phases	CDC intervals	Federal indicators for CDC intervals	State/local indicators for CDC intervals
Interpandemic: Period between influenza pandemics **Alert:** Influenza caused by a new subtype has been identified in humans	**Investigation:** Investigation of novel influenza A infection in humans or animals	Identification of novel influenza A infection in humans or animals anywhere in the world with potential implications for human health	Identification of novel influenza A infection in humans or animals in the United States with potential implications for human health
	Recognition: Recognition of increased potential for ongoing transmission of a novel influenza A virus	Increasing number of human cases or clusters of novel influenza A infection anywhere in the world with virus characteristics, indicating increased potential for ongoing human-to-human transmission	Increasing number of human cases or clusters of novel influenza A infection in the United States with virus characteristics indicating increased potential for ongoing human-to-human transmission
Pandemic: Global spread of human influenza caused by a new subtype	**Initiation:** Initiation of a pandemic wave	Confirmation of human cases of a pandemic influenza virus anywhere in the world with demonstrated efficient and sustained human-to-human transmission	Confirmation of human cases of a pandemic influenza virus in the United States with demonstrated efficient and sustained human-to-human transmission
	Acceleration: Acceleration of a pandemic wave	Consistently increasing rate of pandemic influenza cases identified in the United States, indicating established transmission	Consistently increasing rate of pandemic influenza cases identified in the state, indicating established transmission
	Deceleration: Deceleration of a pandemic wave	Consistently decreasing rate of pandemic influenza cases in the United States	Consistently decreasing rate of pandemic influenza cases in the state
Transition: Reduction in global risk, reduction in response activities, or progression toward recovery actions	**Preparation:** Preparation for future pandemic waves	Low pandemic influenza activity but continued outbreaks possible in some jurisdictions	Low pandemic influenza activity but continued outbreaks possible in the state

Source: Adapted from Holloway R, Rasmussen SA, Zaza S, Cox NJ, Jernigan DB. 2014. Updated preparedness and response framework for influenza pandemics. *MMWR Recomm Rep.* 63(RR06):1-9.
Note: CDC=Centers for Disease Control and Prevention; WHO=World Health Organization.

Table 12-3. Interventions and Mitigation Strategies by Setting

Setting	Interventions
Home	Many sick individuals who are not critically ill may be managed safely through voluntary isolation at home combined with use of antiviral treatment as available and indicated
	Voluntary quarantine of household members in homes with sick people
School	Social distancing by dismissal of students from schools and school-based programs
	Closure of child care centers
	Reduce social contacts and community meetings
Workplace/Community Social Distancing	Encourage alternatives to in-person meetings (e.g., teleconferences)
	Modify contact at work via telecommuting and staggered schedules
	Postpone or cancel public gatherings where large groups will congregate

Source: Adapted from U.S. Department of Health & Human Services (HHS). 2007. *Interim Pre-pandemic Planning Guidance: Community Strategy for Pandemic Influenza Mitigation in the United States—Early, Targeted, Layered Use of Nonpharmaceutical Interventions.* Table 2. Summary of the community mitigation strategy, by pandemic severity. Washington, DC: HHS. Available at: http://www.flu.gov/professional/community/commitigation.html. Accessed January 23, 2017.

Note: The use of each of these interventions will depend on the phase and severity of the pandemic. Interventions are used in combination with other infection control measures, including hand hygiene, cough etiquette, and personal protective equipment such as face masks. Since HHS developed its interim guidance, the World Health Organization has developed a revised schema for describing the phases of a pandemic (see Table 12-1), which does not use a severity scale.

epidemiologic parameters of transmissibility and severity after a virus has emerged. The PSAF requires a sufficient number of cases and human clusters and is a more reliable indicator of risk when novel viruses have efficient and sustained transmission.

Lessons Learned

During the last century, important lessons were learned about pandemics that should be incorporated into public health preparedness for the next pandemic[2]:

- Pandemics are unpredictable, with great variation in mortality, severity of illness, and patterns of spread.
- Consistently, the number of cases will exponentially increase very quickly, and hospitals need to be prepared for a sudden surge in patients needing medical care.
- The capacity of the virus to cause severe disease in the very young and elderly will determine the pandemic's impact.
- Pandemics occur in waves; subsequent waves can be more severe if the virus mutates to a more virulent form, or the second wave reaches those more at risk of severe disease causing fatal complications.
- Virological surveillance is key to rapidly confirming the onset, alerting health services, isolating and characterizing the virus, and making it available to vaccine manufacturers.
- While the 2009 pandemic started in Mexico, most pandemics have originated in Asia, where surveillance for both influenza among animals and clusters of unusual respiratory disease in humans provides an early warning.
- Public health interventions have delayed but not stopped the spread of past pandemics, and quarantine and travel restrictions have shown little effect, but the temporary banning of public gatherings and closure of schools are potentially effective measures.
- Delaying the spread of the virus is important because with fewer people ill, medical and other essential services are more likely to be maintained.
- Vaccination during a pandemic must be sufficient and timely.
- Health officials must design their communication efforts to reach a diverse audience, including non-English speaking populations.
- Countries that manufacture vaccine will be the first to receive it.

---

2. Adapted from World Health Organization (WHO). 2005. *Avian Influenza: Assessing the Pandemic Threat.* Geneva, Switzerland: WHO. Available at: http://apps.who.int/iris/bitstream/10665/68985/1/WHO_CDS_2005.29.pdf. Accessed January 23, 2017; Holloway R, Rasmussen SA, Zaza S, Cox NJ, and Jernigan DB. 2014. Updated preparedness and response framework for influenza pandemics. *MMWR Recomm Rep.* 63(RR06):1–9. Available at: http://www.cdc.gov/mmwr/preview/mmwrhtml/rr6306a1.htm. Accessed January 23, 2017.

- Since pandemics have been most severe in later waves, there is an extension of the time needed to produce more vaccine for high-risk populations; successive waves may begin as quickly as a month later.
- Although a community's experience in administering yearly vaccination to large groups of people can reduce excess mortality because of their skill at the logistics of vaccination, regions should expect a sudden surge of many sick people and a high demand for medical care during a pandemic.
- Health officials need to incorporate storage of stockpile medical materials into their pandemic planning efforts.

Public Health Planning and Preparedness for Pandemic Flu

Local and state health departments have developed plans to prepare for and respond to an influenza pandemic. Preparing for a pandemic requires both internal and communitywide planning. When a novel strain of flu virus emerges, it is unlikely that there will be time to manufacture sufficient vaccine for the new strain before it spreads widely. As a result, responders (e.g., first responders, public health, and health care professionals) could become ill. A prolonged outbreak will occur over months, impacting the continuity of operations of essential services. Planning for a pandemic should assume that there will be a significant decrease in the available workforce. Regional and federal assets, such as ventilators, may not be available because of both the demand and the difficulty of transporting them with reduced manpower.

HHS[3] identifies the primary strategies for combating influenza as the following:

- Vaccination
- Early treatment of infected individuals and prophylaxis of exposed individuals with influenza antiviral medications
- Implementation of infection control and social distancing measures

Carrying out these tasks requires epidemiology and surveillance; planning mass vaccination, including the receipt of the vaccine, distribution to a broad spectrum of vaccination sites, monitoring doses, and the administration of the vaccination process; the delivery and distribution of antiviral countermeasures; community mitigation through social distancing and quarantine; communicating to the public; and confirmatory laboratory diagnostics.

When response to a pandemic begins, decisions will be made about the use of antiviral medications because of the expected time delays in the availability of effective vaccination

---

3. U.S. Department of Health & Human Services (HHS). 2007. *Interim Pre-pandemic Planning Guidance: Community Strategy for Pandemic Influenza Mitigation.* Washington, DC: HHS. Available at: https://www.cdc.gov/flu/pandemic-resources/pdf/community_mitigation-sm.pdf. Accessed January 30, 2017.

for mass immunization. Additional decisions on how to protect the public using social distancing, such as isolation and quarantine, will be made. All decisions will be based on scientific data, ethical considerations, public opinion on protective measures and their impact on society, and common sense. Key public health tasks include robust surveillance and laboratory testing. Laboratories will be required to handle a surge of specimens and to verify that their testing algorithms are adequate. In an era of technology, traditional "shoe leather" investigative methods will be required for contact tracing. Health departments should prepare by vetting the legality of procedures for the implementation of social distancing in advance of any outbreak. The distribution of vaccine and antiviral medications will be a massive undertaking and coordination with the SNS will be required. Procedures should be in place for (1) acquiring and taking delivery of the drugs, (2) prioritizing the population that will receive available drugs, (3) tracking the distribution and use of supplies, (4) conducting mass vaccination clinics, and (5) tracking adverse events caused by vaccination. If vaccination to a novel virus requires 2 doses of vaccine to achieve maximum immunity, health departments should develop a plan for tracking and recalling individuals who receive a novel flu vaccine. As part of planning, health departments should determine how they will communicate about behaviors that reduce risk, such as social distancing, hand washing, and respiratory etiquette. Further, planning should include communications about seeking care and about vaccine or antiviral distribution. Table 12-4 identifies key actions by pandemic phase. The following lists key behaviors for preventing the spread of flu:

- Cover nose and mouth with a tissue while sneezing.
- Cough into one's sleeve.
- Dispose of tissues in the trash immediately after use.
- Wash hands with soap and water, especially after coughing or sneezing.
- Clean hands with alcohol-based hand sanitizers.
- If sick with influenza, stay home from work or school and limit contact with others to avoid infecting them.
- Avoid touching eyes, nose, or mouth with unwashed hands.
- Stay away from those who are sick.
- Stay away from settings where large groups have gathered when there is illness in the community.
- Clean frequently touched surfaces often (e.g., door knobs, hand rails).
- Get an influenza vaccine every year.

Collection, Storage, Processing, and Testing of Flu Specimens

In 2009, the CDC issued interim guidance on the appropriate collection, storage, processing, and testing of specimens for patients with suspected novel H1N1 virus infection.

Table 12-4. World Health Organization Actions by Pandemic Phases

Phases	Actions
Interpandemic	• Support emergency risk management capacity development
Alert	• Conduct global risk assessment through the International Health Regulation mechanism
	• Provide advice to member states
	• Activate support networks, advisory groups, partner networks
	• Deploy antivirals
	• Intensify regulatory preparedness
Pandemic	• Scale response as indicated by the global risk assessment
	• Declare a pandemic
	• Provide continued support to affected member states
Transition	• Scale response as indicated by the global risk assessment
	• Consider modification of termination of temporary measures and termination of a PHEIC assessments

Source: Based on World Health Organization (WHO). 2013. *Pandemic Influenza Risk Management WHO Interim Guidance*. Geneva, Switzerland: WHO. Available at: http://www.who.int/influenza/preparedness/pandemic/GIP_PandemicInfluenzaRiskManagementInterimGuidance_Jun2013.pdf?ua=1. Accessed January 23, 2017.
Note: PHEIC = public health emergencies of international concern.

As of this writing, this detailed guidance has not been updated and is now archived (available at: http://www.cdc.gov/h1n1flu/specimencollection.htm). All facilities that collect specimens during an outbreak should check with the CDC for any updates.

In the case of H1N1, the novel influenza A virus was confirmed in people with an influenza-like illness by a laboratory test (e.g., real-time reverse transcription test, real-time polymerase chain reaction test, or viral culture). Although isolating the novel influenza virus helps diagnose the infection, lab results may not be returned quickly enough for timely management of clinical symptoms. Furthermore, in 2009, a negative viral culture did not rule out infection with the H1N1 virus.

Because the duration of viral shedding with novel influenza A/H1N1 virus is unknown, the CDC estimated the duration of viral shedding based upon the behavior of seasonal influenza virus. They assumed that infected individuals shed the virus and were potentially infectious from the day prior to the onset of illness until the fever resolved, or up to 7 days from the onset of illness.

Clinicians can test for suspected cases of novel H1N1 by obtaining an upper respiratory specimen. Preferred respiratory specimens should be collected as soon as possible after the onset of illness and include nasopharyngeal swab, nasal aspirate, or a combined nasopharyngeal swab with oropharyngeal swab. A nasal swab or oropharyngeal swab is acceptable. An endotracheal aspirate, bronchoalveolar lavage, or sputum specimens should also be collected from intubated patients.

Respiratory specimens should not be kept longer than 4 days. Specimens should be placed in sterile viral transport media and immediately placed on ice or cold packs or refrigerated at 39.2°F (4°C) for transport to the laboratory. Clinical specimens should be shipped on wet ice or cold packs in appropriate packaging. All specimens should be labeled clearly and include complete information requested by each state's public health laboratory. Specimens from suspected cases shipped from the state public health laboratory to the CDC should include all information required for submitting seasonal influenza surveillance isolates or specimens.

For more details, see recommended infection control guidance for people collecting clinical specimens for influenza in clinical settings (available at: http://www.osha.gov/Publications/OSHA_pandemic_health.pdf) and for laboratory personnel (available at: http://www.cdc.gov/h1n1flu/guidelines_labworkers.htm).

Infection Control

The CDC has published infection control recommendations for suspected or confirmed influenza patients for which treatment involves aerosol-generating procedures, potentially spreading the virus via droplets in the air. These aerosol-generating activities include the collection of clinical specimens, inserting or removing of endotracheal tubes, giving nebulizer treatments, performing bronchoscopy, and performing cardiac pulmonary resuscitation or emergency intubation. Once medically cleared, fit-tested, and trained for respirator use, medical personnel should wear a fit-tested disposable N95 respirator when entering the patient's room. All hospital personnel should follow hand hygiene practices by washing with soap and water or using hand sanitizer immediately after removing gloves and other equipment and after any contact with respiratory secretions. Any personnel providing care to or collecting clinical specimens should wear disposable nonsterile gloves, gowns, and eye protection (such as goggles). Information on comprehensive respiratory protection programs and fit-test procedures can be accessed online (at: http://www.osha.gov/SLTC/etools/respiratory).

Other infection control procedures include the following:

- Patients should be placed in a single-patient room with the door kept closed or an airborne infection isolation room with negative pressure, and suctioning, bronchoscopy, or intubation should be performed in a procedure room with negative-pressure air handling.
- The ill person should wear a surgical mask when outside of the patient room and should be encouraged to wash hands frequently and follow respiratory hygiene practices.
- Routine cleaning and disinfection strategies performed during influenza seasons can be used for the environmental management of swine flu.
- Standard, droplet, and contact precautions should be used for all patient care activities, and maintained for 7 days after the onset of illness or until symptoms have resolved.

Influenza Preparedness for At-Risk Populations

Because flu is a highly contagious respiratory disease that spreads quickly and exponentially, it is critical that preparedness for influenza involve all populations, including those with vulnerabilities that increase their risk during a pandemic. In addition to the large population already identified in Chapter 11 as at-risk from other disasters, many factors such as access to treatment, health literacy, immigration status, and spoken language may increase the number of people who are vulnerable during an influenza pandemic. Immigrants and refugees are at-risk from pandemic influenza as a result of a high prevalence of chronic disease that predisposes them to complications from flu, low rates of seasonal flu vaccination, and numerous social, linguistic, and economic barriers to accessing and using preventive measures. Many immigrants work in low-paying jobs without benefits such as sick leave; this discourages them from staying home when ill. They may also live in crowded conditions, making it difficult to isolate a sick family member. In addition, there are millions of undocumented people living in the United States who may not follow advice for preventive immunization or other actions that could expose them to potential deportation. Some may lack the experience to understand how to carry out the preventive actions being recommended. Some might experience cross-cultural misunderstanding, which acts as a barrier and reduces their ability to take preventive measures or get timely medical care. Further, risk is increased for those who lack the funds to stockpile medications and supplies, lack adequate health insurance, or are not aware of or cannot take preventive measures because of limited emotional and/or financial resources.

Social Distancing

When public health officials want to slow or stop the spread of a highly contagious disease, such as pandemic influenza, they may apply techniques known as social distancing.[4] Since effective vaccine and antiviral drugs may not be available when an influenza pandemic begins, social distancing may be a key strategy for preventing the virus from spreading through droplet, aerosol, or contact transmission through the social contacts limit. Such actions include quarantine or isolation; closing schools or asking ill children to stay home from school; closing workplaces; canceling or postponing meetings, large social or religious gatherings, and athletic events; or prohibiting travel. Social distancing usually involves actions that will maintain a distance of 3 feet or more between people. State laws give health officers the legal authority to carry out such measures within state borders. Since the actions needed to implement social distancing are likely to have considerable

4. While social distancing is discussed as a strategy for influenza, it has also been used with Ebola virus disease and has application for any infectious disease where public health professionals are concerned about spread.

impact on any community, such action is usually coordinated with local agencies such as cities, police departments, and schools, as well as with state and federal partners.

Quarantine and Isolation

Quarantine may be used when a person has been exposed to a contagious disease, is not yet sick, but may become infectious and spread the disease to others. When a person is placed in quarantine, they are separated from others. For example, as a way of isolating household contacts, infectious individuals may be asked to remain in their homes so that they do not come in contact with unexposed people. Isolating household contacts of index cases has been shown to be moderately effective in reducing the caseload and in delaying the peak of pandemic influenza. Other quarantine measures include restricting the travel of individuals who have been exposed to a contagious disease and implementing restrictions on people coming or going into a specific area.

Isolation is used to reduce transmission by reducing contact between a person who is sick with a contagious infection and uninfected people. Isolation is moderately effective, but may be helpful where there is limited access to antiviral medication. The time that an infected person is isolated varies depending on the specific infectious disease. While isolation can occur in hospitals, other health care facilities and in people's homes, hospitals have rooms that are specially equipped with negative air pressure to stop the release of microbes into the environment outside the room. Isolation in hospitals is limited to the number of medically equipped rooms that are available.

School Closure

Closing schools is moderately effective in reducing the transmission of influenza and in delaying the peak of an epidemic. However, just closing schools may not be sufficient to interrupt transmission, so also closing social events and extracurricular activities may be necessary. Such actions have high economic costs (i.e., parents needing to take time off from work and losing income) and should be considered only in a severe pandemic and for the shortest possible interval. Studies suggesting that proactively closing schools can reduce the transmission of influenza by up to 50%, delay the peak of an epidemic by a week or two, and weaken subsequent waves of the epidemic. If closing schools for a long time, it is better to initiate closure as soon as possible after the start of the epidemic.

Closing schools, even when influenza is already present in the community, is moderately effective. To have a significant effect on the overall attack rate, school closure may need to be maintained throughout most of the epidemic (i.e., at least 8 weeks). School closure should be considered when the attack rate of influenza-like illnesses reaches 5%

(e.g., closure in advance of influenza in the community when rate of symptomatic influenza reaches 5% of the population; closure when influenza is present in the community when single-day influenza-related absentee rate in a school reaches 5%).

Workplace Closure

To reduce the transmission of influenza when people have brought the virus to the workplace, closing the place of work and asking employees to work from home are modestly effective. According to Booy and Ward, about a third of workplaces would need to be closed to be successful, potentially causing considerable economic hardship and social distress. Closing workplaces after the virus has been introduced to these environments is worth considering, especially if the community decides on also closing local schools. A decision may be made to temporarily eliminate meetings in the workplace to reduce transmission.

Other social distancing strategies in the workplace might include:

- Limiting the frequency of face-to-face contacts
- Limiting social interactions that normally occur at work
- Asking employees not to report to work if sick
- Asking the employer to schedule staggered break times
- Establishing flexible work hours
- Using text messaging and personal mobile phones to communicate instead of face-to-face contact
- Avoiding conferences and group gatherings

Working From Home

Allowing employees, who may or may not be infectious, to work from home can reduce transmission outside the home. Working from home can be moderately effective in reducing the transmission of influenza.

Cancellation of Mass Gatherings

By canceling mass gatherings (e.g., sporting events, concerts) and thus limiting the number of potentially ill contacts that an individual is exposed to, public health professionals aim to reduce the transmission of infectious disease. The duration of an event, amount of crowding, type of venue, and when the event is held in relation to either side of the peak of the epidemic can affect the risk of transmission of influenza. One consideration is that the costs of canceling a mass gathering could be substantial and potentially controversial.

Communication and Response

Ideally, the public acts as a partner with government officials in taking actions that will prevent infectious disease from spreading in the community. An effective partner must receive and understand the messages being communicated and accept the actions being recommended. To reach diverse groups, targeted communication and response strategies need to be developed that address any potential concerns about receiving vaccination, taking antiviral medications, staying home from work, or potential reprisal for coming forward to seek vaccination or treatment. As discussed in Chapter 7, officials should strengthen their partnerships with trusted members of a targeted population and involve them in development of both the communication strategy and the messages during the pre-pandemic period. The first step is collaboration between public health agencies and the various communities that might be vulnerable. Possible participants include community health centers, school-based clinics, primary care practices, and home health care workers. Faith- and community-based organizations may be helpful in working with immigrants in adopting preventive behaviors, such as cough etiquette and the use of face masks and respirators. Members of vulnerable communities should also be asked to participate in their community's pandemic planning and preparedness activities.

Since pandemic influenza is likely to occur over a period of months or years and to appear and abate in waves, one challenge will be to get the public to trust and act upon messages that might evolve. As a pandemic progresses, public uncertainty may grow; specific strategies should be developed with the targeted communities to deal with any doubts. The public will look to officials to quickly respond to their concerns about the risks inherent in the rapid spread of infection or in any proposed preventive actions. What is communicated should be personally relevant (i.e., expressed in the spoken language of the targeted communities) and reflect a group's cultural beliefs and views about the risk. Communications about unanticipated complications should be timely and ongoing. When mass immunization is being given, providers of mobile clinical vans can reach out and work with the various agencies that serve the targeted communities.

Ebola Virus Disease

EVD, previously known as Ebola hemorrhagic fever, is a rare, severe, and often fatal disease. EVD is caused by infection with a virus of the family *Filoviridae*, genus *Ebolavirus*. There are 5 identified Ebola virus species, 4 of which are known to cause disease in humans: Ebola virus (*Zaire ebolavirus*); Sudan virus (*Sudan ebolavirus*); Taï Forest virus (*Taï Forest ebolavirus*, formerly *Côte d'Ivoire ebolavirus*); and Bundibugyo virus (*Bundibugyo ebolavirus*). The fifth, Reston virus (*Reston ebolavirus*), has caused disease in nonhuman primates, but has yet to present in humans. The natural reservoir host of EVD remains unknown. However, the basis of evidence and the nature of similar viruses have led researchers to believe that the virus is animal-borne with bats being the most likely reservoir. Four of the 5 virus strains occur in an animal host native to Africa.

The EVD pathogen can impede the proper functioning of macrophages and dendritic cells. Dendritic cells are the cells that produce an immune response in the epithelial tissue layers that make up the outer surface of the body and help protect or enclose organs. Most epithelial cells, found throughout the body, produce mucus or other secretions including in the respiratory tract. EVD prevents these epithelial cells from carrying out their antiviral functions but does not interfere with the initial inflammatory response that brings additional cells to the infection site. These additional cells contribute to further distribution of the virus. EVD is transmitted through direct contact (i.e., broken skin or mucous membranes in the eyes, nose, or mouth) with:

- Blood or body fluids (e.g., urine, saliva, sweat, feces, vomit, breast milk, or semen from a person who has recovered from EVD through oral, vaginal, or anal sex);
- Objects (e.g., needles and syringes) that have been contaminated with body fluids from a person who is sick with EVD or from the body of a person who died from EVD; and
- Infected fruit bats or primates.

The incubation period for the virus typically lasts 8–10 days, but can range from 2 to 21 days. Transmission of EVD can occur from the outset of symptoms and extend through the subsequent stages of disease, and into postmortem. Studies of transmission in EVD outbreaks have identified activities like caring for an infected person, sharing a bed, and funeral activities as additional key risk factors for transmission.

There has been much discussion on whether EVD can be aerosolized (also see Chapter 10). Many body fluids, including vomit, diarrhea, blood, and saliva, are capable of creating inhalable aerosol particles in the immediate vicinity of an infected person. The following factors contribute to the need for adequate respiratory protection against EVD:

- Patients and procedures generate aerosols, and EVD remains viable in aerosols for up to 90 minutes.
- All sizes of aerosol particles are easily inhalable both near and far from the patient.
- The probability that health care workers will be exposed to high concentrations of infectious aerosols increases with crowding, limited air exchange in the treatment space, and close interactions with patients.
- Experimental data support aerosols as a mode of disease transmission in nonhuman primates.

Case Definition for Ebola Virus Disease

The CDC requires that a person with the following symptoms and risk factors be considered a person under investigation (PUI) for EVD:

1. Elevated body temperature or subjective fever or symptoms, including severe headache, fatigue, muscle pain, vomiting, diarrhea, abdominal pain, or unexplained hemorrhage; and
2. An epidemiologic risk factor within the 21 days before the onset of symptoms.

High-risk epidemiologic factors include:

- Percutaneous (e.g., needlestick) or mucous membrane exposure to blood or body fluids, including but not limited to feces, saliva, sweat, urine, vomit, and semen from a person with EVD who has symptoms
- Direct contact with a person, or the person's body fluid, who presents with symptoms of EVD, without wearing appropriate PPE
- Laboratory processing of blood or body fluids from a symptomatic person with EVD without wearing appropriate PPE or without using standard biosafety precautions
- Providing direct care in a household setting to a person showing symptoms of EVD
- Residence in or recent travel within the last 21 days from countries with widespread transmission or cases in urban settings with uncertain control measures
- Direct contact with a body of a person who died of EVD without wearing appropriate PPE

Information about other epidemiological risk factors can be found at: http://www.cdc.gov/vhf/ebola/exposure/risk-factors-when-evaluating-person-for-exposure.html.

Public Health Preparedness for Ebola Virus Disease

The response to EVD involves partnering with many disciplines (i.e., public health and health care professionals, emergency medical technicians and paramedics, police, sanitation, medical examiner, airport officials including security and governmental officials). In addition, there are numerous tasks in a response to EVD, many of which are the extension of everyday public health practice, discussed in this chapter and elsewhere in the book.

During the EVD outbreak in the United States in 2014, collaboration between health departments and hospitals was critical in the nation's response. When the first domestic cases of Ebola occurred, local health departments requested assistance from the National Association of County and City Health Officials (NACCHO) to access and implement federal guidance. Urgent issues included the handling of medical waste and choosing appropriate PPE. Given that the public health and health care systems had never previously diagnosed or treated a case of EVD in the United States, confusion over the isolation and quarantine of travelers arriving from West Africa developed. Based on the experience, NACCHO made the following recommendations for local health departments:

- Form partnerships in advance with local and regional health care systems to prepare for and coordinate a response to EVD so that health departments and local health care partners can act quickly to identify and manage potential Ebola cases.
- Communicate information about risk accurately and timely, using materials in the languages spoken in your community and at the appropriate reading levels to mitigate fear and panic caused by misinformation and rumors.
- Assign dedicated staff to interpret federal guidance, work with community partners, respond to information requests, and disseminate risk information.
- Participate in health care coalitions to improve coordination between local health departments and health care facilities to facilitate the community's planning, training, and responding to public health emergencies.
- Work with state health departments to review and test isolation and quarantine plans and plan for the resources needed for future global health threats.
- Learn about global threats that could affect health security.

Health Care Facilities and Emergency Medical Services

The CDC issued guidance for both health care facilities and emergency medical services (EMS).

Following the EVD outbreak of 2014, the CDC created a tiered structure of health care facilities to support the assessment and treatment of person with this highly infectious disease. This tiered structure supports a regionalized approach to treating EVD. All health care facilities are considered "frontline" facilities. Additional requirements have been developed for the smaller number of health care facilities identified and designated as assessment or treatment facilities.

Frontline Health Care Facilities

Frontline health care facilities (e.g., acute care hospitals, other emergency care settings, urgent care clinics, and critical access hospitals), in coordination with local and state health authorities, should be prepared to evaluate a person who presents with EVD-like symptoms and a known potential exposure. To ensure timely care, frontline health care facilities should be prepared to identify and isolate PUIs and inform state and local public health authorities immediately. Frontline health care facilities should have the capability to:

- Rapidly identify and triage patients with relevant exposure history *and* signs or symptoms compatible with EVD as outlined in CDC's guidance for Emergency Department Evaluation and Management for PUIs for EVD (available at: http://www.cdc.gov/vhf/ebola/healthcare-us/emergency-services/emergency-departments.html).
- Immediately isolate any patient with relevant exposure history and signs or symptoms compatible with EVD and take appropriate steps to adequately protect staff caring for the patient, including appropriate use of PPE.
- Immediately notify the hospital/facility infection control program, other appropriate facility staff, and the state and local public health agencies that a patient has been identified who has relevant exposure *and* signs or symptoms compatible with EVD; discuss level of risk, clinical and epidemiologic factors, alternative diagnoses, plan for EVD testing, and plan for possible patient transfer to another facility for further care.
- Work in coordination with state and local health authorities in accordance with the state's plan to consider transferring the patient to an EVD assessment hospital that can provide any necessary testing and care until an EVD diagnosis is either confirmed or ruled out. Patients with mild illness and low probability of EVD based on clinical and epidemiologic factors, but require testing for EVD, may, in some circumstances, remain at the frontline health care facility for the assessment.
- Transfer patients with confirmed EVD to an EVD treatment center.

Ebola Assessment Hospitals

Ebola assessment hospitals are prepared to receive and isolate patients with suspected EVD and provide care until an EVD diagnosis can be confirmed or ruled out. State and local health authorities, consulting with hospital administration, have the authority to designate a facility as an Ebola assessment hospital. The CDC encouraged all states to consider identifying Ebola assessment hospitals to ensure that suspected patients can be appropriately cared for, if Ebola is present in the United States, until an EVD diagnosis is confirmed or ruled out. The Ebola assessment hospitals should be in a location that provides adequate geographic coverage across the state and avoids extended time beyond 1–2 hours to transport patients, particularly in areas where a large number of travelers return from high risk locations.

Ebola assessment hospitals may receive patients transferred from frontline health care facilities or referred by public health authorities if they have traveled to an Ebola-affected area or had potential exposure to someone with EVD within the past 21 days and have developed signs and symptoms of EVD. Patients identified as being at risk for EVD through airport screening will be monitored daily by public health authorities during the 21 days following travel to a country with widespread EVD transmission or exposure (i.e., it will be assumed they had contact with a person with EVD).

State and local public health authorities will coordinate closely with facilities when directing patients to an Ebola assessment hospital. Ebola assessment hospitals should be prepared to promptly test, manage, and treat alternative causes of febrile illness (e.g., malaria, influenza) as clinically indicated. Assessment hospitals should be equipped to use the level of PPE recommended to care for hospitalized patients with EVD and ensure their staff is appropriately trained in the donning and doffing of PPE. While initial isolation and evaluation of clinically stable patients can be carried out using the CDC's guidance for PPE and infection control practices for clinically stable PUIs, the highest level of PPE should be used for patients presenting with more severe symptoms, such as vomiting, copious diarrhea, or bleeding. Consult Chapter 10 for more information on the use of PPE.

Confirming or ruling out an EVD diagnosis in a PUI may take up to 72 hours or longer and may require an additional 12 to 24 hours for specimen transport, testing, and identification of another facility for any needed transfer. Therefore, Ebola assessment hospitals should be prepared to provide care for a PUI, including those with a high level of clinical suspicion for EVD, for up to 96 hours.

Ebola assessment hospitals supplement the state-designated Ebola treatment centers, which care for and manage patients with laboratory-confirmed EVD through the full course of the illness. The decision to transport a PUI from an assessment hospital to a treatment center should be made on a case-by-case basis, informed by the status of the patient, the capacity of the Ebola assessment hospital, and discussions between public health authorities and the referring and accepting physicians. State health officials are responsible for ensuring the readiness of Ebola assessment hospitals in their respective states.

Patient Transfer

When patients are transferred from an assessment hospital to a treatment center, transport providers should be informed of the patient's status and have appropriate training and PPE to safely move the patient. A state's or jurisdiction's plan for transferring patients may include arrangements to move a patient to another state based on the patient's risk, severity of illness and the geographic location of Ebola treatment centers. Once a patient is confirmed to have EVD, and upon the request of the health department and the treatment center, a CDC Ebola Response Team will be deployed to provide technical assistance for infection control procedures, clinical care, and logistics of managing the patient. Table 12-5 summarizes guidance on the minimum capabilities that Ebola assessment hospitals should have in place before receiving PUIs.

Table 12-5. Minimum Capabilities of Ebola Virus Disease Assessment Hospitals

Facility Infrastructure: Patient Room(s)	Hospital has a private room with in-room dedicated bathroom or covered bedside commode, equipped with dedicated patient-care equipment, including separate areas immediately adjacent to patient room: one for putting on (donning) of PPE and one for removing (doffing). These areas must be sufficient to allow a trained observer to safely and effectively supervise donning and doffing of PPE.
Patient Transportation	Joint determination by state and local public health agency, emergency medical services, and hospital of interfacility transport plans (i.e., transfer of patients with confirmed EVD to the designated EVD treatment hospital), including identification of transportation provider(s) (including ground and air transport) with appropriate training and PPE to safely transport a patient. Intrafacility plans for patient transport (e.g., from ambulance entrance to the designated ward or unit for patients under investigation) are developed and in place. Additional information on patient transport is available at: http://www.cdc.gov/vhf/ebola/healthcare-us/emergency-services/ems-systems.html.
Laboratory	Diagnostic laboratory procedures and protocols are in place for testing of specimens for EVD by the nearest LRN laboratory capable of testing for EVD, addressing dedicated space (if possible), possible point-of-care testing, equipment selection and disinfection, staffing, reagents, training, and specimen transport for routine clinical diagnostic testing at the facility, as well as protocols for lab personnel PPE use and training. For more information, see the CDC's Guidance for Collection, Transport, and Submission of Specimens for EVD Testing in the United States (available at: http://www.cdc.gov/vhf/ebola/healthcare-us/laboratories/specimens.html).
Staffing	Readiness plans include input from a multidisciplinary team of all potentially affected hospital departments (including clinical and nonclinical staff). Staffing plans have been developed and scheduled to support 96 consecutive hours of clinical care. Sufficient physician and nursing staff should be available to handle the patient's care needs. The facility has a process for continuous staff input from those who may or may not be directly involved in EVD patient care, including from employee unions, and has addressed employee safety questions and concerns.
Training	All staff involved in or supporting patient care are appropriately trained for their roles, and according to their roles, have demonstrated proficiency in donning and doffing of PPE, proper waste management, infection control practices, and specimen transport. Ongoing training is provided and breaches in infection control are addressed through retraining. Bearing in mind the need to limit the number of staff in direct contact with the patients, hospitals should consider comprehensive cross-training. For more information, see the CDC's EVD information page for U.S. Healthcare Workers and Settings (available at: http://www.cdc.gov/vhf/ebola/healthcare-us/index.html).

(Continued)

Table 12-5. (Continued)

PPE	For patients who are clinically stable and without vomiting, copious diarrhea, obvious bleeding, or a clinical condition that warrants invasive or aerosol-generating procedures (e.g., intubation, suctioning, active resuscitation), PPE and infection control practices according to the CDC's guidance for clinically stable PUIs may be used. For patients with vomiting, copious diarrhea, or obvious bleeding, or patients requiring invasive or aerosol-generating procedures, PPE designated for the care of hospitalized EVD patients should be used. Clinical staff has successfully drilled and demonstrated proficiency in donning/doffing PPE. The overall safe care of EVD patients in a facility must be overseen by an onsite manager at all times, and each step of every PPE donning/doffing procedure must be supervised by a trained observer to ensure proper completion of established PPE protocols. Hospital has selected appropriate PPE for EVD and has at least a 4- to 5-day supply of PPE in stock and a vendor capable of providing re-supply. In the event that a facility does not have sufficient PPE, the facility should work with local health care coalitions, emergency medical services, and local and state public health departments, in collaboration with CDC, to identify additional PPE resources. See CDC's additional information regarding PPE supplies and how to increase access to PPE at: http://www.cdc.gov/vhf/ebola/healthcare-us/ppe/supplies.html.
Waste Management	EVD assessment hospitals should have in place the services of a waste-management vendor capable of managing and transporting Category A infectious substances, have appropriate containers and procedures for the safe temporary storage of Category A infectious waste, and ensure staff are trained in the correct use of PPE and in the proper handling and storage of Category A infectious substances at the facility. If a vendor capable of transporting Category A infectious substances has not been arranged, hospitals may consider sequestering medical waste until the patient's EVD test result becomes known. At that time, if the patient is confirmed to have EVD, arrangements should be made with a vendor capable of managing the waste as a Category A infectious substance; if the patient is ruled out for EVD, waste can be handled according to procedures in compliance with local waste management ordinances. Additional information about Interim Guidance for Environmental Infection Control in Hospitals for EVD is available at: http://www.cdc.gov/vhf/ebola/healthcare-us/cleaning/hospitals.html.
Worker Safety	Worker safety programs and policies are in place. The hospital is in compliance with all federal or state occupational safety and health regulations applicable to reducing employee exposure to the EVD. Hospital has a program for ensuring direct active monitoring of all health care workers involved in direct patient care to ensure monitoring for 21 days since the last known exposure. This monitoring should be done in coordination with local and state public health agencies.

(Continued)

Table 12-5. (Continued)

Environmental Services	Hospital has a program in place to clean and disinfect patient care areas and equipment, including use of an Environmental Protection Agency-registered hospital disinfectant with a label claim of potency at least equivalent to that for a nonenveloped virus (e.g., norovirus, rotavirus, adenovirus, and poliovirus), PPE, and safe practices. Designated staff are trained in correct cleaning and disinfection of the environment, safe practices, and correct use of PPE; and cleaning staff are directly supervised during all cleaning and disinfection. For more information, see the CDC's EVD information page for U.S. Healthcare Workers and Settings (available at: http://www.cdc.gov/vhf/ebola/healthcare-us/index.html).
Clinical Management	Staff who will be involved in managing the patient know the clinical protocols for management of PUIs. For more information, see evaluation and discharge of patients under investigation.
Operations Coordination	The hospital has an emergency management structure, plans and processes for routinely communicating with local and state public health agencies, emergency management authorities, its health care coalition (if appropriate), and hospital employees, patients, and community leadership, to ensure coordination of the response and communication regarding any PUIs for EVD.

Source: Based on Centers for Disease Control and Prevention. 2015. Interim Guidance for Preparing Ebola Assessment Hospitals. Available at: http://www.cdc.gov/vhf/ebola/healthcare-us/preparing/assessment-hospitals.html. Accessed January 23, 2017.

Note: CDC=Centers for Disease Control and Prevention; EVD=Ebola virus disease; LRN=Laboratory Response Network; PPE=personal protective equipment; PUI=person under investigation.

Table 12-6. Minimum Capabilities of Ebola Virus Disease Treatment Centers

EVD Treatment Center Capability	Capability Description
Facility Infrastructure: Patient Room(s)	Hospital has a private room with in-room dedicated bathroom or covered bedside commode, is equipped with dedicated patient-care equipment and has available separate areas immediately adjacent to patient room: one for putting on (donning) of PPE and one for removing (doffing) of PPE. These areas must be large enough to allow a trained observer to safely and effectively supervise donning and doffing of PPE.
Patient Transportation	The state and local public health agency, emergency medical services provider(s), and the hospital have collaborated on the development of interfacility transportation plans that include identification of transport provider(s) with adequate training and PPE to safely transport a patient. Appropriate plans are in place for safe intrafacility patient transfer from ambulance entrance to treatment unit.
Laboratory	Laboratory procedures/protocols, dedicated space, if possible, possible point-of-care testing, equipment, staffing, reagents, training, and specimen transport are in place. See CDC's Guidance for Collection, Transport and Submission of Specimens for EVD Testing (available at: http://www.cdc.gov/vhf/ebola/healthcare-us/laboratories/specimens.html).
Staffing	Readiness plans include input from a multidisciplinary team of all potentially affected facility departments, including clinical and nonclinical departments, and staff. Staffing plans have been developed to manage several weeks of clinical care. Staffing includes dedicated critical care nurses, physicians, environmental services, infection control practitioners, laboratory staff, and respiratory services personnel designed to minimize the number of staff with direct patient contact. The facility has a process for continuous staff input from those who may or may not be directly involved in care of patients with EVD, including from employee unions, and has addressed employee safety questions and concerns.
Training	A limited number of staff should have direct contact with patients. All staff that will be involved in patient care or supporting patient care have been appropriately trained for their role. Staff members who are involved in patient care have demonstrated proficiency in donning and doffing of PPE, proper waste management, infection control, and safe transport of lab specimens. Ongoing training program is in place and breaches in infection control are addressed through retraining. Teams have conducted a functional exercise of core processes. For more information, see U.S. Healthcare Workers and Settings (available at http://www.cdc.gov/vhf/ebola/healthcare-us/index.html).

(Continued)

Table 12-6. (Continued)

EVD Treatment Center Capability	Capability Description
PPE	Given current PPE shortages, hospitals may not be able to procure in advance the amount of PPE needed to care for a patient with EVD. Therefore, at a minimum, to be ready to accept and care for patients with EVD, hospitals will need sufficient PPE for EVD for at least 7 days. If hospitalization is anticipated to exceed 7 days, state and local health authorities, in collaboration with the CDC, may provide or facilitate the procurement of additional PPE supplies. Staff who are involved in patient care or supporting patient care have successfully drilled and demonstrated proficiency on donning/doffing. The overall safe care of patients with EVD in a facility must be overseen by an on-site manager at all times. Each step of every PPE donning/doffing procedure must be supervised by a trained observer to ensure proper completion of established PPE protocols.
Waste Management	Hospital should have secured the services of a waste management vendor capable of managing and transporting Category A infectious substances and have appropriate containers and procedures for the safe temporary storage of Category A infectious substances. Staff are trained in the correct use of PPE and are trained in the proper handling and storage of Category A infectious substances at the facility. If a vendor capable of transporting Category A infectious substances has not been arranged, hospitals may consider sequestering medical waste until the patient's EVD test result becomes known. At that time, if the patient is confirmed to have EVD, arrangements must be made with a vendor capable of managing for the waste as a Category A infectious substance; if the patient is ruled out for EVD, waste can be handled according to routine procedures in compliance with local waste management ordinances.
Worker Safety	Worker safety programs and policies are in place. The hospital is in compliance with all federal or state occupational safety and health standards applicable to reducing employee exposure to the Ebola virus. Hospital has a program for ensuring direct active monitoring of all health care workers involved in direct patient care to ensure monitoring for 21 days since last exposure. This monitoring should be done in coordination with local and state public health agencies.

(Continued)

Table 12-6. (Continued)

EVD Treatment Center Capability	Capability Description
Environmental Services	Hospital has a program in place to clean and disinfect patient care areas and equipment, including use of an Environmental Protection Agency-registered hospital disinfectant with a label claim of potency at least equivalent to that for a nonenveloped virus, such as norovirus, rotavirus, adenovirus, and poliovirus. Hospital has staff trained in correct cleaning and disinfection of the environment, safe practices, and correct use of PPE; and cleaning staff are directly supervised during all cleaning and disinfection.
Clinical Competency	Staff members who will be involved in managing the patient are familiar with the clinical protocols for management of patients with EVD and have access to consultation from experienced clinical EVD specialists.
Operations Coordination	The hospital has a practiced emergency management structure and a plan and methods for routinely communicating with relevant local and state public health agencies, emergency management authorities, its health care coalition (if appropriate), and the hospital's employees, patients, and community to ensure coordination of the response and communication regarding any people under investigation for EVD and patients being treated for EVD in the facility.
State/Hospital Selection as an EVD Treatment Center	The hospital and the state public health department, as the hospital's regulatory authority, have agreed that the facility is ready to serve as an EVD treatment center.

Source: Based on Centers for Disease Control and Prevention. 2014. Interim Guidance for Preparing Ebola Treatment Centers. Available at: http://www.cdc.gov/vhf/ebola/healthcare-us/preparing/treatment-centers.html. Accessed on January 23, 2017.

Note: CDC=Centers for Disease Control and Prevention; EVD=Ebola virus disease; PPE=personal protective equipment

Ebola Treatment Centers

Ebola treatment centers provide comprehensive care to individuals diagnosed with EVD. The decision to designate a facility as an Ebola treatment center should be collaboratively made between the state and local health authorities and the hospital's administrative leadership. Prior to any designation, an interdisciplinary team from the CDC conducts a site visit, once a facility has planned and made preparations to accept patients with EVD. During the site visit, the team assesses a hospital's ability to meet the minimum capabilities in each of the domains outlined in Table 12-6. If critical gaps are identified, the CDC provides technical assistance and regular follow-up consultation to the facility and specialists from the state and local health departments to help ensure that the facility is capable of safely treating a patient with EVD. In the 2014 outbreak in the United States, both the CDC and HHS provided ongoing technical assistance and clinical consultation to facilities that cared for patients infected with EVD. Hospital leaders, state and local health officials, and the site visit team members from the CDC determine whether the capabilities for readiness have been adequately demonstrated and whether caring for patients with EVD will impact the hospital's ability to provide other health care services.

Experts at the CDC are available 24/7 for consultation to treatment centers and state and local health departments. Table 12-7 provides a list of Ebola treatment centers as of September 2016.

Emergency Medical Services

While patients who are symptomatic can be cared for in hospitals, patients may be identified in the community and need to be transported while symptomatic. To ensure provider safety and the proper management of patients, the CDC issued guidance on the management of suspected EVD patients for EMS and first responders. People who may have a history of possible exposure to EVD, or signs and symptoms suggestive of EVD, should be transported to a health care facility prepared to evaluate and manage the patient. In collaboration with the receiving hospital, EMS agencies should establish a supervised donning and doffing process for PPE. The transport protocols should be consistent with the predefined plan developed by public health officials and hospital, medical, and EMS personnel and include:

- Isolating the ambulance driver from the patient compartment; and
- Ensuring that an appropriate disinfectant (e.g., EPA-approved hospital grade disinfectant with a nonenveloped virus claim) is available in spray bottles or as commercially prepared wipes.

Table 12-7. Ebola Virus Disease Treatment Centers as of September 2016

- Maricopa Integrated Health Systems; Phoenix, Arizona
- University of Arizona Health Network; Tucson, Arizona
- Kaiser Los Angeles Medical Center; Los Angeles, California
- Kaiser Oakland Medical Center; Oakland, California
- Kaiser South Sacramento Medical Center; Sacramento, California
- University of California Davis Medical Center; Sacramento, California
- University of California Irvine Medical Center; Orange, California
- University of California Los Angeles Medical Center; Los Angeles, California
- University of California San Diego Medical Center; San Diego, California
- University of California San Francisco Medical Center; San Francisco, California
- Children's Hospital Colorado; Aurora, Colorado
- Denver Health Medical Center; Denver, Colorado
- Emory University Hospital; Atlanta, Georgia
- Grady Memorial Hospital; Atlanta, Georgia
- Ann & Robert H. Lurie Children's Hospital of Chicago; Chicago, Illinois
- Northwestern Memorial Hospital; Chicago, Illinois
- Rush University Medical Center; Chicago, Illinois
- University of Chicago Medical Center; Chicago, Illinois
- Johns Hopkins Hospital; Baltimore, Maryland
- University of Maryland Medical Center; Baltimore, Maryland
- National Institutes of Health Clinical Center; Bethesda, Maryland
- Baystate Medical Center; Springfield, Massachusetts
- Boston Children's Hospital; Boston, Massachusetts
- Massachusetts General Hospital; Boston, Massachusetts
- UMass Memorial Medical Center; Worcester, Massachusetts
- Allina Health's Unity Hospital; Fridley, Minnesota
- Children's Hospitals and Clinics of Minnesota-Saint Paul campus; St. Paul, Minnesota
- Mayo Clinic Hospital-Rochester, Saint Marys campus; Rochester, Minnesota
- University of Minnesota Medical Center, West Bank campus, Minneapolis, Minnesota
- Nebraska Medicine-Nebraska Medical Center; Omaha, Nebraska
- North Shore System LIJ/Glen Cove Hospital; Glen Cove, New York
- Montefiore Health System; New York, New York
- New York-Presbyterian/Allen Hospital; New York, New York
- NYC Health and Hospitals Corporation/HHC Bellevue Hospital Center; New York, New York
- Robert Wood Johnson University Hospital; New Brunswick, New Jersey
- The Mount Sinai Hospital; New York, New York
- MetroHealth Medical Center; Cleveland, Ohio
- Children's Hospital of Philadelphia; Philadelphia, Pennsylvania
- Hospital of the University of Pennsylvania; Philadelphia, Pennsylvania
- Lehigh Valley Health Network-Muhlenberg Campus; Muhlenberg, Pennsylvania
- Penn State Milton S. Hershey Medical Center; Hershey, Pennsylvania
- University of Texas Medical Branch at Galveston; Galveston, Texas
- Texas Children's Hospital; Houston, Texas
- University of Virginia Medical Center; Charlottesville, Virginia
- Virginia Commonwealth University Medical Center; Richmond, Virginia
- Children's Hospital of Wisconsin; Milwaukee, Wisconsin

(*Continued*)

Table 12-7. (Continued)

- Froedtert & the Medical College of Wisconsin-Froedtert Hospital; Milwaukee, Wisconsin
- UW Health-University of Wisconsin Hospital and the American Family Children's Hospital; Madison, Wisconsin
- MedStar Washington Hospital Center; Washington, D.C.
- Children's National Medical Center; Washington, D.C.
- George Washington University Hospital; Washington, D.C.
- Harborview Medical Center; Seattle, Washington
- Seattle Children's Hospital; Seattle, Washington
- Providence Sacred Heart Medical Center; Spokane, Washington
- West Virginia University Hospital; Morgantown, West Virginia

Source: Based on Centers for Disease Control and Prevention. 2015. Current ebola treatment centers. Available at: http://www.cdc.gov/vhf/ebola/healthcare-us/preparing/current-treatment-centers.html. Accessed January 23, 2017.

EMS providers can safely manage a PUI by following the recommendations for use of appropriate PPE and other CDC guidance, including:

- Limiting activities, especially during transport, that may increase the risk of exposure to infectious material;
- Limiting the use of needles and other sharps as much as possible;
- Limiting invasive procedures to only those essential for patient management; and
- Donning and doffing of PPE under the supervision of a trained observer to ensure proper completion of established PPE protocols.

The CDC's guidance for the cleaning or maintaining of EMS vehicles and equipment after transporting a PUI is available at: http://www.cdc.gov/vhf/ebola/healthcare-us/emergency-services/ems-systems.html.

Collection, Storage, Processing, and Testing of Ebola Virus Disease Specimens

Diagnosing EVD in a person who has only been infected for a few days is difficult because the early symptoms, such as fever, are nonspecific to Ebola infection. While the status of a patient suspected to have EVD should be determined as quickly as possible, it may take up to 3 days after symptoms start for the virus to reach detectable levels. The CDC recommends that EVD testing be conducted only for people who meet the criteria for PUIs for EVD. Presumptive testing for EVD is available at over 50 LRN laboratories (discussed below) located throughout the United States and confirmatory testing is available at the CDC. Table 12-8 describes the laboratory tests used in diagnosing EVD.

Hospitals or clinical laboratories concerned about a patient with potential EVD exposure should consult with their local and state public health authorities for guidance and

Table 12-8. Laboratory Tests Used in Ebola Virus Disease Diagnosis

Timeline of Infection	Diagnostic tests available
Within a few days after symptoms begin	• Antigen-capture ELISA testing • IgM ELISA • PCR • Virus isolation
Later in disease course or after recovery	• IgM and IgG antibodies
Retrospectively in deceased patients	• Immunohistochemistry testing • PCR • Virus isolation

Source: Based on Centers for Disease Control and Prevention. 2015. Ebola virus disease: diagnosis. Available at: http://www.cdc.gov/vhf/ebola/diagnosis. Accessed on January 23, 2017.
Note: ELISA=enzyme-linked immunosorbent assay; EVD=Ebola virus disease; IgG=immunoglobulin G; IgM=immunoglobulin M; PCR=polymerase chain reaction.

any decision to test for EVD should only be made in consultation with public health officials. The CDC should be notified immediately if a decision is made to test. Any presumptive positive EVD test result must be confirmed at the CDC.

Collecting Specimens

Specimens should be obtained when a patient meets the criteria for PUI, including the clinical signs, symptoms, and epidemiologic risk factors for EVD. If the PUI symptoms have been present for less than 3 days, a second sample collected 72 hours after onset of symptoms may be required to definitively rule out EVD, such as when the initial tests are negative, but the patient remains symptomatic without another diagnosis. For adults, a minimum volume of 4 milliliter whole blood collected in a plastic tube preserved with EDTA is the preferred sample for testing. For pediatric samples, a minimum of 1 milliliter whole blood should be collected in pediatric-sized collection tubes.

Whole blood preserved with EDTA is preferred, but whole blood preserved with sodium polyanethol sulfonate, citrate, or with clot activator is also acceptable. The technicians running the tests should not separate and remove serum or plasma from the primary collection container.

Transporting Specimens

Specimens should be packaged and kept at 35.6°F to 46.4°F (2°C to 8°C) with refrigerant, such as cold packs, while being transported to the designated test site of the

LRN. Agencies interested in submitting specimens other than blood should consult with the CDC. If short-term storage of any specimens is necessary before shipping, the specimens should be kept at 39.2°F (4°C) or frozen. Specimens cannot be transported or shipped in glass containers or in heparinized tubes.

EVD is classified as a Category A infectious substance by the Department of Transportation (DOT). Therefore, the transport of samples from PUIs or patients confirmed or suspected of having EVD is regulated by the DOT's Hazardous Materials Regulations (HMR) 49 C.F.R., Parts 171–180 (available at: http://www.ecfr.gov/cgi-bin/text-idx?gp=&SID=994e5ed7210bb285ce6a2d21434e652e&mc=true&tpl=/ecfrbrowse/Title49/49CIsubchapC.tpl). Specimens for shipment should be packaged following the basic triple packaging system consisting of (1) a primary container (i.e., a sealable specimen container) wrapped with absorbent material, (2) a secondary container (i.e., watertight and leak-proof), and (3) an outer shipping package. See Figure 12-1 for additional details. In addition, the Occupational Safety and Health Administration has guidance on the handling of blood-borne pathogens (available at: https://www.osha.gov/OshDoc/data_BloodborneFacts/bbfact01.pdf).

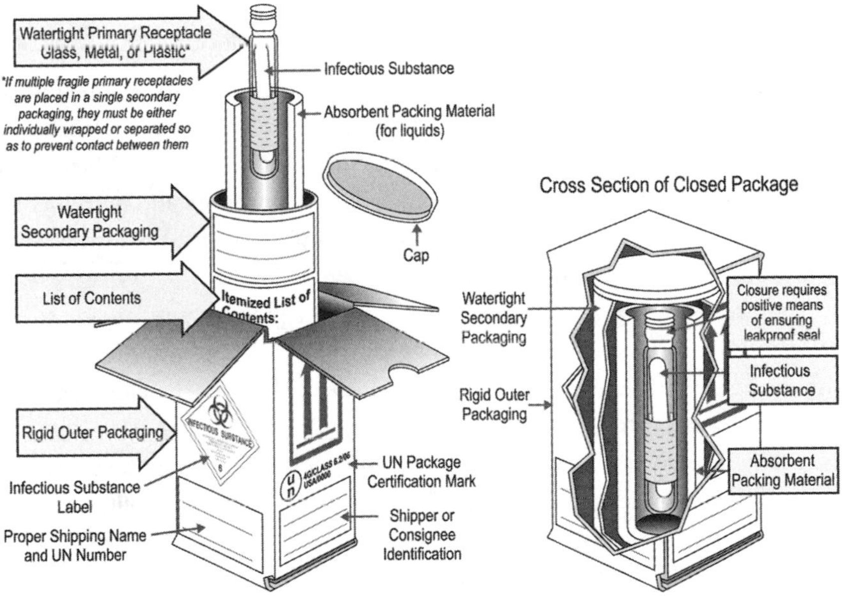

Source: Reprinted from Centers for Disease Control and Prevention. 2014. Packaging and shipping clinical specimens diagram. Available at: http://www.cdc.gov/vhf/ebola/healthcare-us/laboratories/shipping-specimens.html. Accessed January 23, 2017.

Figure 12-1. Packaging and Shipping Clinical Specimens Diagram

Treatment

While an experimental vaccine for EVD has been developed and found effective, as of this writing such a vaccine has not been approved by the Food and Drug Administration (FDA) and no medicine (e.g., antiviral drug) is available.

Symptoms of EVD and complications are treated as they appear. The following basic interventions, when used early, can significantly improve the chances of survival:

- Providing intravenous fluids and balancing electrolytes
- Maintaining oxygen levels and blood pressure
- Treating other infections if they occur

Recovery from EVD depends on good supportive care and the patient's immune response. People who recover from EVD develop antibodies that last for at least 10 years, possibly longer. It is not known if people who recover are immune for life or if they can become infected with a different strain of EVD. Some people who have recovered from EVD have developed long-term complications, such as joint and vision problems.

Infection Control

In 2015, the CDC released updated guidelines on infection prevention and control recommendations for hospitalized PUIs for EVD in U.S. hospitals (available at: http://www.cdc.gov/vhf/ebola/healthcare-us/hospitals/infection-control.html). These recommendations were determined based on the high rate of morbidity and mortality among infected patients, the risk of human-to-human transmission, and the lack of an FDA-approved vaccine and therapeutics.

The CDC recommends a combination of measures to prevent transmission of EVD in hospitals, including the use of the appropriate level of PPE and environmental measures to control infection. (See Chapter 10 for discussion on blood-borne pathogens and the use of PPE and administrative strategies for caring for patients with EVD.)

The role of the environment in the transmission of Ebola has not been established. Limited laboratory studies suggest that the EVD can remain viable on solid surfaces, with concentrations falling slowly over several days. There is no epidemiologic evidence of transmission of EVD via the environment or through fomites that could become contaminated during patient care (e.g., bed rails, door knobs, laundry). However, given the apparent low infectious dose, the potential of high virus titers in the blood of ill patients, and the severity of the disease, all personnel involved in caring for a patient with EVD should use elevated levels of precaution to avoid exposure to contaminated surfaces in the patient care environment.

As part of the care of PUIs or patients with confirmed EVD, hospitals are advised to:

- Ensure that staff providing environmental services wear the recommended level of PPE (see Chapter 10) to protect against direct exposure of skin and mucous membranes to cleaning chemicals, contamination, splashes, or spatters when cleaning and disinfecting the patient environment.
- Use a hospital disinfectant that is registered by the U.S. Environmental Protection Agency (EPA) and is capable of disinfecting environmental surfaces for a nonenveloped virus (e.g., norovirus, rotavirus, adenovirus, poliovirus) in rooms of PUIs or patients with confirmed EVD. Enveloped viruses, such as EVD, are susceptible to a broad range of hospital disinfectants used to clean hard, nonporous surfaces while nonenveloped viruses are more resistant to disinfectants, requiring a higher potency. Since there are currently no products with specific label claims against the Ebola virus, the selection of a disinfectant with a higher potency than what is normally required for an enveloped virus is recommended.
- Remove all possible porous surfaces and materials to avoid contamination. Use only a mattress and pillow with plastic or other covering that fluids cannot penetrate. Do not place PUIs or patients with confirmed EVD in carpeted rooms. Remove all upholstered furniture and decorative curtains from patient rooms before use.
- Routine cleaning of the area where the PPE is removed, by a health care worker wearing clean PPE, should be performed at least once per day and after the doffing of PPE that is significantly contaminated. When cleaning and disinfection are complete, the health care worker should carefully doff the PPE they are wearing and thoroughly wash their hands.
- Rather than launder potentially contaminated products, discard all linens, nonfluid-impermeable pillows or mattresses, and textile privacy curtains using the hospital's waste disposal process for highly infectious materials. Any item that is contaminated or suspected of being contaminated with a Category A infectious substance, as EVD is, must be packaged and transported offsite for disposal in accordance with the HMR. This includes medical equipment, sharps, linens, used health care products such as soiled absorbent pads or dressings, kidney-shaped emesis pans, portable toilets, used PPE (i.e., gowns, masks, gloves, goggles, face shields, respirators, booties), and byproducts of cleaning articles contaminated with a Category A infectious substance.
- Additional infection control measures apply to patient placement and care, equipment used, hand hygiene, and injection practice, which are discussed in more detail in Table 12-9.

Table 12-9. Infection Control Measures for Ebola Virus Disease

Component	Recommendation	Comments
Patient Placement	• Single patient room (containing a private bathroom) with the door closed. • Facilities should maintain a log of all people entering the patient's room.	• Consider posting personnel at the patient's door to ensure appropriate and consistent use of PPE by all people entering the patient room.
PPE	See Guidance on Personal Protective Equipment (PPE) To Be Used By Healthcare Workers during Management of Patients with Confirmed Ebola or Persons under Investigation (PUIs) for Ebola who are Clinically Unstable or Have Bleeding, Vomiting, or Diarrhea in U.S. Hospitals, Including Procedures for Donning and Doffing PPE (available at http://www.cdc.gov/vhf/ebola/healthcare-us/ppe/guidance.html).	
Patient Care Equipment	• Dedicated medical equipment (preferably disposable, when possible) should be used for the provision of patient care. • All nondedicated, nondisposable medical equipment used for patient care should be cleaned and disinfected according to manufacturer's instructions and hospital policies.	
Patient Care Considerations	• Limit the use of needles and other sharps as much as possible. • Phlebotomy, procedures, and laboratory testing should be limited to the minimum necessary for essential diagnostic evaluation and medical care. • All needles and sharps should be handled with extreme care and disposed in puncture-proof, sealed containers.	

(*Continued*)

Table 12-9. (Continued)

Component	Recommendation	Comments
AGPs	• Avoid AGPs for patients with EVD. • If performing AGPs, use a combination of measures to reduce exposures from aerosol-generating procedures when performed on patient with EVD. • Visitors should not be present during AGPs. • Limiting the number of HCP present during the procedure to only those essential for patientcare and support. • Conduct the procedures in a private room and ideally in an AIIR when feasible. Room doors should be kept closed during the procedure except when entering or leaving the room, and entry and exit should be minimized during and shortly after the procedure. • HCP should wear appropriate PPE during AGPs. • Conduct environmental surface cleaning following procedures (see section below on environmental infection control).	• Although there are limited data available to definitively define a list of AGPs, procedures that are usually included are BiPAP, bronchoscopy, sputum induction, intubation and extubation, and open suctioning of airways. • Because of the potential risk to individuals reprocessing reusable respirators, disposable filtering face piece respirators are preferred.
Hand Hygiene	• HCP should perform hand hygiene frequently, including before and after all patient contact, contact with potentially infectious material, and before putting on and upon removal of PPE, including gloves. • Health care facilities should ensure that supplies for performing hand hygiene are available.	• Hand hygiene in health care settings can be performed by washing with soap and water or using alcohol-based hand rubs. If hands are visibly soiled, use soap and water, not alcohol-based hand rubs.
Environmental Infection Control	See Hospital Guidance (available at http://www.cdc.gov/vhf/ebola/healthcare-us/cleaning/hospitals.html).	See Hospital Guidance (available at http://www.cdc.gov/vhf/ebola/healthcare-us/cleaning/hospitals.html).
Safe Injection Practices	• Facilities should follow safe injection practices as specified under Standard Precautions.	• Any injection equipment or parenteral medication container that enters the patient treatment area should be dedicated to that patient and disposed of at the point of use.

(Continued)

Table 12-9. (Continued)

Component	Recommendation	Comments
Duration of Infection Control Precautions	• Duration of precautions should be determined on a case-by-case basis, in conjunction with local, state, and federal health authorities.	• Factors that should be considered include, but are not limited to, presence of symptoms related to EVD, date symptoms resolved, other conditions that would require specific precautions (e.g., tuberculosis,*Clostridium difficile*) and available laboratory information.
Monitoring and Management of Potentially Exposed Personnel	• Facilities should develop policies for monitoring and management of potentially exposed HCP. • Facilities should develop sick leave policies for HCP that are nonpunitive, flexible and consistent with public health guidance that: ○ Ensure that all HCP, including staff who are not directly employed by the health care facility but provide essential daily services, are aware of the sick leave policies. • People with percutaneous or mucocutaneous exposures to blood, body fluids, secretions, or excretions from a PUI should: ○ Stop working and immediately wash the affected skin surfaces with soap and water. Mucous membranes (conjunctiva) should be irrigated with copious amounts of water or eyewash solution. ○ Immediately contact occupational health/supervisor for assessment and access to postexposure management services for all appropriate pathogens (e.g., Human Immunodeficiency Virus, Hepatitis C).	

(Continued)

Table 12-9. (Continued)

Component	Recommendation	Comments
	• HCP who develop sudden onset of fever, fatigue, intense weakness or muscle pains, vomiting, diarrhea, or any signs of hemorrhage should: o Not report to work or should immediately stop working. o Notify their supervisor. o Seek prompt medical evaluation and testing. o Notify local and state health departments. o Comply with work exclusion until they are deemed no longer infectious to others. • For asymptomatic HCP who had an unprotected exposure (not wearing recommended PPE at the time of patient contact or through direct contact to blood or body fluids) to a patient with EVD: o Should receive medical evaluation and follow-up care including fever monitoring twice daily for 21 days after the last known exposure. o Hospitals should consider policies ensuring twice daily contact with exposed personnel to discuss potential symptoms and document fever checks.	

(Continued)

Table 12-9. (Continued)

Component	Recommendation	Comments

Monitoring, Management, and Training of Visitors	• Avoid entry of visitors into the patient's room.
	  ○ Exceptions may be considered on a case by case basis for those who are essential for the patient's well-being.
	• Establish procedures for monitoring managing and training visitors.
	• Visits should be scheduled and controlled to allow for:
	  ○ Screening for EVD (fever and other symptoms) before entering or upon arrival to the hospital.
	  ○ Evaluating risk to the health of the visitor and ability to comply with precautions.
	  ○ Providing instruction, before entry into the patient care area on hand hygiene, limiting surfaces touched, and use of PPE according to the current facility policy while in the patient's room.
	  ○ Visitor movement within the facility should be restricted to the patient care area and an immediately adjacent waiting area.
		• Avoid entry of visitors into the patient's room.
		  ○ Exceptions may be considered on a case by case basis for those who are essential for the patient's well-being.
		• Establish procedures for monitoring managing and training visitors.
		• Visits should be scheduled and controlled to allow for:
		  ○ Screening for EVD (fever and other symptoms) before entering or upon arrival to the hospital.
		  ○ Evaluating risk to the health of the visitor and ability to comply with precautions.
		  ○ Providing instruction, before entry into the patient care area on hand hygiene, limiting surfaces touched, and use of PPE according to the current facility policy while in the patient's room.
		  ○ Visitor movement within the facility should be restricted to the patient care area and an immediately adjacent waiting area.

Source: Based on Centers for Disease Control and Prevention. 2015. Key infection control precautions recommended for preventing Ebola transmission in U.S. hospitals. Atlanta, GA. Available at: http://www.cdc.gov/vhf/ebola/healthcare-us/hospitals/infection-control.html. Accessed January 23, 2017.

Note: AGP=aerosol generating procedures; AIIR=airborne infection isolation room; BiPAP=Bilevel Positive Airway Pressure; EVD=Ebola virus disease; HCP=health care personnel; PPE=personal protective equipment; PUI=person under investigation.

Zika Virus

Our world has seen an uptick in mosquito-borne diseases that are suddenly threatening global health in new and previously unseen ways. Many countries are at risk because they lack a robust public health infrastructure with strong preparedness and response capabilities. One disease that caused great concern is the Zika virus, a mosquito-borne flavivirus that was first identified in Uganda in 1947. Before 2007, only sporadic human disease cases were reported from countries in Africa and Asia. By 2007, almost three-fourths of the population over 3 years of age had been infected in Micronesia. Subsequent outbreaks occurred in Southeast Asia and the Western Pacific. In May 2015, local transmission of the virus was reported in Brazil and the Brazilian Ministry of Health estimated 440,000–1,300,000 suspected cases that year. The following February the WHO declared a Public Health Emergency of International Concern. By July 2016, cases of locally transmitted Zika occurred in Miami, the first on the mainland of the United States. Soon after, the CDC issued travel guidance for the parts of Florida most affected by the virus. By that November, almost 4,500 cases of Zika were reported in the United States.

Transmission

Zika is primarily transmitted to humans through bites by the *Aedes aegypti* and *Aedes albopictus* mosquitoes and has also been confirmed to be sexually transmitted. These mosquitoes bite during the day and night. Intrauterine transmission of Zika from a viremic mother to her newborn has been reported, resulting in congenital infection. Zika during pregnancy can result in microcephaly, other congenital anomalies, and death of the fetus. In addition, there is risk for transfusion-associated transmission.

Although the exact incubation period of Zika has not yet been determined, evidence from case reports and experience from related flavivirus infections indicate that the incubation period likely is 3 days to 2 weeks. Symptoms usually last from several days to a week. Most infections are asymptomatic, generally mild and characterized by 2 or more of the following: acute onset of fever, rash, arthralgia, or nonpurulent conjunctivitis. The rash associated with Zika has been described as pruritic and maculopapular. Guillain-Barré syndrome has been reported following infection with Zika, although a causal link has not been established. The incidence of Guillain-Barré syndrome following infection with Zika may rise with increasing age. However, it is unclear how often the syndrome has resulted from Zika in children. Severe disease requiring hospitalization is uncommon and deaths from Zika appear to be rare in people of all ages.

In June 2016, the Maryland Department of Health and Mental Hygiene reported a woman with laboratory-confirmed Zika infection. However, the woman had not traveled to a region with ongoing transmission of Zika, but did have sexual contact with a male partner who had recently traveled to the Dominican Republic. The male partner reported exposure to mosquitoes while traveling, but no symptoms consistent with Zika either before or after returning to the United States. This was the first report of sexual transmission of Zika from an individual with no symptoms of infection.

Temporary deferral of blood donations from individuals who have recently traveled to an area affected with Zika has been recommended to reduce the risk for transfusion-associated transmission.

Diagnosis

In February 2016, the Council of State and Territorial Epidemiologists (CSTE) approved interim case definitions for Zika virus and Zika congenital infection and added them to the list of nationally notifiable conditions. Subsequent reports of Zika will include cases reported to ArboNET, the national arboviral surveillance system, using the interim CSTE case definitions. Pregnant women who develop a clinically compatible illness during or within 2 weeks of returning from an area where Zika is being transmitted should be tested for the virus. Fetuses and infants of women infected with Zika during pregnancy should be evaluated for possible congenital infection.

The diagnosis of infection is made through molecular and serologic testing. This includes reverse transcription-polymerase chain reaction (RT-PCR) for viral RNA and immunoglobulin M (IgM) enzyme-linked immunosorbent assay and plaque reduction neutralization test (PRNT) for antibodies. Because it is currently not known which type of testing most reliably establishes the diagnosis of congenital infection, the CDC recommends both molecular and serologic testing of infants who are being evaluated for evidence of a congenital infection. Commercial tests are available and confirmatory testing is performed at the CDC and some state and territorial health departments. Health care providers should contact their health department to discuss testing.

Reverse Transcription-Polymerase Chain Reaction Testing

When Zika is suspected, RT-PCR testing should be performed on serum specimens collected from the umbilical cord or directly from the infant within 2 days of birth. In addition, the placenta and cerebrospinal fluid (CSF) should be tested using RT-PCR. PRNT can be performed to measure virus-specific neutralizing antibodies and to discriminate between cross-reacting antibodies from closely related flaviviruses (e.g., dengue or yellow fever viruses). Immunohistochemical staining to detect Zika antigen on fixed placenta and umbilical cord tissues can be considered. In addition to the placenta, testing can be done on the amniotic fluid.

An infant is considered congenitally infected if Zika RNA or viral antigen is identified in any of the tested samples. In addition, evidence of a congenital Zika infection includes the presence of Zika-IgM antibodies with confirmatory neutralizing antibody titers in the infant serum or CSF that are equal to or more than 4-fold higher than neutralizing antibody titers for dengue virus. If the neutralizing antibody titers for Zika are less than 4-fold higher than dengue, the results are considered inconclusive.

Prevention and Treatment

The only way to prevent congenital Zika infection is to prevent maternal infection, either by avoiding areas where the Zika is being transmitted, avoiding sexual relations with someone who might have Zika, or by avoiding mosquito bites. Mosquito bites can be prevented by using air conditioning or window and door screens when indoors, wearing long sleeves and pants, using larvicide that kills young mosquitoes before they grow into biting adults, using permethrin-treated clothing or hats, and using insect repellents. Insect repellents that are registered with the EPA are safe for pregnant and lactating women, when used according to the product label.

Treatment

No specific antiviral treatment or vaccine to prevent Zika infection is available at the time of this writing. Treatment is generally supportive, including rest, fluids, and use of analgesics and antifebrile products. Treatment of congenital Zika infection is also supportive and should include the specific medical and neurodevelopmental needs that an infant requires. Where dengue, a virus also transmitted by mosquitos, may be suspected as an alternate diagnosis or in addition to Zika, aspirin and other nonsteroidal anti-inflammatory drugs should be avoided to reduce the risk of hemorrhage until this alternative diagnosis is ruled out. Febrile pregnant women should be treated with acetaminophen.

Mothers are encouraged to breastfeed infants even in areas where Zika is found since available evidence indicates the benefits of breastfeeding outweigh any theoretical risks associated with Zika transmission through breast milk.

Management of Congenital Zika Infections

The CDC issued guidelines to reduce the risk for travel-associated infections, especially among pregnant women, including recommendations for preventing sexual transmission of Zika from contact with travelers to infected areas (available at: https://www.cdc.gov/zika/prevention/plan-for-travel.html). This guidance includes direction for diagnosing and treating infants and children with possible acute Zika disease (available at: https://www.cdc.gov/zika/parents/what-parents-should-know.html). When the infant is born with a normal head circumference, normal prenatal and postnatal ultrasounds, and normal physical examination, the guidelines recommend that physicians provide routine care for infants born to mothers who traveled to or resided in areas with Zika transmission during pregnancy.

In 2016, the CDC issued an "Alert Level 2" travel notice that encourages travelers to practice enhanced precautions when visiting areas that have reported recent Zika transmission. In addition to mosquito bite precautions for all travelers, the CDC advises that pregnant women postpone travel to affected countries and U.S. territories. The list of current locations where this travel notice is in effect is available at: http://wwwnc.cdc.gov/travel/page/zika-travel-information.

Surveillance

The Puerto Rico Department of Health and the CDC developed a surveillance system called Zika Active Pregnancy Surveillance System/Sistema de Vigilancia Activa de Zika en Embarazos. This surveillance system will be used to evaluate the association between Zika virus infection during pregnancy and adverse outcomes during pregnancy, birth, and early childhood up to 3 years of age. Pregnant women in Puerto Rico with laboratory evidence of Zika infection and prenatally or perinatally exposed infants born to these women will be actively monitored. This information will be used to inform best practices in the care of women infected with Zika during pregnancy and their infants.

In a recent published article from the CDC, 13 infants who were born with normal head size but had laboratory evidence of Zika went on to develop microcephaly. These findings provide evidence that among infants with prenatal exposure to Zika, the absence of microcephaly at birth does not exclude having congenital Zika or the presence of Zika-related brain and other abnormalities. These findings support the recommendation for thorough medical and developmental follow-up of infants prenatally exposed to Zika. In addition, early neuroimaging might identify brain abnormalities related to congenital Zika infection even among infants with a normal head circumference.

For further information, the CDC established a microsite that provides information and current developments in the Zika outbreak, including prevention, symptoms, treatment, and information for pregnant women and travelers (available at: https://tools.cdc.gov/medialibrary/index.aspx#/microsite/id/234558). The HHS also created a page with updated information through the Disaster Information Management Resource Center (available at: https://disasterinfo.nlm.nih.gov/dimrc/zikavirus.html).

Chemical or Biological Warfare

The global recognition of the potential peril from bioterrorism is highlighted by the increase in terrorist activity around the world. With increased terrorist activity, the likelihood of a chemical or biological warfare (CBW) attack is also growing. Of the 15 National Planning Scenarios discussed in Chapter 4, almost one-third are centered on biological attacks, indicating the degree to which this threat is taken seriously. Because the public health and health sectors would have difficulty containing a massive outbreak caused by an intended spread of infectious disease, it is important to understand CBW and be prepared to respond should it occur.

Overt and Covert Releases

Detection of an intentional release of CBW may occur in several different ways. Overt releases of CBW are those where a threat assessment is possible before a response is initiated because the threat is announced. Some announced threats are hoaxes. Public health officials should assume that potential hoaxes are in fact real when threats are accompanied by increased morbidity or mortality, even if the microorganisms have not been confirmed. Communities may choose a limited response to hoaxes based on a sophisticated analysis of the situation and a relatively easy resolution of the incident.

Covert releases are those without prior warning in which a biological agent presents as illness in the community and for which traditional surveillance methods are needed to detect the agent. With covert releases, patients fall ill or die from unknown causes or unusual origins. Covert dissemination of a biological agent in a public place will probably not have an immediate impact because of the incubation period of the disease, resulting in a delay between exposure and onset and subsequent identification.

The covert release of a contagious agent or the appearance of a highly infectious illness has the potential for multinational spread prior to detection. Release in a transportation hub or in a mobile population could disseminate a highly contagious agent such as smallpox across borders before the epidemic is recognized. As person-to-person contact continues, successive waves of transmission could carry infection to other localities around the globe. In a very short time, public health authorities would be asked to determine that an attack has occurred, identify the organism, and prevent more casualties through prevention strategies (e.g., mass vaccination, prophylactic treatment, or universal precautions and quarantine). The ability to detect covert releases depends on enhancing public health infrastructure and increasing the skills of frontline medical practitioners so they recognize and report suspicious syndromes.

Critical Biological Agents

The CDC has identified several high-priority agents: high priority because of high impact, those that are easily spread that require enhanced diseases surveillance, and a third group of emerging agents that could be mass produced.

High-Priority Agents

High-priority agents include organisms that pose a risk to national security because they:

- can be easily disseminated or transmitted from person to person;
- result in high mortality rates and have the potential for major public health impact;
- might cause public panic and social disruption; and
- require special action for public health preparedness.

These agents include 9 of the highest priority agents. Although the occurrence of these diseases is relatively infrequent, their impact is high because of the speed with which they spread. The highest priority agents pose a risk to national security because they can be easily disseminated or transmitted person to person; cause high mortality, with the potential for major public health impact; could cause public panic and social disruption; and require special action for public health preparedness.

Bacillus anthracis: Anthrax, an acute bacterial disease affecting the skin, chest, or intestinal tract is considered to be a highly efficacious biological warfare agent, because it forms spores (providing stability in aerosol form), is relatively easy to disseminate using off-the-shelf technology, and is frequently fatal if inhaled. Its incubation period is 1 to 7 days, but postexposure disease is possible up to 60 days later. Transmission from person to person is very rare.

Clostridium botulinum: Botulism is poisoning by a toxin produced by a common environmental organism that can be easily cultured from soil. Victims of the toxin often require intensive supportive medical care. Food-borne botulism results from ingesting contaminated food. Botulism in wounds occurs when the organism grows in a deep wound and forms toxin, which is carried to the bloodstream. Intestinal botulism occurs mostly in infants, less than 1 year old, from the ingestion of spores that grow in their intestines. The case-fatality rate for infants is less than 1%.

The public health response to botulism is complicated. If paralysis occurs in a large number of individuals, the current supply of respiratory ICU beds and ventilators may not be enough. The immunoglobulin used in the routine treatment of both wound and food-borne botulism can be lifesaving if given early, but is limited in both supply and availability. Public health preparedness requires a major stockpiling effort to cover possible bioterrorism response needs resulting from botulism.

Variola major: Smallpox, for which dissemination requires person-to-person transmission, is highly contagious in unimmunized populations and has a mortality rate as high as 35%. Smallpox has a cycle time of 10 to 14 days, an attack rate of up to 90%, and a secondary attack rate among the unvaccinated of 50%.

Yersinia pestis: Pneumonic plague is a respiratory-acquired illness that is spread from person to person through sneezing or coughing. It is diagnosed by culturing bacteria from sputum, blood, spinal fluid, or infected glands. Pneumonic plague is almost 100% fatal if not treated quickly. Bubonic plague is the form characterized by severely swollen and infected lymph nodes in the groin or axilla, called buboes. Plague occurs as an enzootic disease of rodents in the United States, making it relatively easy to obtain an isolate for use as a terrorist agent. Infected rats and their fleas transfer bacterial infection to animals and humans through bites or via scratches from infected cats. Symptoms occur 2 to 7 days after exposure. If untreated, bubonic plague has a 50% to 60% mortality.

Francisella tularensis: Tularemia is a zoonotic bacterial disease with varying clinical manifestations related to the route of transmission. It can be transmitted from rabbit, tick, or fly bites, or by handling infected animal carcasses. Tularemia can also be disseminated in water. Tularemia is not transmissible person to person. In aerosol form, the organism produces a severely debilitating pneumonia with a lower mortality rate than anthrax. The incubation period, related to strain, can range from 1 to 14 days but is commonly 3 to 5 days.

Filoviruses, bunyaviruses, flaviviruses, and arenaviruses: The remaining high-priority agents are:

- 2 filoviruses—EVD and Marburg virus disease
- 3 bunyaviruses—hantavirus pulmonary syndrome, Rift Valley fever, and Crimean-Congo hemorrhagic fever
- 1 flavivirus—dengue fever
- 6 arenaviruses—Lassa fever, Machupo virus, Junin virus, Guanarito virus, Chapare virus, and Lujo virus

Easy to Disseminate Needing Enhanced Surveillance

These agents are considered the second highest priority because they are moderately easy to disseminate, cause moderate morbidity and low mortality, and require specific enhancements of the CDC's diagnostic capacity as well as enhanced disease surveillance. The agents include the following:

- Brucellosis (*Brucella* species)
- Epsilon toxin of *Clostridium perfringens*

- Glanders (*Burkholderia mallei*)
- Melioidosis (*Burkholderia pseudomallei*)
- Psittacosis (*Chlamydia psittaci*)
- Q fever (*Coxiella burnetii*)
- Ricin toxin from *Ricinus communis* (castor beans)
- Staphylococcal enterotoxin B
- Typhus fever (*Rickettsia prowazekii*)
- Viral encephalitis (e.g., Venezuelan equine encephalitis, eastern equine encephalitis, western equine encephalitis, and West Nile virus)

A subset of agents that are easy to disseminate and need enhanced surveillance include pathogens that are food- or waterborne. These pathogens include but are not limited to the following:

- *Salmonella species*
- *Shigella dysenteriae*
- *Escherichia coli* O157:H7
- *Vibrio cholerae*
- *Cryptosporidium parvum*

Emerging Pathogens

The third highest priority agents, include emerging pathogens that could be engineered for mass dissemination because of their availability; ease of production and dispersion; and potential for high morbidity, mortality, and public health impact. Preparedness for these agents requires ongoing research to improve disease detection, diagnosis, treatment, and prevention. These agents include, but are not limited to, infectious diseases such as Nipah virus, highly pathogenic coronaviruses (including SARS-CoV and MERS-CoV), additional hantaviruses, and many antimicrobial-resistant pathogens.

Table 12-10 summarizes the information contained in the current CDC fact sheets on known bioterrorism agents (available at: https://emergency.cdc.gov/bioterrorism/factsheets.asp).

Biological Incident Response Plan

Chapter 4 describes general principles that apply to disaster planning for natural hazards or technological events. Tasks related to threats from biological agents that require similar preparation include interorganizational coordination, sharing information, resource management, triage, casualty distribution, using the media to communicate to the

Table 12-10. Bioterrorism Agent Summary

	Inhalational Anthrax	Brucellosis	Botulism	Tularemia	Pneumonic Plague	Smallpox	Viral Hemorrhagic Fever
Infective dose	8,000–50,000 spores	10–100 organisms	0.001 g/kg (type A)	10–50 organisms	<100 organisms	10–100 particles	1–10 particles
Incubation	1–6 days	5–60 days	6 hours to 10 days	1–21 days	2–3 days	7–17 days	4–21 days
Duration	3–5 days	Weeks to months	24–72 hours	~2 weeks	1–6 days	~4 weeks	7–16 days
Mortality untreated	~100%	~5%[a]	1st case 25% Subsequent cases 4% Overall 5%–10%	33%	40%–70%	Variola minor: 1% Variola major: 20%–50%	53%–88%
Mortality treated	~40%	<1%	1st case 25% Subsequent cases 4% Overall 5%–10%	<4%	5%	Variola minor: 1% Variola major: 20%–50%	53%–88%
Person-to-person transmission[b]	No	No	No	No	Yes (high)	Yes (high)	Yes (moderate)
Isolation precautions[c]	Standard	Standard	Standard	Standard	Droplet[d]	Airborne[d]	Airborne and contact[d]
Persistence	40 years in soil	10 weeks in water/soil	Weeks in food/water	Months in moist soil	1 year in soil	Very stable	Unstable

Source: Adapted from National Center for Preparedness. 2016. General fact sheets on specific bioterrorism agents. Available at: https://emergency.cdc.gov/bioterrorism/factsheets.asp. Accessed January 23, 2017.

[a]Endocarditis accounts for the majority of brucellosis-related deaths.

[b]For inhalational anthrax, brucellosis, botulism, or tularemia, no evidence of person-to-person transmission exists; for pneumonic plague, for 72 hours following initiation of appropriate antimicrobial therapy or until sputum culture is negative; for smallpox, approximately 3 weeks, which usually corresponds with the initial appearance of skin lesions through their final disappearance, though most infections during the first week of rash via inhalation of virus released from oropharyngeal-lesion secretions of the index case; for viral hemorrhagic fever, varies with virus but at minimum, all of the duration of illness and for Ebola/Marburg, transmission via semen may occur up to 7 weeks after clinical recovery.

[c]Graner JS. 1996. Guidelines for isolation precautions in hospitals. The hospital infection control practices advisory committee. *Infect Control Hosp Epidemiol.* 17(1):53–80.

[d]In addition to standard precautions that apply to all patients.

public, and patient tracking. Because of the potential for the rapid spread of disease, however, planning to mitigate the impacts of emerging infections or biological agents relies heavily on skills that are uniquely those of public health and health care systems, and include additional functions that are not normally included in a community's comprehensive emergency plan.

Federal Planning and Response Overview

The federal response to bioterrorism or to a naturally occurring disease outbreak with a known or novel pathogen is found in the Biological Incident Annex (BIA), a document that supplements the National Response Framework. BIA describes federal actions, roles, and responsibilities in response to a human disease outbreak of known or unknown origin. The federal actions described in BIA can occur whether or not there has been a presidential Robert T. Stafford Disaster Relief and Emergency Assistance Act of 1988 declaration or the secretary of HHS has declared a public health emergency. The response actions in the BIA include detection and assessment of threat through disease surveillance and environmental monitoring, procedures for identifying and notifying the population(s) at risk, laboratory testing, procedures for joint investigation and response, controlling any possible epidemic, augmenting local public health and medical services, and recovery activities.

Planning Assumptions

A biological incident may be identified in multiple jurisdictions concurrently causing public health and medical emergencies at numerous sites. Contemporaneous biological incidents require a highly coordinated response between numerous agencies at all levels of government and with the private sector across many jurisdictions. The biological incident may also affect other countries, necessitating extensive coordination with the international health community. Finally, local officials may be the first to identify the threat or disease outbreak.

Federal Response

HHS leads the federal effort for the public health and emergency medical planning, and the response to a biological terrorism attack or naturally occurring outbreak. This outbreak could result from either a known or novel pathogen, including an emerging infectious disease. HHS also provides guidance on the proper handling of materials related to a disease outbreak, and collaborates with other federal departments and agencies to determine the level of public health and medical response required. If environmental contamination occurs, HHS also collaborates with the EPA. The Department of Homeland Security (DHS) coordinates all nonmedical activities, and the Federal Bureau of Investigation (FBI) coordinates the investigation of any suspected criminal activities. In addition, for a significant outbreak of zoonotic disease or human food-borne pathogen, HHS collaborates with the U.S. Department of Agriculture (USDA). Finally, the LRN tests samples for the presence of biological threat agents and the original samples may be sent to the CDC for confirmation of LRN analyses.

Once notified that there is a credible threat of a biological incident or a disease outbreak, HHS assembles the agency partners who provide support under Emergency Support Function #8. Officials from the impacted jurisdiction(s) are involved in the coordination of assessment and response activities. Their task is to assess the situation and determine the appropriate public health and medical actions. An investigation into intentional biological threats or incidents will likely require the initiation of a joint criminal and epidemiological investigation. The FBI will coordinate any criminal investigation activities with appropriate state, local, and federal partner agencies, such as DHS, HHS, and USDA.

The first task following notification is to identify the affected population and the geographic scope of the incident. Figure 12-2 shows the flow of communication when the

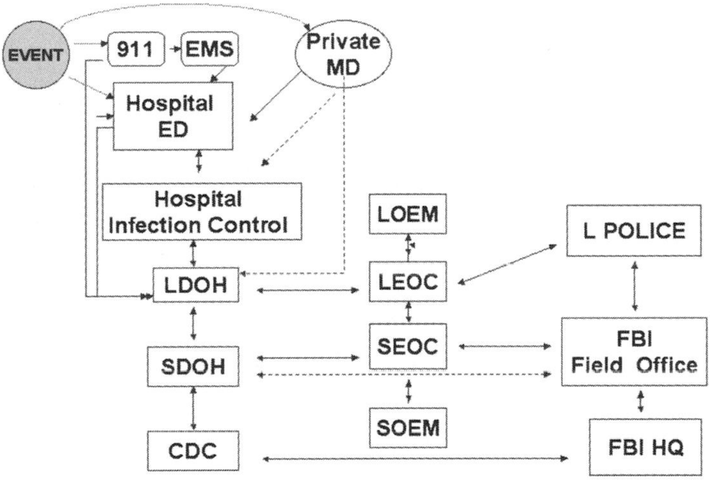

Note: CDC=Centers for Disease Control and Prevention; ED=emergency department; EMS=emergency medical services; FBI=Federal Bureau of Investigation; HQ=headquarters; L Police=local police; LDOH=local department of health; LEOC=local emergency operations center; LOEM=local office of emergency management; MD=medical doctor; SDOH=state department of health; SEOC=state emergency operations center; SOEM=state office of emergency management.

Figure 12-2. When Medicine or Public Health Identifies an Event

public health system is the first to learn that a bioterrorism event has occurred. The local public health system initiates appropriate measures for everyone affected, including first responders and other workers engaged in incident-related activities. These measures may include mass vaccination or prophylaxis for populations at risk but not yet exposed, including exposure from secondary transmission or through environmental contact. The public health and medical response also includes the following:

- Targeted epidemiological investigation (e.g., contact tracing)
- Dissemination of key safety information and necessary medical precautions
- Intensified syndromic surveillance with health care settings, provider offices, laboratory test orders, school absences, over-the-counter pharmacy sales, unusual increase in sick animals, wildlife deaths, or decreased commercial fish yields
- Organization and potential deployment of federal public health and medical response assets (e.g., personnel, medical, and veterinary supplies, SNS, and the National Veterinary Stockpile)

Controlling the Epidemic

HHS will assist public health and medical authorities with epidemic surveillance and coordination in the affected region and will assess whether increased surveillance is needed in locales not initially involved in the outbreak. If necessary, HHS will notify public health officials in the additional jurisdictions.

HHS makes recommendations regarding the need for isolation, quarantine, or shelter in place to prevent the spread of disease. Using the legal authorities of a state or locality, the governor of an affected state implements isolation, quarantine, or social-distancing requirements. Under tribal legal authorities, the leader of a federally recognized tribe may also order a curfew, isolation, social distancing, and quarantine. Federal actions to prevent interstate spread are authorized in Titles 42 and 21 of the U.S. Code (42 C.F.R., Parts 70 and 71, and 21 C.F.R., Part 1240).

Although DHS coordinates the release of public messages regarding a biological incident, public health and medical messages to the public should be communicated by a recognized health authority (e.g., the U.S. surgeon general). Table 12-11 lists the numerous agencies that cooperate in responding to a biological incident.

Regional Planning

Regional planning can improve a community's response in preventing the spread of disease. Regional agreements should specify how coordination will work, including roles, chain of command, reimbursement, distribution of scarce resources, information

Table 12-11. Cooperating Agencies in a Biological Incident

Department of Agriculture
Department of Commerce
Department of Defense
Department of Energy
Department of Homeland Security
Department of the Interior
Department of Justice
Department of Labor
Department of State
Department of Transportation
Department of Veterans Affairs
Environmental Protection Agency
General Services Administration
U.S. Agency for International Development
U.S. Postal Service
American Red Cross

Source: Adapted from Federal Emergency Management Agency (FEMA). 2008. *Biological Incident Annex, National Response Framework.* Washington, DC: FEMA. Available at: https://www.fema.gov/pdf/emergency/nrf/nrf_BiologicalIncidentAnnex.pdf. Accessed January 23, 2017.

management strategies, and the maintenance, inventory, and supply of response equipment. For a coordinated effort between and within agencies it is recommended to utilize the National Incident Management System so that communication and operations are synchronized, uniform, and not redundant (see Chapter 3 for more on the National Response Framework).

Following a bioterrorism attack, a community needs the following:

An emergency management program: A comprehensive plan, coordination with emergency management and health care coalitions, training, and drills

Personnel: Clinicians, public health officials, logisticians, and pharmacists

Material: Pharmaceuticals, isolation facilities, sites for mass vaccination, PPE, decontamination showers, and supplies with backup for mass care

Monitoring and providing information: Prevention guidelines, home care instructions for patients, and information regarding characteristics of the infectious agent to aid decision making about quarantine, isolation, social distancing, and evacuation

Communication system: Redundant equipment tested regularly

Security: Identification badges, restricted vendor access, security patrol, access control for entire facility, mail handling procedures

Financial support: Sufficient financial resources for each of the above

At the local or regional level, public health preparation for a biological incident can be modeled after planning paradigms for pandemic influenza because many biological agents present as flu-like illness. A planning committee should be established with key representatives from the health and public health, emergency management, and public safety sectors. This committee is responsible for establishing an overall command and control structure (see Chapter 3 on incident command); overseeing the prevention, planning, response, and recovery activities; and ensuring that a jurisdiction's plan is developed, reviewed, and revised when needed. Because the response to a biological incident will require cooperation from a broad variety of community groups, it is important to identify who the stakeholders are and solicit their support. Participation from the community should involve personnel knowledgeable about communicable disease and immunization, hospitals, laboratories, specialists in information systems, the media, citizen band radio groups, social service agencies, the Red Cross, law enforcement, fire and EMS, the medical community, the medical examiner and coroner, funeral directors, local utilities, local veterinary facilities capable of handling affected animals, and local government officials, among others. The planning committee will ask that stakeholders develop the components of the plan for which they have expertise.

Local health departments interested in obtaining "Project Public Health Ready" recognition need to develop comprehensive all-hazards preparedness and response plans, develop the capacity to respond within their workforce, and demonstrate the department's readiness through exercises or response to actual events. Each year's planning guidance for local public health agencies is available online from the NACCHO. (The Project Public Health Ready is available at: http://www.naccho.org/topics/emergency/pphr/index.cfm.)

Communities or regions should plan for 3 levels of response to an incident involving biological agents. Examples of this 3-tiered approach include separate plans for incidents with up to 100 victims, for incidents with 100 to 10,000 victims, and for incidents with more than 10,000 victims. An important part of each plan will be the logistics of obtaining and distributing vaccines and antibiotics. Plans should identify the location of local or federal depositories, designate distribution sites, and establish priorities for distribution. Stockpiles will most likely be flown into commercial airports or trucked from private vendors. A protocol must be established for off-loading antibiotics and supplies, and a site located for repackaging the materials into smaller units. In addition, a system must be established for ensuring that the antibiotics are used before their shelf life expires. If a push pack is predeployed in anticipation of an event, permission is required to open it.

Planning for surge capacity[5] should consider higher estimates for the morbidity and mortality resulting from a release of highly contagious agents such as smallpox or pneumonic plague. (Surge capacity planning is discussed in Chapter 4.) Attempts should be made to direct patients to alternative sites and away from hospitals that could become quickly overwhelmed. To ensure adequate staffing, prepare contingency plans for

5. The CDC developed software to assist local planners in estimating the potential impact of large flu outbreaks that can be adapted to planning for bioterrorism events. The software can be downloaded online (available at: http://www.cdc.gov/flu/pandemic-resources/tools/fluaid.htm).

replacements for essential personnel, such as reassignment of personnel from nonessential programs within the local agencies, or calling up retired personnel or private-sector personnel with relevant expertise. Establish a protocol for the protection of public safety personnel early in the outbreak through inoculation or the distribution of PPE. Further, to ensure the maintenance of a healthy workforce, those wearing PPE in order to decontaminate victims can only remain in PPE for about 15 minutes. Multiple teams need to be trained and these responders should be required to prehydrate themselves. Although estimates vary widely for those who might seek care because they think they are sick, a comprehensive plan should arrange to triage a large number of unaffected patients (i.e., the worried well). In major metropolitan regions, a conservative estimated ratio of worried well to affected patients was as high as 30 to 1, yet more than 30,000 people nationwide received prophylaxis for anthrax in 2001, far exceeding this ratio. Large numbers of potential patients will require the rapid establishment of alternative care facilities. Because patients will likely seek health care from locations at which they regularly receive care, alternative care facilities should be set up as close in proximity to hospitals as possible.

Public Health Community Plan for Biological Incident Response

Many of the activities for response to a novel influenza virus or other emerging disease and to a bioterrorism attack are similar.[6] In addition to a description of a unified command and control, a management structure, and responsibilities (including protocols for coordinating activities of the health care coalition with those of the emergency management sector), a public health community plan for biological incidents includes the following:

- Protocols for large-scale outbreak investigation and infection control that detail duties of personnel
- Notification and response protocols for suspected and confirmed cases
- Protocols for field decontamination and transfer to hospitals
- Assessment of staffing and maintenance of health care and essential community functions during periods of high absenteeism, including outreach criteria, guidelines for worker safety, and training needs
- Protocols on the handling of laboratory specimens to ensure rapid diagnostic testing, including collection, transfer and laboratory confirmation of samples, safe disposal, labeling, and appropriate chain of custody of samples related to suspected

6. For specific guidance on responding to bioterrorism, see *The Public Health Response To Biological and Chemical Terrorism: Interim Planning Guidance for State Public Health Officials* (available at: https://emergency.cdc.gov/documents/planning/planningguidance.pdf).

terrorism and referrals to reference or national laboratories, as well as whether laboratory reports require the attention of the local health department

- Assessment of facility needs, type/availability/location of drugs, vaccines, beds, and equipment
- Stockpiling and monitoring of expiration dates of pharmaceutical inventories for a range of potential agents
- Plans for mass medical care
- Resolution of legal issues
- Protocols for both external communication to the public and internal communication among those coordinating the response
- Measures to ensure environmental decontamination, biosafety, arrangements for mass burials, and mortuary management
- Protocols for management of mental health issues
- Coordination with civic organizations and other volunteers to provide food, medical, and other essential support for people confined to their homes
- Baseline data with scheduled updates on the following:
    - Hospital admissions
    - Acute bed occupancy
    - ICU bed occupancy
    - Emergency room visits for infection
    - Ambulatory department utilization
    - Influenza-like illness
    - Flu cases in patient billing and emergency department visit data
    - Unexplained deaths
    - Unusual syndromes in ambulatory patients
    - 911 calls
    - Diarrheal disease
    - Weekly sales of antidiarrheal medicine from a regional distributor
    - Daily number of stool samples submitted to labs
    - Daily incidence of gastrointestinal illness in nursing home populations
    - Calls to poison control centers
    - Antibiotic and other pharmaceutical supplies
    - Total number of respirators
    - Workforce and school absenteeism

Initial tasks during an infectious disease emergency include:

- Activate response plan, emergency operations centers, and an incident command system in departments of health.
- Interface with appropriate state and federal counterparts.

- Activate communications plan: disseminate information on the infectious disease emergency, prevention, and control.
- Increase surveillance at hospitals and clinics and other appropriate sites.
- Initiate vaccine/pharmaceutical distribution if appropriate.
- Coordinate activities with neighboring jurisdictions.
- Notify key government officials and legislators of the need for additional resources where needed.

Table 12-12 summarizes the supplies and antidotes that should be stockpiled and monitored for a response to a range of potential agents.

Defining, Detecting, and Responding to Biological Events

A possible bioterrorism event includes one of the following:

- A single, definitively diagnosed or strongly suspected case of an illness caused by a recognized bioterrorism agent occurring in a patient without a plausible explanation for his or her illness
- A cluster of patients presenting with a similar clinical syndrome with either unusual characteristics (e.g., age distribution) or unusually high morbidity or mortality without an obvious etiology or explanation
- An unexplained increase in the incidence of a common syndrome above seasonally expected levels

A biological event or emerging disease would most likely present as one of the above, with initial detection likely to take place at the local level. Because most agents that could be used for biological agents have incubation periods, an attack may not be apparent until days or even weeks after the attack has occurred. During the early stages of illness, many related diseases have vague, nonspecific symptoms making them difficult to

Table 12-12. Supplies and Antidotes for Potential Chemical or Biological Warfare Agents

Agent	Supplies Needed
Bacterial agents	Ciproflaxin, doxycycline, penicillin, chloramphenicol, and azithromycin
Botulinum toxin	Mechanical respiratory ventilators and associated supplies
Burn/vesicants	Sterile bandages, intravenous fluids, and broad spectrum antibiotics
Cyanide	Cyanide antidote kits containing amyl nitrate, sodium nitrate, and sodium thiosulfate
Lewisite	British anti-lewisite, nerve agent atropine, pralidoxime chloride, and diazepam
Radiological exposure	Potassium iodide
All	Resuscitation equipment and supplies, vasopressors

differentiate from numerous naturally occurring diseases. Primary health care providers in the local medical community may be the first to recognize unusual disease caused by a covert attack, with state and local health departments most likely to initiate a communitywide response. A potential biological incident might be a group of patients with a similar clinical syndrome with unusual characteristics, such as age distribution, unusually high morbidity or mortality without obvious explanation for the illness, unusual concurrence of geographic exposure, unusual disease not previously found in the region, a case of inhalation anthrax or smallpox, or unexplained increase in a common syndrome above seasonally expected levels (e.g., cluster flu epidemic in summer with negative virology, food poisoning without a single source).

Veterinarians should also be encouraged to report suspicious illness in their patients. The beginning of the West Nile epidemic in the United States was marked by the avian veterinarian at the Bronx Zoo in New York reporting birds dying around the time that a community physician called the New York City Department of Health and Mental Hygiene about an unusual cluster of meningitis cases.

Because accurate diagnosis of diseases caused by the most likely bioterrorism agents may be delayed because of the initial flu-like presentation and the several days needed for positive laboratory identification, public health officials cannot depend on passive surveillance systems (see Chapter 5). Labor-intensive active surveillance requires outreach and can be costly, but will be essential in identifying when the flu is not "the flu." Flu-like symptoms usually come on suddenly and may include the following:

- High fever
- Headache
- Tiredness/weakness (can be extreme)
- Dry cough
- Sore throat
- Runny nose
- Body or muscle aches
- Diarrhea and vomiting (more common in children)

A full mobilization of public health efforts includes sending suspected samples to reference laboratories for rapid confirmation of bioterrorism agents, deploying active surveillance and epidemiological teams to identify the source of initial exposure (e.g., review charts of suspected patients), ensuring appropriate isolation and universal precautions where indicated, initiating treatment and prophylaxis to reduce morbidity and mortality, assessing geographic spread, identifying unexpected features of the outbreak, and the launching of preestablished communication protocols among many medical community and emergency management agencies and between government and the public. The public health team should be organized to respond to potential biological, chemical, or radiological events and include professionals from multiple disciplines, such as laboratory scientists, emergency management, emergency medical technicians and paramedics, environmental health scientists, epidemiologists, hazardous material response teams, health physicists, industrial hygienists, infectious disease specialists, medical examiners, occupational health physicians, public health laboratory designees, toxicologists, and veterinarians.

An effective surveillance system will be able to rapidly track changes in disease trends, be based on clinical syndromes, and be generated by data that are collected continually, reviewed daily, and remain geographically representative. An alert in these systems prompts an epidemiological investigation to determine if there is an outbreak and to identify the potential microbial etiology and the source of transmission. Sources of data for biological and emerging disease include the following:

- Biosurveillance
- Hospital reports (admissions to ICUs of previously healthy people with unexplained febrile illnesses)
- Infectious disease and laboratory reports
- Diagnostic categories with trends and unusual patterns from emergency departments
- Outbreaks in institutional settings (e.g., skilled nursing facilities)
- Workforce and school absenteeism
- Prescription and over-the-counter medication sales
- Animal outbreaks and deaths
- Police and EMS reports
- Geographic analyses of 911 calls categorized by disease syndrome (e.g., codes for difficulty breathing, respiratory distress, and other markers for influenza-like disease)

Although medical examiner reports are useful, a 2- to 3-day delay often occurs between the time of death and the filing of the death certificate. In addition, it is difficult to identify clusters using death certificates. Optimally, electronic death reporting can be instituted so that this information is more timely. In addition, epidemiologists will want to examine environmental factors such as food, the presence of vectors (e.g., ticks, fleas, flies, rodents, cats, mosquitoes, bats), and trends in animal populations and food crops.

Early detection of a covert release is designed to occur through autonomous detection systems, which include focused active surveillance and diagnostic laboratory testing. In the environmental surveillance system known as BioWatch, vacuum cleaner-like machines, operating both indoors and outdoors, continuously collect air samples. BioWatch may detect the presence of a biological agent in the environment. This detection triggers environmental sampling; samples are tested in public health laboratories 7 days a week. In addition, clinical surveillance is intensified to rule out or confirm an incident. If confirmed, the early detection through environmental surveillance systems such as BioWatch prompts a mobilized response by public health professionals, health care institutions, and law enforcement agents before too many clinical cases are identified.

Active Surveillance and Epidemiological Investigations

To activate a rapid surveillance, materials must be prepared in advance. Essential tools include preplanned instruments of generic questions designed to determine case and risk exposure, a sampling strategy, a centralized database with fields defined, and a mechanism to call up and deploy teams to conduct the surveillance around the clock. The instrument might pose questions about location of residence, travel, and work, usual commuter routes, and a detailed diary of the patient's activities during the incubation period of the suspected agent.

If there is a confirmed bioterrorism event, health departments will be responsible for tracking the cases and performing epidemiological investigations to determine the source and sites of exposure. Public health officials will implement active hospital-based and enhanced passive surveillance, including hard-to-reach populations (such as the homeless), contact tracing similar to that used for measles or syphilis, and coordination with local poison control centers. This information will be essential in determining who else might have been exposed and will require prophylaxis. Epidemiological investigations will help identify the determinants, distribution, and frequency of disease in both human and animal populations. Epidemiology will detect possible vector control requirements and the likelihood of secondary spread. These investigations will be coordinated with neighboring health departments as well as interstate and international agencies.

Mass Medical and Mortuary Care

In addition to baseline surveys that provide information about a community's capacity to care for patients exposed to bioterrorism agents, guidelines are needed for the care of exposed patients. Community care guidelines should include distributing protocols and disease-specific information to the health care community on identifying cases, medical management of those exposed, initiating mass medical care including triage and surge capacity with trained personnel, turning shelters or schools into hospitals, establishing patient isolation in many locations including homes, distributing pharmaceuticals to large numbers of the population, transporting patients, and mortuary care.

Managing the media and keeping the general public accurately informed is a crucial component of a mass care plan. Communication is accomplished with providers through the HAN, broadcast alerts, and communication hotlines. Consider establishing 3 separate hotlines: one for physicians, one for people requiring the services at a point of distribution (POD) center, and one for the general public with staff being given prepared scripts to answer questions. Use the media to issue warnings to the public and for public service announcements on how to prevent exposures and distinguish symptoms, control measures, who may need antibiotics, and local effects of disease.

A plan for mass antibiotic prophylaxis or immunization of the population should include the following:

- Description of the decision making process that would be used to initiate a mass immunization campaign
- Method of identifying the affected population
- Communication plans to reach the identified affected population, with language-appropriate considerations
- Adjustable distribution plans to provide vaccine or antibiotics to high-priority target groups and the general population where there is a severe vaccine shortage, moderate vaccine shortage, or an adequate vaccine supply
- Plans for transporting the Strategic National Stockpile to distribution points
- Designated personnel who will manage the arrival, distribution, and local dissemination of vaccines and antibiotics; ensure the smooth flow of clients into POD; and translate when needed, including sign language
- Plans for the storage, transportation, and handling of pharmaceuticals; one refrigerated tractor trailer would be adequate to handle the storage of 12 million doses of vaccine
- Clinical algorithm and preprinted instruction sheets for different prophylactic regimens, including procedures for immunization of differing age groups
- Procedures for record keeping and strict accountability, including a log for recording the manufacturer, lot number, expiration date, and quantity of vaccine received and distributed in compliance with federal vaccine administration guidelines
- Plans for the availability of protective clothing by personnel
- Plans for ensuring community participation
- Development of information sheets in all relevant languages
- Regional coordination of proposed pharmaceutical distribution plan
- Procedures for monitoring compliance with medication protocols, symptoms or illness attributable to the vaccine, illness following immunization attributable to vaccine failure, and adverse events

Hospitals

For both pandemic influenza and releases of biological agents, hospitals should prepare for a dramatic increase in patients visiting the emergency department and requiring hospitalization. Even a mild pandemic could produce a dramatic increase in demand for inpatient and ICU beds and ventilators. With high attack rates, assume staff absenteeism will be high, resulting in limited availability of critical resources. Hospital preparations should address the following:

- Surge capacity
- Management of triage, volunteers, and home care
- Infection control guidelines
- Resource allocation
- Mass mortality
- Support for staff and their families
- Management and tracking of hospital resources

Although hospitals are required to have a disaster plan to be accredited by The Joint Commission, a sequence of stand-alone facility plans do not prepare a community to respond to a biological incident. The hospitals in a community or region must coordinate their efforts, including the transport of patients, communications during the event, handling of bodies, and other major tasks. The coordination of resources is all the more important as more hospitals practice "just-in-time" delivery of supplies and pharmaceuticals. Designating the delivery of services to certain hospitals in advance (e.g., limiting high-cost specialty care to those hospitals with the most experience in treating severely injured patients) and formalizing protocols for coordination between prehospital and hospital care (e.g., establishing protocols for first responders to rapidly transport patients) have been shown to contribute to improved patient outcomes. The regional plan should ensure that all hospitals participate in multihospital drills.

Hospitals plans for responding to a large infectious disease outbreak include provisions for triaging large numbers of patients in the emergency department, patient decontamination and patient overflow, increasing bed capacity, calling in additional staff, and establishing isolation units on short notice, including airborne, contact, and universal precautions. Staff should be educated about their specific roles in the hospital incident command system and instructed to continue with their regular duties if they are not involved in the hospital's own incident command structure. Hospital staff should know whom to notify if they are the first to learn about the event, what questions to ask (e.g., where is it and what is happening), and how to use universal precautions. Multilingual information sheets and consent forms should be prepared. In addition, instructional sheets on the methodology for administering vaccines should be ready for use.

Hospital plans establish the medical protocols that will be followed, the distribution of medications or vaccines, and whether to set up community-based mass prophylaxis clinics. If a patient presents where the providers suspect an infectious disease, at a minimum the emergency department protocol should include the following:

- Contacting the department of health with specifics of the case
- Rapid screening of individuals in waiting room
- Checking for supply of isolation equipment, particulate respirators, isolation rooms for negative pressure
- Triage and isolation in negative-pressure rooms for those with known contact with the index case or with fever or suspicious rash
- Contacting hospital infection control and disease experts
- Standard precautions, including fit-tested N95 or N100 masks
- Rapid screening and gathering of contact information for all in waiting area

Point of Distribution

When large numbers of people require prophylaxis by medication or vaccine, it is necessary to establish a POD. POD activities include registration, triage, taking swab samples, medical evaluation or screening, dispensing antibiotics or vaccine, reassuring the worried well, briefing clients about the infectious disease and POD operations, collecting information for surveillance or investigative purposes, transferring individuals to a medical facility (when needed), counseling, managing client flow, and maintaining security. Preplanning is essential because once an event occurs necessitating mass distribution of medication, there is little time between the decision to open a POD and the initiation of operations. Prior arrangements should be made with other community agencies and medical volunteers so that issues of credentialing, medical-legal responsibility, and reimbursement are worked out in advance.

Experience, such as that of the New York City Department of Health and Mental Hygiene, suggests that the services within PODs may be organized or function differently depending on the type and scope of event. Allocate sufficient time to ensure that supplies have arrived and trained staff are ready before opening a POD. Adequate staffing is essential, including a dedicated physician in charge, liaison, supplies coordinator, and clinic manager. In New York's experience, approximately 50 to 55 people per shift are needed for round-the-clock coverage in 12-hour shifts to provide antibiotic prophylaxis to up to 10,000 people in 72 hours. In selecting a site for a POD, choose a place convenient to members of the community who have to use it and one that is large enough to distribute antibiotics or vaccine to the necessary population. To dispense antibiotics to 500 to 10,000 people over a 72-hour period, a space of at least 2,500 square feet is needed. Software to help plan for PODs, such as AnyLogic, uses simulation modeling to determine how many PODs with the number of staffing personnel would be needed.

Establishing good communication is critical from the incident command center to POD, from the health department to the public, and from the health department to community medical providers. When events do not indicate immunizing or prophylaxing large segments of the population, it will be necessary to establish a plan for triaging the worried well. Figures 12-3 and 12-4 show schemata of a model POD layout.

When an event involves bioterrorism—a criminal act—law enforcement agencies require separate space for investigation away from the POD to minimize concerns about confidentiality. The FBI and CDC developed a guide that describes the role of public health and law enforcement in these investigations.

Point of Distribution Functional Areas

A typical POD includes space for these types of functions (see Figures 12-3 and 12-4):

Screening station: Verify eligibility; provide writing tools, information sheets, epidemiologic interview forms, law enforcement interview forms, and medical record forms.

Client registration: Logbook or spreadsheet on a laptop, or data entry screens and wireless connections to an on-site server.

Triage area: Assess if people go to the dispensing station, need to be medically evaluated, or need further evaluation and transfer to a health care facility; provide printed material (e.g., medication fact sheets, epidemiological interviews); staff at triage: physicians, nurses, and physician assistants. Where potentially ill people can be separated from healthy to minimize exposure of the well population.

Briefings on risks of exposure, symptoms, and side effects of antibiotics

Specimens collection as needed (e.g., nasal swabs)

Screening station for determining which drugs should be dispensed

Dispensing station for antibiotic distribution. Staff: nurses, physicians, pharmacists

Counseling staff: behavioral health, medical advisers, and public health educators at POD entrance, near POD exit, and as consultation for referring people to hotlines and Web sites

Security at the entrance, exit, and pharmaceutical supplies

Clerical area for medical charting

Space for filling out forms and conducting interviews

Box 12-1 lists key information collected in a medical chart at a POD.

Laboratory Response Network

The LRN was established in 1999 by the Association of Public Health Laboratories, the CDC, and the FBI to assist in the U.S. response to biological and chemical terrorism.

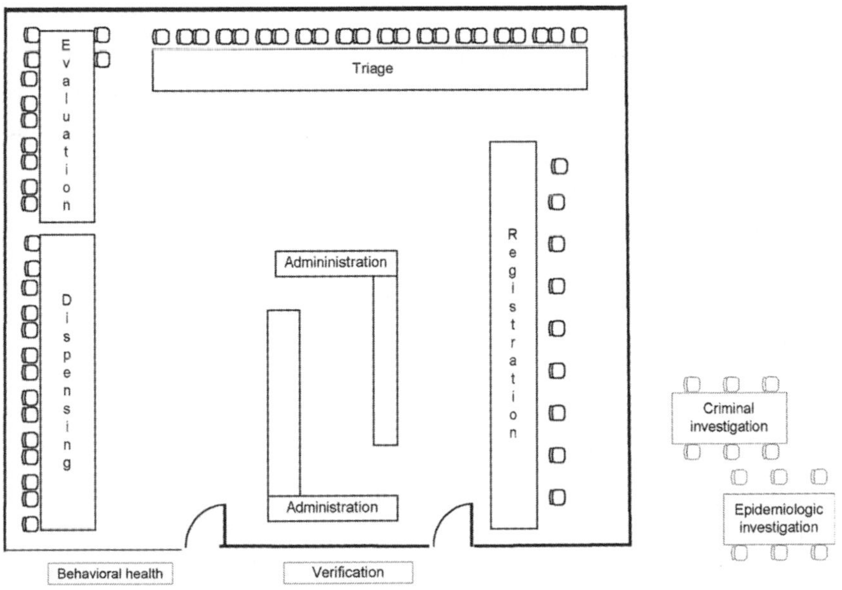

Figure 12-3. Template Point of Distribution Layout: Reception Area

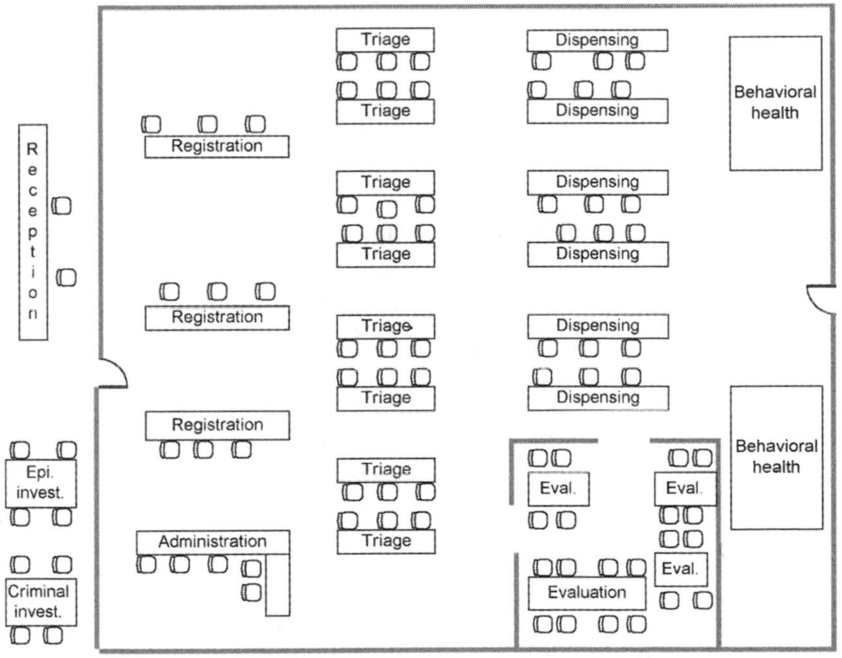

Figure 12-4. Template Point of Distribution Layout: Delivery Area

Box 12-1. Point of Distribution Medical Chart

Use a two-sided, one-sheet, self-administered questionnaire as a medical chart, limited to information relevant to the rapid distribution of antibiotics (similar medical record for pediatrics) which includes the following:

Contact information:
- Address
- Telephone numbers
- Emergency contacts
- Age

Signed consent form for testing and treatment

Brief medical history:
- Presence or absence of current symptoms
- Relevant drug allergies
- Use of specific medications known to interact with drugs of choice (e.g., doxycycline or ciprofloxacin for anthrax) and pregnancy status

Place to document:
- Specimen collection
- Dispensing and receipt (or refusal) of antibiotics/vaccine
- Antibiotic/vaccine lot numbers

Source: Adapted from Blank S, Moskin LC, Zucker JR. 2003. An ounce of prevention is a ton of work: mass antibiotic prophylaxis for anthrax, New York City, 2001. *Emerg Infect Dis.* 9(6):615–622.

The LRN is now an integrated national and international network of about 150 biological and 53 chemical laboratories with the capacity to respond to acts of CBW, emerging infectious diseases, and other public health threats and emergencies. These laboratories produce high-confidence test results that are the basis for threat analysis and intervention by both public health and law enforcement authorities.

LRN includes the following types of labs:

- Federal (the CDC, U.S. Army Medical Research Institute for Infectious Diseases [USAMRIID], and other federally run facilities)
- State and local public health laboratories
- Military
- Food testing (the FDA, USDA, and state food testing laboratories)
- Environmental (testing water and other environmental samples)
- Clinical (local hospitals and other larger clinical laboratories)
- Veterinary (the USDA [animal testing], veterinary diagnostic laboratories)
- International (labs in Canada, the United Kingdom, Australia, and Mexico)

The LRN supports surveillance and epidemiological investigations by identifying disease, providing direct and reference services, and conducting environmental, rapid, and specialized testing. Five of the major threats (botulism, plague, anthrax, tularemia, and poxvirus illnesses) occur naturally in the United States, and specimens for these diseases are routinely evaluated by public health laboratories. In addition, the standard techniques for detecting bacterial agents (e.g., gram stain, culture on selective media, visual colony morphology, growth after heat shock, and confirmatory methods using phage and direct immunofluorescence) are well recognized for establishing definitive diagnoses. Methods such as isolation in cell culture, inoculation of animals, direct fluorescence, and electron microscopy are considered definitive methods in virology.

The personnel who work in public health laboratories are highly skilled and familiar with following complex identification algorithms. The procedures used can be readily adapted to environmental samples that might be collected after an overt threat, or in the attribution of the source of a sample. Further, the public health laboratories are all certified under the Clinical Laboratory Improvement Act of 1967 as employing appropriate quality assurance and quality control procedures. Although definitive identification requires a few days, preliminary results can be available in hours. In particular, the minimum response time for a definitive negative result with a rapidly growing organism such as anthrax may be 16 hours. Slower growing organisms or complex procedures may take 48 hours or more. Furthermore, many methods require a fixed facility with traditional lab techniques not readily adaptable to a field situation.

The Laboratory Network for Biological Terrorism has 3 levels of organization designated as sentinel, reference, or national. Designation depends on the types of tests a laboratory can perform and how it handles infectious agents to protect workers and the public. Membership in the LRN is not automatic. State lab directors determine the criteria and whether public health labs in their states should be included in the network. In addition to regulatory requirements, prospective reference labs must have the equipment, trained personnel, properly designed facilities, and must demonstrate testing accuracy.

Sentinel labs (formerly Level A) represent the thousands of hospital-based clinical labs that are on the front lines. In an unannounced or covert bioterrorism attack, sentinel labs could be the first to identify a suspicious specimen and screen out a presumptive case during routine patient care. A sentinel laboratory's responsibility is to recognize, rule out, and refer a suspicious sample to the right reference lab. Laboratory personnel use Biosafety Level 2 (BSL-2) techniques for agents that can cause human disease, but with limited potential for human transmission.[7]

Reference labs (formerly Levels B and C) can perform tests to detect and confirm the presence of a threat agent. Approximately 90% of the U.S. population lives within 100 miles of a reference lab. These labs ensure a timely local response in the event of a

7. Laboratory personnel use work practices and safety equipment in a facility designed to minimize exposures to infectious agents. This combination of containment practices is known as a Biosafety Level (BSL). The CDC specifies 4 levels of containment, which range from the lowest (BSL-1) to the highest (BSL-4).

terrorist incident or other emergency. Rather than having to rely on confirmation from labs at the CDC, reference labs are capable of producing conclusive results. Reference labs can be city, county, or major state public health laboratories that perform direct fluorescence or phage testing such as molecular diagnostics. Using BSL-3 techniques for agents that may be transmitted by the respiratory route and can cause serious infection, reference labs have the safety and proficiency to confirm and characterize susceptibility and to probe, type, and perform toxigenicity testing.

National laboratories (formerly Level D) are part of the CDC and USAMRIID and can perform research on and development of new techniques that are disseminated to other levels of the network. National labs have unique resources to handle highly infectious agents and are responsible for definitive high-level characterization (e.g., seeking evidence of molecular chimeras) or identifying specific agent strains. The CDC and USAMRIID national labs, operating at BSL-4, handle the most dangerous agents that have the highest risk of life-threatening disease, are transmitted by as aerosols, and for which there is no vaccine or treatment.

If a covert event occurs that is not recognized immediately, the incidence of disease in the community would trigger public health agencies to submit samples to the laboratory and report to the surveillance network. With an announced threat or an overt event, the situation would be reported to the FBI, which would in turn determine what level of laboratory is required and transport samples to the nearest appropriate laboratory resource in the network. Figure 12-5 shows the chain of events if law enforcement is the first to recognize an event.

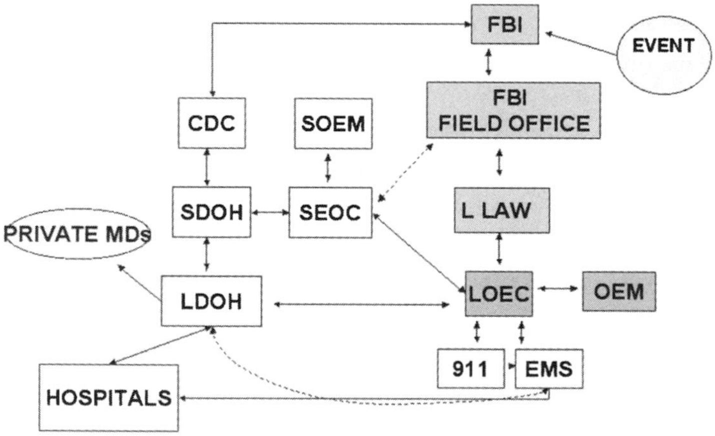

Note: CDC=Centers for Disease Control and Prevention; EMS=emergency medical services; FBI=Federal Bureau of Investigation; L LAW=local law enforcement; LDOH=local department of health; LEOC=local emergency operations center; MD=medical doctor; OEM=office of emergency management; SDOH=state department of health; SEOC=state emergency operations center; SOEM=state office of emergency management.

Figure 12-5. When Law Enforcement Identifies an Event

Legal Issues

As legal authority varies from state to state, it is necessary for public health to investigate specific state laws regarding emergency preparedness. Legal questions that may arise regarding the powers of the health commissioner upon a declaration of emergency must be clarified and include the following:

- The ability to remove legal barriers relative to dispensing of medicines
- Licensing of out-of-state physicians and nurses
- Transfer of patients between hospitals during the emergency
- Emergency credentialing of providers who are not credentialed through the federal response
- Isolation, quarantine, social distancing, blockade, zone perimeters, requisitions, curfews, governance, restricted access, and due process under different scenarios
- The power to define diseases deemed dangerous to public health
- Control and prevention
- Reportable disease
- The liability of hospitals in the reporting of information
- The process of declaring a state of emergency in a locale

Public health authorities should identify who has the authority, what criteria must be met, what legal mechanism must be followed, and who is responsible for enforcement. Once the legal mechanism is defined, contingency plans to quarantine patients and protocols for implementation and enforcement should be established. Finally, although the Health Insurance Portability and Accountability Act Privacy Rule regulates how "covered entities" use and disclose "protected health information" (PHI), PHI disclosures without patient authorization may occur if the disclosure was required by law, authorized by the individual, for treatment purposes, or to legally authorized public health entities for public health activities. Public health activities include surveillance, investigation, and intervention.

CHAPTER 13

PUBLIC HEALTH CONSIDERATIONS IN RECOVERY AND RECONSTRUCTION

Disaster preparedness plans must also consider the long-term process of recovery and reconstruction. Public health professionals are key players in recovery because those who lose power, water, and their source of food have increased morbidity and mortality. This chapter examines the federal guidance and support structure for federal agencies to aid recovery, factors influencing recovery, 3 postimpact phases of disaster and the priorities in planning for each. Particular attention is paid to providing services immediately post-impact, such as shelters, and caring for those with functional and medical needs.

Public Health Role

- Restore the public health and health care delivery infrastructures.
- Organize communitywide programs for delivery of health care and public health services, including functional needs and medical shelters.
- Provide community education to enhance public awareness (e.g., injury control), aid community adjustment, form the basis for future disaster mitigation, and educate the community about likely health risks and how to deal with them.
- Assess health needs in the community to determine necessary services to meet the long-term physical and behavioral health needs of affected populations, including continuity of care.

Principles of Disaster Recovery and Reconstruction

The federal government is obligated to assist states and localities in their recovery from disasters as provided for in the Robert T. Stafford Disaster Relief and Emergency Assistance Act of 1988. Specific federal guidance for recovery is found in the National Disaster Recovery Framework (NDRF).[1] The NDRF provides a structure for unified and

1. Initially, the National Response Framework included an annex, Emergency Support Function (ESF) #14: Long-Term Community Recovery Annex (available at: http://www.fema.gov/pdf/emergency/nrf/nrf-esf-14.pdf), that described the federal role in recovery and designated the lead agency for each task. This guidance was replaced by the NDRF. State and local plans, which have not been updated to reflect the principles of the NDRF, may include references to ESF #14.

collaborative federal activities to help communities recover from disasters significant enough to have received federal support through the Stafford Act. Some elements of the framework may also be used for significant non-Stafford Act incidents, such as major oil spills. The NDRF defines principles of disaster recovery, identifies the roles and responsibilities of recovery coordinators and others, provides a coordinating structure to facilitate communication and collaboration, and guides pre- and post-disaster recovery planning.

The NDRF describes the tasks required to recover from a disaster in its Recovery Support Functions (RSF). The RSF structure is similar to and builds upon the ESF discussed in Chapter 3. When a community's resources and efforts for recovery are insufficient to meet the needs of the disaster, the RSFs guide the identification, coordination, and delivery of federal assistance needed to supplement local efforts. With federal support, local officials must set the priorities and direct the use of resources.

Because recovery activities are different than those required to respond to a disaster (i.e., rebuild vs. cleanup), RSFs have different objectives, approaches, time spans, and organizational structure, as well as new partners. The partners involved in recovery may have different skill sets than those who help with response and include organizations that have experience with financing for permanent housing, economic development, advocacy for underserved populations and long-term community planning. At the federal level, each RSF is led by a designated federal coordinating agency. The RSFs and the lead agency for each are:

- Community Planning and Capacity Building (Federal Emergency Management Agency [FEMA])
- Economic (U.S. Department of Commerce)
- Health and Social Services (U.S. Department of Health & Human Services [HHS])
- Housing (U.S. Department of Housing and Urban Development)
- Infrastructure Systems (U.S. Army Corps of Engineers)
- Natural and Cultural Resources (U.S. Department of Interior)

The RSFs are activated as the level of response activities declines and recovery activities accelerate. When indicated, the federal disaster recovery coordinator (FDRC) will call upon the RSF agencies to organize and coordinate the federal recovery assistance. During this early recovery phase, there is some overlap between the ESF and RSF missions, and there is close coordination between the FDRC, RSF, and ESF. The timing of the transition from ESF to RSF depends on the nature of the disaster and may vary considerably. The federal coordinating officer (FCO) determines when a specific ESF is no longer required. As the coordinating agency for the function of health and social services, HHS assists the locally led recovery efforts as they work to restore public health, health care and social services in the affected communities. Data can be used to signal when recovery has begun. By looking at health care utilization before and after the disaster and at patterns of multiple health outcomes, public health agencies will be able to tell when the community has returned to their usual pattern of health care utilization. (See Table 13-1 below for more information).

Congress set restrictions on reimbursements available to states and localities after a disaster. In the event that an exception is made to previously set limits, it is very important that agencies involved in response and recovery can account for all resources lost in a disaster and all funds spent in recovery, regardless of how miniscule the amounts. Without documentation, opportunities for reimbursement may be lost.

Influencing Factors

Community participation is essential for planning the recovery and reconstruction phase because local residents better understand their own needs and the problems that create those needs. Factors that influence recovery planning and policy include the accuracy of needs assessments, intense pressure by citizens to rebuild as soon as possible, the amount of time and resources allocated to problem solving and recovery, and the many and often conflicting preferences of affected groups. In the recovery following Hurricane Sandy, the region experienced a lot of inter-organizational engagement, with interaction of both individual and community resources. Residents should be the direct beneficiaries of recovery projects, since they will be responsible for monitoring development that continues after relief workers have left.

In planning each activity, aid agencies and the community must consider both short- and long-term positive and negative impacts. For example, aid should be provided in such a way that allows people to stay at home when possible, continue their normal lives, and resume normal activities when possible. Integrated recovery programs may include work schemes to repair community facilities that pay residents cash to replace lost possessions. This injection of money will stimulate local markets and help speed recovery. To aid recovery further, loans or grants can be made available to small businesses.

Phases of Recovery and Reconstruction

Three phases categorize the types of activities that occur postimpact in the affected community: emergency, transition or recovery, and reconstruction. During the emergency phase, activity focuses on saving lives through search and rescue, first aid, emergency medical assistance, and overall disaster assessment. Efforts immediately begin to repair critical facilities, restore communications and transportation networks, and, in some cases, to evacuate residents from areas still vulnerable to further disaster. When evacuating patients from hospitals or long-term care facilities, it is critical to track the patients

Table 13-1. Health and Social Services Recovery Support Functions by Phase

Pre-Disaster	Post-Disaster	Outcomes
• Plan for the transition from response to recovery as part of preparedness and operational plans (collaborating with ESFs #3, #6, #8, and #11). • Plan for the transition from post-incident recovery to community preparedness and operational plans. • Develop strategies to address recovery issues for health, behavioral health and social services, particularly for response and recovery workers and vulnerable populations. • Promote the principles of sustainability, resilience, and mitigation as part of preparedness and operational plans.	• Maintain situational awareness to identify and mitigate potential recovery obstacles during the response phase. • Expedite recovery during the response phase by leveraging response, emergency protection measures, and hazard mitigation resources. • Provide technical assistance and support recovery planning of public health, health care, and human services infrastructure. • Conduct Health and Social Services Recovery Support Function assessments with primary agencies. • Deploy in support of the health and social services recovery support function when activated by the federal disaster recovery coordinator. • Establish communication and information-sharing forum(s) for health and social services with the state and/or community. • Coordinate and leverage applicable federal resources for health and social services. • Develop and implement a plan to transition from federal health and social services recovery operations back to daily operations. • Identify and coordinate with other governmental partners to assess food, animal, water, and air conditions to ensure safety. • Evaluate the effectiveness of health and social services recovery efforts.	• Restore the capacity and resilience of essential health and social services to meet ongoing and emerging post-disaster community needs. • Encourage behavioral health systems to meet the behavioral health needs of affected individuals, response and recovery workers, and the community. • Promote self-sufficiency and continuity of the health and well-being of affected individuals (particularly vulnerable populations). • Assist in the continuity of essential health and social services, including schools. • Reconnect displaced populations with essential health and social services. • Protect the health of the population and response and recovery workers from the longer-term effects of a post-disaster environment. • Promote clear communications and public health messaging to provide accurate, appropriate, and accessible information; ensure information is developed and disseminated in multiple mediums, multilingual formats, alternative formats, is age-appropriate and user-friendly and is accessible to underserved populations.

Source: Adapted from Federal Emergency Management Agency. 2011. *National Disaster Recovery Framework*. Health and Social Services Recovery Support Function. Available at: http://www.fema.gov/pdf/recoveryframework/health_social_services_rsf.pdf. Accessed January 24, 2017.

with their medical information. The New York State Office of Information Technology Services developed a web-based tracking system called e-FINDS (Evacuation of Facilities in Disasters System). Each patient receives preprinted wristbands with bar codes and identifying numbers. Hospital and ambulance personnel use handheld scanners, a mobile app, and optional paper tracking to track patients and residents in real time across facilities.

During the transition or recovery phase, people return to work, repair damaged buildings and infrastructure, and initiate other actions that allow the community to return to normal as soon as possible. The priorities during the recovery phase include the assurance of adequate shelter, medical services, infrastructure, utilities, business, economic activity, and social networks. Victims begin their emotional recovery and some may experience depression or post-traumatic stress disorder (see Chapter 8). External assistance is provided in the form of cash and credit. Construction projects and other types of job creation are common types of aid.

The reconstruction phase is characterized by physical reordering of communications, utilities, roads, and the general physical environment. Residents repair or rebuild their housing, and agricultural activities resume. Reconstruction may span years, especially for the restoration of housing and other buildings.

The timing of each phase varies with the nature of the disaster, its location, and the capacity of the affected community to mend. This process often occurs in 4 stages, which are not necessarily sequential. Different parts of a community can be moving forward at different paces, depending on the extent of devastation and resources available. The stages are as follows:

- Emergency response (i.e., debris removal, provision of temporary housing, establishment of emergency medical clinics)
- Restoration of public services (e.g., electricity, water, and telephone)
- Replacement and reconstruction (e.g., health and behavioral health infrastructure and/or systems that have been disrupted or destroyed)
- Initiation of improvements and reconstruction that stimulate economic growth and local development

Factors affecting recovery time include the environment (e.g., risk of secondary disasters, availability of communications, general economy); the economy (e.g., cash flow, cost and supply of materials); technical aspects (e.g., availability of technical assistance, existence of conflicts in technical advice, ability to reuse salvaged materials, process of dealing with irrelevant aid); politics (e.g., public rejection of recovery plans, bureaucracy in government and other responding agencies, efforts by interest groups to channel aid to rebuild their areas first); and community motivation. Table 13-1 identifies the health and social services support functions carried out by public health professionals by phase of recovery.

Post-Disaster Assessments

Needs assessments conducted postimpact provide the information required to begin recovery. Emergency needs are more apparent than are long-term needs, and long-term needs vary over time. Working with neighboring jurisdictions (i.e., across state or county lines) can help identify at-risk populations. Sharing information between health care systems could facilitate the distribution of regional assets and capabilities. Communication about the findings and the next steps must be established between responding jurisdictions and organizations and those affected by the disaster.

The first step in such an assessment is to assess community capacities and vulnerabilities, including physical environment (e.g., intact infrastructure and resources), social conditions (e.g., existing organizations and support networks), and the population's attitude toward recovery and their motivation to recover. Needs are determined by visiting representative areas, talking to selected groups in affected communities, and conducting rapid health assessments (see Chapter 6). The needs of patients in evacuation zones can be an early indicator of medical and nonmedical needs so that public health can plan a geographically targeted response.

When possible, needs should be quantified (e.g., percentage of families without running water, number of patients served by pharmacies that were destroyed), even if the number is determined by extrapolation. Public health workers should highlight gaps in the community's emergency response that impact public health and health care services. Once the baseline capacities and vulnerabilities have been assessed, this information must be continuously gathered and reevaluated to determine progress toward recovery and identify what remains to be done.

The use of technology can be an essential tool in determining where public health and health care services are needed following disaster. Technological structures and systems can be made operational in a disaster so responders can more easily locate people in need. In the days following Hurricane Sandy, public health planners used geographic mapping techniques linked with insurance claims data (i.e., Medicare and Medicaid) to identify clusters of individuals who might need care. Geospatial analysis of community factors (e.g., neighborhoods, resources, access, functional needs) has shown clear patterns of who is vulnerable. Analyzing big datasets can help communities watch for shifts in health care utilization, especially by at-risk populations. Collect Smart and CASPER are discussed in Chapter 6 and HAZEL is discussed below. Another system is called FRED (Framework for Reconstructing Epidemiological Dynamics), an open-source modeling system located at the University of Pittsburgh (available at: http://fred.publichealth.pitt.edu). FRED has been used to conduct research on the spread of infectious disease in order to determine changes to health behavior that can be made to alter the spread of the infection.

Reestablishing Local Business and Economic Activity

When reestablishing lost infrastructure, communities should take the opportunity to make improvements and reduce future vulnerability to disaster. Local efforts can influence the pace, location, type, density, design, and cost of redevelopment. In addition to providing guidance on disaster-resistant building techniques, community leaders can aid reconstruction by ensuring optimal urban planning, permitting families to rebuild housing according to their tastes and incomes, and financing the delivery of electricity, water, and sewer lines.

A major disaster usually causes a decline in income and employment, thus reducing the resources of the population at the time of its greatest need. This income reduction reduces the tax base when increased government resources are most needed. Jobs, economic activity, and reestablishing schools give people a sense of returning to normalcy. Jobs, economic growth, and housing repair influence long-term recovery more than do immediate disaster relief efforts.

Social Environment

To aid in social recovery, local leaders must be familiar with basic family structure, economic patterns, governmental structure, religious affiliations, customs and practices, and power relationships within their community before disaster strikes. Each community has a variety of internal social structures that help individuals and families through difficult periods. Coping mechanisms exist at the level of the individual, family, community, and region. Effective intervention after a disaster requires an understanding of these coping mechanisms.

Strengthening horizontal community ties provides a means of redevelopment and preparation for future disasters. In some cases, the disaster may provide an opportunity for the community to work together in ways it previously has not, resulting in a stronger community—and a stronger sense of community—than existed before the crisis.

Emphasis on reestablishing community means that where options exist, leaders should choose the option that strengthens or maintains the community. For example, disaster recovery plans should avoid building camps or large shelters whenever possible and instead provide aid in such a way that people can stay at home or in their neighborhoods, which will allow residents to rely on preexisting social connections and promote resumption of normal activities.

Incorporating Disaster Preparedness Into Recovery

Vulnerability assessments require a review of land use based on post-disaster needs. Vulnerability assessments can also be used to predict the effects (both positive and negative) of redevelopment by projecting the impact of anticipated changes. The assessment of vulnerabilities should be used to avoid or reduce negative outcomes from future disasters. Encouraging communities to rebuild and commit to their communities in the long term requires attracting investment and demonstrating that the community has worked to reduce the negative impact if disaster recurs. For example, if housing is needed following a flood, a vulnerability assessment can tell officials where to build new houses to reduce the risk of damage from future flooding. Reconstruction should use improved designs and standards that reduce the vulnerability of structures. Reconstruction may also involve the erection of structures to reduce future mortality, such as hurricane shelters, and to detect possible future events, such as early warning systems.

Access to Primary Care

A key goal during disaster recovery is to ensure that people with chronic disease are able to get continuity of care and needed medicine lost in the disaster, in order to keep them from being hospitalized or sent to an emergency departments when they don't need to be there. This is often difficult because natural disasters commonly interrupt power, communication, and transportation, creating a deficit in primary care for the impacted communities. With the loss of infrastructure, primary care providers and facilities (i.e., hospitals, ambulatory centers, clinics and pharmacies) may be unable to deliver needed care to patients. This creates an *access deficit*, the gap between the ability of health care providers to deliver primary care services and the increased health care needs of the population following disasters. An access deficit might result in interruptions of treatment for dialysis and numerous unmet medical needs (e.g., asthma exacerbations, medication refills and supplemental oxygen). Continuity of care is impaired if computers and phones don't work and coordination between hospitals and community-based organizations is interrupted or temporarily impossible. Following Hurricane Sandy, many centers providing the WIC program for women, infants, and children closed because of lost infrastructure and clients couldn't get services, redeem vouchers for nutritional supplementation, or receive referrals for other services.

Identifying Need

Several strategies have been used to facilitate the continued deliver of primary care following disasters. The first type of strategy involves the use of technology. Following Hurricane Sandy, public health professionals used HAZEL (Hazard Zone Primary Care Locator; available at: http://fred.publichealth.pitt.edu/HazelWeb). HAZEL is a decision support application that was used to assess the impacted population (e.g., demographics, location, household income, type of insurance, status), storm parameters (e.g., evacuation patterns), and primary care need (e.g., primary care sites, pharmacies, chronic disease prevalence, primary care and health care utilization). This data enabled them to identify where the patient need was, match that to provider capacity and identify where there was an excess or deficit of primary care access. A second strategy is to use prehospital data as a real-time metric to measure the potential volume of patients needing care and predict what areas are most likely to have patients seeking care. Utilizing geographic information systems to map the home addresses of staff, administrators were able to identify which staff would have difficulty getting to work. By combining the population data and provider data, officials knew where likely deficits of primary care could occur. As a result, hospitals and clinics cross-trained staff and volunteers in multiple tasks and reassigned employees from closed offices to other functions. A third strategy, with the fastest and largest impact, was the deployment of mobile medical vans. These vans went to where the patents were located while increasing the capacity of individual medical offices and clinics. Finally, the uninsured can replace lost or damaged prescriptions and some durable medical equipment (DME) through the Emergency Prescription Assistance Program (EPAP). EPAP, a joint program of FEMA and the HHS, allows pharmacies to process claims for prescriptions and DME in areas with a presidential disaster declaration.

Mass Care

Just as the National Response Framework describes the federal government's role in recovery, it also details the roles of agencies and organizations, including public health, participating in or supporting the operations of shelter, or congregate care facilities in the ESF #6 Annex. ESF #6 provides guidance on the delivery of what are known as mass care services and includes mass care, emergency assistance, housing, human services, and temporary housing (available at: https://www.fema.gov/media-library-data/1470149820826-7bcf80b5dbabe158953058a6b5108e98/ESF_6_MassCare_20160705_508.pdf).

Within ESF #6, the HHS is responsible for human services, public health and medical services, and veterinary medical service. Table 13-2 details the responsibilities of HHS in the delivery of mass care under ESF #6.

Local governmental agencies, including human services and the health department, coordinate with the American Red Cross (Red Cross) and other voluntary agencies in the provision of mass care. The Red Cross, a nongovernmental organization, has primary responsibility for disaster sheltering in the United States. During presidentially declared disasters, federal agencies may provide support and coordination, in collaboration with the Red Cross. To provide direction to individuals who operate shelters in a disaster, FEMA and the Red Cross developed the *Shelter Field Guide*, with input from local and state emergency management representatives. The handbook is a comprehensive

Table 13-2. Responsibilities of Department of Health & Human Services in Mass Care Under Emergency Support Function #6

Support Agency	Actions
Department of Health & Human Services	Human Services • Executes requirements defined in the Crisis Counseling Assistance and Training Program. • Executes requirements defined in the Disaster Case Management Program, assist survivors with developing and carrying out a disaster recovery plan. • Provides subject matter expertise, consultation, and technical assistance to ESF #6 partners on disaster human services issues (e.g., accessing HHS programs that address human services needs in an emergency, effective human services delivery to children, people with disabilities and others with access and functional needs, economically disadvantaged people, and other individuals and families served by HHS programs). • Provides requested assistance to agencies that administer emergency human services programs. • Assists in the provision of medical pharmaceuticals, supplies, and services, including durable medical equipment, through the Emergency Prescription Assistance Program. • Coordinates with ESF #6 in disaster planning for human services to promote seamless transition to HHS-led Health and Social Services Recovery Support Function under the National Disaster Recovery Framework. Public Health and Medical Services • Provides HHS medical workers to augment health services personnel. • Provides medical care and mental/behavioral health services for impacted populations either in or outside the shelter locations using guidelines of local health agencies. • Provides technical assistance for shelter operations related to food, vectors, water supply, and waste disposal. • Assists in the provision of medical supplies and services, including durable medical equipment. • Coordinates requested emergency medical care in shelters using guidelines of local health agencies. • Coordinates with the National Center for Missing and Exploited Children to facilitate the expeditious reunification of children displaced as a result of disaster. • Provides technical expertise in issues related to the assessment of health and medical needs of shelter occupants. • Assists with monitoring of public health conditions that can affect the health of all shelter occupants including shelter workers. Veterinary Medical Services • Identifies and provides personnel for events requiring veterinary medical services or public health support for household pets and service animals. • Coordinates and provides emergency and disaster-related veterinary medical care services to impacted animal populations and provides veterinary public health, zoonotic disease control, environmental health, and related services.

Source: Adapted from U.S. Department of Homeland Security, Federal Emergency Management Agency (FEMA). 2016. *Emergency Support Function #6: Mass Care, Emergency Assistance, Temporary Housing, and Human Services Annex*. Washington, DC: FEMA. Available at: https://www.fema.gov/media-library-data/1470149820826-7bcf80b5dbabe158953058a6b5108e98/ESF_6_MassCare_20160705_508.pdf. Accessed January 24, 2017.

reference for setting up and managing such shelters (available at: http://www.nationalmasscarestrategy.org/wp-content/uploads/2015/10/Shelter-Field-Guide-508_f3.pdf). In addition, FEMA has a catalog of items commonly used in shelters (available at: http://www.nationalmasscarestrategy.org/wp-content/uploads/2014/07/cusi-catalog-as-of-march-2013-v2.pdf).

Public Health and Mass Care Shelters

Mass care is provided through temporary shelters, fixed or mobile feeding stations, and direct distribution of relief supplies. Local public health professionals may be involved in the following:

- Selection of the shelter site
- Organization and layout of shelter
- Assuring food safety
- Assuring adequate safe water for drinking and food preparation
- Provision of toilets, sinks for hand washing, soap, disposable towels, showers, and laundry
- Ensuring proper management of wastewater and solid waste
- Protecting indoor air quality (e.g., temperature control, humidity, odors, dust)
- Identifying and assuring general safety
- Monitoring housekeeping and cleaning
- Identifying and controlling vector- or pest-related concerns
- Monitoring outside grounds (e.g., playgrounds, debris, and physical hazards)
- Monitoring and intervening in operations of shelter (e.g., address needs of people in long lines)
- Care for pets

The Centers for Disease Control and Prevention (CDC) developed a shelter assessment tool to assist environmental health practitioners in conducting a rapid assessment of shelter conditions during emergencies and disasters. Designed as a checklist that facilitates the documentation of immediate needs in shelters, the tool covers key areas of environmental health, including status of facility structure, food safety, water quality, solid waste and sanitation, childcare and sleeping area, health/medical, and companion animals.

Shelter Specifics

While securing permanent shelter is a top priority, postimpact shelter may be provided as emergency or temporary housing. Emergency or temporary shelters should be located in a facility capable of withstanding a disaster and that has communication capabilities, power, running water, and an area to care for those who have functional needs. The ideal general population shelter would have separate zones for registering residents, conducting physical examinations, offering mental and behavioral health treatment, childcare, sleeping, eating, and recreation. All shelters must comply with state and local codes and all standards related to accessibility. When selecting a shelter location, if the chosen facility has features that are inaccessible, a plan must be in place to make the shelter accessible before use.

When establishing an emergency shelter, the Red Cross allocates 40 square feet per person for sheltering longer than 72 hours. Routes through the shelter and around cots must be accessible to people using wheelchairs, crutches, or walkers. People who use wheelchairs, lift equipment, service animals, and personal assistants can require up to 100 square feet. Accessible cots must be available. An accessible cot is 17 to 19 inches high (without a mattress) and at least 27 inches wide. It can hold 350 pounds and is constructed with flexible head and feet positioning. If the accessible cot has side rails, the rails must be movable so that a wheelchair user can access the cot. Red Cross shelters do not permit pets but do allow service animals (e.g., seeing eye or hearing dogs).

One toilet for every 20 people is recommended or a minimum of 1 toilet for every 6 people must be accessible for people with disabilities. If the shelter has only 1 toilet, it must be accessible for people with disabilities. Planners should include 1 shower for every 25 people, and a minimum of 1 shower for every 6 people must be accessible for people with disabilities. If the shelter has only 1 shower, it must be accessible for people with disabilities.

Individuals who come to shelters during disasters bring with them the breadth of health and behavioral health issues reflected in their communities. Public health and health care professionals will be asked to assess and provide care for many of these problems while these people are residents in the shelters. Table 13-3 describes common health and behavioral health issues in shelters and suggests potential solutions, and Table 13-4 provides information about the physical requirements of shelters.

Finally, shelters are responsible for feeding everyone housed there. Table 13-5 identifies key components of feeding stations.

Functional Needs Support Services

A body of federal law[2] mandates that people with disabilities have equal opportunities in disaster response and recovery, including support services for individuals with

2. Stafford Act; Post-Katrina Emergency Reform Act, Section 689; and Title VIII of the Civil Rights Act of 1968 (Fair Housing Act) as amended.

Table 13-3. Health and Behavioral Health Services in Shelters

Issue	Suggested Solutions
Common Health Issues	**Potential Solutions**
Communicable conditions (e.g., flu, lice)	Provide areas of isolation for individuals with identified infections.
Health and mental health issues	Arrange for screening and referral if required for health and mental health conditions.
Lack of medications and/or prescriptions	• Maintain current list of pharmacies near the shelter. • Ask pharmacies if they will support medication/prescription needs of the residents. • If access to a local pharmacy is not available, contact supporting agency or the local Emergency Operations Center.
Restricted dietary requirements	Accommodate the dietary needs of people with restricted diets by ensuring that alternate food is available.
Maternity	Confirm maternity delivery plans, including location.
Common Behavioral Health Issues	**Potential Solutions**
Symptoms of anxiety, anger and depression	• Promote feelings of calm and hope. • Provide accurate information about the situation. • Listen. • Make connections to support systems and resources. • Provide realistic reassurance. • Provide psychological first aid.
Preexisting behavioral health issues such as substance abuse or addiction	Ensure that access to appropriate needed medications and support services is available.
Preventing Contagious Disease Outbreaks	
Prevention	Remind residents and staff to follow proper personal hygiene.
Personal Hygiene	• Develop a personal hygiene outreach plan to ensure that the shelter population practices proper personal hygiene. • Cover mouth when coughing and sneezing. • Wash hands often with soap and warm water and use hand sanitizer. • Avoid touching eyes, nose, or mouth to prevent the spread of germs. • Try to avoid close contact with sick people. • Keep areas clean, especially living areas. • Promptly report illnesses or other medical concerns to shelter staff.

(*Continued*)

Table 13-3. (Continued)

Issue	Suggested Solutions
Food Preparation	
Prevention	Use gloves when packaging food and/or serving or handling uncooked, prepared foods. Use fresh water for consumption and in food preparation. Separate raw and cooked foods. Cook food thoroughly. Ensure that food is kept within the temperature safety zone (above 140°F or below 40°F). Follow proper hand washing procedures. Ensure that food preparation and serving surfaces and equipment are sanitized properly.
Contagious Disease Outbreak	Promote personal hygiene measures. Report any outbreak to the local public health department and the local Emergency Operations Center. Request medical assistance as necessary. Ask residents who feel they may be affected to self-report to shelter staff. With medical personnel or other agencies, identify residents who may be affected and speak with them privately. • Increase the distance between people. • When possible, place groups or families in individual rooms or in separate areas of the facility. • Place cots head-to-toe. Perform additional environmental cleaning. • Implement strategies to ensure infection prevention and control during food service. • Serve food cafeteria-style. • Pay special attention to children. • Encourage parents and caregivers to monitor children for symptoms of illness and report immediately to shelter staff. Isolate staff, residents, and their caregivers or family members if they are ill. If individual rooms are not available, designate a separate area. • Regularly and frequently clean all areas where children play, particularly items that are more likely to have frequent contact with the hands, mouths, or body fluids of children (e.g., toys).

(*Continued*)

Table 13-3. (Continued)

Issue	Suggested Solutions
	Coordinate with local health departments, hospitals, ambulance services, crisis counseling services, and local behavioral health agencies to establish their capabilities and protocols for support. Have emergency phone numbers in an easily viewable location, and make a phone available for staff and residents to call for help. Identify qualified staff that can administer first aid/CPR, and have a fully stocked first aid kit available.

Source: Based on Federal Emergency Management Agency (FEMA), American Red Cross. 2015. *Shelter Field Guide: FEMA P-785.* Washington, DC: FEMA. Available at http://www.nationalmasscarestrategy.org/wp-content/uploads/2015/10/Shelter-Field-Guide-508_f3.pdf. Accessed January 24, 2017.

Note: CPR = cardio-pulmonary resuscitation.

Table 13-4. Shelter Requirements

	Provision	Requirement
Spacing	Toilets	One toilet for every 20 people
	Showers	One shower for every 15 people
	Hand washing	One hand washing fixture with clean water for every 15 people (hand sanitizers are not a replacement for hand washing fixtures)
	Cots/beds	Minimum floor space of 30 square feet per person, spaced 3 feet apart, alternating head-to-toe
	Ventilation	40 to 50 cubic feet of air space per person
Waste management	Containers	One 30-gallon plastic container per 10 people
		Containers should have plastic liner bags and lids and be emptied daily
	Sharps container	Approved sharps containers at designated areas
		Arrange for approved medical waste transporter to collect, transport, and dispose of sharps
Food and food equipment safety	Food storage, preparation, handling, and distribution	Follow local food safety guidelines
	Dishwashing	At least 1 dishwashing machine for baby bottles, nipples, and pacifiers
	Refrigerators	Dedicate refrigerator(s) for storage of baby formulas and opened baby foods
		Equip refrigerators with thermometers and keep temperatures at or below 40°F
Housekeeping	Cleaning	All floors should be mopped or vacuumed daily
Insect and rodent control	Food	No food in sleeping areas of shelter
	Reporting	Alert staff and residents to immediately report insect or rodent sightings or droppings
	Integrated pest management program	Should be developed and implemented by pest control specialist
	Prevention	Screen all openings with at least 16 mesh screen materials and close any crawl spaces with wire mesh
Soiled linen and clothing	Hampers	Provide hampers for soiled towels and other clothing
	Procedures	Provide residents with procedures for handling soiled and clean linen (e.g., with posters in shower rooms or other strategic locations)

(*Continued*)

Table 13-4. (Continued)

	Provision	Requirement
Childcare facilities	Diaper changing	Provide posters near diaper changing stations with sanitary procedures
	Sanitary supplies	Provide sanitary wipes, disposable diaper changing pads, sanitizing solution, and hand washing facilities at each diaper changing station
	Other supplies	All lotions, creams, and ointments applied to children's skin should be dispensed from single-use containers or containers designated for use on an individual child
	Safety	All electrical outlets should be covered by protective caps or similar child safety devices
Toilet and shower facilities	Supplies	Provide soap dispensers with soap, paper towel dispensers with paper towels, and trash receptacles at hand washing stations
	Signage	Provide hand washing signs in relevant languages at hand washing stations
	Safety	Provide watertight, slip-resistant floors in all lavatories and showers
General safety	Maintenance	Follow local building code regulations
		Fire exits must comply with local fire code regulations

Source: Adapted from Golob BR. 2007. *Environmental Health Emergency Response Guide*. Hopkins, MN: Twin Cities Metro Advanced Practice Center. Available at http://www.cdc.gov/nceh/ehs/docs/eh_emergency_response_guide.pdf. Accessed January 24, 2017.

Table 13-5. Elements Needed at Mass Feeding Stations

Water supplies
Toilets for staff and others: at least 1 toilet for every 20 people
Hand washing facilities: at food handler stations and near toilets
Facilities for liquid wastes from kitchens: grease trap or strainer is a must
Facilities for solid wastes from kitchens: dispose in rubbish bins that are tightly covered
Basins, tables, chopping blocks: thoroughly disinfect with strong chlorine solution after each meal
Facilities for dishwashing: separate basins for washing, eating, and cooking
Adequate materials for cooking/refrigeration: prepare food sufficient for 1 meal
Layout to prevent cross-contamination: adequate space and separation of raw food and animal products
Adequate serving pieces: use disposables if no facilities to thoroughly wash and rinse
Control of rodents and other pests: use traps for flies, screen kitchen areas, dispose of sullage and waste; never place rodenticides on surfaces used for food preparation
Food safety information: place posters in full view by those in the food preparation areas

Source: Based on Wisner B, Adams J, eds. 2002. *Environmental Health in Emergencies and Disasters: A Practical Guide*. Box 9.2. Facilities needed at mass-feeding centres. Page 155. Geneva, Switzerland: World Health Organization.

functional needs. Historically, shelters may not have met the standards of the Americans With Disabilities Act for accessible design (28 C.F.R. Part 36), resulting in difficulties in providing appropriate care to those with access and functional needs.

FEMA issued guidelines (FEMA guidance)[3] to help communities plan to meet the access and functional needs of vulnerable populations within general population shelters. The FEMA guidance recommends activities, the so-called Functional Needs Support Services (FNSS), that change the way general population shelters have traditionally been established and operated. FNSS is defined as "services that enable children and adults to maintain their usual level of independence in general population shelters." The services include reasonable modifications to policies, procedures, and practices, and the provision of DME, consumable medical supplies (CMS), personal assistance services (PAS), and other goods and services as needed. DME is medical equipment used in the home to aid in a better quality of living and is a benefit included in most insurance plans, including Medicaid and Medicare. CMS are nondurable supplies and items that enable activities of daily living. PAS are services provided to assist children and adults with activities of daily living (e.g., bathing, eating, toileting). The regulatory foundation for FNSS is found in the Americans With Disabilities Act of 1990, the Rehabilitation Act of 1973, and the Fair Housing Act of 1968. FEMA has courses on integrating access and functional needs into emergency planning and response that provide details on implementation.

3. Federal Emergency Management Agency (FEMA). 2010. *Guidance on Planning for Integration of Functional Needs Support Services in General Population Shelters.* Washington, DC: FEMA. Available at: http://www.fema.gov/pdf/about/odic/fnss_guidance.pdf. Accessed April 10, 2017. This publication includes Guidance, Operational Tools, and Appendices.

Planning the Shelters

Public health professionals should be involved in planning for shelters because they bring skills and knowledge that can facilitate the appropriate preparations for the broadest health needs of the community. Specialized shelters that can provide medical care following a disaster are scarce resources. Where feasible, communities should plan for the integration of FNSS in general population shelters to preserve this precious medical resource for those who truly need it. With better planning, more people can be safely accommodated in general population shelters. Some elements of FNSS are already in place. Currently, the Red Cross operates a health services unit that is responsible for replacing medications and other items at general population shelters.

Even with the integration of FNSS, there will still be the need for medical shelters. The responsibility for setting up medical shelters following a disaster varies from state to state—sometimes it lies with the local health department, sometimes a private agency. Medical shelters may be colocated with general population shelters. Planners can use processes identified in Chapters 5, 6, and 11 for the estimation and identification of the medical and functional needs of a community's residents. To facilitate the development of a system to triage patients who require medical shelters when the disaster strikes, it is helpful to identify endemic medical needs in the region as part of community planning. If plans are in place when evacuation is required, officials can notify residents through emergency alerts and direct them to the appropriate shelter (medical or general population) with the supplies and resources to match their needs.

Radiation Emergencies[4]

While many communities already have plans to shelter populations in the aftermath of natural disasters (e.g., tornadoes, hurricanes, floods, and wildfires), these plans may not be adequate for caring for people in a radiation emergency. Because the displaced population in a radiation emergency is potentially contaminated with radioactive material and may be at risk for developing radiation sickness, shelter operators should anticipate modifying routine services or adopting new services to protect residents from the radiation hazard. Advance planning is needed for shelter operations in radiation emergencies. Planning should include partner agencies, such as the state radiation control authority, emergency management officials, and public health planners.

To help communities prepare, the National Center for Environmental Health at the CDC developed *A Guide to Operating Public Shelters in a Radiation Emergency*. The

4. This topic requires in-depth technical guidance that is beyond the scope of this chapter. Interested readers should consult the resources listed in the reference section for more information.

shelters discussed in this guide are long-term, public shelters that house people evacuated from an area impacted by a radiation emergency. These shelters provide the same range of services discussed elsewhere in this chapter, with the core services the same in a radiation emergency. However, additional precautions are needed to protect against radiation hazards.

Public health professionals will be involved in assessing and monitoring people potentially exposed to radiation or contaminated with radioactive material. This process, called population monitoring, will be conducted in community reception centers (CRCs). Ideally, people will process through CRCs and receive screening for contamination, decontamination, registration, and limited medical evaluation and care before reporting to shelters. However, there may be situations in which CRCs are not available and special considerations will be needed to ensure the health and safety of shelter residents and staff in a radiation emergency. The CDC document provides guidance on the planning, operating, or working at shelters during a radiation emergency.

Planning for Functional Needs Support Services

When planning for the integration of FNSS in general population shelters, communities should coordinate with stakeholders, including the following:

- Individuals requiring FNSS
- Agencies and organizations that provide FNSS
- Advocates for FNSS
- Providers of DME, CMS, PAS, and communication services

These stakeholders can help identify the types of DME and CMS that may require emergency replacement. Table 13-6 lists typical DME and CMS items.

FEMA recommends that planning includes arrangements for a credentialed team that assesses the needs of children and adults who have access or functional needs when they arrive at a shelter. The Functional Assessment Service Team (FAST)[5] is a program developed in California that determines what resources are necessary to support identified needs in a general population shelter and enable them to maintain their independence. FAST members may come from governmental agencies or community-based organizations that have broad experience working with individuals with disabilities. FAST members should be knowledgeable about the services required and the vendors who can supply the needs of this population quickly. Memorandums of understanding should be established in advance with the individuals or organizations that will participate in FAST.

5. FAST is a California-only model. More information can be found online (at: http://www.cdss.ca.gov/dis/PG1909.htm). Another model is used in Louisiana through their Louisiana Volunteers in Action (LAVA) program (information available at: https://www.lava.dhh.louisiana.gov).

Table 13-6. Typical Durable Medical Equipment and Consumable Medical Supplies

Durable Medical Equipment	Consumable Medical Supplies
Blood glucose monitors	Blood-testing strips
CPAP machines	Bandages and dressings
Crutches	Catheters and electrodes
Hospital beds	Forceps
Knee braces	Gloves
Orthotics and prosthetic devices	Plasters and bandage grips
Oxygen tents	Swabs
Nebulizers	Syringes and needles
Walkers	Wooden tongue depressors
Wheelchairs	

Note: CPAP=continuous positive airway pressure.

FEMA guidelines also direct the staffing patterns in shelters. General population shelters include assistants for personal care, communications support for those with hearing or visual impairments, and translators. Shelters should prepare to track the numerous providers who may deliver services. The list includes the following:

- Communication (e.g., interpreters, computer services, and text telephones)
- FNSS equipment (e.g., DME and CMS)
- Food services (including special diets)
- Medical staffing (e.g., on-site nursing, dental, pharmaceutical)
- Personal assistance (e.g., basic personal care and activities of daily living)
- Resource suppliers (e.g., blood sugar monitoring, dialysis, oxygen, power source)
- Service animals (e.g., veterinarians)
- Transportation (e.g., paratransit)

To care for those who arrive at a shelter without DME, supplies, or medications but who need them, planners should arrange for the provision and maintenance of equipment and supplies through memorandums of understanding. The list should include the needs of children and adults with and without disabilities who have access and functional needs. Appendices 3 and 4 of the FEMA guidance provide a sample list of the estimated DME and CMS needed in a shelter for 100 people for 1 week.

Medications

State and local laws differ about the storage, preparation, administration, documentation, and disposal of medications. Planners should consult with state and local authorities to determine if and how they can obtain, store, and dispense medications in a general

Table 13-7. Medication Considerations in General Population Shelters

Procedure or Program	Considerations
Filling prescriptions	Chain pharmacies may have information about a shelter resident's medications in a centralized site away from the disaster location
Storage	Residents are usually responsible for safeguarding, storing, and administering their own medication If refrigeration is needed or residents can't self-medicate, keep prescription medications in locked container used only for storing medications at first aid station
Disposal	All medications kept at first aid station should be returned to residents at discharge Needles or hypodermic syringes with needles attached must be disposed of in biohazard containers
Emergency Preparedness Assistance Program, a joint program of Federal Emergency Management Agency and the Department of Health & Human Services	Provides a 30-day supply of pharmaceuticals and DME lost in disaster, or lost or damaged in transit to the designated shelter facility Permits pharmacies to process claims for prescription medications and limited DME for uninsured individuals from area with a presidential disaster declaration

Source: Adapted from Federal Emergency Management Agency (FEMA). 2010. *Guidance on Planning for Integration of Functional Needs Support Services in General Population Shelters.* Washington, DC: FEMA. Available at: http://www.fema.gov/pdf/about/odic/fnss_guidance.pdf. Accessed January 24, 2017.
Note: DME=durable medical equipment.

population shelter. To ensure that shelter residents have access to medications, agreements should be established with pharmacies to supply needed medications to shelters. Table 13-7 describes key medication considerations in general population shelters.

Medical Shelters

Disaster victims who cannot be evacuated to a general population shelter include those with certain health or medical conditions, such as an infectious disease requiring isolation, a serious injury, or intensive postsurgical care. Although community planning may vary, patients for whom a dedicated shelter is appropriate may include those who require infusion therapy, complex sterile dressing changes, hyperalimentation, intensive care, or life support equipment. Medically complex, unstable, and terminally ill patients with "do not resuscitate" orders should be cared for in a hospital-level setting where possible.

For these patients, communities may choose to continue establishing plans for alternative care facilities referred to as *medical shelters.* These facilities may be associated with a hospital so that requiring medical management but not hospital-level care can be safely housed. Bedridden and total-care patients who go to medical shelters must bring a responsible caregiver and not actually require a hospital bed. Medical shelters are generally intended to operate for a limited period (1 to 4 days). Plans should detail how bedridden patients will be moved if additional evacuation is necessary (e.g., using flatbed trucks).

For patients needing the services provided in medical shelters, public health officials are advised to make arrangements with providers and hospitals as part of global community planning. In the event of natural disasters such as hurricanes, earthquakes, and tornadoes, hospitals may be damaged or may receive large numbers of severely injured patients, necessitating the discharge of stable medical patients and the inability to handle medical patients whose conditions have become acute.

Protocols and Procedures

Communities should establish protocols for staff assistance and procedures for triage, supportive care, and universal precautions (e.g., no smoking, proper handling of body fluids and medical waste, continuous monitoring of patients by caregivers). Nurses and other staff at medical shelters can offer supportive care while patients and their caregivers manage routine needs. Caregivers focus on helping with activities of daily living, administering medications, and providing oxygen and other medical support. Medical shelter nurses offer supervision and assistance, if needed, when patients or caregivers assume responsibility for their own procedures.

The community plan must anticipate medical staffing requirements, including the types of personnel (e.g., medical director, nurses, emergency medical technicians, social workers, and support staff), credentialing process, scheduling, and on-site recruitment, registration, and supervision of volunteers. Plans for medical shelters must ensure cultural and linguistic competence among staff members. Protocols must be established for admitting and registering patients and caregivers and for acquiring and storing supplies. Staff members must be capable of handling a range of medical and nursing requirements, including labor in pregnant women, violent situations, and deaths. Procedures for closing down the medical shelter and relocating patients as needed must be established as part of the overall plan.

Dialysis Centers

Individuals who require dialysis need to know what to do in an emergency. Dialysis centers should develop a plan for each patient. This plan should include prepared statements or messages that communicate the circumstances that make the centers unavailable to provide care. Centers should provide the names, locations, and contact information for available treatment facilities. Finally, if no other dialysis centers are operating, patients should receive detailed directions on the procedures they should follow to stretch the time before another dialysis treatment is needed.

CHAPTER 14

EVALUATION METHODS FOR ASSESSING PUBLIC HEALTH AND MEDICAL RESPONSE TO DISASTERS

Evaluating disaster response is essential for preparedness planning. In this chapter, we review the fundamental principles involved in the assessment of disaster plans and the development of tools to evaluate both plans and response, and introduce a newly developed framework for evaluating disaster research.

Public Health Role

- Conduct assessments of planning and emergency response to provide continuing feedback to improve an organization or community's preparedness.
- Conduct systematic reviews of public health and medical aspects of disaster response to improve the reduction of morbidity and mortality.
- Use professionally recognized measures of process and outcome to monitor public health and medical programs and to direct resources in all phases of disaster response and recovery.
- Use information revealed through evaluation to make decisions about a community's emergency management needs or improve future response.
- Determine whether emergency plans and disaster response are effective and efficient.

Evaluation in Disasters

Emergency management has traditionally been a response-oriented field. As a result, advancements in practice do not often come from scientific evaluation. Emergency preparedness and response have improved through analysis of what are known as *after action reports,* application of institutional knowledge, establishment of guidelines and protocols, and self-initiation by thinking "it *can* happen to me."

Despite the nature of any particular disaster, there are numerous and similar challenges in conducting disaster research. During a disaster, there is a small window of time to identify, collect, and analyze critical and time-sensitive data necessary to protect the health and safety of first responders and communities. Most fields advance by incorporating scientific evidence of what works. In emergency response, one cannot evaluate how well things have gone or identify areas for improvement through experimentation, such as through the use of case-control studies. Evaluation of disaster response cannot use scientific methods for data collection or analysis unless assessment teams are in place with prepared methods and instruments because the exact timing of most disasters cannot be predicted. Because public health is a science-based field, public health principles can be applied to the evaluation of disaster preparedness and response in a manner that will advance both practice and policy.

Unfortunately, scientific evidence on the health and public health impacts of a disaster tends to accumulate slowly, long after the events have ended. Further, regardless of methodology, the quality of initial data is frequently flawed and conflicting across studies. In contrast, the process and timeline for policy formation in response to a disaster often involves rapid decision making to address immediate and long-term needs, as seen in the prompt passage of federal legislation following the flawed response to Hurricane Katrina and the expansive needs caused by Hurricane Sandy. Because policy decisions can have a major impact on the pace of recovery and service delivery, public health professionals face the dual challenges of generating quality evidence on the burden and causes of health outcomes in a timely fashion and keeping policy makers abreast of what is known and not known over time.

Due to the importance of data and assessments in improving disaster response, evaluation has a direct impact on policy development both pre- and post-event. The Pandemic and All-Hazards Preparedness Act of 2006 mandated that research centers conduct evaluations to improve public health preparedness and response. Preparedness and Emergency Response Research Centers (PERRCs) were established at designated schools of public health in 2008. The PERRCs continue to conduct critical research to develop evaluation methods, metrics, and modeling approaches that can be used to both measure a community's capabilities and inform planning to minimize variability in how systems perform in the future.

Evaluation Methods

Evaluation has several purposes, the most fundamental of which is to determine the extent to which an organization, program, or unit achieves its clearly stated and measurable objectives in responding to a disaster. Evaluations are used to adjust disaster plans, focus practice drills and preparedness, improve planning for rapid assessment and management of daily response operations, provide input for the refinement of measures of effectiveness, and collect data for hypothesis-driven research. Evaluations often provide objective information for managers to formulate and revise policy through a retrospective and descriptive design for capturing information. Administrators can improve their management of health care systems affected by disasters by drawing information systematically from a variety of sources. For example, collecting information from broad categories of personnel and lay informants could be used in lieu of probability sampling.

Disaster evaluation research seeks to obtain information that can be used in preparation for future disasters by:

- Developing profiles of victims and types of injuries to inform the revision of existing or preparation of enhanced disaster plans (e.g., disaster epidemiology).
- Assessing whether program adjustments can reduce disability and save lives (e.g., effectiveness of community collaborations).
- Determining whether better methods to organize and manage a response exist, including the use of resources in a relief effort (i.e., effectiveness of Incident Command Systems and Emergency Operations Center, improvements in drills and exercises, and reaching diverse audiences with critical information about emergencies).
- Determining best practices (e.g., effectiveness of preparedness and emergency response systems, improvements in training).
- Identifying measures that can be implemented to reduce harm to communities and residents (e.g., communications to at-risk populations).
- Assessing the long-term physical and emotional effects of a disaster on individuals and communities (e.g., ability to prepare for and respond to behavioral health needs of victims and responders).

Evaluations should examine the structure of the public health and health care system's response to the disaster, the allocation of medical and public health resources, the sequence of events, the impact of the program at each stage, issues that arose during the public health and health care system's response to the disaster, the limitations of the response, and policy lessons. Key steps in developing and implementing an evaluation plan[1] include:

- Defining goals of what is being evaluated
- Selecting measures
- Determining how the data will be collected
- Collecting and reviewing the data

Designing Evaluation Studies

A structured evaluation, which might look at preparedness activities and how participants carry them out or the capacity to conduct rapid surveillance, must begin before the

1. Adapted from RAND Corporation 2010. *Enhancing Public Health Emergency Preparedness for Special Needs Populations: A Toolkit for State and Local Planning and Response*. Chapter 8. Arlington, VA: RAND Corp. Available at: http://www.rand.org/pubs/technical_reports/2009/RAND_TR681.pdf. Accessed January 24, 2017.

disaster occurs. If evaluating a disaster response, the evaluators would assess elements of the response, such as equipment needs, strategies for medical and public health interventions, and the chain of command among participating response organizations. Internal and external communication methods and participants should also be examined. All personnel who participate in disaster response must be evaluated for the timing and execution of duties in relation to their planned assignments and actual implementation in the field.

Define Goals and Measures

Evaluations begin by reviewing the plan for disaster response and its measurable objectives. Without measurable objectives, a disaster response plan cannot be evaluated. To ensure accurate measurement, the first step is to identify the core outcome that is desired. For example, when evaluating a center that is distributing mass vaccination, the focus of the evaluation might be the efficiency of operations (i.e., how many people received vaccination per hour), the communication during operations (i.e., what types of methods were used to communicate with individuals who are visually or hearing impaired), or the actual distribution process (i.e., actions taken to prepare, vaccinate, and discharge).

Once the specific goals are defined, determining how to measure them is the next important step. Continuing with the previous example, to measure how many people received vaccination per hour, each consent form could be time stamped. Other goals could result in requiring users to sign a log to collect information about the equipment or using navigators or interpreters to communicate with individuals who are visually or hearing impaired. The distribution process for vaccination could be described through interviews at each step. The key is to follow the principles of research methods as vigorously as possible given the events.

Data Collection

During the impact and postimpact phases of a disaster, a record of important medical, environmental, and social events is usually created and searchable in journalistic features, photographs, videos, official records, recollections of participants, and other reports. To study these events, information must be obtained from a variety of informants, documents, and records. Thorough preplanning of the evaluation is essential to ensure that the evaluation will yield valid findings. Multidisciplinary teams must design studies, collect data, and interpret the findings. A typical postimpact team consists of a physician, emergency medical services specialist, social or behavioral scientist, epidemiologist, and disaster management specialist. This research team should hold daily debriefings to discuss issues and problems related to the implementation of the evaluation protocol.

Although record keeping during a disaster is difficult and gaps in the record will often occur, some written accounting on a case-by-case basis is usually available. Public health officials can look for data in hospital e-codes, electronic health records, emergency department records, field station logs, and autopsy reports. Impressions of patient treatment can be made by reviewing available patient records, supplemented by interview data. Other sources of evaluation data include journalistic accounts and interviews with injured survivors, public health and medical professionals, search and rescue personnel, relief workers, lay bystanders, and disaster managers.

For interviews, a series of questions designed to probe the effectiveness of the disaster relief operation can be incorporated into an administered questionnaire. In such a questionnaire, questions should be structured, calling for a fixed response, although a small number of open-ended questions can provide useful information. In addition, medical record abstract forms can be used to collect hospital and autopsy data. The data should be validated by cross-checking multiple sources.

Conducting an Evaluation

In the process of conducting an evaluation, assessments are directed for five domains of activity: structure, process, outcomes, response adequacy, and costs.[2] The following sections describe each domain and provide sample questions that might be asked in order to evaluate the response to a disaster involving a large number of casualties.

Structure

Evaluation of structure examines how the medical and public health response was organized, what resources were needed, and what resources were available. Questions used to evaluate structure for the response to mass casualty incidents may include the following:

- Were ambulances, hospital emergency departments, and critical care units sufficiently equipped and supplied to meet the demands of the disaster?
- Were sufficient numbers of properly trained staff available, especially volunteers, first responders, ambulance personnel, emergency department nurses, critical care physicians, and communications staff?

2. The Agency for Healthcare Research and Quality provides a model to evaluate hospital disaster drills designed to identify specific weaknesses that can be improved to strengthen hospital preparedness (available at: https://archive.ahrq.gov/prep/drillelements).

- Did staff receive prior training in methods specific to the provision of public health and medical care during a disaster?
- Did the communications system have sufficient capacity, flexibility, and backup capabilities during the disaster for both internal and external communications?
- How were patients transported to the hospital? To what extent was the ambulance system overloaded? What equipment shortages were experienced?
- How well did the following functions operate during the impact and postimpact phases: resource management (e.g., dispatch, coordination with emergency medical services and public services), medical supervision, and communication among hospitals, mobile units, and other services?

Process

Process assessments identify how the system (both medical and public health components) functioned during the impact and postimpact, how well individuals were prepared, and what problems occurred. The process questions should be sorted into those that probe the operation of the disaster response system and those that assess the process of treating patients. Process questions to ask for a mass casualty incident include the following:

- Were medical staff available during the search and rescue of patients? How soon after the response was initiated did they arrive?
- Did medical staff trained in detection and extrication possess the skills and knowledge required to perform their functions during the disaster?
- Were medical staff trained in detection and extrication able to apply their medical knowledge under disaster conditions? What factors, if any, prevented optimum performance?
- How effectively was the triage function performed? What, if any, factors interfered?
- Was there adequate control over the management and deployment of resources during the postimpact response? Was responsibility for decision making clear? Were appropriate decisions made concerning the process of patient triage, transfer, and treatment?
- What first aid was provided to victims, by whom, and when? Was this appropriate and effective?
- How were patients transferred from the scene of the disaster to treatment sites?
- Did effective coordination and communication among agencies occur?
- How did the hospital respond to the volume of patients?
- How did volunteers function? Was their participation supportive, or did it interfere with the treatment of patients? What controls, if any, were exercised?
- Did any compromises in standard medical care occur? Were these compromises necessary and acceptable?

- Was the public prepared to act appropriately when the disaster occurred? Should the plan to provide public education and information be modified to facilitate a future public health or medical response?

Outcomes

Outcomes assessments identify what was and was not achieved as a result of the medical and public health response. This assessment focuses on the impact of care provided to patients during the disaster. Outcome assessment can be achieved using either implicit (understood or implied) or explicit (specifically stated) criteria through a review of patient records. If implicit standards and criteria are used, a panel of critical care and emergency care specialists can review a sample of patient records and make judgments about the appropriateness of treatment related to patient outcomes. If explicit standards and criteria are employed, the reviewer uses written guidelines to determine the adequacy of treatment. Forms for summarizing patient treatment and outcome data should be developed well in advance of their use, and evaluated for completeness once filled out. Data to be collected should include, at a minimum, the following:

- Personal characteristics of patient (e.g., age, sex, residence)
- Medical condition/status prior to injury
- Principal diagnosis, secondary diagnosis, type of injury
- Body location of injury (e.g., extremities, back, chest, head, neck, abdomen)
- Whether (and what) prehospital care was provided and by whom
- Method of transportation to hospital
- Hospital treatment provided
- Patient status on discharge
- Cause of death, if applicable

Response Adequacy

Assessing the adequacy of the disaster response examines the extent to which the responding systems were able to meet the needs of the community during the disaster. The analysis of the adequacy of the response is valuable in planning for future disasters. The main concern is, *overall, how much death and disability occurred that could have been prevented?* To assess this dimension of the response for a mass casualty incident, information should be obtained about the following:

- Were responders able to rescue vulnerable patients so that they could get needed care?

- To what extent was the prehospital system able to function as designed?
- What types of victims were cared for and what types were the hospital and prehospital systems unable to treat? For what reasons?
- How many victims were transported to more than one hospital because of limitations in hospital beds, intensive care beds, supplies, or staff?
- How effectively did hospitals cooperate to distribute patients to share the burden of treatment and to refer patients in need to specialty care?

Costs

Disaster response costs can be measured in several ways: the total cost of the relief effort, the cost per each life saved, the cost for various subsystems that operated during the response phase, and the costs of preparedness. Questions to ask include the following:

- What were each of the previously defined costs?
- What portion did the state pay? The federal government? The local community?
- How well did the local community capture reimbursable costs?
- Did the cost of the program correlate with the benefits to the community?

Science Preparedness: A New Approach to Evaluation

The extensiveness of public health impacts following Hurricane Sandy, which struck 24 states and the entire Eastern Seaboard in October 2012, motivated a new approach to evaluations of disaster effects and response. The Office of the Assistant Secretary for Preparedness and Response (ASPR), the Centers for Disease Control and Prevention, and the National Institute of Environmental Health Sciences (NIEHS) joined together to make funding for disaster research available in a new science preparedness program. (More information is available at: www.phe.gov/sciencepreparedness.) The science preparedness program provides a framework for conducting scientific research before, during, or after a disaster. This approach encourages building a strong foundation of knowledge about disasters based on evidence to support decision making and policy development that can guide recovery and future preparedness efforts.

The Need for Science Preparedness

Evidenced-based decision making requires the identification, collection, and analysis of critical and time-sensitive data in order to protect the health and safety of first responders and communities. Science preparedness provides the mechanisms necessary to characterize the response and collect critical information for such scientific analysis and evidence-based decision making. Through science preparedness, public health and community leaders are equipped with evidence-based information to make important short- and long-term decisions regarding community health and safety. Preparedness and response will be strengthened through the integration of scientific research in disaster management because based on expanding evidence, activities will be geared toward those populations that data show need them the most.

When a disaster occurs, there is only a small window of time to get organized and secure the data. During the January 2010 earthquake in Haiti, real-time collection and analysis of data would have allowed for the development of timely clinical guidelines to treat complex fractures in resource-strained environments. Such data may have led to improved patient outcomes. In addition, lacking the essential infrastructure has implications for post-disaster research. The events surrounding the nuclear leak following the massive Japanese earthquake and tsunami in 2011 drove the United States to assess its capability to respond to a similar event. The analysis underscored that the United States had a limited number of experts in radiation exposure, limited laboratory capacity to manage radiation disasters, and inconsistent guidelines on the use of potassium iodide. The ability to do this important review was hindered by their needing to start from scratch with the elements necessary to complete it. Lacking a pre-prepared roster of experts, identification of knowledge gaps, and research that is pre-integrated into the protocols for response would make research about a similar event in the United States a challenge.

Current efforts are underway to enable the rapid expansion of available evidence. The first initiative facilitates the ability to conduct research rapidly. An effective response to public health emergencies or disasters requires the speedy collection of data to assess the impact on individuals, populations, and communities. All research requires both compliance with federal protections for human subjects and approval by an institutional review board (IRB) before investigators can begin field work. This process does not normally happen immediately when an investigator wants to conduct a study. A rapid IRB evaluation and approval process during a public health emergency can play a critical role in advancing evidence-based decision making while protecting the health and safety of people who volunteer to participate in the studies. The Public Health Emergency Research Review Board (PHERRB) is a specialized IRB established under the auspices of the National Institutes of Health (NIH) to carry out ethical reviews of research protocols involving human subjects during public health emergencies. PHERRB-reviewed protocols are conducted, supported, or regulated by the U.S. Department of Health & Human Services and subject to 45 C.F.R. § 46 and/or 21 C.F.R. §§ 50 and 56. Through this central IRB, investigators can work on multicenter studies. In addition, the ASPR is creating a dataset so investigators do not have to start from scratch.

The second group of initiatives involves the infrastructure for conducting research. The NIH introduced the Disaster Research Response Project (DR2) in 2015. Developed by NIEHS and the National Library of Medicine (NLM), DR2 is a pilot project creating a system for disaster research consisting of a network of trained research responders and the tools to collect real-time data. In addition, the NLM Disaster Lit Web site offers a central repository for data collection tools and research protocols (available at: http://dr2.nlm.nih.gov/tools-resources). NIEHS is also developing an Intramural Fast Data Collection Team that will be mobilized in a disaster to collect baseline epidemiology data and biospecimens, using preexisting IRB-approved protocols.

Science Preparedness Methods

The approach of science preparedness is similar to traditional evaluation methods used in disaster research and discussed in this chapter. The science preparedness framework provides the basic components required to build a robust examination of disasters, based on the scientific rules of investigation. Unlike more traditional evaluation methods, science preparedness is distinguished by its collaborative effort to establish and sustain a research framework, based on scientific procedures. Incorporating a research framework enables emergency planners, responders and communities to better prepare for, respond to, and recover from major public health disasters because they will have real-time data about what works, who needs services most, and what might have been previously overlooked because of lack of information. Further, science preparedness describes how to operationalize each component (see Table 14-1).

Science preparedness is not a practice in and of itself. Rather, science preparedness is a system with 5 core elements:

- **Coordination and Integration:** Leverages a "whole community" and an "all-hazards" approach to bring together the scientific research, public health, and emergency management communities. Science preparedness encourages government agencies, private sector, academic institutions, and community organizations to collaborate in conducting studies. Further, it provides a forum for improving the preparedness, response, and recovery efforts of public health and medical professionals through communication, coordination, and the incorporation of the findings.
- **Scientific Research:** Access to accurate, timely, and reliable information is critical to improving health outcomes and saving lives following a disaster. The advancement of scientific research enables researchers to operate within a limited time period and to identify, collect, and analyze critical and time-sensitive data that may only be available during or immediately after the event.
- **Research Infrastructure:** The existence of a solid infrastructure to conduct research is the foundation of science preparedness and is critical to carrying out

scientific studies in advance of, during, and after disasters. Major components of the research infrastructure include rapid IRB approval, a pool of scientific researchers and research networks identified in advance, pre-scripted research protocols and data collection tools, and reliable and accessible data sources.

- **Public Health Practice:** Federal, state, and local public health agencies routinely collect and analyze health data to perform a number of activities including surveillance, outbreak and exposure investigations, community health assessments, and population-based clinical care. The types of activities conducted by public health professionals during an emergency response are often characterized as public health practice and nonresearch because these activities are intended to address and ameliorate an immediate health or medical issue. Such public health practice areas (e.g., public health preparedness, epidemiology, environmental health, and occupational health and safety) are key participants in science preparedness because these domains are the core areas where scientific evidence can inform future policies and practice.
- **Emergency Management:** Science preparedness is the critical component needed to align and integrate applied measures of effectiveness and scientific research efforts into a community's preparedness, response and recovery efforts as required in the National Planning Frameworks (i.e., National Response Framework, and National Disaster Recovery Framework).

Table 14-1. Components of a Robust Science Response

Components	Making It Operational
Listed experts in research design, technology, and topical areas of concern	Identify experts and include on roster; experts are on "ready reserve" to be contacted in case their expertise in required in a disaster
Scientific research integrated into response plans	Ensure that scientific research is a formal component of planning documents and incident command structure
Identification of knowledge gaps and research questions	Explicitly review, prioritize, and recommend which research to pursue
Generic and scenario-specific templates and protocols	Develop preapproved core survey documents; pre-scripted clinical protocols; minimum dataset
Rapid-review mechanism for human subjects research	Advance approval, national review board for emergencies
Rapid funding	Implement administrative mechanism to enable receipt of funding
Registries and networks for studies	Pre-prepared registries of incidents
Involvement of impacted communities	Establish mechanism to directly engage community to discuss concerns and share findings

Source: Reprinted with permission from Institute of Medicine. 2015. Science preparedness: conducting research during public health emergencies. *Enabling Rapid and Sustainable Public Health Research During Disasters: Summary of a Joint Workshop by the Institute of Medicine and the U.S. Department of Health and Human Services*. Washington, DC: The National Academies Press. 13.

CHAPTER 15

ETHICAL CONSIDERATIONS IN PUBLIC HEALTH EMERGENCIES

Why are ethics important in times of emergencies? The ethical implications of how public health services are delivered during disaster response and recovery need to be considered to avoid serious consequences for society. Our ability to provide the fairest treatment may be hindered if ethical decisions are not determined before an emergency occurs. Failure in ensuring ethical considerations when establishing these processes can lead to the loss of public trust, confusion about roles and responsibilities, low staff morale, and unnecessary loss of life. The continuing disruption of many victims' lives following Hurricane Sandy exemplifies the shortcoming of a lack of ethical planning. Further, the recent tenth anniversary of Hurricane Katrina highlighted the long-term individual and community impact of a lack in ethical planning.

Public Health Role

- Understand the decision areas where ethical principles should be incorporated into preparedness and response activities.
- Collaborate with ethicists in identifying potential issues and applying ethical principles in determining the criteria used in the planning and response phases of a disaster.
- Balance the limitation of individual freedom with doing the greatest good for the larger community.
- Communicate regularly with community partners to build trust to ensure acceptance of necessary decisions.

The Ethical Dilemma

Historically, disasters have had a more catastrophic impact on developing countries where infrastructure is poor or nonexistent and resources are not always well organized. For those countries, international preparedness to care for vulnerable populations is commonplace. We saw the importance of an ethical international response when the rapid spread of the Ebola virus disease quickly overwhelmed local health care resources, and the region relied on outside humanitarian efforts to curtail the epidemic.

As natural disasters have had an increasingly catastrophic effect on at-risk populations in the United States, our nation has been confronted with the necessity of ethical planning. During the aftermath of Hurricane Katrina and the subsequent flooding, the elderly and the poor were disproportionately affected by this tragic storm. Although planners had evacuation plans for the region, many elderly and poor residents lacked the resources to vacate the coastal regions before the hurricane struck land. The elderly, who are often frail, isolated, or afraid to leave everything they own, accounted for nearly half of the deaths due to the storm and its aftermath.

Although the federal government has developed stockpiles of pharmaceuticals and medical supplies (see Chapters 3 and 11) and has organized the capacity to create a surge in workforce, it is likely that the availability of medical personnel, equipment, and supplies will be limited in a catastrophic natural disaster or highly infectious pandemic disease. Limited resources could result in some individuals receiving care and others not. Without planning that has carefully deliberated the ethical considerations of providing care, public health workers may find themselves forced to deny treatment to patients without guidance, policy, or protocol in the middle of an emergency response. The ethical dilemmas faced by medical personnel, in the post-Katrina flooding, who found themselves providing care without adequate resources in isolated health care facilities is an example of what professionals must grapple with in the absence of protocols.

In order to assure public safety, public health professionals may have to make difficult decisions that affect individuals but benefit the community, region, or country. As example, clinical decision making by triage during an emergency is based on the principle of the common good—what is best for the greatest number of individuals. Those who are affected are more likely to cooperate if they know that public health workers' actions are based on ethical principles. Good planning may minimize the need for tough choices if adequate resources and effective arrangements are in place before a disaster strikes. Even with good planning, using ethical principles to predetermine the criteria that will be used in any triage process and having a protocol to follow, can relieve individual workers from the burden of making these decisions while trying to deliver care.

Developing an ethical framework as part of a community's emergency response plan can:

- Improve the quality and management of care during a surge of patients requiring medical care.
- Establish a uniform and fair allocation of resources.
- Minimize legal liability for providers.
- Increase clinician compliance with triage protocols.

What Are the Ethical Principles That Apply to Emergencies?

Preparing for emergencies has inherent ethical goals, including the protection of the lives and health of those impacted. To accomplish these goals during a disaster, it may be necessary to limit the individual freedom inherent in U.S. culture in order to do the most good for the community. Response to public health emergencies often requires the setting of priorities, rationing of supplies or care, and triage of the services to be performed. Any of these may necessitate the use of coercive measures that override individual liberty and property rights.

The Humanitarian Charter, first drafted in 1997 by a group of nongovernmental organizations (NGOs) and the International Red Cross and Red Crescent, identified minimum standards for disaster assistance. This guidance is based on principles of international humanitarian law, international human rights law, refugee law, and the Code of Conduct for the International Red Cross and Red Crescent and NGOs in Disaster Relief (available at: http://www.ifrc.org/Docs/idrl/I259EN.pdf). The core principles assert that populations impacted by disaster have the right to protection and assistance. As emergency planners have come to understand that disasters disproportionately affect those who are most vulnerable and that the poorest communities may need help the most because they have fewer resources, it is particularly important that planning includes special consideration for at-risk populations. It is also essential to recognize the differing needs of at-risk groups, to understand how they are affected in different disaster contexts, and to formulate a response accordingly.

Public Health Principles

Public health ethics are based on a set of principles that will ensure fairness and respect for all individuals even when it is necessary to adopt utilitarian methods during an emergency. One of the first principles for ethical practice in public health were codified by the Public Health Leadership Society in 2002 following a "town hall" assembly at the 2000 American Public Health Association Annual Meeting in Boston, Massachusetts. Many of the highlighted values are delineated in a document called *Principles of Public Health Ethics* and are applicable during a public health emergency. Table 15-1 describes some of these ethical principles and how each applies to public health emergencies.

Ethical goals for public health response were developed in 2008 when the Ethics Subcommittee of the Advisory Committee to the Director at the Centers for Disease

Table 15-1. The Application of Ethics to Public Health Emergencies

Ethical Principle	Impact/Action in Emergencies
Prevent adverse health outcomes by addressing fundamental causes of disease	Emergencies can disrupt and destroy the protective barriers that ensure health.
Respect the rights of individuals in the community	Public health response should be equitable in a public health emergency. Restrictions should be necessary, relevant, and proportional.
Ensure input from community members in development and evaluation of policies, programs, and priorities	Solidarity and trust are essential in ethical response, such as in vetting an emergency response plan with the community. For example, the U.S. Department of Health & Human Services conducted town hall meetings when developing vaccine allocation guidelines.
Ensure that basic resources and conditions necessary for health are accessible to all, including disenfranchised community members	Apply fairness principle by ensuring that preparedness and response activities reach all who are affected.
Provide information needed for decisions on policies or programs	Actions that impinge on liberty may be required but should be clearly explained.
Conduct public health actions in a timely manner with information and resources at hand	Ethical decisions can be made in an emergency with limited information when a delay in additional information can lead to greater harm.
Incorporate a variety of approaches that anticipate and respect diverse values, beliefs, and cultures in the community	In an emergency, public health agencies need to communicate with all who live in the impacted area.
Protect the confidentiality of information	Individual privacy may be compromised during emergency conditions.
Build the public's trust and the institution's effectiveness through collaboration and affiliation	Confidence in the choice being made requires transparency and careful communication.

Source: Based on Public Health Leadership Society. 2002. *Principles of the Ethical Practice of Public Health.* Version 2.2. Washington, DC: American Public Health Association. Available at: https://nnphi.org/wp-content/uploads/2015/08/PHLSposter-95321.pdf. Accessed January 24, 2017.

Control and Prevention (CDC) released a white paper titled "Ethical Guidance for Public Health Emergency Preparedness and Response." In the document, the subcommittee outlined 7 ethical targets that should guide both the content of preparedness plans and the process by which they are created, updated, and implemented in disaster situations. The 7 ethical goals are:

- **Harm reduction and benefit promotion:** Disaster preparedness activities should protect public safety, health, and well-being. They should minimize the extent of death, injury, disease, disability, and suffering during and after an emergency.
- **Equal liberty and human rights:** Disaster preparedness activities should be designed to respect the equal liberty, autonomy, and dignity of all people.
- **Distributive justice:** Disaster preparedness activities should be conducted so as to ensure that the benefits and burdens imposed on the population by emergency response measures and mitigations are shared equitably and fairly.
- **Public accountability and transparency:** Disaster preparedness activities should be based on and incorporate decision making processes that are inclusive, transparent and encourage public trust.
- **Community resiliency and empowerment:** A principal goal of disaster preparedness should be to develop resilient, as well as safe communities. Disaster preparedness activities should strive toward the long-term goal of developing community resources that will make them more hazard-resistant and allow them to recover appropriately and effectively after emergencies. Resilient communities have robust internal support systems and networks of mutual assistance and solidarity. They also maintain sustainable and risk mitigating relationships with their local ecosystems and their natural environment.
- **Public health professionalism:** Disaster preparedness activities should recognize the special obligations of certain public health professionals and promote competency of and coordination among these professionals.
- **Responsible civic response:** Disaster preparedness activities should promote a sense of personal responsibility and citizenship.

Making Ethical Decisions

Judgments that determine the deployment and allocation of resources are made both in preparation for and in response to disasters. Public health professionals are trained to take actions that reduce harm and promote the health and safety of communities and inherently understand how ethical principles are incorporated into preparedness and response activities. Seven tasks identified by the University of North Carolina Gillings School of Global Public Health highlight the decision areas in which ethical considerations should be incorporated. The tasks where ethics should be considered include:

- **Coordination and collaboration:** Responders from diverse professional backgrounds, whose motivation and perception of the tasks may conflict, need to work together in a regional response. Use of the National Incident Management System reduces the opportunity for ethical differences by establishing a clear and mutual understanding of how services will be organized and delivered.
- **Decision making:** While some response activities are planned, the unpredictability of events results in decisions being made in real time and reality may not be anything like what was expected. As a result, those in charge determine priorities, policies, and protocols in an accelerated time frame and a course of action may be determined without the best or necessary information.
- **Protection and response of emergency responders:** Disaster response can be dangerous work. Employers have an ethical duty not to put responders in danger, both physically and psychologically, yet health workers have a duty to provide care, which includes during a highly infectious disease outbreak. It is likely that responders and organizations will have conflicting duties, such as medical providers to their patients and their own families, even when they are clear on their duties and responsibilities.
- **Informing the public:** When possible, public health professionals inform their communities of preventive actions in advance of a known emergency, during the emergency, and during the recovery period. In all of these phases, the public needs to receive timely and accurate information in order to mitigate harm.
- **Resource constraints:** In many disasters, an expected surge in demand for health and public health services stresses resources. Even with the deployment of national stockpiles and additional manpower through volunteers, potentially challenging ethical decisions may be needed regarding the availability of limited resources (e.g., ventilators) and their assignment to which patients. Limited resources will increase the urgency of making such decisions in an ethical manner.
- **Isolation and quarantine:** To limit the spread of infectious disease, public health professionals use *social distancing,* where distance or a barrier is established between individuals. (For a full discussion see Chapter 12.) Social distancing techniques that limit mobility, such as isolation and quarantine, can be considered constraints of civil liberty. Other prevention strategies are mechanical (e.g., requesting that individuals wear personal protective equipment such as masks). Sometimes it may be necessary to restrict liberty in the interest of protecting the public's health. Public health professionals have been preparing for emergencies that require social distancing and have had the opportunity to discuss strategies to reduce the spread of infection. The mandatory quarantine, during the 2014 outbreak, of some

providers returning from caring for patients with Ebola virus disease reminded us that there is not universal acceptance of when to use social distancing techniques.

- **Timeliness and responsiveness:** Because emergencies involving highly infectious medical conditions and public health threats require accelerated actions in a condensed time frame, it may not be possible to prevent negative health effects.

Ethical Guidelines in Epidemics and Pandemics

Ethical decisions while a disaster is unfolding can be challenging. The gravity is further compounded during an epidemic or pandemic, in which a highly infectious disease may spread faster than already strained resources can contain the impact. Recognizing the challenge, the U.S. Bioethics Committee and the CDC released guidance documents to assist in the planning, management, and response phases of an epidemic or pandemic.

Ebola Virus Disease Epidemic

The Ebola virus disease epidemic in western Africa demonstrated that public health ethics is of global, and not merely local, relevance. At the height of the 2014 epidemic, many U.S. citizens feared that the United States would join affected countries in western Africa in confronting a serious domestic outbreak of the deadly Ebola virus disease. In response to the arrival of Ebola virus disease on U.S. soil, some called for travel bans, quarantine of health care workers, and stigmatization of and discrimination against western Africans. To respond ethically to the Ebola virus disease epidemic, to prepare for and to facilitate coordinated efforts during this and future public health emergencies, the Presidential Commission for the Study of Bioethical Issues (Bioethics Commission) delineated 7 recommendations focused on engagement, infrastructure, communications, and integration. The Bioethics Commission considered lessons learned about ethical preparedness of the U.S. response to the Ebola virus disease epidemic in western Africa and examined the ethical dimensions of restrictive public health measures, the use of placebos for treatment and vaccines trials, and the collection and sharing of biospecimens for future research.

Briefly, the 7 recommendations issued by the Ebola Bioethics Commission are:

- The U.S. government has a responsibility to engage in global preparedness and to participate in coordinated international responses to public health emergencies. Such preparedness requires strong international and federal public health infrastructures for responding effectively to emergencies and their short- and long-term public health consequences.

- The United States should reinforce key elements of its domestic and global response capabilities for health and public health emergencies. These include strengthening the capacity of the World Health Organization to respond to a global health disaster, identifying and authorizing a single U.S. health official to be accountable for all federal response activities involving public health, and strengthening the deployment capabilities of the U.S. Public Health Service.
- Public officials have a responsibility to support public education and communication regarding the nature and justification of the response of public health organizations. Communication efforts should provide the public with useful, clear, accessible, and accurate information about the response; provide those most directly affected by public health policies and programs with the reasoning behind their implementation; and mitigate stigmatization and discrimination associated with public health emergencies.
- Ethical principles should be integrated into timely decision making by public health officials in response to rapidly unfolding epidemics. Qualified experts in public health ethics should be readily available to identify the ethical considerations relevant to any response to public health emergencies using available real-time evidence.
- Governments and public health organizations should employ the least restrictive means necessary based on the best available scientific evidence in implementing public health measures that involve social distancing. Governments and public health organizations should be prepared to clearly communicate the rationale for actions intended to control the spread of infectious disease, such as quarantines and travel restrictions. Restrictive measures must meet a high standard of justification that establishes that they are necessary to curb the epidemic. Officials should provide regular updates to the public about the implementation of social distancing strategies, with particular attention to the needs of those most directly affected.
- Research during the Ebola virus disease epidemic should provide all participants with the best supportive care available in the community in which the research is conducted. Trial designs should be methodologically rigorous and capable of generating results that are clearly interpretable, acceptable to the host communities, and, to the extent possible, minimize delays to completing the research. Clinical research conducted during an Ebola virus disease epidemic should be designed to provide the greatest possible benefit to those currently affected, both in terms of supportive care and access to experimental interventions. The clinical research should also minimize the time necessary to obtain results and yield reliable evidence of the safety, efficacy, and effectiveness of experimental interventions for future patients.
- The U.S. government should ensure that biospecimens of Ebola virus disease are obtained ethically, including addressing the challenges of obtaining informed

consent during a public health emergency and ensuring adequate privacy protections. The U.S. government should facilitate access to the benefits that result from related research to the broadest group of people possible. This can be achieved by engaging in dialogue with global partners and working collaboratively with local scientists whenever possible to develop effective strategies for ensuring equitable distribution of the benefits of research both in the United States and abroad.

Local emergency public health planners can incorporate the recommendations issued by the Bioethics Commission into their own regional planning efforts.

Pandemic Influenza

In 2007, the CDC issued a report entitled *Ethical Guidelines in Pandemic Influenza* to guide decision making in preparing for and responding to pandemics. The 2015 Bioethics Commission report, discussed above, leveraged many of the same principles that were discussed in the CDC's document on pandemics. The guidance released by the CDC focused on 2 primary tasks that are likely to be relevant in any epidemic, as the world saw in the 2014 spread of Ebola virus disease in western Africa. The 2 tasks are: (1) distribution and prioritization of vaccine and antiviral drug and (2) development of interventions that would limit individual freedom and social distancing.

Distribution and Prioritization of Vaccine and Antiviral Drug

The 2007 CDC report emphasized that a classic utilitarian approach to defining priorities for distributing medical resources, "the greatest good for the greatest number," is not a morally adequate platform for pandemic influenza planning. Instead, they recommend an approach to ethical justification that, like utilitarianism, evaluates the rightness or wrongness of actions or policies primarily by their consequences. The report further recommended that planning should take into account additional checks grounded in the ethical principles of respect for people, nonmaleficence, and justice. For example, a classic utilitarian approach, which might accept imposing suffering on the few for the greater benefit of all, would be tempered by such principles as:

- Refraining from harming or injuring individuals and communities
- Assuring equal opportunity to access resources to those included in agreed upon priority groups
- Respecting individual autonomy by employing the least restrictive interventions that are likely to be effective

The ethical allocation of resources should be guided by criteria specified well in advance of any need to apply them. The primary goals of an ethical distribution system should be clearly specified, such as determining how to allocate a limited supply of vaccine during an expected outbreak. Further criteria for the distribution of vaccine and/or antiviral drugs should be evaluated according to an organization's ability to contribute to the realization of the primary goals. Organizations with limited manpower or geographical reach might plan differently than those with massive resources and comprehensive mutual aid agreements. These further criteria should be directed at maximizing fairness (or equity) in the distribution process. For example, if the elderly and young children are most vulnerable to a strain of influenza, would they be given the first doses of vaccine?

With the goal of preserving the functioning of society, distribution plans should specify:

- Names of individual vaccines or classes of goods (e.g., antivirals for the purpose of treating or preventing influenza) that will be included (or not included) in the distribution plan
- Names of specific agencies or individuals who will decide about prioritization and distribution
- Clearly stated guidelines for eligibility to be a recipient and exceptions
- Morally relevant criteria that will be employed to assign higher or lower priorities to groups of individuals or individuals

Development of Interventions That Would Limit Individual Freedom and Social Distancing

In the management of a pandemic of influenza or other highly infectious disease, public health officials may employ procedures and interventions that will limit the freedom of movement of individuals or create conditions of social distancing. Where public health officials propose the voluntary use of such interventions and procedures, these recommendations are most likely to be accepted by the public. Mandatory interventions that limit liberty or require isolation are less likely to be accepted and should be imposed only in cases in which voluntary actions seem unlikely to be effective or the infectious agent is so virulent that voluntary action is unlikely to contain it.

Mandatory Liberty-Limiting and Social Distancing Intervention

Per the CDC, sound guidelines should be based on the best available scientific evidence. While the ideal method of validating the effectiveness of interventions would be established through evidence-based research, given the ethical complications of conducting studies on liberty-limiting or required-isolation policies, it is unlikely that this will be possible, particularly during a pandemic. In the absence of methods validated by evidence-based research, public health officials have turned to *evidence-informed* decision making, which uses the best available evidence from research, context, and experience. Evidence-informed decision making suggests that liberty-limiting and social-distancing interventions should include the following:

- Isolating individuals infected with or ill with influenza
- Quarantining those thought to have already been exposed, including family members and others in close contact
- Closing schools, canceling public events (e.g. sports events, concerts), and closing public venues (e.g., shopping malls, restaurants, museums, theaters) as mechanisms to decrease social contact that may lead to the spread of influenza or other highly infectious disease
- Restricting access to public venues deemed more "essential" such as grocery stores, public transportation, and gasoline stations
- Providing guidance on personnel practices and/or flexible work scheduling that decreases potential for exposure in the work environment
- Limiting travel within or between cities and regions

How to Use the Ethical Process

Decisions during the planning stage should be based on the ethical principles discussed previously. Underlying these principles are professional and societal values that include the following:

- Professional duty to provide care
- Every patients' right to receive needed medical care equally
- Any restrictions to individual liberty should be necessary and relevant to protect the common good
- Protection of individual privacy when possible
- Proportional actions to restrict individual liberty as necessary to benefit the community
- Support provided to those facing a disproportionate risk of disease or injury
- Solidarity in communication and collaboration across systemic and institutional boundaries
- Allocation of resources using ethical behavior and decision making process

In planning for disasters, it is important and necessary to build trust with the community before an emergency occurs. Obtaining the cooperation of the public is a critical

Table 15-2. Analysis of Tasks Involved in Ethical Decision Making

Analyze Ethical Issues	Evaluate Ethical Dimensions	Justify Decision
Identify stakeholders and their particular interest	Identify moral norms and moral considerations	Present sufficient reasons for course of action
Understand inherent public health risks and potential harms	Action produces balance of benefits over harms	Base actions on moral norms, ethical principles, professional codes, and history
Identify public health goals	Benefits and burdens are distributed fairly	Goal is likely to be accomplished
Identify any legal authority being questioned	Affected groups have opportunity to participate in decision	Probable benefits outweigh any moral infringements
Identify any precedence or historical context	Action respects individual's autonomy, liberty, and privacy	Action is least restrictive and intrusive
Identify alternative courses of action	Action respects professional roles and values	Public justification for action or policy exists that is acceptable to those most affected
Professional code of ethics provides guidance	Ethical principles provide guidance	By following ethical principles, guarantee fairness

goal of preparedness. Although public health officials can use legal remedies during a disaster, it is far better to gain the cooperation and collaboration of a population by their acceptance of the actions being taken. Ensuring that public health workers and health care providers know and adhere to the tenets of public health ethics makes it more likely that the community will accept necessary decisions. Through transparent communication and participation in decisions, members of a community can be assured that public health decisions are made fairly.

The CDC describes a process for making ethical determinations in its Public Health Law 101 course. The 3-step process includes analyzing the ethical issues, evaluating the ethical dimensions, and justifying a decision. In thinking through these steps, public health workers should look to the professional code of ethics for guidance. Table 15-2 identifies the tasks involved in each step.

BASICS

APPENDIX A

COMMON TERMS USED IN DISASTER PREPAREDNESS AND RESPONSE

Access-based needs—ensuring that resources, such as human services, housing, information, transportation, and medications to maintain health, are accessible to all individuals.

Access deficit—the gap between the ability of health care providers to deliver care and the increased health care needs of the population following disasters that disrupt primary care services.

Accessible—having the legally required elements to ensure that individuals with a wide variety of disabilities can enter and use places, programs, services, and activities.

Active surveillance—utilizes designated staff members to regularly contact health care providers, laboratories, hospitals, the affected population, and others to seek out information about specific health conditions.

Adaptive equipment—equipment that helps a person move, groom, or eat independently such as mobility aids, grooming aids, feeding aids, and similar devices used to offset functional limits.

Administrative preparedness—a term coined during the H1N1 influenza response, is the process of ensuring that fiscal and administrative authorities and practices (e.g., funding, procurement, contracting, hiring, and legal capabilities) used in public health emergency response and recovery are effectively managed throughout all levels of government.

Advanced life support—provided by paramedics; includes much more sophisticated diagnosis of patient conditions followed by protocol-driven, on-site initial medical treatment for conditions that will receive definitive treatment in hospitals.

Aerosol generating procedures (AGP)—procedures that stimulate coughing and promote the generation of aerosols, which are airborne particles. Additional infection prevention and control precautions are required for some AGP where an increased risk of infection has been identified.

Aerosal transmissible—pathogens that can transmit disease via infectious particles suspended in air.

After Action report—document that summarizes and reviews all aspects of an agency's preparations for, immediate response to, and initial recovery from a disaster.

Alarm procedure—alerting every concerned party as part of disaster management; various optical and acoustical means of alarm are possible: flags, lights, sirens, radio, telephone.

All-hazards—grouping all types of emergencies together for purposes of preparedness and response; types of hazards include natural disasters, accidental human actions, terrorism, or any chemical, biological, radiological, nuclear, or explosive accident.

Analysis-epidemiologic measures—descriptive statistics, specific disease and death rates, secular trends, tests for sensitivity, and predictive value positive, if appropriate.

Antemortem—information about a dead or missing person that can be used for identification.

Antigen—any substance (such as a toxin or enzyme) that stimulates an immune response in the body (particularly the production of antibodies).

Antigenic drift—mutational changes in viruses that occur, rendering immune responses against previous strains ineffective and enabling the virus's spread throughout a partially immune population; occurs in both influenza A and influenza B viruses.

Antigenic shift—sudden shift in viral proteins in influenza A, through a recombination of the genomes of 2 strains, that produces a novel virus; that may result in a pandemic or a worldwide epidemic.

Assessments—short- and long-term "snapshots" of disaster situations that help with decision making and enhance monitoring; the goal of conducting assessments is to convey information quickly in order to recalibrate a system's response.

Augmentative communication device—device used to help a person communicate by voice.

Avalanche—sudden slide of a large mass of snow and ice, usually carrying with it earth, rocks, trees, and other debris.

Average throughput time—time from a client's entry into a point-of-distribution site until exit.

Basic life support—noninvasive measures (such as elimination of airway obstruction, cardiopulmonary resuscitation, hemorrhage control, wound care, and immobilization of fractures) used to preserve the lives of unstable patients.

Becquerel (Bq)—unit of nuclear activity that has replaced the curie; 1 Bq represents the amount of radioactive substance for which disintegration occurs per second.

Bioterrorism—unlawful release of biological agents or toxins targeted at humans, animals, or plants/crops with the intent to intimidate or coerce a government or civilian population in furtherance of political or social objectives.

Blast wave—intense over-pressurization impulse created by a detonated high explosive; injuries incurred by such an impulse are characterized by anatomical and physiological changes caused by the direct or reflective over-pressurization force impacting the body's surface. Should be distinguished from the forced super-heated air flow of a "blast wind."

Blindness/visual disability—visual condition that interferes with a person's ability to see, occasionally resulting in a person's complete loss of vision.

Blogs—frequently updated Web site with chronological entries. A **microblog** is a short form of blogging in which users write brief messages up to 140 characters on their Web site.

Cache—predetermined tools, equipment, or supplies stored in a designated location.

Capabilities—the operational capacity and ability to execute preparedness tasks aimed at prevention, mitigation, response, and recovery.

Capability target—describes what a community wants to achieve for each core capability, with measurable desired outcomes, in response to a given threat or hazard context. Part of the Threat and Hazard Identification and Risk Assessment (THIRA) process.

Case—unit of observation in the surveillance system regarding the health condition of interest.

Case definition—standardized criteria used in investigations and comparing potential cases for deciding whether a person has a particular disease or health-related condition; provide the basis for deciding which disaster-specific health conditions should be monitored through an emergency information surveillance system.

Casualty—any person suffering physical or psychological damage as a result of outside violence that leads to death, injuries, or material losses.

Casualty clearing station—collection point for victims in the immediate vicinity of the disaster site at which further triage and basic and advanced life support can be provided.

Catastrophic incident—any natural or man-made incident that results in extraordinary amounts of mass casualties, damage, or disruption.

Centers for independent living—community-based, nonresidential organizations that work with people who have disabilities.

Central holding area—location at which ambulances assemble and leave to pick up patients from a casualty clearing station or a neighboring hospital, according to a victim distribution plan.

CHEMTREC—Established in 1971, CHEMTREC (CHEMical TRansportation Emergency Center) provides around-the-clock, chemical-specific information to emergency responders.

Closed captions—visual text displays hidden in video signals that are used to display information for those who are deaf or hearing impaired; can be accessed through a television remote control, an onscreen menu, or a special decoder. All televisions with a 13-inch or larger screen manufactured after 1993 have the needed circuitry. Open captions are an integral part of the television picture, like subtitles in a movie, and cannot be turned off. Text that advances very slowly across the bottom of the screen is referred to as a *crawl*; displayed text or graphics that move up and down the screen are said to *scroll*.

Cognitive impairment—medical condition or injury that affects a person's ability to understand spoken or written information.

Common alerting protocol—created by FEMA; standardizes the formatting of messages to allow consistent digital messaging to be disseminated simultaneously over different communications systems.

Communication disability—medical condition or injury that interferes with a person's ability to communicate by using one's voice.

Community profile—characteristics of the local environment prone to natural disasters or technological accidents, including population density, age distribution, roads, railways, waterways, types of dwellings and buildings, and the relief agencies locally available.

Community Reception Centers (CRCs)—A place, apart from hospitals and shelters, where health care professionals can evaluate and triage people for further care in order to ease the burden on hospitals and manage scarce medical resources during a radiation emergency. Their services include contamination screening, decontamination and limited medical care.

Comprehensive emergency management—integrated approach to organizing multiple emergency programs and activities; 5 phases comprise the "life cycle" of emergency management: prevention, mitigation, preparedness, response, and recovery.

Comprehensive Preparedness Guide 101: Developing and Maintaining Emergency Operations—guide that describes the intersection of federal, state, tribal, and local emergency planning.

Contamination—accidental release of hazardous chemical or nuclear materials leading to pollution of the environment and that places humans at risk for exposures, potentially affecting populations externally (skin and mucous membranes), internally (by inhalation or ingestion), or both.

Context—A community or region-specific description of an incident, including location, timing, and other important circumstances. Part of the THIRA process.

Context descriptions—Part of the THIRA process in which the planner describes how the identified threats and hazards may affect a given community.

Contingency plan—anticipatory emergency plan to be followed during an expected or eventual disaster, based on risk assessment, availability of human and material resources, community preparedness, and local and international response capability.

Contingency planning—site-specific plan that recognizes a disaster could occur at any time.

Covered entity—defined in the Health Insurance Portability and Accountability Act of 1996 rules as health plans, health care clearinghouses, and health care providers who electronically transmit any health information in connection with transactions for which the U.S. Department of Health & Human Services has adopted standards (generally, those concerning billing and payment for services or insurance coverage).

Covert releases—unannounced releases of a biological agent that present as illness in the community. Since detection of the released agent is dependent on traditional surveillance methods, the potential for large-scale spread is high.

Cracker—individual who uses computer programming to gain unauthorized or illegal access to a computer network or file.

Crisis-crowd—where the people located at the site provide information about emergencies happening in a community.

Crisis standards of care—substantial change in the delivery of health care necessitated by a catastrophic disaster and formally declared by a state government; such a declaration legally protects health care providers in the event of scarce medical resource allocation and implementation of alternative operations at their facilities.

Data collection—accumulation of information conducted by various media, such as e-mail or facsimile, or by regular pickup and delivery by an assigned person to an assigned place.

Datacasting—the process of delivering Internet Protocol data over a traditional broadcast television signal. Most often, the data is supplemental information sent along with digital television, but may also be applied to digital signals on analog TV or radio.

Deafness/hearing disability—medical condition or injury that interferes with a person's ability to hear sounds.

Decontamination—removal of hazardous chemical or nuclear substances from the skin and mucous membranes by showering, washing with water, or rinsing with sterile solutions.

Demobilization—orderly, safe, and efficient return of a resource to its original location and status.

Disability—physical or mental impairment that substantially limits one or more major life activities of an individual.

Disaster—any occurrence (typically a sudden one) that causes damage, ecological disruption, loss of human life, deterioration of health and health services, *and* that exceeds the adjustment capacity of the affected community on a scale sufficient to require outside assistance; may include such events as earthquakes, floods, fires, hurricanes, cyclones, major storms, volcanic eruptions, spills, air crashes, droughts, epidemics, serious food shortages, and civil strife.

Disaster continuum—life cycle of a disaster event; also referred to as emergency management cycle.

Disaster epidemiology—study of disaster-related deaths, illnesses, or injuries in humans and of the factors impacting those events; methods involve identification of risk factors and comparison of affected people with those not affected. May provide informed advice regarding probable health effects.

Disaster informatics—theoretical and practical aspects of information processing and communication based on knowledge and experience derived from processes in medicine and health care in disaster settings.

Disaster-prone—measure of risk that an individual, community, population, or area faces in regards to a particular hazard or disaster or disaster agent; determined by a history of past events and the risks of new events. Also referred to as *at-risk*.

Disaster recovery center—facility established in a centralized location within or near the disaster area at which victims can apply for disaster aid.

Disaster Severity Scale—the classification of disasters by a number of criteria (radius of disaster site, number of dead, number of wounded, average severity of injuries sustained, impact time, and rescue time), the attribution of a numeric value between 0 (least severe) and 2 (most severe) to each of the variables, and the totaling of all numeric values to provide a number between 0 and 18 that indicates the severity of an event.

Disaster vulnerability—ability to absorb and recover from the effects of an extreme event or situation; varies from one society to another or from one place to another.

Dispatch communications system—system used to assign ambulance personnel and other first responders to respond to people in need.

Drills—supervised activities designed to test one or more components of an overall emergency management plan; a drill may be a step toward an exercise or may be an actual field response.

Durable medical equipment—certain medical equipment for use in the home, such as walkers, wheelchairs, and scooters.

Earthquake measures—scales used to measure earthquake intensity or magnitude. Most common are the Richter scale and the Modified Mercalli Intensity (MMI) scale. The MMI scale is a subjective measure of the intensity of an earthquake, whereas the Richter scale is an objective and numerical measurement based on readings taken by seismometers. A correlation between the magnitude and intensity of an earthquake can be made by correlating the measurements of the Richter and MMI scales.

Aftershocks—sequence of smaller earthquakes that can follow a larger-magnitude earthquake by day, months, or years, exacerbating damage.

Intensity—a subjective measure of earthquakes quantified by the MMI scale, which describes the physical effects of an earthquake to a specific location, people, or man-made structures.

Magnitude—numerical quantity that characterizes earthquakes in terms of the total energy released after adjusting for difference in epicentral distance and focal depth. Magnitude differs from intensity in that magnitude is determined on the basis of instrumental records; whereas intensity is determined on the basis of subjective observations of the damage.

Modified Mercalli Intensity scale—Subjectively applied measurement system that indicates the intensity of an earthquake; a measure of the degree of damage from a particular location. Measurement is denoted by Roman numerals from I to XII. Intensity VI denotes the threshold for potential ground failure, such as liquefaction. Intensity VII denotes the threshold for architectural damage. Intensity VIII denotes the threshold for structural damage. Intensity IX denotes intense structural damage. Intensities X to XII denote various levels of destruction up to total destruction. An earthquake has many intensities, but only one magnitude.

Richter scale—Devised by Charles F. Richter, the Richter scale has a logarithmic formula for calculating the magnitude of earthquake from the instrument readings, and ranges from 0 to excess of 10 in numerical magnitude. Minor earthquakes measure 0–4.9, moderate earthquakes 5–5.9, strong earthquakes 6–6.9, and the most destructive earthquakes 7 and greater. The energy increases exponentially with magnitude; thus, a magnitude 6.0 earthquake releases 31.5 times more energy than a magnitude 5.0 earthquake or approximately 1,000 times more energy than does a magnitude 4.0 earthquake.

Emergencies—any occurrence that requires an immediate response that may be a result of epidemics, technological catastrophes, strife, or other natural or man-made causes.

Emergency Information Form—a concise, single-sheet medical summary that describes a child's medical condition(s), medications, and special health care needs to inform those providing health care during disasters so that optimal emergency medical care can be provided.

Emergency Management Assistance Compact—congressionally ratified organization that facilitates interstate mutual aid by establishing written agreements regarding liability and reimbursement.

Emergency Medical Services System—organizational structure that includes prehospital (e.g., public access, dispatch, emergency medical technicians/paramedics, and ambulance services) and in-hospital (e.g., emergency departments, hospitals, and other definitive care facilities and personnel) support for victims of emergencies who require medical support.

Emergency medical technicians—commonly referred to as EMTs; emergency medical responders trained to identify and field-treat the most common medical emergencies and injuries, and to provide medical support to victims while en route to the hospital.

Emergency Support Functions—standardized concepts of resource management used by the federal government to organize and provide assistance following an emergency.

Emergency Support Function Annexes—describe the missions, policies, structures, and responsibilities of federal agencies in response to an emergency.

Emergency Support Function #6: Mass Care, Emergency Assistance, Temporary Housing, and Human Services—concept that includes the tasks of sheltering, feeding, emergency first aid, family reunification, and distribution of emergency relief supplies to disaster victims; the National Response Framework designates the Department of Homeland Security and FEMA as the coordinating agencies responsible for this function.

Emergency Support Function #8: Public Health and Medical Services—basis of federal preparedness, response, and recovery actions in regards to the health needs of disaster victims; coordinated by the Office of the Assistant Secretary for Preparedness and Response. The lead agency is the Department of Health & Human Services.

Epidemic—occurrence of a number of cases of a disease, known or suspected to be of infectious or parasitic origin, that is unusually large or unexpected for the given place and time. A **threatened epidemic** occurs when the circumstances are such that a specific disease may reasonably be anticipated to occur in unusually large or unexpected numbers.

Evacuation—organized removal of people from dangerous or potentially dangerous areas.

Evacuation assistive equipment—equipment or devices used to help people leave a building in an emergency.

Evaluation—detailed review of a program; purpose is to determine whether the program met its objectives, to assess its impact on the community, and to generate "lessons learned" for the design of future projects; conducted during the program, at the completion of important milestones, or at the end of a specific period.

Evaluation research—application of scientific methods to assess the effectiveness of programs, services, or organizations designed to improve health or prevent illness.

Exposure surveillance—search for exposure variable. In disaster settings, exposure may be based on physical or environmental properties of the disaster event.

Exposure variable—characteristic of interest, also known as risk factor or predictor variable.

Famine Early Warning System—established by the U.S. Agency for International Development to monitor climate and meteorology, availability of food in the market, and morbidity related to nutrition to predict the occurrence of famine.

Far-field—following a nuclear accident at a nuclear plant, the area outside the immediate (or near-field) vicinity in which effects of the incident are still noticeable.

Federal coordinating officer—person appointed by the Federal Emergency Management Agency (FEMA) following a presidential declaration of a severe disaster or of an emergency to coordinate federal assistance. He or she initiates immediate action to assure that federal assistance is provided in accordance with the disaster declaration, any applicable laws or regulations, and the FEMA-state agreement. The federal coordinating officer is also the senior federal official appointed in accordance with the provisions of Public Law 93-288 (the Stafford Act), as amended, to coordinate the overall consequence management response and recovery activities and to represent the president by coordinating the administration of federal relief activities in the designated disaster area. Additionally, the federal coordinating officer is delegated responsibilities and performs those for the FEMA director as outlined in Executive Order 12148 and those responsibilities delegated to the FEMA regional director in the Code of Federal Regulations, Title 44, Part 205.

Federal on-scene commander—official designated upon the activation of the Joint Operations Center who ensures appropriate coordination of the U.S. government's overall response with federal, state, and local authorities. The on-scene commander maintains this role until the U.S. attorney general transfers the lead federal agency role to FEMA.

Federal-to-federal support—coordination of additional assistance, such as interagency or intra-agency reimbursable agreements, in accordance with the Economy Act of 1933 or other applicable authorities.

First responder—local police, fire, and emergency medical personnel who arrive first on the scene of an incident and take action to save lives, protect property, and meet basic human needs.

Food defense—protection of food products from intentional adulteration by biological, chemical, physical, or radiological agents.

Food safety—protection of food products from intentional or unintentional contamination.

Function-based needs—restrictions or functional limitations that interfere with an individual's ability to perform fundamental physical and mental tasks or activities of daily living, such as eating, toileting, or bathing. This definition reflects the capabilities of the individual, not the condition, label, or medical diagnosis.

Functional model of public health response in disasters—paradigm for identifying disaster-related activities for which each core area of public health has responsibility; interface between the core components of professional public health training and the 5 phases identified in the National Preparedness Goal that correspond to the type of activities involved in preparing for and responding to a disaster: prevention, protection, mitigation, response and recovery.

Functional needs populations—formerly referred to as "special needs populations," populations whose members may have additional needs before, during, and after an emergency, including but not limited to maintaining independence, communication, transportation, supervision, and medical care. May include those with disabilities or living in institutionalized settings, the elderly, children, people from nonnative cultures, those with limited English proficiency or who are non-English speaking, or who are transportation disadvantaged.

Functional needs support services—services that enable individuals to maintain their independence in a general care shelter.

Fujita scale—classification system used to measure the strength of tornadoes; assesses the damage caused by the tornado after it has passed over a man-made structure. The scale ranges from F0 (breaks tree branches with winds 40–72 mph) to F5 (steel reinforced concrete structures badly damaged with winds 261–318 mph). (An F6 tornado has been classified but is considered "inconceivable" with winds at 319–379 mph.)

Geographic Information System[1]—commonly referred to as GIS; a collection of computer hardware, software, and geographic data for capturing, storing, updating,

1. Reprinted with permission from Kennedy H, ed. 2001. *Dictionary of GIS Terminology*. Redlands, CA: ESRI Press.

manipulating, analyzing, and displaying all forms of geographically related information.

Access rights—privileges given to a user for reading, writing, deleting, and updating files on a disk or tables in a database. Access rights are stated as "no access," "read only," and "read/write."

Address—point stored as an x and y location in a geographic data layer, referenced with a unique identifier.

Address geocoding—Assigning x- and y- coordinates to tabular data such as street addresses or zip codes so they can be displayed as points on a map.

Altitude—elevation above a reference datum, usually sea level, of any point on the earth's surface or in the atmosphere, or the *z* value in a three-dimensional coordinate system.

Area chart—chart that emphasizes the difference between 2 or more groups of data; for example, the changes in a population from one year to the next. The area of interest is usually shaded in a different color.

Attribute—information about a geographic feature in a GIS, generally stored in a table and linked to the feature by a unique identifier.

Base data—map data over which other information is placed.

Basemap—map depicting geographic features used for locational reference and often including a geodetic control network as part of its structure.

Cell—smallest square in a grid. Each cell usually has an attribute value associated with it.

Clean data—data that are free from error.

Connectivity—how geographic features in a network of lines are attached to one another functionally or spatially.

Database—includes data about the spatial locations and shapes of geographic features recorded as points, lines, areas, pixels, and grid cells, as well as their attributes.

Data dictionary—set of tables containing information about the data stored in a GIS database, such as the full names of the attributes, meanings of codes, scale of source data, accuracy of locations, and map projections used; also referred to as metadata.

Geocode—code representing the location of an object, such as an address, census tract, postal code, or x- and y- coordinates.

Global Positioning System—commonly referred to as GPS, a constellation of 24 satellites developed by the U.S. Department of Defense that orbit the earth at an altitude of 20,200 kilometers (12,552 miles) and transmit signals that allow a receiver anywhere on earth to calculate its own location. GPS is used for navigation, mapping, surveying, and other applications for which precise positioning is necessary.

Hierarchical database—database that stores related information in a structure similar to that of a tree, where records can be traced to parent records that in turn can be traced to a root record.

Lookup table—tabular data file that contains additional attributes for records stored in an attribute table.

Managed data—data that has been standardized, compared with U.S. postal street data, verified, and corrected so that it precisely identifies locations of each address.

Overlay—superimposed series of 2 or more maps registered to a common coordinate system, either digitally or on a transparent material, in order to show the relationships between features that occupy the same geographic space.

Raster—spatial data model of rows and columns of cells that share the same value representing geographic features.

Relational database—data stored in tables that are associated with shared attributes, which can be arranged in different combinations.

Shapefile—vector file format for storing location, shape, and attributes of geographic features; stored in a set of related files and contains one feature class.

Spatial analysis—study of the locations and shapes of geographic features and the relationships between them; traditionally includes overlay and contiguity analysis, surface analysis, linear analysis, and raster analysis.

Unmanaged data—commercially available data that provides household level information without an extensive effort to ensure that the coordinates match the physical address.

Vector—data structure used to represent linear geographic features. Features are made of ordered lists of x- and y- coordinates and represented by points, lines, or polygons; points connect to become lines, and lines connect to become polygons. Attributes are associated with each feature (as opposed to a raster data structure, which associates attributes with grid cells).

Golden hour—principle that a victim whose airway, breathing, or circulation is erratic must be stabilized as soon as possible or within one hour following injury or he or she will die.

Governor's authorized representative—individual empowered by a governor who executes documents for disaster assistance on behalf of the state, represents the governor in the Unified Coordination Group, coordinates the disaster assistance program for states, and helps identify state's critical information needs.

Hardiness—psychological state, characterized by belief that one can exert control over events, viewing stressful events as challenges that can be overcome, and strong commitment and purpose.

Hazard—probability of the occurrence of a disaster caused by a natural phenomenon (e.g., earthquake, tropical cyclone), failure of man-made sources of energy (e.g., nuclear reactor, industrial explosion), or uncontrolled human activity (e.g., conflicts, overgrazing).

Hazard identification and risk assessment—process to identify hazards and associated risk likely to occur in a specified region or environment (e.g., earthquakes, floods, industrial accidents).

Hazard surveillance—assessment of the occurrence of, distribution of, and the secular trends in levels of hazards (e.g., toxic chemical agents, physical agents, biomechanical stressors, as well as biological agents) responsible for disease and injury.

Health care coalition—groups of local health care and responder organizations that collaborate to prepare for and respond to emergencies.

Impact phase—phase during a disaster event when activities of warning and preparedness occur.

Incident—occurrence or event, natural or human-caused, that requires an emergency response to protect life or property.

Catastrophic incidents—comparable with presidentially declared major disasters.

Incident Action Plan—written document developed by the incident commander or the planning section of the Incident Command System that details actions that will be conducted through the Incident Command System in response to an incident; developed for specific time periods, referred to as *operational periods*, based on the needs of the incident. The incident commander is responsible for overseeing and implementing the plan.

Incident Command System—model for command, control, and coordination of a response that provides a means to coordinate the efforts of individual agencies.

Area Command—activated when complexity of the incident requires oversight of multiple incidents for which multiple incident management teams are involved.

Branch—organizational level having functional or geographic responsibility for major parts or incident operations. The incident commander may establish geographic branches to resolve span-of-control issues or may establish functional branches to manage specific functions (e.g., law enforcement, fire, emergency medical).

Chain of command—series of command, control, executive, or management positions in hierarchical order of authority.

Command—act of directing, ordering, or controlling by virtue of explicit statutory, regulatory, or delegated authority.

Division—organizational level with responsibility for operations within a defined geographic area; the organizational level between single resources, task forces or strike teams, and the branch level.

Emergency Operations Center—location where department heads, government officials, and volunteer agencies coordinate the response to an emergency event.

Function—one of the 5 major activities in the Incident Command System: command, operations, planning, logistics, and finance/administration.

Group—organizational level having responsibility for a specified functional assignment at an incident (e.g., perimeter control, evacuation, fire suppression); managed by a group supervisor.

Incident commander—person with overall authority and responsibility for conducting incident operations and managing all incident operations.

Integrated communications—system using a common communications plan, standard operating procedures, clear text, common frequencies, and common terminology.

Resource management—functional area that maximizes use, consolidates control, reduces communication barriers, provides accountability, and ensures safety for personnel.

Section—organizational level with responsibility for a major functional area of the incident; located organizationally between branches and the incident commander.

Sizeup—problem identification and an assessment of the possible consequences; is initially the responsibility of the first officer to arrive at the scene, but continues throughout the response to update continually the nature of the incident, hazards that are present, the size of the affected area, whether the area can be isolated, if a staging area is needed and the best location, and where to establish entrance and exit routes for the flow of personnel and equipment.

Span of control—number of individuals that one supervisor manages; a manageable span of control for one supervisor ranges between 3 to 7 resources, with 5 being optimal.

Staging area—place where resources are kept awaiting assignment.

Strike team—group of resources of the same size and type.

Task force—combination of single resources assembled for a particular operational need, with common communications and a leader.

Top-down—command function that is established by the first arriving officer, who becomes the incident commander.

Unified Area Command—command system established when incidents under an Area Command are multijurisdictional.

Unified Command—within an Incident Command System, used when more than one agency has incident jurisdiction or when incidents cross political jurisdictions. Agencies work together through the designated members of the Unified Command to establish a common set of objectives and strategies and a single Incident Action Plan.

Unity of command—concept that each person within an organization reports to only one designated person.

Incident Command Post—field location at which the primary response functions are performed.

Incident Coordination Plan—plan approved and published by the Emergency Management Group for the support of response operations.

Incident management—way in which incidents are managed across all Department of Homeland Security activities, including prevention, protection, response, and recovery.

Incident Management Assistance Team—interagency nationally or regionally based team composed of subject-matter experts and incident management professionals from multiple federal departments and agencies.

Incubation period—time between when a person is exposed to an infectious disease and when they start to have symptoms.

Integrated recovery programs—balanced recovery programs that respond to a variety of community needs; characterized by stimulation of activity in various sectors, sequencing of activities at appropriate times, and the use of both indirect and direct methods.

International assistance—assistance provided by one or more countries or international and voluntary organizations to a country in need, usually for development or for an emergency. The 4 main elements of assistance within the international community are: intergovernmental agencies such as the United Nations and the European

Union, nongovernmental organizations, the International Red Cross, and bilateral agreements.

Interoperable communications—ability to exchange and use information through different types of equipment.

Isolation—sequestration of symptomatic patients either in their homes or in the hospital so that they will not infect others.

Joint Field Office—temporary federal facility that provides a central location for the coordination of federal, state, tribal, and local governments and private-sector and nongovernmental organizations with primary responsibility for response and recovery.

Joint Information Center—interagency hub that coordinates and disseminates information for the public and media concerning an incident.

Jurisdiction—the territory over which a governmental agency has authority for public health legal, or other similar matters. The jurisdiction of health departments is either state, county, municipal, or territorial.

Jurisdictional agency—agency having jurisdiction and responsibility for a specific geographical area or function.

Landslide—the most common and widespread type of ground failure that is characterized by massive and more or less rapid toppling, sliding, falling, spreading, or flowing of soil and rock down unstable slopes.

Latrines—holes in the ground, usually with a covering platform and privacy wall, designed to capture and contain excreta; may be dug as a trench with multiple platforms across it, or can be a solitary pit with a self-standing structure.

Limited English proficiency—classification of people who have a limited ability to read, speak, write, or understand English and who may be entitled to language assistance in order to access a particular type of service, benefit, or encounter.

Liquefaction—when wet soil behaves like liquid and temporarily loses bearing strength; occurs mainly in young, shallow, loosely compacted, water-saturated sand and gravel deposits when subjected to ground shaking.

Local transmission—when mosquitoes in an area have been infected with a virus and are spreading it to people in that locale or region.

Logistician—individual skilled at calculating and arranging for the various tasks involved in moving and providing personnel, supplies, and so on as part of a response.

Long-term evolution—next-generation wireless technology for mobile broadband networks that provides high bandwidth and accelerates the transfer of information.

Long-term recovery—process of recovery that may continue for months or years, depending on the severity and extent of the damage sustained.

Loss—range of adverse consequences impacting communities and individuals that includes but is not limited to damage; decrease in economic value, function, natural resources, or ecological systems; environmental impact; health deterioration; mortality; and morbidity.

Major disaster—under the Robert T. Stafford Disaster Relief and Emergency Assistance Act of 1988, any natural catastrophe or, regardless of cause, any fire, flood, or explosion in the United States that, in the determination of the president, causes damage of sufficient severity and magnitude to warrant major federal disaster assistance to supplement the efforts and available resources of states and local governments.

Man-made or technological disasters—technological events that are not caused by natural hazards but that occur in human settlements, such as fire, chemical spills and explosions, and armed conflict.

Mass casualty incident—incident that generates a large number of patients in a relatively short period, usually as the result of a single occurrence, such as an aircraft accident, hurricane, flood, or earthquake, that exceeds the local capacity to respond.

Measures of biological effects—human health effects that indicate impacts of disasters, including but not limited to age-specific injury and death rates, laboratory typing of organisms, biochemical testing of exposures to toxic chemicals, and anthropometric measurements, such as height-to-weight ratios.

Measures of physical effects—used to indicate magnitude of disaster; examples include the height of a river above flood stage, the level of pollutants in the air after a forest fire, and the level of toxic chemicals in drinking water or sediment.

Measuring environmental hazards—assessment of the occurrence, distribution, and trends in the level of environmental hazards responsible for disease and injury; examples of hazards include biomechanical stressors, biological agents, and toxic chemicals.

Medical coordination—coordination between prehospital and hospital phases of medical care; characterized by simplification and standardization of materials and methods utilized.

Mission assignment—work order issued to another federal agency directing completion of a specific task or provision of a service in anticipation of, or in response to, a presidential declaration of a major disaster or emergency.

Mitigation—measures taken to reduce the harmful effects of a disaster by attempting to limit impacts on human health and economic infrastructure.

Mobile Web sites—Web sites designed to display on mobile devices, such as smartphones, capable of accessing the Internet.

Mobility disability—medical condition or injury that impedes a person's ability to move.

Mobilization—process and procedures used for activating, assembling, and transporting all resources that have been requested to respond to or support an incident.

Monitoring—process of observing response and recovery programs to determine performance by measuring them against their stated objectives; used to identify bottlenecks and obstacles that cause delays or require reassessment.

Mortality data—information regarding the number of deaths caused by a disaster; used to assess the magnitude of an event, evaluate the effectiveness of disaster preparedness and the adequacy of warning systems, and identify high-risk groups for contingency planning.

Mortality surveillance—process that identifies the number of deaths caused by a disaster and the key information regarding those deaths; such information is collected through disaster mortuary teams, medical examiners, coroners, hospitals, nursing homes, and funeral homes.

Multiagency coordination group—team of administrators or their representatives authorized to commit agency resources and funds that coordinates decision making and allocation of resources, establishes the disaster priorities, and provides strategic guidance and direction to support incident management.

Multiagency coordination system—mechanism for assisting agencies and organizations during a response by coordinating prioritization, critical resource allocation, communications systems integration, and information coordination.

Multijurisdictional incident—incident requiring action from multiple agencies that each have jurisdiction to manage certain aspects of the incident. In the Incident Command System, these incidents will be managed under Unified Command.

Mutual aid and assistance agreement—written or oral agreement between and among agencies, organization, or jurisdictions that provides a mechanism to quickly obtain emergency assistance in the form of personnel, equipment, materials, and other associated services.

National Capital Region Interconnection Network—a private, high-speed fiber optic network interconnecting 24 regional jurisdictions and municipalities as well as the Metropolitan Washington Council of Governments; represents one of the most sophisticated approaches to regional interoperability currently in effect in the United States.

National Disaster Recovery Framework—one of the National Planning Frameworks. Describes how the whole community works together to restore, redevelop and revitalize the community following a disaster.

National Mitigation Framework—one of the National Planning Frameworks. Describes the fostering of a culture of preparedness centered on risk and resilience and how mitigation efforts relate to all other parts of national preparedness.

National Operations Center—primary national hub for coordination of disaster response operations across the federal government; provides the secretary of the Department of Homeland Security and other principals with information necessary to make national-level incident management decisions.

National Planning Scenarios—scenarios that depict the range of potential emergencies as the basis for coordinated federal planning, training, and exercises.

National Preparedness Goal—the core capabilities required to achieve the goal of "a secure and resilient nation with the capabilities required across the whole community to prevent, protect against, mitigate, respond to, and recover from the threats and hazards that pose the greatest risk."

National Preparedness Guidelines—guidance for national preparedness that provides a systematic approach for prioritizing preparedness efforts across the United States.

National Preparedness System—the process used to build, sustain, and deliver core capabilities in order to achieve the goal of a secure and resilient nation.

National Preparedness Vision—concise statement of the core preparedness goal for the United States.

National Prevention Framework—one of the National Planning Frameworks. Provides context for how the whole community works together and how prevention is an important part of national preparedness. Provides roles and examples of prevention-related activities.

National Protection Framework—one of the National Planning Frameworks. Describes activities necessary to secure the homeland against acts of terrorism and man-made or natural disasters.

National Response Coordination Center—component of the National Operations Center that serves as the primary operations center responsible for national incident response, recovery, and resource coordination.

National Response Framework—one of the National Planning Frameworks. Document that provides the key principles, roles, and structures that organize national response to disasters; how all partners coordinate by applying these principles; and defines circumstances in which the federal government has a larger role.

National Voluntary Organizations Active in Disaster—consortium of more than 30 national organizations active in disaster relief that provide capabilities to assist in incident management and response efforts at all levels. During major incidents, the consortium typically sends representatives to the National Response Coordination Center to represent the voluntary organizations and assist in response coordination.

Natural disasters—rapid, acute onset phenomena with profound effects, such as earthquakes, floods, tropical cyclones, tornadoes.

Natural-technological disasters—natural disasters that create technological emergencies, such as urban fires resulting from seismic motion or chemical spills resulting from floods.

Nongovernmental organization—organization that works cooperatively with governmental agencies to provide relief services to disaster victims, including specialized services to disabled people.

Notifiable disease—any disease that is required by law to be reported to health authorities (e.g., local and/or state health departments).

Outbreak—the occurrence of cases of disease that exceed what is normally expected and may occur in a geographical area, over a region or national borders. Outbreaks can last a few days, weeks, or years. An outbreak can be a single case of a communicable disease that has not appeared in a population for a long time, has not previously been found in that community or area, or is a previously unknown disease.

Outcome surveillance—monitoring for a health outcome or event of interest, usually illness, injury, or death.

Outcome variable—health event, usually illness, injury, or death; also known as response variable, dependent variable, or effect variable.

Overt release—announced release of a biological agent, by terrorists or others; this type of release often allows treatment before the onset of disease.

Pandemic—epidemic over a wide geographic area or one that affects a large proportion of the world's population.

Paramedic—highly trained EMT capable of providing advanced life support functions to victims in a disaster or emergency setting.

Paratransit—transportation services used by the mobility impaired or transportation disadvantaged. Includes taxis, carpools, vanpools, minibuses, jitneys, demand-responsive bus services, and specialized bus services.

Passive surveillance—involves the routine reporting of disease data by health institutions to health authorities.

Patient Under Investigation (PUI)—a person who has both clinical features and an epidemiologic risk of a particular disease.

Personal assessment—Written list of what an individual needs and the resources for meeting those needs following a disaster.

Personal assistance services—formal and informal services provided by paid personnel, personal attendants, friends, family, and volunteers that enable those in general population shelters to maintain their usual level of independence.

Personal space—area immediately surrounding a person, including the objects within that space.

Personal support network—group of people who help those with disabilities at home, school, workplace, volunteer site, or any other location; can include roommates, relatives, neighbors, friends, and coworkers. Such a network must know that individual's capabilities and needs, be able to check if an individual needs assistance, and be able to help within minutes.

Phases of the functional model—model composed of 5 phases that correspond to the type of activities that public health professionals are involved in preparing for in the event of a disaster.

Public Health Information Network (PHIN)—an initiative developed by the Center for Disease Control and Prevention (CDC) to establish and implement a framework for sharing public health information electronically.

Messaging System (PHIN MS)—CDC-provided software that enables public health information systems to reliably exchange critical and sensitive data among their disparate systems.

Public Health Directory (PHIN Dir)—repository of information about people, organizations, and jurisdictions that are important to public health programs, and includes the roles that people play within organizations.

Vocabulary Access and Distribution System (PHIN VADS)—provides standard vocabularies to the CDC and its public health partners in one place.

Planning—working cooperatively with other disciplines in advance of a disaster event to initiate prevention and preparedness.

Podcast—Web-based audio or video file that users download to portable listening devices.

Point of distribution—area established in which mass distribution of antibiotics or vaccine is performed and patients are registered, are triaged, have swab samples taken, are medically evaluated, and are provided with antibiotics or vaccine.

Post-disaster surveillance—conducted by health authorities primarily to monitor health events, detect sudden changes in disease occurrence, follow long-term trends of specific diseases, identify changes in agents and host factors for the diseases of interest, and recognize changes in health practices for treating relevant diseases.

Postimpact phase—period after a disaster event when activities of response and recovery occur.

Power-dependent equipment—equipment that requires electricity to operate.

Predictive value positive—ability to detect that cases considered positive have the health event being assessed under surveillance.

Preimpact phase—period before a disaster strikes during which activities of mitigation or prevention occur.

Preparedness—aggregate of all measures and policies taken by humans before an event occurs that allows mitigation of the impact caused by the event through responses to the impact of the event; includes contingency plans and responses, warning systems, evacuation, relocation of dwellings, stores of food and water, temporary shelter, energy, management strategies, disaster drills and exercises, and laying a framework for recovery; also includes prevention, mitigation, and readiness.

Prepositioned resources—resources moved to an area near the expected incident site in response to anticipated resource needs.

Pre-scripted mission assignment—mechanism used by the federal government to facilitate a rapid response of federal resources. Pre-scripted mission assignments identify resources or capabilities that federal departments and agencies, through various emergency support functions, commonly provide during incident response.

Presidential Directives—U.S. government policy decisions on foreign affairs and national security that occur after the National Security Council gathers facts, conducts analyses, determines alternatives, and presents policy choices to the president for decision. These directives have been given different names by different presidential administrations. Bill Clinton used the Presidential Decision Directive (PDD) series to promulgate presidential decisions on national security matters. George W. Bush issued the first of a new series of Homeland Security Presidential Directives (HSPDs) governing homeland security policy. In the Barack Obama administration, the directives used to promulgate presidential decisions on national security matters were designated Presidential Policy Directives (PPDs).

Prevention—primary, secondary, and tertiary efforts to avert a disaster; includes the activities that are commonly thought of as "mitigation" in the emergency management model, and in public health terms, refers to actions that may prevent further loss of life, disease, disability, or injury.

Primary prevention—averting occurrence of deaths, injuries, or illnesses related to a disaster event (e.g., evacuation of a community in a flood-prone area, sensitizing warning systems for tornadoes and severe storms).

Secondary prevention—mitigating health consequences of disasters (e.g., use of carbon monoxide detectors when operating gasoline-powered generators after loss of electric power after ice storms, employing appropriate occupant behavior in multistory structures during earthquakes, building a "safe room" in dwellings located in tornado-prone areas); may be instituted when disasters are imminent.

Tertiary prevention—minimizing the effects of disease and disability among the already ill or injured; employed in people with preexisting health conditions and in whom the health effects from a disaster event may exacerbate those health conditions. Examples include appropriate sheltering of people with respiratory illnesses and those prone to such conditions, particularly the elderly and young children, from haze and smoke originating from forest fires, and sheltering elderly who are prone to heat illnesses during episodes of extreme ambient temperatures.

Principal federal official—may be appointed to serve as the secretary of the Department of Homeland Security's primary representative in the federal management of catastrophic or unusually complex incidents.

Public access system—911 emergency telephone system by which the public notifies the authorities that a medical emergency exists.

Public health surveillance—ongoing and systematic collection, analysis, and interpretation of health data used for planning, implementing, and evaluating public health interventions and programs; used to determine the need for public health action and to assess the effectiveness of programs.

Quarantine—separation of asymptomatic people who may have been exposed to infection from the general community.

Radiation

Acute radiation exposure—single large dose or a series of lesser but substantial doses over a short period.

Acute radiation syndrome—radiation illness associated with an acute radiation exposure.

Alpha particle—positively charged subatomic particle consisting of 2 protons and 2 neutrons, identical with the nucleus of the helium atom; the most energetic alpha particle is incapable of penetrating the skin.

As Low As Reasonably Achievable (ALARA)—concept and administrative program meant to keep workers' exposures to ionizing radiation "as low as reasonably achievable." This specific action program, which takes economic and social factors into account, is expected to reduce collective medical and occupational doses (person-rems) while maintaining an individual worker's dose at 10% or less of the dose limits contained in 10 C.F.R. § 20.

Background radiation—ionizing radiation that is a natural part of a person's environment; primarily, cosmic rays and that emitted by natural materials.

Beta particle—charged particle that is ejected from the nucleus of an atom; it has a mass and charge equal in magnitude to that of the electron.

Buffer zone—intermediate area between a radioactively contaminated zone and the rest of a "clean" building.

Cytogenetic dosimetry—estimation of radiation dose based on typical radiation-induced chromosomal aberrations as calibrated against standard exposures.

Film bandage—type of personal radiation monitor, or dosimeter, that records the extent of one's radiation exposure by means of sensitized photographic film.

Gamma ray—high-energy radiation of short wavelength emitted during the radioactive decay of many radioactive elements. Similar in properties to X-rays, gamma rays are of nuclear origin, whereas X-rays are formed by the excitation of orbital electrons.

High-level radiation dose—defined as being from 150 to 350 rems, per the National Council on Radiation Protection and Measurements Report No. 64.

International Commission on Radiological Protection—group, founded in 1928, whose function is to recommend international standards for radiation protection.

Ionizing radiation—form of radiation that is able to cause a neutral atom or molecule to gain or lose orbital electrons and thereby acquire a net electrical charge.

Isotope—one of 2 or more atoms with the same atomic number (and thus, similar chemical properties) but with different atomic weights and somewhat different physical properties.

Low-level radiation dose—generally considered for occupational purposes to be less than 5 rems per year, or 20 rems of a single dose, of uniform whole body radiation.

National Council on Radiation Protection and Measurements—nonprofit corporation chartered by Congress in 1964 to develop information and recommendations for the United States regarding radiation protection and measurements.

Personal monitor—device for measuring a person's exposure to a physical or chemical agent in the environment, such as radiation; information on the dose-equivalent of ionizing radiation to biological tissue is derived from film badges, ionization chambers, and thermoluminescent devices; determinations based on whole-body counting and analysis of biological specimens; and area monitoring and special surveys. Also referred to as a personnel dosimeter or monitor.

Rad—special unit for an absorbed dose of ionizing radiation.

Radionuclide—radioactive nuclide.

Rem—roentgen/radiation equivalent man; a special unit of dose equivalent based on biological effect and numerically equal to the absorbed dose in rad units multiplied by a modifying factor; however, for simplicity and for the types of radiation most often encountered environmentally, it is numerically equivalent to both the rad and roentgen.

Roentgen (R)—special unit of radiation exposure based on measurement in air or before radiation strikes the body.

Sealed source—radioactive store that is contained within an impervious and durable package so as to prevent contact with or release and dispersal of the radioactive items.

Thermoluminescent dosimeter—personnel monitor in which orbital electrons are displaced or trapped within a crystal such as manganese-activated calcium or lithium fluoride as a result of the crystal's exposure to ionizing radiation; when the crystal is later heated to a certain point, the stored energy of the electron displacement is released as light, which is then measured and related to radiation dose.

Transuranic elements—those elements with an atomic number greater than 92, or heavier than uranium (e.g., americium and plutonium); all are radioactive and not naturally occurring.

Radio bands—collection of neighboring frequencies allocated on different bands. Each two-way radio is designed for a specific band and will not work on other bands.

Rapid needs assessment—collection of techniques (e.g., epidemiologic, statistical, anthropological) designed to provide information about an affected community's needs after a disaster.

Readiness—links preparedness to relief; reflects the current capacity and capability of organizations involved in relief activities.

Real Simple Syndication (RSS) feeds—message that notifies users when a Web site is updated.

Reasonable accommodation/modification—any change to the rules, policies, procedures, or environment that enables an individual with a disability to participate. A requested accommodation is unreasonable if it poses an undue financial or administrative burden or a fundamental alteration in the program or service.

Recovery—actions for returning the community to normal after an emergency but before the reconstruction phase, including the stimulation of community and government cohesion and involvement, such as repair of infrastructure, damaged buildings, and critical facilities; has policy, political, and social implications that are both short and long term.

Red Cross—general term used for one or all the components of the worldwide organization active in humanitarian work. The official overall name is the International Red Cross and Red Crescent Movement, which has 3 components: the International Committee of the Red Cross, which acts mainly in conflict disasters as a neutral intermediary in hostilities and for the protection of war victims; the League of the Red Cross and Red Crescent Societies, which serves as the international federation of the National Societies and is active in nonconflict disasters and natural calamities; and the individual National Red Cross or Red Crescent Society of every country.

Regional Response Coordination Center—multiagency coordination center in a FEMA region staffed by emergency support personnel in anticipation of a serious incident in the region or immediately following an incident; operates under the direction of the FEMA Regional Administrator and is responsible for coordinating federal regional response efforts with state and local efforts.

Rehabilitation or reconstruction—efforts to reconstruct a system or infrastructure to the level that existed before an emergency through long-term development; during this time, attempts should be made to construct a system or infrastructure using the positive aspects of the previous system while at the same time attempting to correct the past problems and add improvements as a "reconstruction plus" approach.

Relief—period in which attention is focused on saving lives via such actions as search and rescue, first aid, and restoration of emergency communications and transportation systems, and attention to immediate care and basic needs of survivors, such as food, clothing, and medical or emotional care.

Report format—instrument on which data, such as surveillance data, are reported.

Reporting unit for surveillance—institution that provides information for the surveillance system, such as a hospital, clinic, health post, mobile health unit, or other unit determined after a case is defined.

Representativeness—accuracy of data in measuring the occurrence of a health event over time and its distribution by person and place.

Resilience—ability of a community or its members to rapidly and effectively rebound from events that are psychologically or behaviorally unsettling.

Resistance—ability of community or its members to resist clinical distress, impairment, or dysfunction associated with the range of disasters; psychological/behavioral immunity to distress and dysfunction.

Resource description framework—standard model for data interchange on the Web.

Response—phase of a disaster that encompasses relief and recovery and addresses the short-term, direct effects of an incident; includes immediate actions to save lives, protect property, and meet basic human needs; includes both the delivery of services and the management of activities.

Reunification—the process of assisting displaced disaster survivors, including children, and reestablishing contact with family and friends after a period of separation.

Risk assessment—systematic process used to determine the likelihood of adverse effects in a population following exposure to a specified hazard; endpoints or consequences depend on the hazard and include damage, loss of economic value, loss of function, loss of natural resources, loss of ecological systems, environmental impact, and deterioration of health, mortality, and morbidity.

Risk indicator—descriptor that briefly denotes a risk that may cause a disaster.

Risk management—public process of deciding what to do when risk assessments indicate that risk, or the chance of loss, exists. Risk management encompasses choices and actions for communities and individuals (e.g., prevention, mitigation, preparedness, and recovery) that are designed to stop increasing the risk to future elements that will be placed at risk to hazards, start decreasing the risk to existing elements already at risk, and continue planning ways to respond to and recover from an extreme situation or catastrophic event.

SAFECOM—group managed by by the U.S. Department of Homeland Security Office of Emergency Communications to create key documents to assist emergency responders nationwide with improving communications and interoperability.

Saffir-Simpson Hurricane Wind Scale—used to alert the public about the possible intensity of a hurricane. The scale categorizes a hurricane's intensity on a 1-to-5 scale to give an estimate of the potential property damage and flooding expected along the coast where the hurricane makes landfall. In general, damage from the hurricane increases by a factor of 4 for every category increase.

Science preparedness—a framework for conducting scientific research before, during or after a disaster. This approach encourages building a strong foundation of knowledge about disasters based on evidence to support decision making and policy development that can guide recovery and future preparedness efforts.

Secure Digital (SD)—memory card format used in portable devices.

Self-efficacy—psychological state characterized by the belief that one can organize and carry out necessary tasks to reach a goal.

Sentinel surveillance—an active or passive surveillance system that collects data about specific health events from a limited number of recruited participants or providers.

Service animal—specially trained animal used by a disabled person to help with daily living; these animals are allowed by law to accompany their owners anywhere they go.

Short-term recovery—process of recovery that is immediate and overlaps with response; includes such actions as providing essential public health and safety services, restoring interrupted utilities, reestablishing transportation routes, and providing food and shelter for those displaced by a disaster. Although called "short term," some of these activities may last for weeks.

Situational awareness—ability to identify, process, and comprehend the critical elements of information about an incident. Knowing what is going on around you during an emergency or disaster.

Social capital—connections within and between social networks that provide access to resources; social relationships that have productive benefits.

Social distancing—range of measures used to impede the spread of infectious disease in a community; does not involve quarantine but can reduce contact between and among people, such as closing schools or prohibiting large gatherings.

Social media—Web sites and applications that allow users to create and disseminate information or to participate in social networking.

Social networking sites—online communities in which users interact and exchange information.

Social vulnerability—susceptibility of individuals or organizations to the adverse impacts that accompany disasters.

Specific Area Message Encoding—protocol used to encode the Emergency Alert System for broadcast stations in the United States.

Stafford Act—the Robert T. Stafford Disaster Relief and Emergency Assistance Act of 1988, P.L. 93-288, as amended, describes the programs and processes by which the federal government provides disaster and emergency assistance to state and local governments, tribal nations, eligible private nonprofit organizations, and individuals affected by a declared major disaster or emergency. The act covers all hazards, including natural disasters and terrorist events.

State coordinating officer—individual appointed by the governor to coordinate state disaster assistance efforts with those of the federal government. The state coordinating officer plays a critical role in managing state response and recovery operations following Stafford Act declarations.

Stockpile—a store of material, medicines, equipment and other supplies needed for emergency relief in disaster that is kept in a specific place.

Stress—physical, mental, or emotional strain or tension.

SUMA—also known as "supply management program"; computer-based system developed by the Pan-American Health Organization that provides a mechanism for sorting, classifying, and preparing an inventory of relief supplies sent to a disaster-stricken country.

Support annexes—describe how federal departments and agencies, the private sector, volunteer organizations, and nongovernmental organizations coordinate and execute the common support processes and administrative tasks required during any type of incident.

Surge capacity—health care system's ability to rapidly expand and deliver services beyond what is required during normal care.

Surveillance—ongoing and systematic collection, analysis, and interpretation of health data essential to the planning, implementation, and evaluation of public health practice, closely integrated with the timely dissemination of data to those who need to know; includes both data collection and monitoring disease.

Syndromic surveillance—collection of data describing actions that precede diagnosis such as laboratory test requests, emergency department chief complaints, ambulance run sheets, prescription and over-the-counter drug use, school or work absenteeism and looks for clusters of medical signs and symptoms that may signal a sufficient probability of an outbreak to warrant further public health response.

Target capabilities list—defined specific capabilities that all levels of government should possess in order to respond effectively to incidents.

Technological hazard—potential threat to humans caused by technological factors, accidents, or failures of systems or structures (e.g., chemical release, nuclear accident, dam failure); natural hazards can trigger technological hazards.

Telecommunications relay service—telephone service that uses operators, called communications assistants, to facilitate telephone calls between people with hearing and speech disabilities and voice telephone users.

Text messaging—short messages exchanged between mobile devices.

Tiger team—military term for a group that probes security to find weaknesses that can be remedied.

Timeliness—how quickly information needed within a quick time frame can be made available.

Toxicological disaster—serious environmental pollution and illness caused by the massive accidental escape of toxic substances into the air, soil, or water.

Toxin—substance secreted by certain living organisms that are capable of causing harmful effects in other organisms.

Transportation to definitive medical care—use of ground ambulances, helicopters, boats, and snowcats for transport of patients to a higher level of medical care, usually at a hospital.

Traumatic stress—somewhat undefined category of stress caused by events and circumstances that are both extreme and outside of the realm of everyday experiences; this type of stress is often the result of dangerous, overwhelming, and sudden events and typically causes fear, anxiety, withdrawal, and avoidance in people who experience them.

Triage—selection and categorization of disaster victims for appropriate treatment according to the degree of severity of illness or injury and the availability of medical and transport facilities.

Tsunami—oceanic tidal wave generated by an underwater upheaval such as an earthquake or volcanic eruption. Waves move out in all directions over many miles, causing great destruction.

Tsunami run-up—measurement of the height of the water when a peak in the tsunami wave travels onto shore, much like very strong and fast-moving tides.

Unified Coordination Group—comprises specified senior leaders representing identified jurisdictions that provides leadership within a Joint Field Office; typically consists of the principal federal official (if designated), federal coordinating officer, state coordinating officer, and senior officials from other entities with primary statutory or jurisdictional responsibility and significant operational responsibility for an aspect of an incident.

Victim—person who has been affected by a disaster. There are 3 classes of victims: primary victims, who are affected by the physical impact of the disaster; secondary victims, who reside within an affected community or on the border of an affected area and suffer economic loss as a result of the disaster or actions taken by relief operations; and tertiary victims, who are indirectly affected and who may live in the same country but not necessarily in the affected area.

Victim distribution—plan established to define transport and distribution of victims among neighboring hospitals according to their hospital treatment capacity; the plan often involves avoiding the hospital nearest the disaster site since walking victims will overcrowd it.

Video relay—form of telecommunications service that enables people who are deaf, hard of hearing, or have speech disabilities and who use American Sign Language to communicate with voice telephone users through video equipment rather than through typed text.

Virtual private network—network that uses a public telecommunications infrastructure, such as the Internet, to provide remote offices or individual users with secure access to their organization's network.

Voluntary agency—nonprofit, nongovernmental, private association maintained and supported by voluntary contributions that provides assistance in emergencies and disasters.

Volunteer—any individual accepted to perform services without compensation.

Vulnerability—susceptibility of a given element to a given adverse event at a given intensity; the factors that influence vulnerability include demographics, age and resilience of the built environment, technology, social differentiation and diversity, regional and global economies, and political arrangements.

Vulnerability analysis—assessment of an exposed population's susceptibility to the adverse health effects of a given hazard.

Warning—indication that a severe weather event is presently happening, is going to happen, or has been observed on radar.

Watch—indication that a severe weather is threatening and may occur in an area; a watch indicates that citizens should listen to the radio or watch television for information and advice.

Whole community—includes individuals, families, and households; communities; the private and nonprofit sectors; faith-based organizations; and local, state, tribal, territorial, and federal governments who participate in national preparedness activities in conjunction with the participation of federal, state, and local governmental partners in order to foster better coordination and working relationships

White hat tools—security tools used to protect systems.

Widgets—small software applications on a Web page or program that have a specific function (e.g., clocks, event countdowns, auction-tickers, stock market tickers, flight arrival information, daily weather alerts).

Wi-Fi—trademark of the Wi-Fi Alliance that manufacturers use to brand products that belong to a class of wireless local area network.

Worried well—individuals who are not ill but seek medical treatment for reassurance.

APPENDIX B

COMMON ACRONYMS USED IN DISASTER PREPAREDNESS, RESPONSE, AND RECOVERY

AAR/IP	After-Action Report/Improvement Plan
ACIP	Advisory Committee on Immunization Practices
ACPHP	Academic Center for Public Health Preparedness
ADA	Americans With Disabilities Act
ADS	Automatic Detection System
AED	Automated External Defibrillator
AHRQ	Agency for Healthcare Research and Quality
ALS	Advanced Life Support
AMA	American Medical Association
APHL	Association of Public Health Laboratories
ASPR	Office of the Assistant Secretary for Preparedness and Response
ASTHO	Association of State and Territorial Health Officials
ATSDR	Agency for Toxic Substances and Disease Registry
AVA	Anthrax Vaccine Adsorbed
AVRP	Anthrax Vaccine Research Program
BARDA	Biomedical Advanced Research and Development Authority
BLS	Basic Life Support
BSL	Biosafety Level
CAP	Common Alerting Protocol
CAT	Crisis Action Team
CBO	Community-Based Organization
CBRNE	Chemical, Biological, Radiological/Nuclear, and High-Yield Explosives
CCP	Casualty Collection Point
CCRF	Commissioned Corps Readiness Force
CDC	Centers for Disease Control and Prevention
CDRG	Catastrophic Disaster Response Group
CEPPO	Chemical Emergency Preparedness and Prevention Office
CERCLA	Comprehensive Environmental Response, Compensation, and Liability Act

CFR	Code of Federal Regulations
CHEMTREC	Chemical Transportation Emergency Center
CHI	Consolidated Health Informatics
CINC	Commander-in-Chief
CLIA	Clinical Laboratory Improvement Act
CMAS	Commercial Mobile Alert System
CMHS	Center for Mental Health Services
CMS	Consumable Medical Supplies
CMT	Crisis Management Team
CONOPS	Concept of Operations Plan
COOP	Continuity of Operations (Plan)
CPHP	Centers for Public Health Preparedness
CPR	Cardiopulmonary Resuscitation
CRC	Crisis Response Cell
CRCs	Community Reception Centers
CSG	Counterterrorism Security Group
CSTE	Council of State and Territorial Epidemiologists
CWA	Clean Water Act
DAE	Disaster Assistance Employee
DCO	Defense Coordinating Officer
DFO	Disaster Field Office
DFSG	Disaster Financial Services Group
DHS	U.S. Department of Homeland Security
DMAT	Disaster Medical Assistance Team
DME	Durable Medical Equipment
DMORT	Disaster Mortuary Response Team, National Disaster Medical System
DPO	Disaster Psychiatry Outreach
DRC	Disaster Recovery Center
DRM	Disaster Recovery Manager
DWI	Disaster Welfare Inquiry
EAP	Emergency Action Plan
EAS	Emergency Alert System
EBS	Emergency Broadcast System
EC	Emergency Coordinator
ECS	Emergency Communications Staff/System
EEI	Essential Elements of Information
EICC	Emergency Information and Coordination Center
EIS	Epidemic Intelligence Service
EISO	Epidemic Intelligence Service Officer
ELR	Electronic Laboratory-Based Reporting

EMAC	Emergency Management Assistance Compact
EMG	Emergency Management Group
EMS	Emergency Medical Services
EMT	Emergency Medical Technician
EOC	Emergency Operations Center
EPA	Environmental Protection Agency
EPAP	Emergency Prescription Assistance Program
EPI-x	Epidemic Information Exchange
EPO	Epidemiology Program Office
ERC	Emergency Response Coordinator
ERCG	Emergency Response Coordination Group
ERT	Emergency Response Team
ERT-A	Emergency Response Team-Advance Element
ESAR-VHP	Emergency Service Advanced Registration of Volunteer Healthcare Providers
ESF	Emergency Support Function
EST	Emergency Support Team
FAA	Federal Aviation Administration
FACT	Family Assistance Center Team
FAST	Functional Assessment Service Team
FBI	Federal Bureau of Investigation
FCC	Federal Communications Commission/Federal Coordinating Center
FCO	Federal Coordinating Officer
FDA	Food and Drug Administration
FECC	Federal Emergency Communications Coordinator
FEMA	Federal Emergency Management Agency
FERC	FEMA Emergency Response Capability
FESC	Federal Emergency Support Coordinator
FHWA	Federal Highway Administration
FMO	Financial Management Office
FMS	Federal Medical Station
FNS	Food and Nutrition Service
FNSS	Functional Needs Support Services
FRCM	FEMA Regional Communications Manager
FRERP	Federal Radiological Emergency Response Plan
FRP	Federal Response Plan
GAR	Governor's Authorized Representative
GIS	Geographic Information System
GMPCS	Global Mobile Personal Communication System
GPMRC	Global Patient Movement Requirements Center

GSA	General Services Administration
HAN	Health Alert Network
HAZMAT	Hazardous Material
HAZWOPER	Hazardous Waste Operations and Emergency Response Standard
HET-ESF	Headquarters Emergency Transportation-Emergency Support Function
HHS	U.S. Department of Health & Human Services
HICPAC	Healthcare Infection Control Practices Advisory Committee
HICS	Hospital Incident Command System
HIPAA	Health Insurance Portability and Accountability Act
HIRA	Hazard Identification and Risk Assessment
HLT	Hurricane Liaison Team
HPP	Hospital Preparedness Program
HQUSACE	Headquarters, U.S. Army Corps of Engineers
HRSA	Health Resources and Services Administration
HSAS	Homeland Security Advisory System
HSPD	Homeland Security Presidential Directive
HUD	U.S. Department of Housing and Urban Development
HWC	Health and Welfare Canada
IAEA	International Atomic Energy Agency
IAP	Incident Action Plan
ICC	Interagency Coordinating Committee on Emergency Preparedness and Individuals with Disabilities
ICP	Incident Command Post
ICPAE	Interagency Committee on Public Affairs in Emergencies
ICRC	International Committee of the Red Cross
ICS	Incident Command System
IMAT	Incident Management Assistance Team
IMS	Incident Management System
IMSurT	International Medical Surgical Team
IPAWS	Integrated Public Alert and Warning System
IRAT	Immediate Response Assessment Team
IRCT	Incident Response Coordination Team
IT	Information Technology
JFO	Joint Field Office
JIC	Joint Information Center
JIS	Joint Information System
JOC	Joint Operations Center
JPAKS	Joint Patient Assessment Tracking System
LRAT	Logistical Response Assistance Team

LRN	Laboratory Response Network
LTE	Long-Term Evolution
MAC	Multi-Agency Coordination
MACS	Multi-Agency Coordination System
MANETS	Mobile Ad Hoc Network
MARS	U.S. Army Military Affiliate Radio System
MASF	Mobile Aeromedical Staging Facility
MERC	Mobile Emergency Response Support
MMWR	*Morbidity and Mortality Weekly Report*
MOA	Memorandum of Agreement
MOU	Memorandum of Understanding
MRC	Medical Reserve Corps
MRE	Meals Ready to Eat
MSEHPA	Model State Emergency Health Powers Act
NACCHO	National Association for City and County Health Officials
NBC	Nuclear, Biological, Chemical
NCBDDD	National Center on Birth Defects and Developmental Disease
NCC	National Coordinating Center
NCCDPHP	National Center for Chronic Disease Prevention and Health Promotion
NCEH	National Center for Environmental Health
NCHS	National Center for Health Statistics
NCHSTP	National Center for HIV, STD, and TB Prevention
NCID	National Center for Infectious Disease
NCIPC	National Center for Injury Prevention and Control
NCP	National Contingency Plan (National Oil and Hazardous Substances Pollution Contingency Plan)
NCS	National Communications System
NCS/DCA-OC	National Communications System/Defense Communication Agency-Operations Center
NDMOC	National Disaster Medical Operations Center
NDMS	National Disaster Medical System
NDMSOSC	National Disaster Medical System Operations Support Center
NDRF	National Disaster Recovery Framework
NECC	National Emergency Coordination Center
NEDSS	National Electronic Disease Surveillance System
NEIS	National Earthquake Information Service
NEMP	National Emergency Management Plan
NFDA	National Funeral Directors Association
NGO	Nongovernmental Organization

NHPP	Division of National Healthcare Preparedness Program
NHSN	National Healthcare Safety Network
NHSS	National Health Security Strategy
NIC	NIMS Integration Center
NICC	National Infrastructure Coordinating Center
NIFCC	National Interagency Fire Coordination Center
NIH	National Institutes of Health
NIMH	National Institutes of Mental Health
NIMS	National Incident Management System
NIOSH	National Institute for Occupational Safety and Health
NIP	National Immunization Program
NLTN	National Laboratory Training Network
NNRT	National Nurse Response Team
NOAA	National Oceanic and Atmospheric Administration
NOC	National Operations Center
NPD	National Preparedness Directorate
NPLT	National Pharmacy Logistics Teams
NPPTL	National Personal Protective Technology Laboratory
NPRT	National Pharmacy Response Team
NRC	Nuclear Regulatory Commission
NRCC	National Response Coordinating Center
NPF	National Planning Frameworks
NRF	National Response Framework
NRT	National Response Team
NSEP	National Security Emergency Preparedness
NSF	National Strike Force
NTIA	National Telecommunications and Information Administration
NTSP	National Telecommunications Support Plan
NTU	Nephelometric Turbidity Units
NVOAD	National Voluntary Organizations Active in Disaster
NVRT	National Veterinary Response Team
NWR	National Oceanic and Atmospheric Administration Weather Radio
NWS	National Weather Service
OAMCG	Office of Acquisition Management, Contracts and Grants
OCHAMPUS	Office of Civilian Health and Medical Program of the Uniformed Services
OCR	Office of Civil Rights
OEP	Office of Emergency Preparedness
OET	Office of Emergency Transportation
OFDA	Office of U.S. Foreign Disaster Assistance

OFPA	Office of Financial Planning and Analysis
OFRD	Office of Force Readiness and Deployment
OHS	Office of Health and Safety
OIG	Office of Inspector General
OPEO	Office of Preparedness and Emergency Operations
OPHPR	Office of Public Health Preparedness and Response
OPLAN	Operations Plan
OPP	Office of Policy and Planning
OSC	On-Scene Coordinator
OSEP	Office of Security and Emergency Preparedness
OSG	Office of the Surgeon General
OSHA	Occupational Safety and Health Administration
OTPER	Office of Terrorism Preparedness and Emergency Response
OVAG	Organic Vapor/Acid Gas
PAHO	Pan-American Health Organization
PAHPA	Pandemic and All-Hazards Preparedness Act
PAS	Personal Assistance Services
PDA	Preliminary Damage Assessment
PFO	Principal Federal Official
PHA	Public Health Advisor
PHEMCE	Public Health Emergency Countermeasure Enterprise
PHEP	Public Health Emergency Preparedness
PHI	Protected Health Information
PHICS	Public Health Incident Command System
PHIN	Public Health Information Network
PHPPO	Public Health Practice Program Office
PIO	Public Information Officer
PKEMRA	Post-Katrina Emergency Management Reform Act
POD	Point of Distribution
PPACA	Patient Protection and Affordable Care Act
PPE	Personal Protective Equipment
PSAP	Public Safety Answering Points
PTSD	Post-Traumatic Stress Disorder
PUI	Person Under Investigation
PVO	Private Voluntary Organization
PVS	Pre-Event Vaccination System
RACES	Radio Amateur Civil Emergency Services
RD	Regional Director
RDC	Office of Research and Development Coordination
RDF	Resource Description Framework

REACT	Radio Emergency Associated Communication Team
REC	Regional Emergency Coordinator
RECC	Regional Emergency Communications Coordinator
RECP	Regional Emergency Communications Plan
REP	Regional Evacuation Point
RET	Regional Emergency Transportation
RETCO	Regional Emergency Transportation Coordinator
RFA	Request for Assistance
RHA	Regional Health Administrator
RISC	Regional Inter-Agency Steering Committee
RRC	Ready Reserve Corps
RRCC	Regional Response Coordinating Center
RSS	Really Simple Syndication
SAME	Specific Area Message Encoding
SAMHSA	Substance Abuse and Mental Health Services Administration
SAP	Select Agent Program
SAR	Search and Rescue (National Urban)
SARA	Superfund Amendments and Reauthorization Act
SCBA	Self-Contained Breathing Apparatus
SCC	Secretary's Command Center
SCO	State Coordinating Officer
SD	Secure Digital (Card)
SEMO	State Emergency Management Office
SFLEO	Senior Federal Law Enforcement Officer
SHO	Senior Health Official
SO	Senior Official
SLPP	State and Local Preparedness Program
SLPS	State and Local Programs and Support Directorate
SNS	Strategic National Stockpile
SOC	Secretary's Operations Center
SOP	Standard Operating Procedure
SUMA	Supply Management System
SVP	Smallpox Vaccination Program
TARU	Technical Advisory Response Unit
TCL	Target Capabilities List
TED	Training, Education, and Demonstration Package
THIRA	Threat and Hazard Identification and Risk Assessment
TOPOFF	Top Officials
TRPLT	Terrorism Response and Preparation Leadership Team
TTY	Text Telephone

24/7	Twenty-Four Hours a Day/Seven Days a Week
UC	Unified Command
UCG	Unified Coordination Group
UNDRO	United Nations Disaster Relief Organization
UNHCR	United Nations High Commission for Refugees
UNICEF	United Nations International Children's Education Fund
USACE	U.S. Army Corps of Engineers
USAID	U.S. Agency for International Development
USCG	U.S. Coast Guard
USDA	U.S. Department of Agriculture
USGS	U.S. Geological Survey
USPHS	U.S. Public Health Service
US&R	Urban Search and Rescue
VA	U.S. Department of Veterans Affairs
VAERS	Vaccine Adverse Effects Reporting System
VANET	Vehicular Ad-Hoc Network
VHA	Veterans Health Administration
VIG	Vaccinia Immune Globulin
VMAT	Veterinary Medical Assistance Team
VMI	Vendor Managed Inventory
VOAD	Voluntary Organizations Active in Disaster
VPA	Volunteer Protection Act
VPN	Virtual Private Network
VRS	Video Relay Service
WHO	World Health Organization
WISER	Wireless Information for Emergency Responders
XML	Extensible Markup Language

APPENDIX C

THE LANGUAGE OF DISASTERS, EMERGENCIES, HAZARDS, AND INCIDENTS

Numerous terms are used to describe disasters. These terms include "major disaster," "emergency," "incident," and "catastrophic incident." These terms are derived from 2 documents: the Stafford Act as amended (major disaster and emergency) and the National Response Framework (NRF; incident and catastrophic incident).

Disasters and Hazards

As defined in the the Stafford Act as amended, a *major disaster* is:

> Any natural catastrophe (including any hurricane, tornado, storm, high water, winddriven water, tidal wave, tsunami, earthquake, volcanic eruption, landslide, mudslide, snowstorm, or drought), or, regardless of cause, any fire, flood, or explosion, in any part of the United States, which in the determination of the president causes damage of sufficient severity and magnitude to warrant major disaster assistance under this act to supplement the efforts and available resources of states, local governments, and disaster relief organizations in alleviating the damage, loss, hardship, or suffering caused thereby.

The Stafford Act, as amended, defines *emergency* as:

> Any occasion or instance for which, in the determination of the president, federal assistance is needed to supplement state and local efforts and capabilities to save lives and to protect property and public health and safety, or to lessen or avert the threat of a catastrophe in any part of the United States.

As defined by the NRF, a hazard is "something that is potentially dangerous or harmful, often the root cause of an unwanted outcome." The earthquake that struck Japan on March 11, 2011, was a disaster, although earthquakes in general are hazards.

Incidents

The NRF uses the term "incident" in a broader and more inclusive manner than it uses the terms "disaster" and "emergency." According to the NRF, an incident is "an occurrence or event, natural or human-caused that requires an emergency response to protect life or property." As defined, thousands of incidents across the United States occur every year. Most do not involve public health and are handled by first responders. Only a small number are of the magnitude that requires federal assistance, including catastrophic incidents.

Catastrophic incidents are comparable with presidentially declared major disasters and are described as:

> Any natural or man-made incident, including terrorism, that results in extraordinary levels of mass casualties, damage, or disruption severely affecting the population, infrastructure, environment, economy, national morale, and/or government functions.

The NRF includes a Catastrophic Incident Annex that can only be implemented by the secretary of the Department of Homeland Security or a designee. The annex covers both natural and man-made disasters that do significant harm and that overwhelm the response capabilities of local and state governments.

Details of the 2 Documents

Full Name	Robert T. Stafford Relief and Emergency Act of 1988 (as amended)	National Response Framework
Short Name	Stafford Act or 42 USC §§ 5121-5206	NRF
Date	1988; effective May 1989	January 2016
Creator	U.S. Congress	U.S. Department of Homeland Security
Purpose	"To provide an orderly and continuing means of assistance by the Federal Government to State and local governments in carrying out their responsibilities to alleviate the suffering and damage which result from ... disasters."	"The NRF is a guide to how the Nation responds to all types of disasters and emergencies. It is built on scalable, flexible, and adaptable concepts identified in the National Incident Management System (NIMS) to align key roles and responsibilities across the Nation. The NRF describes specific authorities and best practices for managing incidents that range from the serious but purely local to large-scale terrorist attacks or catastrophic natural disasters."
Lead Agency	Federal Emergency Management Agency	U.S. Department of Homeland Security

Source: Based on Federal Emergency Management Agency (FEMA). 2013. *The Stafford Act: Robert T. Stafford Disaster Relief and Emergency Assistance Act, as Amended.* Washington, DC: FEMA. Available at: https://www.fema.gov/media-library-data/1383153669955-21f970b19e8eaa67087b7da9f4af706e/stafford_act_booklet_042213_508e.pdf. Accessed January 25, 2017; Department of Homeland Security (DHS). 2016. National Response Framework. Washington, DC: DHS. Available at: https://www.fema.gov/media-library-data/1466014682982-9bcf8245ba4c60c120aa915abe74e15d/National_Response_Framework3rd.pdf. Accessed January 25, 2017.

STANDARDS, CAPABILITIES, AND RESPONSIBILITIES

APPENDIX D

KEY ELEMENTS OF A PUBLIC HEALTH PREPAREDNESS PROGRAM

System Characteristics

Resiliency, capacity to maintain continuity of activities

Ability to effectively manage the response to a disaster

Ability to recover or return to normal as quickly as possible

Advance Preparedness

Identify hazards and vulnerabilities to inform planning

Conduct advanced planning for emergencies and build capabilities necessary for coordinated and effective response

Integrate planning so local, state, and federal partners in emergency management and public health know how they will work together during disaster response

- Community determines gaps in local assets
- Plan compares available assets to likely needs
- Community, state, and federal partners identify what gaps will be filled by state or federal resources
- Regularly exercise plans to test roles and responsibilities and to ensure integration of all responding agencies and organizations

Develop an integrated Incident Command System for decision making and response capability, which clearly defines and assigns individual and agency roles and responsibilities in all sectors, at all levels of government, and with all individuals

Develop capacity to deliver essential services

- Identify critical resources for public health emergency response and arrange for delivery of these resources throughout the supply chain

Ensure reliable communication systems

- Ensure capability to provide accurate and credible information to the public in culturally appropriate ways
- Ensure capacity and reliability of health information infrastructure

Develop capacity for early detection and identification of health threats

- Maintain and improve systems to monitor, detect, and investigate potential hazards (e.g., environmental, radiological, toxic, or infectious)
- Ensure laboratory capacity

Develop community mitigation strategies (e.g., isolation and quarantine, social distancing) and countermeasure distribution strategies

Identify and address issues of legal authority and liability barriers in monitoring, preventing, or responding to a public health emergency

Coordinated Rapid-Response Capability

Use an integrated Incident Command System for decision making and response capability

Identify nature of disaster and public health concerns via surveillance, epidemiological investigation, and laboratory diagnosis

Deliver essential services (i.e., mass health care) postimpact to the affected community

Implement prevention and containment strategies

- Implement community mitigation strategies and distribute appropriate countermeasures
- Educate and mobilize the public by rapidly providing accurate and credible information in culturally appropriate ways

Distribute essential resources needed for public health interventions

Trained Workforce

Develop and maintain a public health and health care workforce that has the skills and capabilities needed in a public health emergency

Train, recruit, and develop public health leaders who can mobilize resources, engage the community, develop interagency relationships, and communicate with the public

Accountability and Quality Improvement

Test operational capabilities through real public health events, drills, and exercises

Develop financial systems to track resources used and services delivered to ensure adequate and timely reimbursement

Source: Based on Nelson C, Lurie N, Wasserman J, Zakowski S. 2007. Conceptualizing and defining public health emergency preparedness. *Am J Public Health*. 97(Suppl 1):S9–S11.

APPENDIX E

PUBLIC HEALTH PREPAREDNESS CAPABILITIES: NATIONAL STANDARDS FOR STATE AND LOCAL PLANNING

Capability Definitions, Functions, and Associated Performance Measures

Capability 1: Community Preparedness

Definition

Community preparedness is the ability of communities to prepare for, withstand, and recover—in both the short and long term—from public health incidents. By engaging and coordinating with emergency management; health care organizations (private and community-based); mental/behavioral health providers; community and faith-based partners; and state, local, and territorial governments, public health's role in community preparedness is to do the following:

Support the development of public health, medical, and mental/behavioral health systems that support recovery.

Participate in awareness training with community and faith-based partners on how to prevent, respond to, and recover from incidents of public health significance.

Promote awareness of and access to medical and mental/behavioral health resources that help protect the community's health and address the functional needs (e.g., communication, medical care, independence, supervision, transportation) of at-risk individuals.

Engage public and private organizations in preparedness activities that represent the functional needs of at-risk individuals as well as the cultural, socioeconomic, and demographic components of the community.

Identify those populations that may be at higher risk for adverse health outcomes.

Receive and integrate the health needs of populations that have been displaced as a result of incidents that have occurred in their own or distant communities (e.g., improvised nuclear device or hurricane).

Functions and Associated Performance Measures

This capability consists of the ability to perform the functions listed below. At present, there are no performance measures defined by the Centers for Disease Control and Prevention (CDC) for these functions.

Function 1: Determine risks to the health of the jurisdiction

Function 2: Build community partnerships to support health preparedness

Function 3: Engage with community organizations to foster public health, medical, and mental/behavioral health social networks

Function 4: Coordinate training or guidance to ensure community engagement in preparedness efforts

Capability 2: Community Recovery

Definition

Community recovery is the ability to collaborate with community partners (e.g., health care organizations, business, education, and emergency management) to plan and advocate the rebuilding of public health, medical, and mental/behavioral health systems to a level of functioning comparable with pre-incident levels at a minimum and improved levels where possible.

This capability supports National Health Security Strategy Objective 8: Incorporate Post-Incident Health Recovery Into Planning and Response. Post-incident recovery of the public health, medical, and mental/behavioral health services and systems within a jurisdiction is critical for health security and requires collaboration and advocacy by the public health agency for the restoration of services, providers, facilities, and infrastructure within the public health, medical, and human services sectors. Monitoring the public health, medical, and mental/behavioral health infrastructure is an essential public health service.

Functions and Associated Performance Measures

This capability consists of the ability to perform the functions listed below. At present, there are no CDC-defined performance measures for these functions.

Function 1: Identify and monitor public health, medical, and mental/behavioral health system recovery needs

Function 2: Coordinate community public health, medical, and mental/behavioral health system recovery operations

Function 3:	Implement corrective actions to mitigate damages from future incidents

Capability 3: Emergency Operations Coordination

Definition

Emergency operations coordination is the ability to direct and support an event or incident with public health or medical implications by establishing a standardized, scalable system of oversight, organization, and supervision consistent with jurisdictional standards and practices and with the National Incident Management System.

Functions and Associated Performance Measures

This capability consists of the ability to perform the functions listed below. Associated CDC-defined performance measures are also listed below.

Function 1:	Conduct preliminary assessment to determine need for public activation
Function 2:	Activate public health emergency operations
Measure 1:	Time for pre-identified staff covering activated public health agency incident management lead roles (or equivalent lead roles) to report for immediate duty. Performance Target: 60 minutes or less
Function 3:	Develop incident response strategy
Measure 1:	Production of the approved Incident Action Plan before the start of the second operational period
Function 4:	Manage and sustain the public health response
Function 5:	Demobilize and evaluate public health emergency operations
Measure 1:	Time to complete a draft of an After Action Report and Improvement Plan

Capability 4: Emergency Public Information and Warning

Definition

Emergency public information and warning is the ability to develop, coordinate, and disseminate information, alerts, warnings, and notifications to the public and incident management responders.

Functions and Associated Performance Measures

This capability consists of the ability to perform the functions listed below. Associated CDC-defined performance measures are also listed below.

Function 1:	Activate the emergency public information system
Function 2:	Determine the need for a joint public information system
Function 3:	Establish and participate in information system operations
Function 4:	Establish avenues for public interaction and information exchange
Function 5:	Issue public information, alerts, warnings, and notifications
Measure 1:	Time to issue a risk communication message for dissemination to the public

Capability 5: Fatality Management

Definition

Fatality management is the ability to coordinate with other organizations (e.g., law enforcement, health care, emergency management, medical examiner/coroner) to ensure the proper recovery, handling, identification, transportation, tracking, storage, and disposal of human remains and personal effects; certify cause of death; and facilitate access to mental/behavioral health services to the family members, responders, and survivors of an incident.

Functions and Associated Performance Measures

This capability consists of the ability to perform the functions listed below. At present, there are no CDC-defined performance measures for these functions.

Function 1:	Determine role for public health in fatality management
Function 2:	Activate public health fatality management operations
Function 3:	Assist in the collection and dissemination of antemortem data
Function 4:	Participate in survivor mental/behavioral health services
Function 5:	Participate in fatality processing and storage operations

Capability 6: Information Sharing

Definition

Information sharing is the ability to conduct multijurisdictional, multidisciplinary exchange of health-related information and situational awareness data among federal, state, local, territorial, and tribal levels of government and the private sector. This capability includes the routine sharing of information as well as issuing of public health alerts to federal, state, local, territorial, and tribal levels of government and the private sector in preparation for, and in response to, events or incidents of public health significance.

Functions and Associated Performance Measures

This capability consists of the ability to perform the functions listed below. At present, there are no CDC-defined performance measures for these functions.

Function 1: Identify stakeholders to be incorporated into information flow

Function 2: Identify and develop rules and data elements for sharing

Function 3: Exchange information to determine a common operating picture

Capability 7: Mass Care

Definition

Mass care is the ability to coordinate with partner agencies to address the public health, medical, and mental/behavioral health needs of those impacted by an incident at a congregate location. This capability includes the coordination of ongoing surveillance and assessment to ensure that health needs continue to be met as the incident evolves.

Functions and Associated Performance Measures

This capability consists of the ability to perform the functions listed below. At present, there are no CDC-defined performance measures for these functions.

Function 1: Determine public health role in mass care operations

Function 2: Determine mass care needs of the impacted population

Function 3: Coordinate public health, medical, and mental/behavioral health services

Function 4: Monitor mass care population health

Capability 8: Medical Countermeasure Dispensing

Definition

Medical countermeasure dispensing is the ability to provide medical countermeasures (including vaccines, antiviral drugs, antibiotics, antitoxins) in support of treatment or prophylaxis (oral or vaccination) to the identified population in accordance with public health guidelines and recommendations.

Functions and Associated Performance Measures

This capability consists of the ability to perform the functions listed below. Associated CDC-defined performance measures are also listed below.

Function 1: Identify and initiate medical countermeasure dispensing strategies

Function 2: Receive medical countermeasures

Function 3: Activate dispensing modalities

Measure 1: Composite performance indicator from the Division of Strategic National Stockpile in the CDC's Office of Public Health Preparedness and Response

Function 4: Dispense medical countermeasures to identified population

Measure 1: Composite performance indicator from the Division of Strategic National Stockpile in the CDC's Office of Public Health Preparedness and Response

Function 5: Report adverse events

Capability 9: Medical Materiel Management and Distribution

Definition

Medical materiel management and distribution is the ability to acquire, maintain (e.g., cold chain storage or other storage protocol), transport, distribute, and track medical materiel (e.g., pharmaceuticals, gloves, masks, ventilators) during an incident and to recover and account for unused medical matriel, as necessary, after an incident.

Functions and Associated Performance Measures

This capability consists of the ability to perform the functions listed below. Associated CDC-defined performance measures are also listed below.

Function 1: Direct and activate medical materiel management and distribution

Measure 1: Composite performance indicator from the Division of Strategic National Stockpile in the CDC's Office of Public Health Preparedness and Response

Function 2: Acquire medical materiel

Measure 1: Composite performance indicator from the Division of Strategic National Stockpile in the CDC's Office of Public Health Preparedness and Response

Function 3: Maintain updated inventory management and reporting system

Measure 1: Composite performance indicator from the Division of Strategic National Stockpile in the CDC's Office of Public Health Preparedness and Response

Function 4: Establish and maintain security

Measure 1: Composite performance indicator from the Division of Strategic National Stockpile in CDC's Office of Public Health Preparedness and Response

Function 5: Distribute medical materiel

Measure 1: Composite performance indicator from the Division of Strategic National Stockpile in CDC's Office of Public Health Preparedness and Response

Function 6: Recover medical materiel and demobilize distribution operations

Measure 1: Composite performance indicator from the Division of Strategic National Stockpile in CDC's Office of Public Health Preparedness and Response

Capability 10: Medical Surge

Definition

Medical surge is the ability to provide adequate medical evaluation and care during events that exceed the limits of the normal medical infrastructure of an affected community. It encompasses the ability of the health care system to survive a hazard impact and maintain or rapidly recover operations that were compromised.

Functions and Associated Performance Measures

This capability consists of the ability to perform the functions listed below. At present, there are no CDC-defined performance measures for these functions.

Function 1: Assess the nature and scope of the incident

Function 2: Support activation of medical surge

Function 3: Support jurisdictional medical surge operations

Function 4: Support demobilization of medical surge operations

Capability 11: Nonpharmaceutical Interventions

Definition

Nonpharmaceutical interventions are the ability to recommend to the applicable lead agency (if not public health agency) and implement, if applicable, strategies for disease, injury, and exposure control. Strategies include the following:

Isolation and quarantine

Restrictions on movement and travel advisory/warnings

Social distancing

External decontamination

Hygiene

Precautionary protective behaviors

Functions and Associated Performance Measures

This capability consists of the ability to perform the functions listed below. At present, there are no CDC-defined performance measures for these functions.

Function 1: Engage partners and identify factors that impact nonpharmaceutical interventions

Function 2: Determine nonpharmaceutical interventions

Function 3: Implement nonpharmaceutical interventions

Function 4: Monitor nonpharmaceutical interventions

Capability 12: Public Health Laboratory Testing

Definition

Public health laboratory testing is the ability to conduct rapid and conventional detection, characterization, confirmatory testing, data reporting, investigative support, and laboratory networking to address actual or potential exposure to all-hazards. Hazards include chemical, radiological, and biological agents in multiple matrices that may include clinical samples, food, and environmental samples (e.g., water, air, soil). This capability supports routine surveillance, including pre-event or pre-incident and postexposure activities.

Functions and Associated Performance Measures

This capability consists of the ability to perform the functions listed below. Associated CDC-defined performance measures are also listed below.

Function 1: Manage laboratory activities

Measure 1: Time for sentinel clinical laboratories to acknowledge receipt of an urgent message from the CDC Public Health Emergency Preparedness (PHEP)-funded Laboratory Response Network biological (LRN-B) laboratory

Measure 2: Time for initial laboratorian to report for duty at the CDC PHEP-funded laboratory

Function 2: Perform sample management

Measure 1: Percentage of Laboratory Response Network (LRN) clinical specimens without any adverse quality assurance events received at the CDC PHEP-funded LRN-B laboratory for confirmation or rule-out testing from sentinel clinical laboratories

Measure 2: Percentage of LRN nonclinical samples without any adverse quality assurance events received at the CDC PHEP-funded LRN-B laboratory for confirmation or rule-out testing from first responders

Measure 3: Ability of the CDC PHEP-funded Laboratory Response Network chemical (LRN-C) laboratories to collect relevant samples for clinical chemical analysis, package, and ship those samples

Function 3: Conduct testing and analysis for routine and surge capacity

Measure 1: Proportion of LRN-C proficiency tests (core methods) successfully passed by CDC PHEP-funded laboratories

Measure 2: Proportion of LRN-C proficiency tests (additional methods) successfully passed by CDC PHEP-funded laboratories

Measure 3: Proportion of LRN-B proficiency tests successfully passed by CDC PHEP-funded laboratories

Function 4: Support public health investigations

Measure 1: Time to complete notification between CDC, on-call laboratorian, and on-call epidemiologist

Measure 2: Time to complete notification between CDC, on-call epidemiologist, and on-call laboratorian

Function 5: Report results

Measure 1: Percentage of pulsed field gel electrophoresis (PFGE) subtyping data results for *E. coli* O157:H7 submitted to the PulseNet national database within 4 working days of receiving isolate at the PFGE laboratory

Measure 2: Percentage of PFGE subtyping data results for *Listeria monocytogenes* submitted to the PulseNet national database within 4 working days of receiving isolate at the PFGE laboratory

Measure 3: Time to submit PFGE subtyping data results for *Salmonella* to the PulseNet national database upon receipt of isolate at the PFGE laboratory

Measure 4: Time for CDC PHEP-funded laboratory to notify public health partners of significant laboratory results

Capability 13: Public Health Surveillance and Epidemiological Investigation

Definition

Public health surveillance and epidemiological investigation is the ability to create, maintain, support, and strengthen routine surveillance and detection systems and epidemiological investigation processes, as well as to expand these systems and processes in response to incidents of public health significance.

Functions and Associated Performance Measures

This capability consists of the ability to perform the functions listed below. Associated CDC-defined performance measures are also listed below.

Function 1: Conduct public health surveillance and detection

Measure 1: Proportion of reports of selected reportable diseases received by a public health agency within the jurisdiction-required time frame

Function 2: Conduct public health and epidemiological investigations

Measure 1: Percentage of infectious disease outbreak investigations that generate reports

Measure 2: Percentage of infectious disease outbreak investigation reports that contain all minimal elements

Measure 3: Percentage of acute environmental exposure investigations that generate reports

Measure 4: Percentage of acute environmental exposure reports that contain all minimal elements

Function 3: Recommend, monitor, and analyze mitigation actions

Measure 1: Proportion of reports of selected reportable diseases for which initial public health control measure(s) were initiated within the appropriate time frame

Function 4: Improve public health surveillance and epidemiological investigation systems

Capability 14: Responder Safety and Health

Definition

The responder safety and health capability describes the ability to protect public health agency staff responding to an incident and the ability to support the health and safety needs of hospital and medical facility personnel, if requested.

Functions and Associated Performance Measures

This capability consists of the ability to perform the functions listed below. At present, there are no CDC-defined performance measures for these functions.

Function 1: Identify responder safety and health risks

Function 2: Identify safety and personal protective needs

Function 3: Coordinate with partners to facilitate risk-specific safety and health training

Function 4: Monitor responder safety and health actions

Capability 15: Volunteer Management

Definition

Volunteer management is the ability to coordinate the identification, recruitment, registration, credential verification, training, and engagement of volunteers to support the jurisdictional public health agency's response to incidents of public health significance.

Functions and Associated Performance Measures

This capability consists of the ability to perform the functions listed below. At present, there are no CDC-defined performance measures for these functions.

Function 1: Coordinate volunteers

Function 2: Notify volunteers

Function 3: Organize, assemble, and dispatch volunteers

Function 4: Demobilize volunteers

Source: Adapted from Office of Public Health Preparedness and Response. 2011. *Public Health Preparedness Capabilities: National Standards for State and Local Planning.* Atlanta, GA: Centers for Disease Control and Prevention. Available at: http://www.cdc.gov/phpr/capabilities/dslr_capabilities_july.pdf. Accessed January 25, 2017.

APPENDIX F

EMERGENCY SUPPORT FUNCTION #8: PUBLIC HEALTH AND MEDICAL SERVICES

ESF Coordinator:	Department of Health & Human Services (HHS)
Primary Agency:	HHS
Support Agencies:	Department of Agriculture
	Department of Commerce
	Department of Defense
	Department of Energy
	Department of Homeland Security
	Department of the Interior
	Department of Justice
	Department of Labor
	Department of State
	Department of Transportation
	Department of Veterans Affairs
	Environmental Protection Agency
	General Services Administration
	U.S. Agency for International Development
	U.S. Postal Service
	American Red Cross

Purpose

Emergency Support Function (ESF) #8: Public Health and Medical Services provides the mechanism for federal assistance to supplement local, state, tribal, territorial, and insular area resources in response to a disaster, emergency, or incident that may lead to a public health, medical, behavioral, or human service emergency, including those that have international implications.

Scope

ESF #8 provides planning and coordination of federal public health, health care delivery, and emergency response systems to minimize and/or prevent health emergencies from occurring; to detect and characterize health incidents; to provide medical care and human services to those affected; to reduce the public health and human service effects on the community; and to enhance community resiliency to respond to a disaster. These actions are informed through integrated biosurveillance capability, assessment of health and human service needs, and maintenance of the safety and security of medical products, as well as the safety and defense of food and agricultural products under the Food and Drug Administration's (FDA) regulatory authority.

Public health and medical services (e.g., patient movement, patient care, and behavioral health care) and support to human services (e.g., addressing individuals with disabilities and others with access and functional needs) are delivered through surge capabilities that augment public health, medical, behavioral, and veterinary functions with health professionals and pharmaceuticals. These services include distribution and delivery of medical countermeasures, equipment and supplies, and technical assistance. These services are provided to mitigate the effects of acute and longer-term threats to the health of the population and maintain the health and safety of responders. ESF #8 disseminates public health information on protective actions related to exposure to health threats or environmental threats (e.g., to potable water and food safety).

Jurisdictional medico-legal authorities are assisted in carrying out fatality management responsibilities by providing specialized teams and equipment to conduct victim identification, grief counseling and consultation, and reunification of human remains and effects to authorized person(s). ESF #8 may continue providing services and ensure a smooth transition to recovery while the community rebuilds their capability and assumes administrative and operational responsibility for services. ESF #8 provides supplemental assistance to local, state, tribal, territorial, and insular area governments in the following core functional areas:

Assessment of public health/medical needs

Public health surveillance

Medical surge

Health/medical/veterinary equipment and supplies

Patient movement

Patient care

Outpatient services

Victim decontamination

Safety and security of drugs, biologics, medical devices

Blood and tissues

Food safety and defense

Agriculture safety and security

All-hazards public health and medical consultation, technical assistance, and support

Behavioral health care

Public health and medical information

Vector control

Guidance on potable water/wastewater and solid waste disposal

Mass fatality management, victim identification, and mitigating health hazards from contaminated remains

Veterinary medical support

Relationship to the Whole Community

This section describes how ESF #8 relates to other elements of the whole community.

Local, State, Tribal, Territorial, and Insular Area Governments

While local, state, tribal, territorial, and insular area officials retain primary responsibility for meeting public health and medical needs, ESF #8 can deploy public health and medical resources to assist as needed. In a major public health or medical emergency, demand for public health and medical resources may exceed local, state, tribal, territorial, and insular area capability. State, tribal, territorial, or insular area jurisdictions may request assistance through the Emergency Management Assistance Compact or may request federal assistance, which may be executed under the Stafford Act or other authorities. When possible, a recognized spokesperson from the affected public health and medical community (e.g., local, state, tribal, territorial, or insular area) delivers relevant health messages.

Private Sector/Nongovernmental Organizations

The vast majority of public health and medical activities and services are provided by the private health care sector. ESF #8 augments the support provided by the private health care sector when requested by local, state, tribal, territorial, or insular area governments. ESF #8 works with retail, wholesale, and other similar private industry associations for information sharing, planning, and exercises that would produce mutually beneficial results in coordinating how, when, where, and by whom critical resources will be provided during all types of incidents. ESF #8 organizations work closely with the private sector (e.g., regulated industries, academic institutions, trade organizations, and advocacy groups); volunteer organizations (e.g., faith-based and neighborhood partnerships); and local and state agencies to coordinate ESF #8 response resources. ESF #8 organizations recognize that leveraging resources from these organizations and individuals with shared interests allows ESF #8 to accomplish its mission in ways that are the least burdensome and most beneficial to the American public and that enhance the resilience of health care systems to deliver coordinated and effective care during public health emergencies and mass casualty events. Nongovernmental organizations, including community-based organizations, are an important partner in recruiting and supporting health professional volunteers and providing medical and counseling services to victims and their families.

Federal Government

Specific information on federal government actions is described in the following sections.

Core Capabilities and Actions

ESF roles aligned to core capabilities. The following table lists the response core capabilities that ESF #8 most directly supports along with the related ESF #8 actions. All ESFs support the following core capabilities: planning, operational coordination, and public information and warning.

Integration with the National Disaster Recovery Framework

ESF #8 is linked closely with the Health and Social Services Recovery Support Functions (RSF) under the National Disaster Recovery Framework. The Health and Social Services RSF may stand up nearly as early as ESF #8, though initially to focus on planning and

Core Capability	ESF #8: Public Health and Medical Services
Public Information and Warning	Public Health and Medical Information • Coordinates the federal public health and medical messaging with jurisdictional officials. • Continuously acquires and assesses information on the incident. • Sources of information may include state incident response authorities; officials of the responsible jurisdiction in charge of the disaster scene; and ESF #8 support departments, agencies, and organizations. • Provides public health, behavioral health, disease, and injury prevention information that can be transmitted to members of the general public and responders who are located in or near affected areas in multiple and accessible formats and languages in a culturally and linguistically appropriate manner that is understandable to all appropriate populations, such as individuals with access and functional needs; those with limited English proficiency; pediatric populations; populations with disabilities and others with access and functional needs; the aging; and those with temporary or chronic medical conditions. • Supports a Joint Information Center in the release of general medical and public health response information to the public.
Critical Transportation	Patient Movement • Transports seriously ill or injured patients and medical needs populations from point of injury or casualty collection points in the impacted area to designated reception facilities. • Coordinates the federal response in support of emergency triage and pre-hospital treatment, patient tracking, distribution, and patient return. This effort is coordinated with federal and local, state, tribal, territorial, and insular area emergency medical services officials. • Provides resources to assist in the movement of at-risk/medically fragile populations to shelter areas and with the sheltering of the special medical needs population that exceeds the state capacity. • Provides private vendor ambulance support to assist in the movement of patients through the National Ambulance Contract. • Provides support for evacuating seriously ill or injured patients though the National Disaster Medical System (NDMS). This is an interagency partnership between the Department of Health & Human Services (HHS), the Department of Homeland Security (DHS), the Department of Defense (DOD), and the Department of Veterans Affairs (VA). • Support may include providing accessible transportation assets; operating and staffing NDMS patient collection points (e.g., aerial ports of embarkation [APOE]); and/or establishing Federal Coordinating Centers (FCCs) that conduct patient reception at ports of debarkation (e.g., aerial ports of debarkation [APOD]). • Federal support may also include processing and tracking patient movement from collection points to their final destination reception. • Facilities through final disposition. (Note: DOD is responsible for tracking patients transported on DOD assets to the receiving FCC.) • Provides patient tracking from point of entry to final disposition. • Provides capability to identify bed capacity for the purposes of bed allocation among health care treatment networks.

(Continued)

Core Capability	ESF #8: Public Health and Medical Services
Environmental Response/ Health and Safety	• Supports the Worker Safety and Health Support Annex; provides technical assistance; and conducts exposure assessments and risk management to control hazards for response workers and the public.
Fatality Management Services	• Assists jurisdictional medico-legal authorities and law enforcement agencies in the tracking and documenting of human remains and associated personal effects; reducing the hazard presented by chemically, biologically, or radiologically contaminated human remains (when indicated and possible); establishing temporary morgue facilities; determining the cause and manner of death; collecting antemortem data in a compassionate and culturally competent fashion from authorized individuals; performing postmortem data collection and documentation; identifying human remains using scientific means (e.g., dental, pathology, anthropology, fingerprints, and, as indicated, DNA samples); and preparing, processing, and returning human remains and personal effects to the authorized person(s) when possible; and providing technical assistance and consultation on fatality management and mortuary affair services. May provide behavioral health support to families of victims during the victim identification mortuary process. • May provide for temporary interment when permanent disposition options are not readily available.
Mass Care Services	• Provides technical expertise and guidance on the public health issues of the medical needs population. • Assists with applications for federal benefits sponsored by HHS and ensures continuity of assistance services in affected states and in states hosting relocated populations. • Provides support for the provision of case management and advocacy services. • Provides support for human and/or veterinary mass care sheltering, as resources are available.
Logistics and Supply Chain Management	Health, Medical, and Veterinary Equipment and Supplies • Arranges for the procurement and transportation of equipment and supplies; diagnostic supplies; radiation detection devices; and medical countermeasures including assets from the Strategic National Stockpile (SNS); in support of immediate public health, medical and veterinary response operations. Blood and Tissues • Monitors and ensures the safety, availability, and logistical requirements of blood, blood products and tissue. This includes the ability of the existing supply chain resources to meet the manufacturing, testing, storage, and distribution of these products.
Public Health, Health Care, and Emergency Medical Services	Health Surveillance • Uses existing all-hazards surveillance systems to monitor the health of the general and medical needs population, as well as that of response workers, and identify emerging trends related to the disaster; carries out field studies and investigations; monitors injury and disease patterns and potential disease outbreaks, behavioral health concerns, blood, blood products, and tissue supply levels; and provides technical assistance and consultations on disease and injury prevention and precautions. Provides support to laboratory diagnostics and through the Laboratory Response Network (LRN) provides a mechanism for laboratories to access additional resources when the capabilities or capacity have been exceeded.

(*Continued*)

Core Capability	ESF #8: Public Health and Medical Services
	Medical Surge • Provides support for triage, patient treatment, and patient movement. • Provides clinical public health and medical care specialists from the NDMS, U.S. Public Health Service, VA, and DOD to fill local, state, tribal, territorial, and insular area health professional needs. • Coordinates with states to integrate federal assets with civilian volunteers deployed from local, state, and other authorities, including those deployed through the Emergency System for Advance Registration of Volunteer Health Professionals and the Medical Reserve Corps. Patient Care • Provides resources to support pre-hospital triage and treatment, inpatient hospital care, outpatient services, behavioral health care, medical-needs sheltering, pharmacy services, and dental care to victims with acute injury/illnesses or those who suffer from chronic illnesses/conditions. • Assists with isolation and quarantine measures as well as with medical countermeasure and vaccine point of distribution operations (e.g., mass prophylaxis). • Ensures appropriate patient confidentiality is maintained, including Health Insurance Portability and Accountability Act privacy and security standards, where applicable. Assessment of Public Health/Medical Needs • Supports national or regional teams to assess public health and medical needs. This function includes the assessment of the health care system/facility infrastructure. Food Safety, Security, and Defense • In coordination with ESF #11, may task HHS components and request assistance from other ESF #8 partner organizations to ensure the safety, security, and defense of federally regulated foods. Agriculture Safety and Security • In coordination with ESF #11, ESF #8 may task components to ensure the health, safety, and security of livestock and food-producing animals and animal feed, as well as the safety of the manufacture and distribution of foods, drugs, and therapeutics given to animals used for human food production. ESF #8 may also provide veterinary assistance to ESF #11 for the care of research animals. Safety and Security of Drugs, Biologics, and Medical Devices • During response, provides advice to private industry regarding the safety and efficacy of drugs; biologics (including blood, blood products, tissues and vaccines); medical devices (including radiation emitting and screening devices); and other products that may have been compromised during an incident and are HHS-regulated products.

(*Continued*)

Core Capability	ESF #8: Public Health and Medical Services
	All-Hazard Public Health and Medical Consultation, Technical Assistance, and Support • Assesses public health, medical, and veterinary medical effects resulting from all hazards. Such tasks may include assessing exposures on the general population, on children, and on those with disabilities and others with access and functional needs; conducting field investigations, including collection and analysis of relevant samples; advising protective actions related to direct human and animal exposures and on indirect exposure through contaminated food, drugs, water supply, and other media; and providing technical assistance and consultation on medical treatment, screening, and decontamination of injured or contaminated individuals. Provides for disaster-related health and behavioral health needs through direct services and/or referrals as necessary. Vector Control • Assesses the threat of vector-borne diseases. • Conducts field investigations, including the collection and laboratory analysis of relevant samples; provides vector control equipment and supplies. • Provides technical assistance and consultation on protective actions regarding vector-borne diseases. • Provides aerial spraying for vector control. • Provides technical assistance and consultation on medical treatment of victims of vector-borne diseases. Public Health Aspects of Potable Water/Wastewater and Solid Waste Disposal • Assists in assessing potable water, wastewater, solid waste disposal, and other environmental health issues related to public health in establishments holding, preparing, and/or serving food, drugs, or medical devices at retail and medical facilities, as well as examining and responding to public health effects from contaminated water; conducting field investigations, including collection and laboratory analysis of relevant samples; providing equipment and supplies as needed; and providing technical assistance and consultation. Veterinary Medical Support • Provides veterinary medical support to treat ill or injured animals and veterinary public health support through HHS National Veterinary Response Team and veterinary medical officers of the Commissioned Corps of the U.S. Public Health Service. • ESF #8 is the primary federal resource for treatment of ill or injured service animals, pets, working animals, laboratory animals, and livestock post-disaster. • Under HHS' statutory authority conduct animal response to zoonotic diseases in order to protect human health. • Support the U.S. Department of Agriculture (USDA) and its authority to manage a foreign animal disease response with the resources listed above for livestock or poultry diseases exotic to the United States that are either not or only mildly zoonotic.

information sharing. The ESFs and RSFs coexist and share information about impacts and assistance provided while focusing on their respective core capability. There will be some overlap between ESF and RSF missions, but as the ESF requirements diminish, the RSFs will examine any outstanding ESF activities that are associated with long-term health and social services recovery and determine subsequent actions consistent with the Recovery Federal Interagency Operational Plan (FIOP). From the earliest period following the disaster, ESF #8 will work closely with the Health and Social Services RSF to synchronize the integration of long-term restoration activities as seamlessly as possible.

Agency Actions

Primary Agency	Actions
Department of Health & Human Services (HHS)	• Possesses statutory authority to take specific actions to prepare for, respond to, and recover from public health and medical emergencies. • Declares a public health emergency through the HHS secretary. • Assumes operational control of federal emergency public health and medical response assets, as necessary, in the event of a public health emergency, except for members of the armed forces, who remain under the authority and control of the secretary of defense. • Leads the federal effort to provide public health and medical assistance to the affected area in an incident requiring a coordinated federal response. • Leads the federal response to international requests for HHS public health and medical assets and coordinates with federal departments/agencies and international partners on the acceptance of international public health and medical assistance. • Maintains primary responsibility for the situational awareness of public health, medical, and behavioral health assistance; determining the appropriate level of response capability based on the requirement contained in the action request form; and developing status updates and assessments. • Requests Emergency Support Function (ESF) #8 organizations to activate and deploy health professional and veterinary personnel, pharmaceuticals, equipment, and supplies in response to requests for federal assistance, as appropriate. • Assigns HHS personnel (i.e., U.S. Public Health Service Commissioned Corps, National Disaster Medical System [NDMS], federal civil service) to address public health, medical, behavioral health, and veterinary needs. • In cooperation with local, state, tribal, territorial, and insular area officials, conducts health surveillance to assess morbidity, mortality, and community needs related to the emergency. • Prepares regional staff to deploy as the Incident Response Coordination Team and to provide initial ESF #8 support to the affected location. • Assists and supports local, state, tribal, territorial, and insular area officials in monitoring for internal patient radiological contamination and administering pharmaceuticals for internal decontamination. • Assists local, state, tribal, territorial, and insular area officials in establishing a registry of individuals potentially exposed to radiation in a radiological/nuclear incident; performing dose reconstruction; and conducting long-term monitoring of this population for potential long-term health effects. • Monitors blood, blood products, and tissue supplies, shortages, and reserves. • Liaises with the American Association of Blood Banks (AABB) Interorganizational Task Force on Domestic Disasters and Acts of Terrorism (AABB Task Force) or the American Red Cross to assist in logistical requirements and to coordinate a national public blood announcement message for the need to donate blood.

(Continued)

Agency Actions (Continued)

Primary Agency	Actions
	• Activates NDMS as necessary to support response operations. • Deploys or redeploys the Strategic National Stockpile (SNS) or other pharmaceutical or medical resources as appropriate. • Coordinates public health and medical support and patient movement requirements with supporting departments, agencies, and governments throughout the incident. • Assures the safety, defense, and security of food in coordination with other responsible federal agencies (e.g., U.S. Department of Agriculture [USDA]). In cooperation with local, state, tribal, territorial, and insular area officials, assesses whether food manufacturing, food processing, food distribution, food service, and food retail establishments in the affected area are able to provide safe food. • Cooperates with local, state, tribal, territorial, and insular area officials as well as the food industry to conduct trace-backs and/or recalls of adulterated products. • Cooperates with local, state, tribal, territorial, insular area, and federal officials to provide guidance regarding the proper disposal of contaminated products and the decontamination of affected food facilities in order to protect public health. Provides public health risk communication messages and advisories that communicate relevant information on health hazards or other situations that could potentially threaten the public in multiple and accessible formats (e.g., visual public announcements, interpreters, etc.) and in a culturally and linguistically appropriate manner. • Disseminates public health information on protective actions related to exposure to health threats or environmental threats. • Notifies or responds to foreign country potential health threats as required by International Health Regulations. • Provides support for public health matters for radiological incidents as a member of the Advisory Team for Environment, Food, and Health. • Consults public health and medical subject matter experts with ESF #8 supporting organizations. This includes partners representing all appropriate populations such as individuals with access and functional needs, which can include pediatric populations, individuals with disabilities, older adults, and individuals with temporary or chronic medical conditions.
Department of Agriculture	• Provides nutrition assistance. • Ensures the safety and defense of the nation's supply of meat, poultry, and processed egg products. • Responds to animal and agricultural health and disease management issues. • Collaborates with HHS and the Department of the Interior (DOI) to deliver effective "one health" response that integrates human, animal, plant, and environmental health. • Supports public health matters for radiological incidents as a member of the Advisory Team for Environment, Food, and Health. • Provides technical expertise in support of animal and agricultural emergency management. United States Forest Service • Provides personnel, equipment, and supplies primarily for communications, aircraft, and base camps for deployed federal public health and medical teams.
Department of Commerce	National Oceanic and Atmospheric Administration • Provides near real-time transport, dispersion, and predictions of atmospheric releases of radioactive and hazardous materials that may be used by authorities in taking protective actions related to sheltering and evacuating affected populations.

(*Continued*)

Agency Actions (Continued)

Primary Agency	Actions
Department of Defense (DOD)	Subject to the availability of resources and the approval of the Secretary of Defense, DOD may perform the following when requested: • Alerts DOD, NDMS, and Federal Coordinating Centers (FCCs) and provides specific reporting instructions to support incident relief efforts. • Alerts DOD, NDMS, and FCCs to activate NDMS patient reception plans in a phased, regional approach, and when appropriate, in a national approach, as determined by HHS. • At the request of HHS and in coordination with interagency partners, provides NDMS support for the aeromedical evacuation and medical management of NDMS patients at DOD patient collection points (i.e., aerial ports of embarkation [APOE]) to patient reception areas (i.e., aerial ports of debarkation [APOD]/FCC). • Coordinates reception, tracking, and management of patients evacuated on DOD assets from the APOE to the APOD, as well as patients received at DOD FCCs and transported to nearby NDMS hospitals and U.S. Department of Veterans Affairs (VA) hospitals that are available and can provide appropriate care. Provides medical regulation of patients moved on DOD transportation assets. • Provides available logistical support (e.g., transportation) to public health/medical response operations. • Deploys available medical, surgical, and behavioral health personnel for casualty clearing and staging, patient management, and treatment. Deploys health care providers in a limited capacity to augment civilian hospital staff and federal deployable teams, and supports points of medical countermeasure distribution. Deploys chemical, biological, radiological, and nuclear (CBRN) medical subject matter experts and/or teams for technical consultation and/or medical support. • Mobilizes and deploys available Active Component, Reserve, and/or National Guard medical units or individuals when authorized for public health and medical response. • Provides deployable units (e.g., Expeditionary Medical Support System, Combat Support Hospitals) and platforms (e.g., U.S. Navy hospital ships, and/or other naval vessels) for patient medical and/or surgical care. • Provides epidemiological and occupational health support, telemedicine, and other specialized medical support. • Provides available military medical personnel to assist ESF #8 in the protection of public health (e.g., food, water, hygiene, wastewater removal, solid waste disposal, and vector control). • Provides available veterinary personnel to assist in the treatment of animals and in food safety, security, and protection activities. Provides available zoonotic and food surveillance data to ESF #8 and ESF #11 partners (e.g., Food and Drug Administration, USDA). • Provides available DOD medical supplies and materiel for use at points of distribution, hospitals, clinics, or medical care locations operated for exposed populations, incident victims, or ill patients. Provides available DOD medical supplies and materiel for mass care centers. • Assists local, state, tribal, territorial, and insular area officials in the provision of emergency medical, surgical, and behavioral health care. • Provides the use of functional DOD military treatment facilities within or near the incident area for medical care of nonmilitary health care system beneficiaries. • Provides available assistance for human fatality management services including remains collection, remains transport, mortuary services, victim identification, autopsy (if appropriate), and consultation and general assistance with temporary interment sites. Provide technical consultation for chemically or radiologically contaminated or infectious remains. Provides support to Victim Information Centers. Tracks decedents transported on DOD assets to fatality management facilities (e.g., mortuary, funeral home).

(*Continued*)

Agency Actions (Continued)

Primary Agency	Actions
	• Provides evaluation and risk management support through use of Defense Coordinating Officers, Emergency Preparedness Liaison Officers, and Joint Regional Medical Plans and Operations Officers. • Provides available blood, blood products, and tissues in coordination with HHS. • Provides public health and medical surveillance, laboratory diagnostics, and confirmatory testing (e.g., U.S. Army Medical Research Institute of Infectious Disease, U.S. Naval Medical Research Center) in coordination with the Laboratory Response Network/HHS and the Integrated Consortium of Laboratory Networks/DHS. U.S. Army Corps of Engineers • Through ESF #3, provides technical assistance, equipment, and supplies in support of HHS to accomplish temporary restoration of damaged public utilities affecting public health and medical facilities. Through ESF #3, provides power (e.g., generators) to medical and public health facilities. Through ESF #3 and in coordination with state and local officials, provides site evaluation and site (e.g., ground) preparation for temporary interment of human remains.
Department of Energy/National Nuclear Security Administration (DOE/NNSA)	• Coordinates federal assets for external monitoring and decontamination activities for radiological emergencies pursuant to criteria established by the state(s) in conjunction with HHS. • Provides, in cooperation with other state and federal agencies, personnel and equipment, including portal monitors to support initial screening; and provides advice and assistance to local, state, tribal, territorial, and insular area personnel conducting screening/decontamination of people leaving a contaminated zone. Radiological Assistance Program • Provides regional resources (e.g., personnel, specialized equipment, and supplies) to evaluate, control, and mitigate radiological hazards to workers and the public. • Provides limited assistance in the decontamination of victims. • Assists local, state, tribal, territorial, and insular area officials in the monitoring and surveillance of the incident area. National Atmospheric Release Advisory Capability • Provides near real-time transport, dispersion, and dose predictions of atmospheric releases of radioactive and hazardous materials that may be used by authorities in taking protective actions related to sheltering and evacuation of people. Federal Radiological Monitoring and Assessment Center (FRMAC) • Assists public health and medical authorities in determining radiological dose information; assists in providing coordinated gathering of environmental radiological information and data; assists with consolidated data sample analyses, evaluations, assessments, and interpretations; and provides technical information. Radiological Emergency Assistance Center/Training Site • Provides medical advice, specialized training, and on-site assistance for the treatment of all types of radiation exposure accidents. • Through the Cytogenetic Biodosimetry Laboratory (CBL), provides for post-exposure evaluation of radiation dose received.
Department of Homeland Security (DHS)	• Provides communications support in coordination with ESF #2. • Maintains situational awareness and the common operating picture via the Homeland Security Information Network. • Assists in providing information/liaison with emergency management officials in NDMS FCC areas.

(*Continued*)

Agency Actions (Continued)

Primary Agency	Actions

	• Identifies and arranges for use of DHS/U.S. Coast Guard (USCG) search and rescue (SAR) aircraft and other assets in providing urgent airlift and other accessible transportation support:
	  ◦ Provides medical assistance to extracted victims.
	  ◦ Assists in coordinating with local emergency medical systems for transfer of victims to appropriate health care facilities.
	  ◦ Conducts search operations for human remains, as mission assigned.
	• Provides location of human remains to facilitate humane recovery and collection of available forensic/ante-mortem data during course of SAR operations.
	• Leads the Interagency Modeling and Atmospheric Assessment Center (IMAAC) to coordinate, produce, and disseminate dispersion modeling and hazard prediction products that represent the federal position during an actual or potential incident to aid emergency responders in protecting the public and environment.
	• Provides enforcement of international quarantines through DHS/USCG, Customs and Border Protection, and Immigration and Customs Enforcement.
	Federal Emergency Management Agency
	• Provides logistical support for deploying ESF #8 medical elements required and coordinates the use of mobilization centers/staging areas; transportation of resources; use of disaster fuel contracts; emergency meals; potable water; base camp services; supply and equipment resupply; and use of all national contracts and interagency agreements managed by DHS for response operations.
	• Provides total asset visibility through the use of global positioning system tracking services to enable visibility of some ESF #8 resources through mapping capabilities and reports.
	• Provides support with the National Ambulance Contract for evacuating patients who are too seriously ill or otherwise incapable of being evacuated in general evacuation conveyances.
	• Provides tactical communications support through Mobile Emergency Response Support, inclusive of all types (i.e., deployable satellite and radio frequency/radio communications).
	Office of Infrastructure Protection
	• Provides situational awareness, cross-sector coordination, and prioritized recommendations regarding critical infrastructure and key resources.

Department of the Interior (DOI)	• If available, provides appropriate personnel, equipment, and supplies primarily for communications, aircraft, and the establishment of base camps for deployed federal public health and medical teams. • Resources will be assigned commensurate with each unit's level of training and the adequacy and availability of equipment. ESF #4 or the DOI Operations Center is the contact for this support.
Department of Justice (DOJ)	• Acts through the Federal Bureau of Investigation (FBI) to conduct evidence collection and analysis of all CBRN-related materials and controls potential crime scenes. • Assists in victim identification, coordinated through the FBI. • Provides local, state, tribal, territorial, and insular area officials with legal advice concerning identification of the deceased consistent with cultural sensitivity practices. • Provides HHS with relevant information of any credible threat or other situation that could potentially threaten public health. This support is coordinated through FBI headquarters. • Provides security for the SNS and secure movement of inbound medical equipment, supplies, blood, and tissues. • As the coordinator for ESF #13, provides crowd control at fixed and deployed health care facilities for the protection of workers and to address public safety and security.

(*Continued*)

Agency Actions (Continued)

Primary Agency	Actions
	• Provides quarantine assistance. • Establishes an adult missing person call center and assists in the disposition of cases. • Shares missing person data with ESF #6, ESF #8, ESF #13, and the American Red Cross in support of identification of the deceased and seriously wounded. • Supports local death scene investigations and evidence recovery. • Provides guidance, promulgates regulations, conducts investigations and compliance reviews, and enforces federal civil rights laws, including their application to emergency management.
Department of Labor	• Coordinates the safety and health assets of federal departments and agencies designated as cooperating agencies under the National Response Framework (NRF) Worker Safety and Health Support Annex and of the private sector to provide technical assistance and conduct worker exposure assessment and responder and worker risk management within the Incident Command System. This assistance may include 24/7 site safety monitoring; worker exposure monitoring; health monitoring; sampling and analysis; development and oversight of the site-specific safety and health plan; and personal protective equipment selection, distribution, training, and respirator fit testing. • Provides personnel and management support related to worker safety and health in field operations during ESF #8 deployments.
Department of State	• Coordinates the diplomatic aspects of international activities related to CBRN incidents and events that pose transborder threats as well as the diplomatic aspects of naturally occurring disease outbreaks with international implications. • Assists with coordination with foreign states concerning offers of support, gifts, offerings, donations, or other aid. This includes establishing coordination with partner nations to identify the immediate support, validated by the United States, in response to an incident. • Acts as the health and medical services information conduit to U.S. embassies/consulates.
Department of Transportation (DOT)	• Collaborates with DOD, the General Services Administration (GSA), and other transportation-providing agencies to provide technical assistance in identifying and arranging for all types of transportation, such as air, rail, marine, and motor vehicle and accessible transportation. • Coordinates with the Federal Aviation Administration for air traffic control support for priority missions. • At the request of ESF #8, provides technical support to assist in arranging logistical movement support (e.g., supplies, equipment, blood supply) from DOT resources, subject to DOT statutory requirements.
Department of Veterans Affairs	Subject to the availability of resources and funding, and consistent with the VA mission to provide priority services to veterans, when requested: • Coordinates with participating NDMS hospitals to provide incident-related medical care to authorized NDMS beneficiaries affected by a major disaster or emergency. • Furnishes available VA hospital care and medical services to individuals responding to, involved in, or otherwise affected by a major disaster or emergency, including members of the armed forces on active duty. • Designates and deploys available medical, surgical, mental health, and other health service support assets. • Provides a Medical Emergency Radiological Response Team for technical consultation on the medical management of injuries and illnesses due to exposure to or contamination by ionizing radiation. • Alerts VA FCCs and provides reporting instructions to support incident relief efforts.

(*Continued*)

Agency Actions (Continued)

Primary Agency	Actions
	• Alerts VA FCCs to activate NDMS patient reception plans in a phased, regional approach and when appropriate, in a national approach. • Buries and memorializes eligible veterans and advises on methods for interment of the dead during national or homeland security emergencies.
Environmental Protection Agency	• Provides technical assistance and environmental information for the assessment of the public health/medical aspects of situations involving hazardous materials, including technical and policy assistance in matters involving water and wastewater systems for critical health care facilities. • Provides support for public health matters for radiological incidents by providing assets to the FRMAC under ESF #10 and to the Advisory Team for Environment, Food, and Health. • Assists in identifying alternate water supplies and wastewater collection and treatment for critical health care facilities. • Provides environmental technical assistance (e.g., environmental monitoring) and information in the event temporary interment is necessary and/or human remains are contaminated.
General Services Administration	• Provides resource support for ESF #8 requirements to meet the needs of the affected population, as requested. • Provides contract support for temporary storage capability of human remains in a catastrophic fatality incident, such as refrigerated trucks, trailers, or rail cars.
U.S. Agency for International Development	Office of Foreign Disaster Assistance • Assists in the tracking and distribution of international support.
U.S. Postal Service	• Assists in the distribution and transportation of medicine, pharmaceuticals, and medical information to the general public affected by a major disaster or emergency, as needed.
American Red Cross	• Provides for disaster-related health and behavior health needs through direct services and/or referrals as necessary. • Assists community health personnel subject to staff availability. • Provides mortality and morbidity information to requesting agencies. • Provides supportive counseling for family members of the dead, injured, and others affected by the incident. • Provides information regarding behavioral health surveillance and behavioral health trends to requesting agencies. • Supports NDMS evacuation through the provision of services for accompanying family members/caregivers in coordination with local, state, tribal, territorial, insular area, and federal officials. • Provides available personnel to assist in temporary infirmaries, immunization clinics, morgues, hospitals, and nursing homes. • Assistance consists of administrative support, logistical support, or health services support within clearly defined boundaries. • At the request of HHS, coordinates with the AABB Task Force to provide blood and services as needed through regional blood centers. • Supports reunification efforts through its Safe and Well Web site and in coordination with government entities as appropriate. • Refers concerns regarding animal health care, safety, or welfare to authority having jurisdiction for animal issues.

Source: Adapted from Federal Emergency Management Agency (FEMA). 2016. *Emergency Support Function #8: Public Health and Medical Services Annex.* Washington, DC: FEMA. Available at: https://www.fema.gov/media-library-data/1470149644671-642ccad05d19449d2d13b1b0952328ed/ESF_8_Public_Health_Medical_20160705_508.pdf. Accessed January 25, 2017.

CORE CAPABILITIES

The National Preparedness Goal (NPG) identifies 32 core capabilities, which identify the tasks needed for the whole community to be prepared. These capabilities are grouped into 5 mission areas. While some capabilities apply to only one mission area, others relate to several. The core capabilities are referenced in many national preparedness efforts, including the National Planning Frameworks.

The following table illustrates how the core capabilities are organized by mission area within the NPG.

Core Capabilities by Mission Area

<table>
<tr><th>Prevention</th><th>Protection</th><th>Mitigation</th><th>Response</th><th>Recovery</th></tr>
<tr><td colspan="5">Planning</td></tr>
<tr><td colspan="5">Public Information and Warning</td></tr>
<tr><td colspan="5">Operational Coordination</td></tr>
<tr><td colspan="2">Intelligence and Information Sharing</td><td></td><td colspan="2">Infrastructure Systems</td></tr>
<tr><td colspan="2">Interdiction and Disruption</td><td></td><td colspan="2"></td></tr>
<tr><td colspan="2">Screening, Search, and Detection</td><td></td><td colspan="2"></td></tr>
<tr><td>• Forensics and attribution</td><td>• Access control and identity verification
• Cybersecurity
• Physical protective measures
• Risk management for protection programs and activities
• Supply chain integrity and security</td><td>• Community resilience
• Long-term vulnerability reduction
• Risk and disaster resilience assessment
• Threats and hazards identification</td><td>• Critical transportation
• Environmental response/ health and safety
• Fatality management services
• Fire management and suppression
• Logistics and supply chain management
• Mass care services
• Mass search and rescue operations
• On-scene security, protection, and law enforcement
• Operational communications
• Public health, health care, and emergency medical services
• Situational assessment</td><td>• Economic recovery
• Health and social services
• Housing
• Natural and cultural resources</td></tr>
</table>

Source: Adapted from U.S. Department of Homeland Security (DHS). 2015. *National Preparedness Goal*. 2nd ed. Page 3. Washington, DC: DHS. Available at: https://www.fema.gov/media-library-data/1443799615171-2aae90be55041740f97e8532fc680d40/National_Preparedness_Goal_2nd_Edition.pdf. Accessed January 25, 2017.
Note: Planning, Public Information and Warning, and Operational Coordination are common to all.

While public health professionals are not responsible for all of the 32 core capabilities in the NPG, those most relevant to public health practice include environmental response/health and safety; fatality management services; health and social services; mass care services; public health, health care, and emergency medical services; public information and warning; and threats and hazards identification.

The Core Capabilities in the NPG, by mission area, are:

PREVENTION—capabilities necessary to avoid, prevent, or stop a threatened or actual act of terrorism. Prevention core capabilities are focused specifically on imminent terrorist threats, including ongoing attacks or stopping imminent follow-on attacks while other mission areas apply to all hazards.

Planning: Conduct a systematic process engaging the whole community as appropriate in the development of executable strategic, operational, and/or tactical-level approaches to meet defined objectives.

Public Information and Warning: Deliver coordinated, prompt, reliable, and actionable information to the whole community through the use of clear, consistent, accessible, and culturally and linguistically appropriate methods to effectively relay information regarding any threat or hazard, as well as the actions being taken and the assistance being made available, as appropriate.

Operational Coordination: Establish and maintain a unified and coordinated operational structure and process that appropriately integrates all critical stakeholders and supports the execution of core capabilities.

Forensics and Attribution: Conduct forensic analysis and attribute terrorist acts (including the means and methods of terrorism) to their source, to include forensic analysis as well as attribution for an attack and for the preparation for an attack in an effort to prevent initial or follow-on acts and/or swiftly develop counter-options.

Intelligence and Information Sharing: Provide timely, accurate, and actionable information resulting from the planning, direction, collection, exploitation, processing, analysis, production, dissemination, evaluation, and feedback of available information concerning physical and cyber threats to the United States, its people, property, or interests; the development, proliferation, or use of weapons of mass destruction (WMDs); or any other matter bearing on U.S. national or homeland security by local, state, tribal, territorial, federal, and other stakeholders. Information sharing is the ability to exchange intelligence, information, data, or knowledge among government or private sector entities, as appropriate.

Interdiction and Disruption: Delay, divert, intercept, halt, apprehend, or secure threats and/or hazards.

Screening, Search, and Detection: Identify, discover, or locate threats and/or hazards through active and passive surveillance and search procedures. This may include the use of systematic examinations and assessments, biosurveillance, sensor technologies, or physical investigation and intelligence.

PROTECTION—capabilities to safeguard the homeland against acts of terrorism and man-made or natural disasters.

Planning: Conduct a systematic process engaging the whole community, as appropriate, in the development of executable strategic, operational, and/or tactical-level approaches to meet defined objectives.

Public Information and Warning: Deliver coordinated, prompt, reliable, and actionable information to the whole community through the use of clear, consistent, accessible, and culturally and linguistically appropriate methods to effectively relay information regarding any threat or hazard and, as appropriate, the actions being taken and the assistance being made available.

Operational Coordination: Establish and maintain a unified and coordinated operational structure and process that appropriately integrates all critical stakeholders and supports the execution of core capabilities.

Access Control and Identity Verification: Apply and support necessary physical, technological, and cyber measures to control admittance to critical locations and systems.

Cyber Security: Protect (and, if needed, restore) electronic communications systems, information, and services from damage, unauthorized use, and exploitation.

Intelligence and Information Sharing: Provide timely, accurate, and actionable information resulting from the planning, direction, collection, exploitation, processing, analysis, production, dissemination, evaluation, and feedback of available information concerning threats to the United States, its people, property, or interests; the development, proliferation, or use of WMDs; or any other matter bearing on U.S. national or homeland security by local, state, tribal, territorial, federal, and other stakeholders. Information sharing is the ability to exchange intelligence, information, data, or knowledge among government or private sector entities, as appropriate.

Interdiction and Disruption: Delay, divert, intercept, halt, apprehend, or secure threats and/or hazards.

Physical Protective Measures: Implement and maintain risk-informed countermeasures, and policies protecting people, borders, structures, materials, products, and systems associated with key operational activities and critical infrastructure sectors.

Risk Management for Protection Programs and Activities: Identify, assess, and prioritize risks to inform Protection activities, countermeasures, and investments.

Screening, Search, and Detection: Identify, discover, or locate threats and/or hazards through active and passive surveillance and search procedures. This may include the use of systematic examinations and assessments, biosurveillance, sensor technologies, or physical investigation and intelligence.

Supply Chain Integrity and Security: Strengthen the security and resilience of the supply chain.

MITIGATION—capabilities necessary to reduce loss of life and property by lessening the impact of disasters.

Planning: Conduct a systematic process engaging the whole community as appropriate in the development of executable strategic, operational, and/or tactical-level approaches to meet defined objectives.

Public Information and Warning: Deliver coordinated, prompt, reliable, and actionable information to the whole community through the use of clear, consistent, accessible, and culturally and linguistically appropriate methods to effectively relay information regarding any threat or hazard and, as appropriate, the actions being taken and the assistance being made available.

Operational Coordination: Establish and maintain a unified and coordinated operational structure and process that appropriately integrates all critical stakeholders and supports the execution of core capabilities.

Community Resilience: Enable the recognition, understanding, and communication of and planning for risk, and empower individuals and communities to make informed risk management decisions necessary to adapt to, withstand, and quickly recover from future incidents.

Long-Term Vulnerability Reduction: Build and sustain resilient systems, communities, and critical infrastructure and key resources lifelines so as to reduce their vulnerability to natural, technological, and human-caused threats and hazards by lessening the likelihood, severity, and duration of the adverse consequences.

Risk and Disaster Resilience Assessment: Assess risk and disaster resilience so that decision makers, responders, and community members can take informed action to reduce their entity's risk and increase their resilience.

Threats and Hazards Identification: Identify the threats and hazards that occur in the geographic area; determine the frequency and magnitude; and incorporate this into analysis and planning processes so as to clearly understand the needs of a community or entity.

RESPONSE—capabilities necessary to save lives, protect property and the environment, and meet basic human needs after an incident has occurred. Response emphasizes saving and sustaining lives, stabilizing the incident, rapidly meeting basic human needs, restoring basic services and technologies, restoring community functionality, providing universal accessibility, establishing a safe and secure environment, and supporting the transition to recovery.

Planning: Conduct a systematic process engaging the whole community as appropriate in the development of executable strategic, operational, and/or tactical-level approaches to meet defined objectives.

Public Information and Warning: Deliver coordinated, prompt, reliable, and actionable information to the whole community through the use of clear, consistent, accessible, and culturally and linguistically appropriate methods to effectively relay information regarding any threat or hazard and, as appropriate, the actions being taken and the assistance being made available.

Operational Coordination: Establish and maintain a unified and coordinated operational structure and process that appropriately integrates all critical stakeholders and supports the execution of core capabilities.

Critical Transportation: Provide transportation (including infrastructure access and accessible transportation services) for response priority objectives, including the evacuation of people and animals, and the delivery of vital response personnel, equipment, and services into the affected areas.

Environmental Response/Health and Safety: Conduct appropriate measures to ensure the protection of the health and safety of the public and workers, as well as the environment, from all-hazards in support of responder operations and the affected communities.

Fatality Management Services: Provide fatality management services, including decedent remains recovery and victim identification, working with local, state, tribal, territorial, insular area, and federal authorities to provide mortuary processes, temporary storage or permanent internment solutions, sharing information with mass care services for the purpose of reunifying family members and caregivers with missing persons/remains, and providing counseling to the bereaved.

Fire Management and Suppression: Provide structural, wildland, and specialized firefighting capabilities to manage and suppress fires of all types, kinds, and complexities while protecting the lives, property, and the environment in the affected area.

Infrastructure Systems: Stabilize critical infrastructure functions, minimize health and safety threats, and efficiently restore and revitalize systems and services to support a viable, resilient community.

Logistics and Supply Chain Management: Deliver essential commodities, equipment, and services in support of impacted communities and survivors, to include emergency power and fuel support, as well as the coordination of access to community staples. Synchronize logistics capabilities and enable the restoration of impacted supply chains.

Mass Care Services: Provide life-sustaining and human services to the affected population, including hydration, feeding, sheltering, temporary housing, evacuee support, reunification, and distribution of emergency supplies.

Mass Search and Rescue Operations: Deliver traditional and atypical search and rescue capabilities, including personnel, services, animals, and assets to survivors in need, with the goal of saving the greatest number of endangered lives in the shortest time possible.

On-Scene Security, Protection, and Law Enforcement: Ensure a safe and secure environment through law enforcement and related security and protection operations for people and communities located within affected areas and also for response personnel engaged in lifesaving and life-sustaining operations.

Operational Communications: Ensure the capacity for timely communications in support of security, situational awareness, and operations by any and all means available, among and between affected communities in the impact area and all response forces.

Public Health, Health Care, and Emergency Medical Services: Provide lifesaving medical treatment via emergency medical services and related operations and avoid additional disease and injury by providing targeted public health, medical, and behavioral health support, and products to all affected populations.

Situational Assessment: Provide all decision makers with decision-relevant information regarding the nature and extent of the hazard, any cascading effects, and the status of the response.

RECOVERY—capabilities necessary to assist communities affected by an incident to recover effectively. Support for recovery ensures a continuum of care for individuals to maintain and restore health, safety, independence and livelihoods, especially those who experience financial, emotional, and physical hardships.

Planning: Conduct a systematic process engaging the whole community as appropriate in the development of executable strategic, operational, and/or tactical-level approaches to meet defined objectives.

Public Information and Warning: Deliver coordinated, prompt, reliable, and actionable information to the whole community through the use of clear, consistent, accessible, and culturally and linguistically appropriate methods to effectively relay information regarding any threat or hazard and, as appropriate, the actions being taken and the assistance being made available.

Operational Coordination: Establish and maintain a unified and coordinated operational structure and process that appropriately integrates all critical stakeholders and supports the execution of core capabilities.

Economic Recovery: Return economic and business activities (including food and agriculture) to a healthy state and develop new business and employment opportunities that result in an economically viable community.

Health and Social Services: Restore and improve health and social services capabilities and networks to promote the resilience, independence, health (including behavioral health), and well-being of the whole community.

Housing: Implement housing solutions that effectively support the needs of the whole community and contribute to its sustainability and resilience.

Infrastructure Systems: Stabilize critical infrastructure functions, minimize health and safety threats, and efficiently restore and revitalize systems and services to support a viable, resilient community.

Natural and Cultural: Protect natural and cultural resources and historic properties through appropriate planning, mitigation, response, and recovery actions to preserve, conserve, rehabilitate, and restore them consistent with post-disaster community priorities and best practices and in compliance with applicable environmental and historic preservation laws and executive orders.

Source: Adapted from U.S. Department of Homeland Security (DHS). 2015. *National Preparedness Goal*. 2nd ed. Pages 6–20. Washington, DC: DHS. Available at: https://www.fema.gov/media-library-data/1443799615171-2aae90be55041740f97e8532fc680d40/National_Preparedness_Goal_2nd_Edition.pdf. Accessed January 25, 2017.

MANAGEMENT STANDARDS

APPENDIX H

REQUIRED ELEMENTS OF RISK ASSESSMENT

The 2016 edition of the National Fire Protection Association (NFPA) 1600 *Standard on Disaster/Emergency Management and Business Continuity Programs* defines the required elements of a risk assessment. Standard 5.2 states that a risk assessment should be conducted "to identify hazards and monitor the likelihood and severity of them occurring over time," assess the "vulnerability of the people," "impacts of the hazards," be aware of the "escalation of impacts over time," "evaluate the potential effects of regional, national, or international incidents that could have cascading impacts," and evaluate the "adequacy of existing prevention and motigation strategies." Although all of the events below do not necessarily meet the definition of a disaster or emergency, the full list is included for reference regarding the NFPA 1600 standard and what it includes.

Risk assessments should identify, evaluate and monitor the vulnerability of the following:

Health and safety of people in the affected area

Health and safety of personnel responding to the incident

Security of information

Continuity of operations

Continuity of government

Property, facilities, assets, and critical infrastructure

Delivery of the entity's services

Supply chain

Environment

Economic and financial condition

Legislated, regulatory, and contractual obligations

Reputation of or confidence in an entity

Work and labor relations.

The risk assessment should be done for the following hazards:

Natural Hazards		
Geological	**Meteorological**	**Biological**
Earthquake	Flood, flash flood, seiche, tidal surge	Emerging diseases (plague, smallpox, anthrax, West Nile virus, foot and mouth disease, severe acute respiratory syndrome, bovine spongiform encephalopathy)
Tsunami	Drought	Animal, insect infestation or damage
Volcano	Fire	
Landslide, mudslide, subsidence	Snow, ice, hail, sleet, avalanche	
Glacier, iceberg movement	Extreme temperatures	
	Lightning strikes	
	Famine	
	Geomagnetic storm	

Human-Caused Events		
Accidents	**Intentional**	**Technological**
Hazardous material spill, release	Terrorism (explosive, chemical, biological, radiological, nuclear, cyber)	Central computer, mainframe, server, software, application failure
Explosion, fire	Sabotage	Ancillary support equipment hazards
Transportation	Civil disturbance, public unrest, mass hysteria, riot	Telecommunications failure
Building, structural collapse	Enemy attack, war	Energy/power/utility failure
Energy/power/utility failure	Insurrection	
Fuel, other resource shortage	Strike or labor dispute	
	Disinformation	
Air or water pollution, contamination	Criminal activity (vandalism, arson, theft, fraud, embezzlement, data theft)	
Water control structure failure	Electromagnetic pulse	
Economic depression, inflation, financial system collapse	Physical or information security breach	
Communication system interruptions	Workplace, school, university violence	
Misinformation	Product defect, contamination	
	Harassment, discrimination	

The following are methodologies and techniques used to conduct a risk assessment:

Methods and Techniques	Functions
What-if	Identify specific hazards or hazardous situations that could result in undesirable consequences Relies on knowledgeable individuals familiar with the area, operations, and processes Value dependent on team and questions asked
Checklist	Specific list of items used to identify hazards and hazardous situations Compare current or projected situations with accepted standards Value dependent on checklist quality and assessor experience and credentials
What-if/checklist	Combines what-if and checklist techniques Uses strengths of both techniques What-if questions are developed and checklists fill in any gaps Value dependent on team and the questions asked
Hazard and operability study	Requires interdisciplinary team that is very knowledgeable of the areas, operations, and processes to be assessed Thorough, time consuming, and costly approach Value depends on team qualifications and experience, quality of reference material available, ability of team to function as a team, and strong, positive leadership
Failure mode and effects analysis	Examines each element in system individually and collectively Determines effect when one or more elements fail Bottom-up approach: elements are examined and effect of failure on overall system is predicted Small interdisciplinary team required Best suited for assessing potential equipment failures Value dependent on credentials of team and scope of system to be examined
Fault-tree analysis	Top-down approach: undesirable event is identified and range of potential causes identified Value dependent on competence in using the fault-tree analysis process, on credentials of team, and depth of team's analysis

Source: Based on National Fire Protection Association (NFPA). 2016. *NFPA 1600 Standard on Disaster/Emergency Management and Business Continuity Programs*. 2016 ed. Section 5.2 and Annex A. Quincy, MA: NFPA.

MORBIDITY

APPENDIX I

COMMON FOOD-BORNE DISEASES

The following table will be helpful when public health professionals require a quick reference to comparative information about food-borne diseases. Professionals can consult this table to review the clinical symptoms for common food-borne diseases, the typical foods associated with each disease, and specific prevention and control measures.

Disease (Causative Agent)	Type of Agent	Principal Symptoms	Typical Foods/Cause	Prevention and Control Measures
Botulism food poisoning (*Clostridium botulinum* and sometimes by strains of *Clostridium butyricum* and *Clostridium baratii*)	Nerve toxin produced by bacteria	Double vision, blurred vision, drooping eyelids, slurred speech, difficulty swallowing, dry mouth, and muscle weakness	Home-canned foods prepared in an unsafe manner	Follow proper canning methods; Inspect commercial and home-canned foods; safely dispose of contaminated food and cans; use a bleach solution to clean spills of contaminated food
Botulism food poisoning: infant infection (*C. botulinum*)	Nerve toxin produced by bacteria	Appears lethargic, feed poorly, constipation, have a weak cry, and have poor muscle tone	Honey, soil	Do not feed honey to children younger than 1 year old
Campylobacteriosis (*Campylobacter jejuni*)	Bacteria	Diarrhea, bloody diarrhea, abdominal pain, fever, nausea, vomiting	Infected food source, animals	Cook animal foods thoroughly, avoid cross-contamination by washing hands, using separate cutting boards and thoroughly clean with soap and hot water, use pasteurized milk
Food poisoning (*Clostridium perfringens*)	Spore-forming gram-positive bacteria	Diarrhea, cramps, rarely nausea and vomiting	Beef, poultry, dried or precooked foods	Cook foods thoroughly maintaining temperature >140°F or <41°F, serve food hot and cool rapidly
E. coli infections, enterohemorrhagic (*Escherichia coli*)	Bacteria	Watery, bloody diarrhea; severe stomach cramps; vomiting	Raw or uncooked beef, raw milk, nonpotable water; unpasteurized apple cider, and soft cheeses made from raw milk	Wash hands thoroughly; cook meats thoroughly, avoid raw milk, unpasteurized dairy products, and unpasteurized juices; prevent cross contamination in food preparation

(*Continued*)

Disease (Causative Agent)	**Type of Agent**	**Principal Symptoms**	**Typical Foods/Cause**	**Prevention and Control Measures**
E. coli infections, enterotoxigenic (*E. coli*)	Bacteria	Profuse watery diarrhea, abdominal cramps, vomiting; Less common: fever, nausea, chills, loss of appetite, headache, muscle aches and bloating	Raw fruits and vegetables, raw seafood or undercooked meat or poultry, unpasteurized dairy products, food from street vendors, and untreated water in areas lacking adequate chlorination	Teach food handlers good hygiene practice, have food handlers wear gloves; avoid or safely prepare foods and beverages that could be contaminated; wash hands with soap frequently
Giardiasis (Giardia)	Parasite	Diarrhea, gas, greasy stools that tend to float; stomach or abdominal cramps; nausea/vomiting; dehydration	Raw fruits and vegetables; food or water that has been contaminated with feces	Avoid eating contaminated food; prevent contact and contamination with feces
Listeriosis (*Listeria monocytogenes*)	Bacteria	Headache, stiff neck, confusion, loss of balance, and convulsions in addition to fever and muscle aches[a]	Raw milk, cheese, vegetables; cooked or processed foods, including certain soft cheeses, processed meats, and smoked seafood	Follow recommendations for safe food preparation, consumption, and storage
Norovirus	Virus	Stomach pain, nausea, diarrhea, vomiting, fever, headache, body aches	Contaminated food or water (i.e., raw fruits and vegetables, oysters and shellfish)	Wash hands carefully with soap and water—after using the toilet, changing diapers, and before eating, preparing, or handling food; carefully wash fruits and vegetables before preparing and eating them; clean and disinfect contaminated surfaces with a chlorine bleach solution
Salmonellosis (*Salmonella species*)	Bacteria	Diarrhea, abdominal pain, chills, fever	Raw, undercooked eggs; raw milk, meat and poultry	Cook foods thoroughly; avoid cross-contamination by washing hands, kitchen work surfaces, and utensils with soap and water immediately after contact with raw meat or poultry
Shigellosis (*Shigella species*)	Bacteria	Diarrhea, fever, abdominal pain, tenesmus	Food contaminated with *Shigella*	Avoid cross-contamination by carefully washing hands with soap before eating and after changing a diaper; avoid swallowing water from ponds, lakes, or untreated swimming pools

(*Continued*)

Disease (Causative Agent)	Type of Agent	Principal Symptoms	Typical Foods/Cause	Prevention and Control Measures
Staphylococcal food poisoning (*Staphylococcus aureus*)	Heat-stable enterotoxin of bacteria	Nausea, vomiting, diarrhea, stomach cramps	Ham, meat, poultry products; unpasteurized milk and cheese products; uncooked food that is handled (i.e., sliced meat, puddings, pastries, and sandwiches)	Food handlers wash hands and under fingernails thoroughly with soap and water before handling and preparing food; wear gloves while preparing food; keep hot foods >140°F and cold foods <40°F
Vibriosis (*Vibrio species*)	Bacteria	Watery diarrhea, abdominal cramps, nausea, vomiting, fever, chills	Raw and undercooked fish and seafood	Cook fish and seafood thoroughly; wash hands with soap and water after handing raw shellfish; avoid contaminating cooked shellfish with raw shellfish and its juices

Source: Based on Centers for Disease Control and Prevention. 2016. Foodborne germs and illnesses. Available at: http://www.cdc.gov/foodsafety/foodborne-germs.html. Accessed January 25, 2017.

[a]Pregnant women typically experience fever and other nonspecific symptoms, such as fatigue and aches. However, infections during pregnancy can lead to miscarriage, stillbirth, premature delivery, or life-threatening infection of the newborn. In older adults and people with immunocompromising conditions, septicemia and meningitis are the most common clinical symptoms. Immunocompetent people may experience acute febrile gastroenteritis or no symptoms.

APPENDIX J

DISEASES AFFECTING DISPLACED PERSONS DURING AND AFTER DISASTERS

Disease	Symptoms	Environmental Risk Factors	Possible Health Hazards
Acute upper respiratory tract infections	Symptoms of common cold; for pneumonia, chest pain and pain between shoulder blades	Crowding, poor hygiene	Influenza and pneumonia can result in severe complications in groups at risk
Cholera	Fever, severe liquid diarrhea, abdominal spasms, vomiting, rapid weight loss, dehydration	Contaminated drinking water or food or poor sanitation	Dehydration, especially in children; dark color of urine, dry tongue, leathery skin
Diarrhea	Watery stools at least 3 times per day; fever, nausea, or vomiting	Contaminated drinking water or food or poor sanitation	Dehydration, especially in children; dark color of urine, dry tongue, leathery skin
Diphtheria	Inflamed and painful throat, coughing	Crowding, poor hygiene	A secretion is deposited in the respiratory tract that can lead to asphyxiation
Heat stress	Elevated body temperatures, nausea, vomiting, headache	Excessive temperatures	Coma
(Viral) hepatitis A	Nausea, slight fever, pale-colored stools, dark-colored urine, jaundiced eyes and skin	Poor hygiene	Long-term disabling effects
Malaria	Painful muscles and joints, high fever with chills, headache, possible diarrhea and vomiting	Breeding of *Anopheles* mosquitoes in stagnant water bodies	Disease may rapidly become fatal unless medical care provided during the first 48 hours
Measles	Fever and catarrhal symptoms, followed by maculopapular rash	Crowding, poor hygiene	High fatality rate
Meningococcal meningitis	Infected people may show no symptoms for a considerable time; headache, fever, and general malaise suggest diagnosis when symptoms are epidemic	Crowding	Only fatal if untreated in early stage; neurological problems in survivors

(*Continued*)

Disease	Symptoms	Environmental Risk Factors	Possible Health Hazards
Rabies	Fatigue, headache, disorientation, paralysis, hyperactivity	Bite from infected animal host	Fatal if untreated
Shigella dysentery	Diarrhea with blood in stool, fever, vomiting, abdominal cramps	Contaminated drinking water or food, poor sanitation, poor hygiene	Case fatality rate may be high
Tetanus	Muscle spasms, starting in the jaws and extending to rest of body over several days	Poor hygiene, injury	Fatal
Typhoid fever	Initial symptoms are similar to malaria; diarrhea, prolonged fever, and delirium are occasional symptoms	Contaminated drinking-water or food or poor sanitation	Without appropriate medical care, can lead to fatal complications in a few weeks
Louse-borne typhus	Prolonged fever, headache, body pains	Unhygienic conditions leading to lice infestations	Potentially fatal without treatment

Source: Based on Wisner B, Adams J, eds. 2002. *Environmental Health in Emergencies and Disasters.* Table 11.1. Control measures for ensuring food safety. Page 170. Geneva, Switzerland: World Health Organization.

BEHAVIORAL HEALTH

APPENDIX K

DSM-5 DIAGNOSTIC CRITERIA FOR POST-TRAUMATIC STRESS DISORDER

Diagnostic Criteria for Posttraumatic Stress Disorder (309.81 [F43.10])

Note: The following criteria apply to adults, adolescents, and children older than 6 years. For children 6 years and younger, see corresponding criteria below.

A. Exposure to actual or threatened death, serious injury, or sexual violence in one (or more) of the following ways:
   1. Directly experiencing the traumatic event(s).
   2. Witnessing, in person, the event(s) as it occurred to others.
   3. Learning that the traumatic event(s) occurred to a close family member or close friend. In cases of actual or threatened death of a family member or friend, the event(s) must have been violent or accidental.
   4. Experiencing repeated or extreme exposure to aversive details of the traumatic event(s) (e.g., first responders collecting human remains; police officers repeatedly exposed to details of child abuse).
      Note: Criterion A4 does not apply to exposure through electronic media, television, movies, or pictures, unless this exposure is work related.

B. Presence of one (or more) of the following intrusion symptoms associated with the traumatic event(s), beginning after the traumatic event(s) occurred:
   1. Recurrent, involuntary, and intrusive distressing memories of the traumatic event(s).
      Note: In children older than 6 years, repetitive play may occur in which themes or aspects of the traumatic event(s) are expressed.
   2. Recurrent distressing dreams in which the content and/or affect of the dream are related to the traumatic event(s).
      Note: In children, there may be frightening dreams without recognizable content.
   3. Dissociative reactions (e.g., flashbacks) in which the individual feels or acts as if the traumatic event(s) were recurring. (Such reactions may occur on a continuum, with the most extreme expression being a complete loss of awareness of present surroundings.)
      Note: In children, trauma-specific reenactment may occur in play.

4. Intense or prolonged psychological distress at exposure to internal or external cues that symbolize or resemble an aspect of the traumatic event(s).
5. Marked physiological reactions to internal or external cues that symbolize or resemble an aspect of the traumatic event(s).

C. Persistent avoidance of stimuli associated with the traumatic event(s), beginning after the traumatic event(s) occurred, as evidenced by one or both of the following:
   1. Avoidance of or efforts to avoid distressing memories, thoughts, or feelings about or closely associated with the traumatic event(s).
   2. Avoidance of or efforts to avoid external reminders (people, places, conversations, activities, objects, situations) that arouse distressing memories, thoughts, or feelings about or closely associated with the traumatic event(s).

D. Negative alterations in cognitions and mood associated with the traumatic event(s), beginning or worsening after the traumatic event(s) occurred, as evidenced by 2 (or more) of the following:
   1. Inability to remember an important aspect of the traumatic event(s) (typically due to dissociative amnesia and not to other factors such as head injury, alcohol, or drugs).
   2. Persistent and exaggerated negative beliefs or expectations about oneself, others, or the world (e.g., "I am bad," "No one can be trusted," "The world is completely dangerous," "My whole nervous system is permanently ruined").
   3. Persistent, distorted cognitions about the cause or consequences of the traumatic event(s) that lead the individual to blame himself/herself or others.
   4. Persistent negative emotional state (e.g., fear, horror, anger, guilt, or shame).
   5. Markedly diminished interest or participation in significant activities.
   6. Feelings of detachment or estrangement from others.
   7. Persistent inability to experience positive emotions (e.g., inability to experience happiness, satisfaction, or loving feelings).

E. Marked alterations in arousal and reactivity associated with the traumatic event(s), beginning or worsening after the traumatic event(s) occurred, as evidenced by 2 (or more) of the following:
   1. Irritable behavior and angry outbursts (with little or no provocation) typically expressed as verbal or physical aggression toward people or objects.
   2. Reckless or self-destructive behavior.
   3. Hypervigilance.
   4. Exaggerated startle response.
   5. Problems with concentration.
   6. Sleep disturbance (e.g., difficulty falling or staying asleep or restless sleep).

F. Duration of the disturbance (Criteria B, C, D, and E) is more than 1 month.
   1. The disturbance causes clinically significant distress or impairment in social, occupational, or other important areas of functioning.

2. The disturbance is not attributable to the physiological effects of a substance (e.g., medication, alcohol) or another medical condition.

Specify whether:

With dissociative symptoms: The individual's symptoms meet the criteria for posttraumatic stress disorder, and in addition, in response to the stressor, the individual experiences persistent or recurrent symptoms of either of the following:

1. **Depersonalization:** Persistent or recurrent experiences of feeling detached from, and as if one were an outside observer of, one's mental processes or body (e.g., feeling as though one were in a dream; feeling a sense of unreality of self or body or of time moving slowly).
2. **Derealization:** Persistent or recurrent experiences of unreality of surroundings (e.g., the world around the individual is experienced as unreal, dreamlike, distant, or distorted).
   Note: To use this subtype, the dissociative symptoms must not be attributable to the physiological effects of a substance (e.g., blackouts, behavior during alcohol intoxication) or another medical condition (e.g., complex partial seizures).

Specify if:

With delayed expression: If the full diagnostic criteria are not met until at least 6 months after the event (although the onset and expression of some symptoms may be immediate).

Posttraumatic Stress Disorder for Children 6 Years and Younger

A. In children 6 years and younger, exposure to actual or threatened death, serious injury, or sexual violence in one (or more) of the following ways:
   1. Directly experiencing the traumatic event(s).
   2. Witnessing, in person, the event(s) as it occurred to others, especially primary caregivers.
      Note: Witnessing does not include events that are witnessed only in electronic media, television, movies, or pictures.
   3. Learning that the traumatic event(s) occurred to a parent or caregiving figure.

B. Presence of one (or more) of the following intrusion symptoms associated with the traumatic event(s), beginning after the traumatic event(s) occurred:
   1. Recurrent, involuntary, and intrusive distressing memories of the traumatic event(s).

Note: Spontaneous and intrusive memories may not necessarily appear distressing and may be expressed as play reenactment.

2. Recurrent distressing dreams in which the content and/or affect of the dream are related to the traumatic event(s).
   Note: It may not be possible to ascertain that the frightening content is related to the traumatic event.
3. Dissociative reactions (e.g., flashbacks) in which the child feels or acts as if the traumatic event(s) were recurring. (Such reactions may occur on a continuum, with the most extreme expression being a complete loss of awareness of present surroundings.) Such trauma-specific reenactment may occur in play.
4. Intense or prolonged psychological distress at exposure to internal or that symbolize or resemble an aspect of the traumatic event(s).
5. Marked physiological reactions to reminders of the traumatic event(s).

C. One (or more) of the following symptoms, representing either persistent avoidance of stimuli associated with the traumatic event(s) or negative alterations in cognitions and mood associated with the traumatic event(s), must be present, beginning after the event(s) or worsening after the event(s):

- Persistent Avoidance of Stimuli
  1. Avoidance of or efforts to avoid activities, places, or physical reminders that arouse recollections of the traumatic event(s).
  2. Avoidance of or efforts to avoid people, conversations, or interpersonal situations that arouse recollections of the traumatic event(s).
- Negative Alterations in Cognitions
  1. Substantially increased frequency of negative emotional states (e.g., fear, guilt, sadness, shame, confusion).
  2. Markedly diminished interest or participation in significant activities, including constriction of play.
  3. Socially withdrawn behavior.
  4. Persistent reduction in expression of positive emotions.

D. Alterations in arousal and reactivity associated with the traumatic event(s), beginning or worsening after the traumatic event(s) occurred, as evidenced by 2 (or more) of the following:

1. Irritable behavior and angry outbursts (with little or no provocation) typically expressed as verbal or physical aggression toward people or objects (including extreme temper tantrums).
2. Hypervigilance.
3. Exaggerated startle response.
4. Problems with concentration.
5. Sleep disturbance (e.g., difficulty falling or staying asleep or restless sleep).

E. The duration of the disturbance is more than 1 month.

F. The disturbance causes clinically significant distress or impairment in relationships with parents, siblings, peers, or other caregivers or with school behavior.
G. The disturbance is not attributable to the physiological effects of a substance (e.g., medication or alcohol) or another medical condition.

Specify whether:

With dissociative symptoms: The individual's symptoms meet the criteria for posttraumatic stress disorder, and the individual experiences persistent or recurrent symptoms of either of the following:

1. **Depersonalization:** Persistent or recurrent experiences of feeling detached from, and as if one were an outside observer of, one's mental processes or body (e.g., feeling as though one were in a dream; feeling a sense of unreality of self or body or of time moving slowly).
2. **Derealization:** Persistent or recurrent experiences of unreality of surroundings (e.g., the world around the individual is experienced as unreal, dreamlike, distant, or distorted).
   Note: To use this subtype, the dissociative symptoms must not be attributable to the physiological effects of a substance (e.g., blackouts) or another medical condition (e.g., complex partial seizures).

Specify if:

With delayed expression: If the full diagnostic criteria are not met until at least 6 months after the event (although the onset and expression of some symptoms may be immediate).

Source: Reprinted with permission from the American Psychiatric Association. 2013. *Diagnostic and Statistical Manual of Mental Disorders*, 5th ed. Arlington, VA: American Psychiatric Association.

APPENDIX L

OVERVIEW OF PSYCHOLOGICAL FIRST AID

Task	Activities
Preparing to Deliver Psychological First Aid	• Preparation • Entering the setting • Providing services • Group settings • Maintain a calm presence • Be sensitive to culture and diversity • Be aware of at-risk populations
Contact and Engagement	• Introduce yourself/ask about immediate needs • Confidentiality
Safety and Comfort	• Ensure immediate physical safety • Provide information about disaster response activities and services • Attend to physical comfort • Promote social engagement • Attend to children who are separated from their parents/caregivers • Protect from additional traumatic experiences and trauma reminders • Help survivors who have a missing family member • Help survivors when a family member or close friend has died • Attend to grief and spiritual issues • Provide information about casket and funeral issues • Attend to issues related to traumatic grief • Support survivors who receive death notification • Support survivors involved in body identification • Help caregivers confirm body identification to a child or adolescent
Stabilization	• Stabilize emotionally overwhelmed survivors • Orient emotionally overwhelmed survivors • The role of medications in stabilization
Information Gathering: Current Needs and Concerns	• Nature and severity of experiences during the disaster • Death of a loved one • Concerns about immediate post-disaster circumstances and ongoing threat • Separations from or concern about the safety of loved ones • Physical illness, mental health conditions, and need for medications • Losses (e.g., home, school, neighborhood, business, personal property, and pets) • Extreme feelings of guilt or shame • Thoughts about causing harm to self or others • Availability of social support

(*Continued*)

Task	Activities
	• Prior alcohol or drug use • Prior exposure to trauma and death of loved ones • Specific youth, adult, and family concerns over developmental impact
Practical Assistance	• Offer practical assistance to children and adolescents • Identify the most immediate needs • Clarify the need • Discuss an action plan • Act to address the need
Connection with Social Supports	• Enhance access to primary support people (i.e., family and significant others) • Encourage use of immediately available support people • Discuss support-seeking and giving • Special considerations for children and adolescents • Model support
Information on Coping	• Provide basic information about stress reactions • Review common psychological reactions to traumatic experiences and ◦ Losses ◦ Intrusive reactions ◦ Avoidance and withdrawal reactions ◦ Physical arousal reactions ◦ Trauma reminders ◦ Loss reminders ◦ Change reminders ◦ Hardships ◦ Grief reactions ◦ Traumatic grief reactions ◦ Depression ◦ Physical reactions • Talk with children about body and emotional reactions • Provide basic information on ways of coping • Teach simple relaxation techniques • Coping for families • Assist with developmental issues • Assist with anger management • Address highly negative emotions • Help with sleep problems • Address alcohol and substance use
Linkage with Collaborative Services	• Provide direct link to additional needed services • Provide referrals for children and adolescents • Provide referrals for older adults • Promote continuity in helping relationships

Source: Adapted from U.S. Department of Veterans Affairs. National Center for PTSD. [n.d.]. *The Psychological First Aid Manual.* Appendix A: Overview of Psychological First Aid. Available at: http://www.ptsd.va.gov/professional/manuals/manual-pdf/pfa/PFA_Appx_AOverview.pdf. Accessed January 25, 2017.

APPENDIX M

BEHAVIORAL INTERVENTIONS

Name of Intervention	Description	Delivery Mode	Delivery Setting	Research Base	Source
Early Interventions (First 4 weeks)					
Assessment, Crisis Intervention, and Trauma Treatment	Three-stage framework and intervention model for acute crisis and trauma treatment services; a sequential set of assessments and intervention strategies; integrates assessment and triage protocols with the 7-stage crisis intervention model and the 10-step acute traumatic stress management protocol.	I, VF, DS	F/C, O	EST, QR	http://btci.edina.clockss.org/cgi/reprint/2/1/1
Cognitive Behavioral Therapy (CBT) for Acute Stress Disorder (ASD)	ASD encompasses post-traumatic stress reactions that are present just after an event until 4 weeks post-trauma. This early intervention treatment manual includes descriptions for 6 sessions of structured CBT, including prolonged exposure.	I, C, VF, DS, RRR, OR	O (clinical setting)	EmST	http://www.istss.org/treating-trauma/treatment-materials/cognitive-behavioral-therapy-for-acute-stress-diso.aspx
Community Emergency Response Teams (CERT)	Initially developed by the Los Angeles City Fire Department, the Federal Emergency Management Agency now teaches this model for all hazards. The CERT program educates people about disaster preparedness for local hazards and trains them in basic disaster response skills. Using the training learned in the classroom and during exercises, CERT members can assist others in their neighborhood or workplace following an event when professional responders are not immediately available to help.	I, F, G, C, VF, DS, RRR, OR	F/C, C, RA	EBBP	http://www.fema.gov/community-emergency-response-teams
Consultation, Outreach, Debriefing, Education, and Crisis Counseling Disaster Mental Health Service Model (CODE-C DMHSM)	Comprehensive, integrated, multiservice model that can be used to address the wide range of survivor mental health needs in communities following disasters; uses a standard nomenclature to facilitate communication between disaster mental health practitioners, emergency managers, and people who will receive services.	I, F, G, C, VF, DS, RRR, OR	F/C	EBBP	http://www.psychceu.com/disaster/disaster.asp

(Continued)

Name of Intervention	Description	Delivery Mode	Delivery Setting	Research Base	Source
Crisis Counseling Assistance and Training Program	Developed by the Federal Emergency Management Agency (FEMA) and the Substance Abuse and Mental Health Services Administration (SAMSHA), this program assists individuals and communities in recovering from the effects of natural and human caused disasters through the provision of community-based outreach and psycho-educational services.	I, C, DS	F/C, O	EBBP	http://www.samhsa.gov/dtac/ccp
Critical Incident Stress Debriefing (CISD)	7-phase, small group, crisis intervention process. it is one of the crisis intervention techniques that fall under the umbrella of critical incident stress management. The process was developed exclusively for small, homogeneous emergency incident responder groups who have encountered a powerful traumatic event, with the goals of reducing distress and restoring group cohesion.	G, C, RRR, OR	F/C	EvST, QR	http://www.info-trauma.org/flash/media-e/mitchellCriticalIncidentStressDebriefing.pdf
Early Psychological Intervention (EPI)	Developed by several national organizations involved in disaster response; focuses on psychological interventions to reduce acute distress while not interfering with the natural recovery process; interventions typically occur within the first month after a traumatic event and have multiple components; includes psychological first aid, triage, needs assessments, consultation, crisis intervention, fostering resilience, and psychological and medical treatments.	I, F, G, C, VF, DS, RRR, OR	FAC, F/C, PH, S, C, FBS, RA	EBBP	http://onlinelibrary.wiley.com/doi/10.1002/14651858.CD007944.pub2/full
The Families' GOALS Project: Going on After Loss	Provides a series of psycho-educational support groups for families that have experienced an event with traumatic loss; has structured curriculum for Pre-K through high school, adults and families; project supported by the New Jersey Department of Human Services Division of Mental Health through funding from SAMHSA and FEMA.	G, VF, F, DS	PH, F/C, FBS, O	EBBP	http://www.mhanj.org/new-jersey-hope-and-healing-emotional-support-for-those-impacted-by-superstorm-sandy-2
Group Crisis Intervention: Public Mental Health Service Delivery Protocols: Group Interventions For Disaster Preparedness and Response	Best practice interventions for use in delivering group-based mental health support services following disasters to population-specific survivors and responders.	I, F, G, C, VF, DS, RRR, OR	F/C, O	EBBP	http://www.agpa.org/home/practice-resources/member-benefit-programs/agpa-at-work-in-the-community/programs-and-services-available

(Continued)

Name of Intervention	Description	Delivery Mode	Delivery Setting	Research Base	Source
Healing After Trauma Skills	Designed for teachers, psychologists, and other counselors working with kindergarten, elementary, and early middle school children who have experienced a disaster or other traumatic event. Includes information about how children are affected by trauma/disaster; tools for enhancing the sharing of experiences, ideas, and thoughts about the trauma or disaster and for building coping skills; can be used with individual children.	I, G, DS	C, S	EBBP	http://www.nctsnet.org/nctsn_assets/pdfs/edu_materials/HATS2ndEdition.pdf
National Organization for Victim Assistance (NOVA) Crisis Response Team (CRT)	CRT members are trained to provide trauma mitigation and education in the aftermath of a emergency or disaster; response is scaled to the need; NOVA CRT provides a minimum of 24 hours of skill-based, field-tested training; teams could be state-based or local.	G, C, DS	F/C	EBBP, EvST	https://www.trynova.org/help-crisis-victims/crisis-training/
Psychological First Aid (PFA)	Modular approach for assisting people in the immediate aftermath of disaster to reduce initial distress, and to foster short- and long-term adaptive functioning; can be used in a variety of settings by first responders, incident commanders, primary and emergency health care providers, school crisis response teams, faith-based organizations, disaster relief organizations, CERT programs, the Medical Reserve Corps, and the Citizens Corps.	I, G, VF, C, DS	FAC, F/C, O	EBBP	http://www.ptsd.va.gov/professional/materials/manuals/psych-first-aid.asp Adaptations of PFA are targeted to specific populations; PFA has been translated into several languages. The following URLs link to PFA models that have been expanded or tailored to specific populations: Homeless families: http://www.nctsn.org/sites/default/files/assets/pdfs/PFA_Families_homelessness.pdf Homeless youth: http://www.nctsn.org/sites/default/files/assets/pdfs/pfa_homeless_youth.pdf Medical Reserve Corps: http://www.nctsn.org/sites/default/files/assets/pdfs/MRC_PFA_04_02_08.pdf Nebraska: http://disastermh.nebraska.edu/education/psychological.php Parents: http://www.ready.gov/sites/default/files/documents/files/PFA_Parents.pdf

(*Continued*)

Name of Intervention	Description	Delivery Mode	Delivery Setting	Research Base	Source
					Schools: http://www.nctsn.org/content/psychological-first-aid-schoolspfa RAPID Model: http://www.jhsph.edu/research/centers-and-institutes/johns-hopkins-center-for-public-health-preparedness/training/PFA.html Religious professionals: http://www.nctsn.org/sites/default/files/assets/pdfs/CRP-PFA_Guide.pdf Teachers: http://www.ready.gov/sites/default/files/documents/files/PFA_SchoolCrisis.pdf Workforce: https://live.blueskybroadcast.com/bsb/client/CL_DEFAULT.asp?Client=354947&PCAT=7365&CAT=9403
Psychological Simple Triage and Rapid Treatment, (PsySTART) Rapid Mental Health Triage and Incident Management System	Strategy for rapid mental health triage and incident management during large-scale disasters and terrorism; can help responders rapidly assess and provide for surge in acute and longer-term mental health impacts; PsySTART has 3 parts: community resilience, rapid triage "tag" (designed for field use by responders without mental health expertise), and an information technology platform to manage the collection and analysis of triage information.	I, VF, DS	F/C, O	EBBP, EvST	http://www.cdms.uci.edu/PDF/PsySTART-cdms02142012.pdf
Screening, Brief Intervention, Referral to Treatment	Early intervention and treatment for people with and those at risk of developing substance abuse disorders; early intervention provided in community settings before more severe consequences occur.	I, DS	FC, O	EvST	http://www.samhsa.gov/sbirt

(Continued)

Name of Intervention	Description	Delivery Mode	Delivery Setting	Research Base	Source
Seeking Safety	Present-focused therapy to help people attain safety from trauma/post-traumatic stress disorder (PTSD) and substance abuse. Conducted in group and individual formats with women, men, and mixed-gender groups; conducted in outpatient, inpatient, residential with substance abuse and dependence.	I, G, DS	PH, F/C, O	EBBP, EvST	http://www.treatment-innovations.org/seeking-safety.html
Wave Riders	After school, intervention offers empowerment, encouragement, positivity, and ongoing resiliency building; developed after Hurricane Sandy, this 6-session, group intervention involves a series of highly structured, expressive-behavioral activities aimed at reducing stress reactions, anxiety, fear, and sadness and developing an increase of hope, self-esteem, self-efficacy, daily functioning, and adaptive skills.	G, DS	C, F/C, O	EBBP	http://www.mhanj.org/new-jersey-hope-and-healing
Intermediate Interventions (6 Months Through the 1-Year Anniversary)					
Cognitive Behavioral Therapy For Post-Disaster Distress	10 session intervention that focuses on identifying and challenging maladaptive disaster-related beliefs; the intervention includes 4 components: psycho-education, breathing retraining, behavioral activation, and cognitive restructuring.	I, F, G, VF, DS, RRR, OR	PH, RA, F/C, FBS	EvST, EBBP, QR	Hamblen JL, Gibson LE, Mueser KT, Norris FH. 2006. Cognitive behavioral therapy for prolonged postdisaster distress. *J Clin Psychol.* 62(8):1043–1052. Hamblen JL, Norris FH, Pietruszkiewicz S, Gibson LE, Naturale AJ, Louis C. 2009. Cognitive behavioral therapy for postdisaster distress: A community based treatment program for survivors of Hurricane Katrina. *Adm Policy Ment Health.* 36(3):206–214.

(*Continued*)

Name of Intervention	Description	Delivery Mode	Delivery Setting	Research Base	Source
Classroom-Based Intervention	4 week, 12 session classroom, clinic, and camp-based group intervention with a series of structured expressive-behavioral activities; activities allow and guide children to play, learn, and engage in creative problem solving; designed and developed for schools and community centers to assist teachers and administrators with stabilization and resiliency building.	I, G, F/C, DS	C, F/C, S, FBS	EBBP, EvST	Tol WA, Komproe IH, Susanty D, Jordans MJ, Macy RD, De Jong JT. 2008. School-based mental health intervention for children affected by political violence in Indonesia: A cluster randomized trial. *JAMA.* 300(6):665–662.
Cognitive Behavioral Intervention In School	10 session group intervention designed for use in an inner-city school mental health clinic with a multicultural population; uses group format (5–8 students per group) to address symptoms of PTSD, anxiety, and depression.	G, DS	S	EmST, EBBP	Stein BD, Kataoka S, Jaycox L, Wong M, Fink A, Escudero P, Zaragoza C. 2002. Theoretical basis and program design of a school-based mental health intervention for traumatized immigrant children: A collaborative research partnership. *J Behav Health Serv Res.* 29(3):318–326. Stein BD, Jaycox LH, Kataoka SH, Wong M, Tu W, Elliott MN, Fink A. 2003. A mental health intervention for schoolchildren exposed to violence: A randomized controlled trial. *JAMA.* 290(5):603–611.

(*Continued*)

Name of Intervention	Description	Delivery Mode	Delivery Setting	Research Base	Source
Mind/Body Therapies	This group includes mindfulness-based cognitive therapy and mindfulness-based stress reduction. Mindfulness-based cognitive therapy includes mindfulness, or paying attention in the present moment, and nonjudgmentally. Mindfulness shifts the individual's perspective in a way that counteracts psychopathological processes. Behavioral and cognitive principles are also strongly incorporated, making these interventions hybrids rather than complementary and alternative medicine (CAM). Mindfulness-based stress reduction is a group intervention that incorporates mindfulness practices, including meditation and yoga. Mindfulness-based interventions show promise for stress reduction in general medical conditions, and initial evidence suggests that they are accepted in trauma-exposed individuals. Overall, the current evidence base does not support the use of CAM interventions as an alternative to current empirically established approaches for PTSD, or as first-line interventions recommended within evidence-based clinical guidelines. Yet, anecdotally, many people report liking mind-body therapies and engaging in them.	I, F, G, C, VF, DS, RRR, OR	FAC, F/C, PH, S, C, FBS, RA	EBBP	Kabat-Zinn J, Massion AO, Kristeller J, Peterson LG, Fletcher KE, Pbert L, Lenderking WR, Santorelli SF. 1992. Effectiveness of a meditation-based stress reduction program in the treatment of anxiety disorders. *Am J Psychiatry*. 149(7):936–943.

Source: Based on Substance Abuse and Mental Health Services Administration. 2015. *SAMHSA Disaster Technical Assistance Center Supplemental Research Bulletin: Disaster Behavioral Health Interventions Inventory*. Rockville, MD: SAMHSA. Available at: http://www.samhsa.gov/sites/default/files/dtac/supplemental-research-bulletin-may-2015-disaster-behavioral-health-interventions.pdf. Accessed January 25, 2017.

Note: **Delivery Mode:** C=Community; DS=Direct Survivors; F=Family (general); G=Group; I=Individual; OR=Other Responders; RRR=Rescue and Recovery Responders; VF=Victim Family. **Delivery Setting:** C=Classrooms; FAC=Family Assistance Centers; FBS=Faith-Based Settings; F/C=Field/Community; O=Other; PH=Private Homes; RA=Responder Agencies; S=Schools (general). **Research Base:** EBBP=Evidence Informed or Evidence Based Behavioral Practice; EmST=Empirically Supported Treatment; EvST=Evidence Supported Treatment; QR=Qualitative Research.

FIRST AID

APPENDIX N

FIRST AID AND EMERGENCY SUPPLY KITS

Basic items that should be assembled and stored in case of emergency include water, food, a first aid kit, tools, and supplies, and special medications and supplies when indicated. First aid supplies should be stored in a fireproof, waterproof box that is easy to carry. As with a first aid kit, all items described below should be inspected regularly and replaced when no longer useable. Important medical information and most prescriptions can be stored in the refrigerator and rotated every 6 months. In addition, copies of important papers (e.g., contact information, copies of most recent social security award letter [if applicable], driver's license, insurance policies, medical plan cards, name and phone number of physician, Social Security card, personal phone book) should be secured and put in a safe place.

Water

Store 1 gallon per person per day in plastic containers. Maintain a 7-day supply that is replaced every 6 months.

Food

Store a 7-day supply of nonperishable food for each person. Rotate the food supply every 6 months.

Baby formula, food

High energy foods: nutrition bars, nuts, peanut butter, trail mix

Juices: canned, boxed, powdered, or crystallized

Milk: boxed, powdered, or canned

Ready-to-eat canned or dried meats, fruits, and vegetables

Soups, bouillon cubes, or dried soups

Vitamins

First Aid Kit

Ace bandages
Adhesive tape roll
Alcohol swabs (individually wrapped)
Antacid
Antibiotic ointment
Antidiarrheal medicine
Antiseptic or hydrogen peroxide
Aspirin and nonaspirin tablets
Assorted sizes of safety pins
Cleansing agent or soap
Cold packs
Cotton-tipped swabs
Dressings
Emetic (to induce vomiting)
Eye drops or eyewash
Hyperallergenic adhesive tape
Latex gloves
Laxative
Moist towelettes
Needle
Prescriptions and any long-term medications
Rolled gauze
Rubbing alcohol
Safety razor blade
Snake bite kit
Sterile adhesive bandages (assorted sizes)
Thermometer
Tweezers

Other First Aid Supplies

Bar soap
First aid book
Needle and thread
Paper cups
Pocket knife
Scissors
Small plastic bags
Splinting materials
Sunscreen

Sanitation Kit

Disinfectant
Facial tissues
Household bleach
Personal hygiene items (e.g., sanitary napkins)
Plastic garbage bags, ties
Soap, liquid detergent
Toilet paper, moist towelettes

Home Survival Tools and Supplies

Adhesive labels
Aluminum foil
Ax
Battery-operated radio
Batteries in various sizes
Blankets or sleeping bags
Broom
Candles
Cash or traveler's checks, coins
Change of clothing
Compass
Disposable dust masks
Facial tissues
Fire extinguisher (multipurpose, dry chemical type)
Flashlight
Food and water for pets
Garden hose (for siphoning and firefighting)
Hammer
Knife
Manual can opener
Map of the area
Medicine dropper
Mess kits or disposable plates, cups, and utensils
Needles, thread
Nylon cord
Paper, pencil
Patch kit and can of seal-in-air
Plastic bucket with tight lid (for indoor toilet)
Plastic sheeting
Plastic storage bags and containers
Pliers
Recreational supplies for children and adults
Rope for towing or rescue
Safety goggles
Scissors
Screwdriver
Shovel
Signal flare
Spray paint
Sturdy shoes
Tape, such as duct tape
Tent
Thick work gloves
Toilet paper
Tools (e.g., crowbar, hammer, nails, pliers, screwdriver, wood screws, adjustable wrench)
Utility knife
Waterproof matches or in a waterproof container
Whistle

Car Survival Kit

Blankets
Bottled water
Change of clothes
Coins for telephone calls
Duct tape
Emergency signal device (light sticks, battery-type flasher, reflector)
Fire extinguisher (multipurpose, dry chemical type)
First aid kit and manual

Flashlight and batteries

Food (nonperishable items such as nutrition bars, trail mix)

Heavy work gloves

Jumper cables

Local map and compass

Moist towelettes

Paper and pencils

Rope for towing and rescue

Small bag or backpack to carry items

Small mirror

Sturdy shoes or work boots

Toilet paper

Tools (e.g., pliers, adjustable wrench, screwdriver)

Whistle

Workplace Survival Kit

Blanket

Bottled water

Essential medications

Extra pair of eyeglasses or contact lens solution

Flashlight

Food (nonperishable items such as nutrition bars, trail mix)

Jacket or sweatshirt

Portable battery-operated radio and batteries

Small first aid kit

Small mirror

Sturdy shoes

Whistle

Disability-Related Supplies and Special Equipment List

Cane(s)

Crutches

Dentures

Dialysis equipment

Dressing device

Eating utensils

Eyeglasses

Flow rate regulator

Grooming utensils

Hearing device

Monitors

Ostomy supplies

Oxygen

Sanitary supplies

Suction equipment

Urinary supplies

Walker

Wheelchair

Wheelchair repair kit

Writing device

AT-RISK POPULATIONS

APPENDIX O

COMMUNITY PLANNING NETWORK FOR AT-RISK POPULATIONS

The following agencies, organizations, and institutions should be involved in disaster planning for at-risk populations:

- Emergency management agencies
- Citizen Corps Councils and program partners (Community Emergency Response Teams, Medical Reserve Corps, fire corps, Volunteers in Police Service, and Neighborhood Watch groups)
- Local emergency planning committees
- First responders (i.e., police, fire and rescue, emergency medical services)
- Metropolitan Medical Response System
- Government and nongovernment disability agencies
- Developmental disabilities networks and service providers
- Protection and advocacy agencies
- Departments of aging and social services
- Hospitals and hospices
- Culturally or language-based community groups
- Voluntary organizations active in disaster such as the Red Cross and Salvation Army
- Departments of health
- Departments of education
- Health and human services agencies (including child welfare)
- Human services information and referral services
- Housing and Urban Development (HUD) or other rent-subsidized multifamily complexes
- HUD or otherwise subsidized nonlicensed supervised living facilities
- Nursing homes
- Media
- Home health care organizations
- Medical service and equipment providers (including durable medical equipment providers)
- Pharmaceutical providers
- Agencies on alcohol and drug addiction

- Job and family service agencies
- Vocational rehabilitation agencies
- Independent living centers
- Behavioral health and mental health agencies
- Commissions on the deaf and hard of hearing and the blind and visually impaired
- Governor's committees on individuals with functional needs and disabilities
- Translation and interpretation service agencies
- Transportation service providers (including those with accessible vehicles)
- Utility providers
- Colleges and universities
- Faith-based organizations
- Schools
- Childcare facilities (both center-based and home-based)
- Veterinary resources
- Individuals with functional needs

Source: Adapted from Federal Emergency Management Agency (FEMA). 2010. *Developing and Maintaining Emergency Operations Plans: Comprehensive Preparedness Guide (CPG) 101*. Version 2.0. Washington, DC: FEMA. Available at: http://www.fema.gov/pdf/about/divisions/npd/CPG_101_V2.pdf. Accessed January 25, 2017.

APPENDIX P

PROTECTION AND DISPOSAL OF MEDICAL DEVICES AND SAFE DRUG USE AFTER A NATURAL DISASTER

The following are a series of guidelines to ensure that medical devices are maintained and remain useable after a natural disaster.

General Safety

- Keep device and supplies clean and dry.
- Notify the local public health authority to request evacuation prior to adverse weather events.
- Check all power cords and batteries to make sure they are not wet or damaged by water. If electrical circuits and electrical equipment have gotten wet, turn off the power at the main breaker.
- Maintain the device in an area with good lighting (e.g., refilling the insulin pump, checking the glucose meter).
- Keep the device in as clean and secure a location as possible.
- Always check the device for pests before use.

Power Outage

- Register with the electric company and fire department as a user who is dependent on a medical device that needs power (e.g., ventilator, apnea monitor).
- Determine if the device can be used with batteries or a generator.
- Locate a generator if possible.
- Do not plug a power cord in an electrical outlet if the cord or the device is wet.
- When power is restored, check to make sure the settings on the medical device have not changed or reset to a default.

Water Contamination

Some medical devices and equipment, such as dialyzers or intravenous pumps, require safe water for their use, cleaning, and maintenance. Disasters involving water, such as hurricanes or flooding, can contaminate the public water supply. Public announcements will be made about the safety of the municipal water supply. In an emergency situation, to ensure that water is safe for use with medical devices:

- Use only bottled, boiled, or treated water until the water supply is tested and found safe.
- If available water cannot be verified as having come from a safe source, it should be boiled or treated before use.
- Boiling water, when practical, is the preferred way to kill harmful bacteria and parasites. Bringing water to a rolling boil for 1 minute will kill most organisms.
- When boiling water is not practical, water can be treated with chlorine tablets, iodine tablets, or unscented household chlorine bleach (5.25% sodium hypochlorite). Follow the directions on the packaging for chlorine or iodine tablets. If household bleach is being used and if the questionable water is clear, add 1/8 teaspoon (~0.75 mL) of bleach per gallon of water; if the water is cloudy, add 1/4 teaspoon (~1.50 mL) of bleach per gallon. Mix the solution thoroughly and let it stand for about 30 minutes before using it. Keep in mind that treating water with chlorine tablets, iodine tablets, or liquid bleach will not kill parasitic organisms.
- Use a bleach solution to rinse water containers before reusing them.
- Use water storage tanks and other types of containers with caution because storage tanks and previously used cans or bottles may be contaminated with microbes or chemicals.

Sterility

- When performing medical procedures, maintain a clean environment by using bleach, alcohol, or a disinfectant in the area in which you are working (e.g., catheter changes, dressing changes, suctioning).
- Check sterile packaging to make sure it is dry and intact (e.g., sterile gauze). If the packaging is wet or damaged, do not use the product inside.
- When purchasing supplies, always check the packaging to make sure it hasn't been damaged.

Reuse of Medical Devices

- Do not reuse a medical device designed for a single use. If you need to reuse a device intended for multiple uses (e.g., infusion tubing, syringes), the device must be cleaned and disinfected or sterilized according to the device manufacturer's instructions. Devices should not be boiled unless explicitly allowed on the product label or instructions for use.
- To clean, disinfect, or sterilize a medical device or its components, make sure the water source is safe first before proceeding.

Heat and Humidity

- Heat and humidity can have an effect on home diagnostic test kits, rendering test results inaccurate. The owner's manual provides instructions to determine if a test kit is working properly.
- Before using a blood glucose meter, check the meter and test strip package insert for information on use during unusual heat and humidity. Store and handle the meter and test strips according to the instructions. Perform quality-control checks to make sure that the home glucose testing is accurate and reliable.
- To protect a device from heat and humidity:
    - Use a dry cloth to wipe off the device regularly.
    - Keep the device out of direct sunlight.
    - Enclose medical products in plastic containers to keep them dry.
    - Use dry ice or instant cold packs to keep devices cool.
    - Do not use disposable devices that are wet.

Source: Adapted from Food and Drug Administration. 2014. FDA offers tips about medical devices and hurricane disasters. Available at: http://www.fda.gov/medicaldevices/safety/emergencysituations/ucm055987.htm. Accessed January 25, 2017.

Checking Medical Devices for Contamination

In determining which medical devices should be discarded, the owner must assess each product's current condition and potential safety risks (as described below). For additional information, see Food and Drug Administration advice about medical devices that have been exposed to unusual levels of heat and humidity (available at: http://www.fda.gov/MedicalDevices/Safety/EmergencySituations/ucm056086.htm).

- Electrical or electronic equipment (e.g., blood pressure measurement devices, glucose meters and digital thermometers)
  - Check packaging for water damage. If the package got wet, the product inside could be damaged or contaminated. Discard the device if the packaging is wet or if it shows signs of having been wet (such as water stains or discoloration).
- Packaged devices, supplies, and test kits
  - Check packaging for water damage, signs of mold or breaks in the package seals. If the package got wet, the product inside could be contaminated. Discard the device if the packaging is wet or if it shows signs of having been wet (such as water stains or discoloration), has mold growth on it, or if the package is torn or damaged in any way that could break its seal.
  - Determine whether and how long the package was exposed to unusually high room temperatures. Many test kit reagents are temperature-sensitive and could perform unreliably if exposed to unusually high storage temperatures for an extended period of time. Discard packaged test kits if the facility had unusually high room temperatures for more than 24 hours.
  - Examples: bandages and gauzes, feminine hygiene products, urinary incontinence pads, contact lens supplies, eye drops, glucometers and test strips, pregnancy tests, fertility prediction tests, glycated hemoglobin test kits, urine dipsticks, drugs-of-abuse tests, pH measurement devices, sperm detection devices, home Protime meters and strips to measure prothrombin time, HIV and hepatitis sample collection kits.
- Refrigerated products (e.g., laboratory reagents, sterilants, and disinfectants)
  - Determine whether the refrigerators in which the products were stored were without power. Because refrigerated devices and supplies could perform unreliably if they were exposed to unusually high temperatures in storage, discard refrigerated devices and supplies if the refrigerator storing them was without power for more than 8 hours.

Source: Adapted from Food and Drug Administration. 2011. Disposal of contaminated devices. Available at: http://www.fda.gov/MedicalDevices/Safety/EmergencySituations/ucm055974.htm. Accessed January 25, 2017.

Protection of Drugs

Concerns about the efficacy or safety of a particular product should be addressed with a pharmacist, health care provider, or the manufacturer's customer service department, but the below guidelines are a general set of parameters for the protection of drugs:

- Drugs exposed to excessive heat, such as fire
  - When lifesaving medication in its original container looks normal, it can be used until a replacement is available.

- Drugs exposed to unsafe water
  - All drugs—even those in their original containers—should be discarded if they have come into contact with flood or contaminated water.
- Lifesaving drugs exposed to water
  - When lifesaving drugs may not be readily replaced, if the container is contaminated but the contents appear unaffected—if the pills are dry—the pills may be used until a replacement can be obtained. However, if a pill is wet, it is contaminated and should be discarded.
- Reconstituted drugs
  - For children's drugs that require water to reconstitute, the drug should only be reconstituted with purified or bottled water. Liquids other than water should not be used to reconstitute these products.
- Drugs that need refrigeration
  - For drugs that require refrigeration (e.g., insulin, somatropin, and drugs that have been reconstituted), the drug should be discarded if electrical power has been off for a long time. If the drug is absolutely necessary to sustain life (e.g., insulin) it may be used until a new supply is available.
  - Temperature-sensitive drugs should be replaced with a new supply as soon as possible. For example, insulin that is not refrigerated has a shorter shelf life than the labeled expiration date.
  - If a contaminated product is considered medically necessary and would be difficult to replace quickly, contact a health care provider (e.g., physician, poison control, health department) for guidance.

Source: Adapted from Food and Drug Administration. 2015. Safe drug use after a disaster. Available at: http://www.fda.gov/Drugs/EmergencyPreparedness/ucm085200.htm. Accessed January 25, 2017.

APPENDIX Q

EMERGENCY POWER PLANNING FOR PEOPLE WHO USE ELECTRICITY- AND BATTERY-DEPENDENT ASSISTIVE TECHNOLOGY AND MEDICAL DEVICES

This emergency power-planning checklist is for people who use electricity- and battery-dependent assistive technology and medical devices. Electricity- and battery-dependent devices include breathing machines (e.g., respirators, ventilators), power wheelchairs and scooters, and oxygen, suction, or home dialysis equipment. Some of this equipment is essential to the independence of those who use it, while other equipment is vital to sustaining life. Persons who are dependent on electricity- and battery-powered equipment (and those responsible for their care) should use the checklist on the pages following to make power-backup plans. Review and update this checklist every 6 months.

The following are Internet sources for more information:

Title	Web Site
Disaster Resources for People With Disabilities, Disability-Related Organizations and Emergency Managers and Planners	June Isaacson Kailes, Disability Policy Consultant home page (http://www.jik.com/disaster.html)
Tips for People With Activity Limitations and Disabilities	Emergency Survival Program home page (http://www.espfocus.org)
American Red Cross Power Outage Checklist	http://www.redcross.org/images/MEDIA_CustomProductCatalog/m4340180_PowerOutage.pdf
Home Generator Advice	Home Generator Advice featured video page (http://www.consumerreports.org/video/view/home-garden/energy-efficiency/2437113716001/home-generator-advice/)
Hazards of Portable Generators	Consumer Product Safety Commission Safety Alert, Portable Generator Hazards page (http://lwd.dol.state.nj.us/labor/forms_pdfs/lsse/Portable%20Generator%20Hazards.pdf)

Source: Based on Kailes JI. 2009. Emergency safety tips for people who use electricity and battery-dependent devices. Available at: http://www.jik.com/Power%20Planning%2010.24.09.pdf. Accessed March 9, 2017.

Emergency Power Planning Checklist

Date Completed	Does Not Apply	*Planning Basics*
		Create a plan for alternative sources of power.
		Read equipment instructions and talk to equipment suppliers about backup power options.
		Get advice from local power company regarding type of backup power planned.
		Regularly check backup or alternative power equipment to ensure it will function during an emergency.
		Ensure many other people know how to operate equipment and use backup systems.
		Keep a list of alternate power providers.
		Ask nearby police and fire departments and hospital it they can be used in the event that personal backup systems tail.
		Label all equipment with name, address, and phone number. Attach simple and clear laminated instruction cards to equipment.
		Keep copies of lists of serial and model numbers of devices, as well as important use instructions in a waterproof container in the emergency supply kit.
Date Completed	**Does Not Apply**	***Life-Support Device Users***
		Contact power and water companies about needs for life-support devices in advance of a disaster.
		Contact the customer service department of your utility companies to ask to be put on a "priority reconnection service" list, if possible.
		Keep in mind that even if you are on the "priority reconnection service" list, power could still be out for many days following a disaster, so maintain power backup options for equipment.
		Let local fire department know about your dependency on life-support devices.
		All ventilator users should keep a bag-valve mask handy.
		If you receive dialysis or other medical treatments, ask your providers what to do in case of emergency.
Date Completed	**Does Not Apply**	***Oxygen Users***
		Check with health care provider to determine if you can use a reduced flow rate in an emergency to extend the life of the system. Record on your equipment the approved reduced flow numbers so that you can easily refer to them.
		Be aware of oxygen safety practices: • Avoid areas where gas leaks or open flames may be present. • Post "Oxygen in Use" signs. • Always use battery powered flashlights or lanterns rather than gas lights or candles when oxygen is in use. • Keep the shut-off switch for oxygen equipment nearby in case of emergency.

Date Completed	Does Not Apply	*Generator Users*
		Determine whether use of a generator is appropriate and realistic.
		Operate generators in open areas to ensure good airing.
		Safely store fuel (note: this can be challenging when living in an apartment) and a siphon kit.
		Test it occasionally to make sure it will work when needed.
		Some generators can connect to the existing home wiring systems; always contact utility company regarding critical restrictions and safety issues.
Date Completed	**Does Not Apply**	***Rechargeable Batteries***
		Check with vendor/supplier to find alternative ways to charge batteries (e.g., connecting jumper cables to a vehicle battery, using a converter that plugs into a vehicle's cigarette lighter).
		If primary mode of transportation is a motorized wheelchair or scooter, store a lightweight manual wheelchair for emergency use.
		If your survival strategy depends on storing batteries, closely follow a recharging schedule.
		Know the working time of any batteries necessary for systems.
		When possible, choose equipment that uses batteries easily purchased from nearby stores.
Date Completed	**Does Not Apply**	***Other Backup Plans***
		When power is restored, check to make sure the settings on medical device have not changed.

Note: A 2000- to 2500-watt gas-powered portable generator can power a refrigerator and several lamps. (A refrigerator needs to run only 15 minutes per hour to stay cool if the door is kept closed. Therefore, it can be unplugged to allow operation of other devices.)

APPENDIX R

CULTURAL COMPETENCE CHECKLIST

Competencies	Tasks
Recognize the importance of culture and respect diversity.	Complete a self-assessment to determine your own beliefs about culture. Assess capabilities of counselors to understand and respect the values, customs, beliefs, language, and interpersonal style of the disaster survivor. Seek evidence of personnel respect for the importance of verbal and nonverbal communication, space, social organization, time, and environment controls within various cultures.
Maintain a current profile of the cultural composition of the community.	Develop and periodically update a community profile that describes composition of race, ethnicity, age, gender, religion, refugee and immigrant status, housing status, income and poverty levels, percent living in rural and in urban areas, unemployment rate, language and dialects, literacy level, and number of schools and businesses. Include information about values, beliefs, social and family norms, traditions, practices, politics, and historic racial relations or ethnic issues. Gather information in consultation with community cultural leaders who represent and understand local cultural groups.
Recruit disaster workers who are representative of the community or service area.	Review community profile when recruiting volunteers and recruit from the ethnic and cultural groups impacted by the disaster. If workers are not available from the impacted groups, recruit from similar backgrounds and spoken language. Assess workers' personal attributes, knowledge, and skills.
Provide ongoing cultural competence training to staff and volunteers.	Include language and sign interpreters and temporary staff.
Ensure that services are accessible, appropriate, and equitable.	Identify and take steps to overcome resistance to use services. Identify and take steps to eliminate service barriers. Involve representatives of diverse cultural groups in program committees, planning boards, policy-setting bodies, and decision making.
Recognize the role of help-seeking behaviors, customs, and traditions and natural support networks.	Identify cultural patterns that may influence help-seeking behavior. Build trusting relationships and rapport with disaster survivors. Recognize that survivors may find the procedures used in providing emergency assistance and traditional relief confusing or difficult. Recognize customs and traditions for healing, trauma, and loss and identify how these influence an individual's receptivity to and need for assistance. Acknowledge cultural beliefs about healing and recognize their importance to disaster survivors. Help survivors establish rituals and organize culturally appropriate anniversary activities. Recognize that outreach efforts focused only on the individual may not be effective for those whose cultures are centered around family and community. Determine who is significant in survivor's families and social networks.

(*Continued*)

Competencies	Tasks
Involve community leaders and organizations representing diverse cultural groups as cultural brokers.	Collaborate with trusted leaders (e.g., spiritual leaders, clergy and teachers). Invite organizations representing cultural groups to participate in program planning and service delivery. Collaborate with community-based organizations to communicate with cultural groups they represent. Identify ways to work with informal culture-specific groups. Coordinate with other public and private agencies in your cultural outreach.
Ensure that services and information are culturally and linguistically competent.	Identify indigenous workers who speak the language of the survivors; use interpreters only when necessary. Identify trained interpreters who share the survivors' background. Determine the dialect of the survivor before asking for an interpreter. Assess the level of acculturation on the interpreter relative to the survivors. Establish a plan to provide written materials in relevant languages at the literacy level of the target population. Provide means to reach people who are deaf or hard of hearing. Consult with cultural groups to determine the most effective outreach. Use existing resources (e.g., multicultural television and radio stations) to enhance outreach.
Assess and evaluate the program's level of cultural competence.	Continuously assess the program. Involve representatives of various cultural groups in the evaluation. Communicate evaluation findings to key informants and cultural groups engaged in the program.

Source: Adapted from Substance Abuse and Mental Health Services Administration, U.S. Department of Health & Human Services (HHS). 2003. *Developing Cultural Competence in Disaster Mental Health Programs.* Washington, DC: HHS. Available at: https://store.samhsa.gov/shin/content/SMA03-3828/SMA03-3828.pdf. Accessed January 25, 2017.

APPENDIX S

STANDARDS AND INDICATORS FOR DISASTER SHELTER AND TEMPORARY RESPITE CARE FOR CHILDREN

The following guidelines are intended to ensure that children have a safe and secure environment during and after a disaster:

- Typically, a parent, guardian, or caregiver will be the primary resource for their children, 18 years old and younger.
- When children are not with parents or guardians, local law enforcement personnel and local child protective and welfare services should be contacted to help reunite families.
- Children should be sheltered together with their families or caregivers.
- Families should have a designated area apart from the general shelter population.
- Family areas should have direct access to bathrooms.
- Parents, guardians, and caregivers are to be notified that they should accompany their children when they use the bathrooms.
- Space should be set aside for family interaction that provides:
    - Reduction of a child's repeated exposure to news coverage of the disaster.
    - Age-appropriate toys, with play supervised by parents, guardians, or caregivers.
- Regular cleaning and disinfecting of shared environmental surfaces with a bleach solution or similar commercial product, including diaper changing surfaces, communal toys, sinks, toilets, doorknobs, and floors. Local health department authorities can provide information about infection control.
- Staff will refer children who show signs of illness to on-site or local health services personnel for evaluation. Parents will be asked for consent.
- Staff will refer children who show signs of emotional stress to on-site or local health services personnel for evaluation. Parents will be asked for consent.
- Age-appropriate and nutritious food (including baby formula and baby food) and snacks should be available and offered to children.

- Diapers should be available for infants and children. Infants and toddlers need up to 12 diapers a day.
- Age-appropriate blankets should be available.
- A private and safe space for breastfeeding women should be available (e.g., curtained-off area or provision of blankets for privacy).
- Basins and supplies for bathing infants should be readily available.

Those caring for children may benefit from a period during which they are temporarily relieved of that responsibility. This temporary respite should be provided in a secure, supervised, and supportive location in which children have a play experience. This may be located in a disaster recovery center, assistance center, shelter, or other service delivery site. Parents, guardians, or caregivers are required to stay on site or designate an on-site adult to be responsible for their children. The following standards and indicators apply to the provision of temporary respite care:

- Temporary respite care for children is provided in a safe, secure environment following a disaster.
- The location, hours of operation, and other information about temporary respite care for children is provided and easy for parents, guardians, and caregivers to understand.
- The site follows all applicable local, state, and federal laws, regulations, and codes.
- The area is fully accessible to all children.
- The area has enclosures or dividers to protect children from hazards and ensure that children are supervised in a secure environment.
- The area is located close to restrooms and a source of drinking water and hand-washing or hand-sanitizing stations are available in the area.
    - Procedures are in place to sign children in and out of the area and ensure that children are only released to the person or people listed on their registration form.
- Attendance records, registration forms, and injury or incident report forms include identifying information, parent, guardian, or caregiver names and contact information, information about allergies, and other special needs; this information must be provided, maintained, and available to staff at all times.
- Toys and materials in the area are safe and age-appropriate.
- All shelter staff members receive training and orientation and undergo a satisfactory criminal and sexual offender background check prior to working in the shelters. Spontaneous volunteers are not permitted. While working, staff must visibly display proper credentials at all times.
- At least 2 adults are present at all times. No child should be left alone with one adult who is not his or her parent, guardian, or caregiver.

- All staff members must be aged 18 years or older and the supervisor must be aged 21 years or older.
- An evacuation plan is developed with a designated meeting place outside the center. The evacuation plan should be posted and communicated to parents, caregivers, and guardians when registering their children.
- The child-to-staff ratio is appropriate to the space available and to the ages and needs of the children in the area at any given time.

Source: Adapted from National Commission on Children and Disasters. 2010. *2010 Report to the President and Congress.* Appendix B: Standards and Indicators for Disaster Shelter Care for Children. AHRQ Publication No. 10-M037. Rockville, MD: Agency for Healthcare Research and Quality.

APPENDIX T

MANUFACTURERS OF EMERGENCY EVACUATION DEVICES AND EMERGENCY PRODUCTS

AOK Global Products, Ltd.
634 Motor Parkway
Brentwood, NY 11717
Toll free: (800) 649-4265
Direct: (631) 242-1642
E-mail: sales@rescuechair.com
Web site: http://www.rescuechair.com

Evac+Chair
3000 Marcus Ave., Suite #3E6
Lake Success, NY 11042
Direct: (516) 502-4240
E-mail: sales@evac-chair.com
Web site: http://www.evac-chair.com

Ferno-Washington, Inc.
70 Weil Way
Wilmington, OH 45177
Toll free: (800) 733-3766
Web site: http://www.ferno.com/index.htm

Frank Mobility Systems, Inc.
1003 International Drive
Oakdale, PA 15071
Phone: (844) 562-8034
Fax: (724) 695-1593
E-mail: info@frankmobility.com
Web site: http://www.frankmobility.com

Garaventa Accessibility
P.O. Box 1769
Blaine, WA 98231
Toll free: (800) 663-6556
E-mail: customerrelations@garaventalift.com
Web site: http://www.garaventalift.com

Junkin
3121 Millers Lane
Louisville, KY 40216
Toll free: (888) 458-6546
Direct: (502) 775-8303
Fax: (502) 772-0548
E-mail: junkinsafety@aol.com
Web site: http://www.junkinsafety.com

LifeSlider, Inc.
25553 61st Road
Arkansas City, KS 67005
Toll free: (888) 442-4543
Fax: (620) 442-2320
E-mail: aaron@lifeslider.com
Web site: http://www.lifeslider.com

MAX-Ability, Inc.
1275 Fourth Street, Suite 304
Santa Rosa, CA 95404
Toll free: (800) 577-1555
Direct: (707) 575-5558
Fax: (707) 575-3856
Web site: http://www. http://max-ability.com
E-mail: info@max-ability.com

Safety Chairs
4307 Hickory Point
Panora, IA 50216
Phone: (707) 479-8586
E-mail: kfoote@safetychairs.net
Web site: http://www.safetychairs.net

Stryker EMS
3800 E. Centre St.
Portage, MI 49002
Toll free: (800) 327-0770
Direct: (269) 389-6260
Fax: (866) 795-2233
Web site: http://www.ems.stryker.com

INFECTIOUS DISEASE AND CBRNE

APPENDIX U

MAINTAINING AND MANAGING THE VACCINE COLD CHAIN

Vaccine Storage Temperature Requirements

Temperature	Instructions	Vaccine
35°F–46°F (2°C–8°C)	Do not freeze or expose to freezing temperatures. Set temperature at mid-range (40°F). Use a continuous temperature monitor that gives a visual record of the temperature fluctuations in the refrigerator. Contact state or local health department or manufacturer for guidance on vaccines exposed to temperatures above or below the recommended range.	Diphtheria, tetanus, or pertussis-containing vaccines *Haemophilus* conjugate vaccine Hepatitis A and hepatitis B vaccines[a] Inactivated polio vaccine Measles, mumps, and rubella vaccine (MMR) in the lyophilized (freeze-dried) state[b] Meningococcal polysaccharide vaccine Pneumococcal conjugate vaccine Pneumococcal polysaccharide vaccine Trivalent inactivated influenza vaccine Smallpox vaccine Anthrax Vaccine Absorbed[c]
≤5°F (−15°C)	Maintain in continuously frozen state with no freeze/thaw cycles. Contact state or local health department or manufacturer for guidance on vaccines exposed to temperatures above the recommended range.	Live attenuated influenza vaccine Varicella vaccine

Source: Adapted from Centers for Disease Control and Prevention (CDC). 2003. Notice to readers: guideline for maintaining and managing the vaccine cold chain. Table 1. Vaccine storage temperature requirements. *MMWR Morb Mortal Wkly Rep.* 52(42):1023–1025; CDC. 2003. *Guidelines for Smallpox Vaccine Packing and Shipping*. Atlanta, GA: CDC. Available at: https://emergency.cdc.gov/agent/smallpox/vaccination/pdf/packing-shipping.pdf. Accessed January 25, 2017; Emergent BioSolutions Inc. 2002. BioThrax. Available at: http://www.biothrax.com. Accessed January 25, 2017.

[a]ActHIB (Aventis Pasteur, Lyon, France) in the lyophilized state is not expected to be affected detrimentally by freezing temperatures, although no data are available.

[b]MMR in the lyophilized state is not affected detrimentally by freezing temperatures.

[c]BioThrax (Emergent BioSolutions, Rockville, MD) is not to be used after expiration date given on the package.

Comparison of Thermometers Used to Monitor Vaccine Temperatures

Thermometer Type	Advantages	Disadvantages
Standard fluid-filled	Inexpensive and simple to use Thermometers encased in biosafe liquids can reflect vaccine temperatures more accurately	Less accurate (+/−1°C) No information on duration of out of specification exposure No information on min/max temperatures Cannot be recalibrated Inexpensive models might perform poorly
Min/max	Inexpensive Monitors temperature range	Less accurate (+/−1°C) No information on duration of out of specification exposure Cannot be recalibrated
Continuous chart recorder	Most accurate Continuous 24-hour readings of temperature range and duration Can be recalibrated at regular intervals	Most expensive Requires most training and maintenance

Source: Adapted from Centers for Disease Control and Prevention. 2003. Notice to readers: guideline for maintaining and managing the vaccine cold chain. Table 2. Vaccine storage temperature requirements. *MMWR Morb Mortal Wkly Rep.* 52(42):1023–1025.

APPENDIX V

INTERNATIONAL NUCLEAR AND RADIOLOGICAL EVENT SCALE

The International Nuclear and Radiological Event Scale (INES) below is a tool used when communicating the safety significance of reported nuclear and radiological incidents and accidents to the media and the public. The scale can be applied to any event associated with nuclear facilities, as well to as the transport, storage, and use of radioactive material and radiation sources. INES is not intended for naturally occurring phenomena, such as radon.

Level	Event Description
1 (anomaly)	Minor problems with safety; does not involve spread of contamination or overexposure of members of the community.
2 (incident)	Significant failure of safety provisions resulting in exposure of a worker to a dose exceeding statutory limit, exposure of a member of the public in excess of 10 mSv,[a] or significant contamination within the facility in areas where not expected by design. Requires corrective action.
3 (serious incident)	Exposure in excess of 10 times the statutory annual limit for workers, nonlethal health effects (e.g., burns), or severe contamination within the facility in areas where not expected by design with a low probability of significant public exposure.
4 (accident with local consequences)	Minor release of radioactive material unlikely to result in implementation of planned countermeasures other than local food controls, at least one death from radiation, or release of significant quantities of radioactive material with a high probability of significant public exposure.
5 (accident with wider consequences)	Limited release of radioactive material likely to require implementation of countermeasures, significant damage to reactor core, release of large quantities of radioactive material with high probability of significant public exposure, could be caused by accident or fire, several deaths from radiation (e.g., the 1979 accident at Three Mile Island).
6 (serious accident)	Significant release of radioactive material likely to require full implementation of planned countermeasures (e.g., the 1957 accident at Kyshtym, Soviet Union).

(Continued)

Level	Event Description
7 (major accident)	Major release of radioactive material with widespread health and environmental effects requiring implementation of planned and extended countermeasures (e.g., the 1986 accident at Chernobyl and the 2011 crisis at Japan's Fukushima plant).

Source: Based on International Atomic Energy Agency. 2016. International Nuclear and Radiological Event Scale. Available at: http://www-ns.iaea.org/tech-areas/emergency/ines.asp. Accessed March 9, 2017.

[a]A sievert (Sv) is a unit of "dose equivalent" radiation. One sievert is a large dose as the recommended Threshold Limit Values (TLVs) established by the American Conference of Governmental Industrial Hygienists is an average annual dose of 0.05 Sv or 50 millisievert (mSv) for occupational exposures. The term *rem* is more commonly used in the United States; 1 rem equals 0.01 Sv, which equals 10 mSv. The International Commission on Radiological Protection recommends an annual dose limit of 1 mSv for the general public. The effects of being exposed to large doses of radiation at one time vary with the dose. As examples: 10 Sv: Risk of death within days or weeks; 1 Sv: Risk of cancer later in life (5 in 100); 100 mSv: Risk of cancer later in life (5 in 1,000); 50 mSv: TLV for annual dose for radiation workers in any 1 year; and 20 mSv: TLV for annual average dose, averaged over 5 years.

WORKER HEALTH AND SAFETY

APPENDIX W

SITE SAFETY CHECKLIST

- Assign key personnel and alternates responsible for site safety.
- Describe risks associated with each operation conducted.
- Confirm that personnel are adequately trained to perform jobs.
- Assign key person to handle volunteers.
- Describe the protective clothing and equipment to be worn by personnel during site operations.
- Describe site-specific medical surveillance requirements.
- Describe needed air monitoring, personnel monitoring, and environmental sampling.
- Describe actions to be taken to mitigate existing hazards (e.g., containment) to make the work environment less hazardous.
- Define site control measures (e.g., secure the area) and include a site map.
- Establish decontamination procedures for personnel and equipment.
- Establish site access and exit control requirements.
- Establish site food, water, shelter, and sanitation requirements.
- Establish site electrical safety requirements.
- Perform exit interviews or surveys regarding adverse health outcomes and exposures during the response.
- Identify those responders who should receive medical referral and possible enrollment into a long-term medical surveillance program, based on concerning exposures or signs and symptoms of physical or emotional ill health.

Source: Adapted from National Institute for Occupational Safety and Health. 2016. Guidance for Supervisors at Disaster Rescue Sites. Available at: http://www.cdc.gov/niosh/topics/emres/emhaz.html. Accessed January 25, 2017.

APPENDIX X

POTENTIAL HAZARDS AND GENERAL RECOMMENDATIONS FOR PROTECTING WORKERS' HEALTH

Hazard 1: Massive piles of construction and other types of debris, unstable work surfaces

Risks: Traumatic injuries, including serious fall injuries, from slips trips and falls or collapsing materials.

General Recommendations:

- Ensure that surfaces are as stable as possible.
- Use alternative methods, such as bucket trucks, to access work surfaces that are unstable.
- Ensure scaffolding is erected on a stable surface; anchor scaffolding to a structure capable of withstanding the lateral forces generated.
- Ensure that workers have a full array of personal protective equipment (PPE), including safety shoes with slip-resistant soles, cut-resistant gloves, eye protection, and hard hats.
- Ensure that workers use fall protection equipment with lifelines tied off to suitable anchorage points, including bucket trucks, whenever possible.

Hazard 2: Excessive Noise

Risks: Communication and temporary hearing loss.

General Recommendations:

- Use hearing protection devices whenever noisy equipment (e.g., saws, earth-moving equipment, Hurst tools) is used. This will prevent temporary hearing loss that can interfere when listening for cries, moans, and other sounds from victims buried in the rubble.

Hazard 3: Breathing dust containing asbestos (from pulverized insulation and fire-proofing materials) and silica (from pulverized concrete), which are toxic

Risks: Short term: irritation of eye, nose, throat, and lung.
Long term: Chronic effects may depend on the extent and the duration of exposure.

General Recommendations:

- Workers should be protected from breathing dust.
- Respiratory protection: An N95 or greater respiratory protection is acceptable for most activities, including silica and portland cement dust.
- If there is reason to believe there is an asbestos exposure, at not more than 10 times the safe level, use a half mask elastomeric respirator with N100-, R100-, or P100-series filters.
- If airborne contaminants are causing eye irritation, full face respirators with P100 OV/AG combination cartridges should be used.
- Respirators must fit properly to protect workers.
- Surgical masks should not be used because they do not provide adequate protection.
- Dust concentrations in the air must be appropriately monitored.
- If dust concentrations are elevated, limit entry to only person with adequate respiratory protection.
- If symptoms of chest pain or chest tightness are present, or if shortness of breath, or rapid breathing persists following a rest break, then medical attention should be sought.
- Respiratory equipment maintenance program should be maintained for the proper cleaning, repair, and storage of reusable respirators.
- Workers should be aware of the risks of "take-home toxic contaminants" and be supervised to ensure end of shift safety compliance.

Hazard 4: Heat stress from wearing encapsulating/insulating bunker gear or doing heavy work in a hot, humid climate

Risks: Significant fluid loss that frequently progresses to clinical dehydration, raised core body temperature, impaired judgment, disorientation, fatigue, and heat stroke.

General Recommendations:

- Adjust work schedules, rotate personnel, add additional personnel to work teams.
- Replenish fluids (1 cup water/sports drink every 20 minutes) and food (small frequent carbohydrate meals).
- Monitor heart rate. If over 180 beats per minute minus age for more than a few minutes, stop work and rest immediately.
- Provide frequent medical evaluation for symptoms and signs of heat stress, such as altered vital signs, confusion, profuse sweating, excessive fatigue.
- Provide shelter in shaded areas and the ability to unbutton and remove bunker gear.

- Make available a cooling station that contains water misting capability, fans, and ice packs.

Hazard 5: Confined Spaces (limited openings for entry and exit, unfavorable natural ventilation)

Risks: Low oxygen, toxic air contaminants, explosions, entrapment, death by strangulation, constriction, or crushing.

General Recommendations:

- Purge, flush, or ventilate the space.
- Monitor the space for hazardous conditions.
- Lock out/tag out procedures for power equipment in or around the space.
- Use appropriate PPE—such as a self-contained breathing apparatus (SCBA).
- Light the area as much as possible.
- Establish barriers to external traffic such as vehicles, pedestrians, or other hazards.
- Use ladders or similar equipment for safe entry and exit in the space.
- Use good communications equipment and alarm systems.
- Have rescue equipment nearby.

Specific Recommendations: Confined Space Attendant

- Provide at least 1 person (attendant) outside the confined space to be in communication with entrant for the duration of the operation.
- Maintain an accurate count of individuals entering the space.
- Evacuate the space if any hazards that could danger the entrants is detected.
- Monitor the behavior of entrants for any effects that suggest they should be evacuated.
- Perform no other duties that may interfere with their primary responsibilities.

Specific Recommendations: Confined Space Entrant

- Use a chest or full body harness with retrieval line attached at the center of entrant's back with the other end of line attached to mechanical device designed for immediate rescue.
- Notify attendant if they experience any warning signs or symptoms of exposure or detect a dangerous condition.
- Exit the permit space when instructed by the attendant or if warning signs indicate an evacuation.

Hazard 6: Potential Chemical Exposures From Fire Scene

Exposure to the following chemicals must be anticipated:

- Metals (dust and fume)

- Hydrogen cyanide
- Inorganic acids (particularly sulfuric acid)
- Aldehydes (including formaldehyde)
- PAHs (polycyclic aromatic hydrocarbons)
    - Benzo(a)anthracene
    - Benzo(b)fluoranthene
    - Benzo(a)pyrene
- VOCs (volatile organic chemicals)
- Aliphatic hydrocarbons
- Acetone
- Acetic acid
- Ethyl acetate
- Isopropanol
- Styrene
- Benzene
- Touene
- Xylene
- Furfural
- Phenol
- Napthalene
- PCBs (polychlorinated biphenyls) may be present in older buildings with electrical equipment manufactured prior to 1977

Risks: Eye, nose, throat, upper respiratory tract, and skin irritation; flu-like symptoms; central nervous system depression, fatigue, loss of coordination, memory difficulties, sleeplessness, mental confusion. Chronic effects depend on the extent and the duration of exposure.

General Recommendations:

- *Firefighting*: Use SCBA with full face piece in pressure demand or other positive pressure mode.
- *Entry into unknown concentration*: Use SCBA gear.
- *Rescue operations with fumes present*: Use gas mask with front mounted organic vapor canister (OVC) or any chemical cartridge respirator with an organic vapor cartridge.
- *Dusty environments*: Use combination HEPA/OVC.

Warning! A surgical or a dust mask will not protect you from chemical vapors.

Hazard 7: Electrical, overhead power lines, downed electrical wires, cables

Risk: Electrocution

General Recommendations:

- Use appropriately grounded low-voltage equipment.

Hazard 8: Carbon Monoxide Risk from gasoline- or propane-powered generators or heavy machinery

Risk: Headache, dizziness, drowsiness, or nausea; progressing to vomiting, loss of consciousness, and collapse, coma or death under prolonged or high exposures.

General Recommendations:

- Locate temporary generators downwind and away from sheltering sites and mass gathering locations.
- Use CO warning sensors when using or working around combustion sources.
- Shut off engine immediately if symptoms of exposure appear.

Warning! Do not use gasoline generators or portable fuel driven tools in confined spaces or poorly ventilated areas.

Warning! Do not work in areas near exhaust (CO poisoning occurs even outdoors if engines generate high concentrations of CO and worker is in the area of the exhaust gases). With symptoms of exposure, shut off the engine.

Hazard 9: Eye Injuries from dust, flying debris, blood

Risk: Blood borne pathogen infection, eye injury.

General Recommendations: Protective Eyewear

- Use goggles or face shield and mask for those handling human remains, recovering deceased. Make sure to cover the nose and mouth to protect the skin of the face and the mucous membranes.
- Use safety glasses with side shields as a minimum by all workers. An eyewear retainer strap is suggested.
- Consider safety goggles for protection from fine dust particles, or for use over regular prescription eyeglasses.
- Any worker using a welding torch for cutting needs special eyewear for protection from welding light, which can cause severe burns to the eyes and surrounding tissue.
- Only use protective eyewear that has an ANSI Z87 mark on the lenses or frames.

Hazard 10: Flying Debris; particles; handling a variety of sharp, jagged materials

Risk: Traumatic injuries, ranging from minor injuries requiring first aid to serious, even disabling or fatal, traumatic injury.

General Recommendations:

- Use safety glasses with side shields as a minimum. An eyewear retainer strap is suggested.
- Consider safety goggles for protection from fine dust particles, or for use over regular prescription eyeglasses.
- Any worker using a welding torch for cutting needs special eyewear for protection from welding light, which can cause severe burns to the eyes and surrounding tissue.
- Only use protective eyewear that has an ANSI Z87 mark on the lenses or frames.
- Educate workers regarding safe work procedures before beginning work.
- Provide workers with a full array of personal protective equipment, including hard hats, safety shoes, eyeglasses, and work gloves.
- Ensure that workers do not walk under or through areas where cranes and other heavy equipment are being uses to lift objects.

Hazard 11: Work with numerous types of heavy equipment, including cranes, bucket trucks, skid-steer loaders, etc.

Risks: Traumatic injury, including serious and fatal injuries, due to failure or improper use of equipment, or workers being struck by moving equipment.

General Recommendations:

- Train workers to operate equipment correctly and safely.
- Ensure operators are aware of the activities around them to protect workers on foot from being struck by moving equipment.
- Ensure operators do not exceed the load capacity of cranes and other lifting equipment.
- Ensure that workers do not walk under or through areas where cranes and other heavy equipment are being used to lift objects.
- Ensure that workers do not climb onto or ride loads being lifted or moved.
- Ensure operators do not exceed site speed limits and obey traffic lane safety when travel on and exiting the site.

Hazard 12: Rescuing Victims, Recovering Deceased, Handling Human Remains, Contact with surfaces contaminated with blood and body fluids

Risk: Blood, bloody fluids, body fluids, and tissues are potential sources of blood-borne infections from pathogens including hepatitis B, hepatitis C, and HIV.

- Route of exposure: Through the skin via a cut or puncture wound; through mucous membranes (eye, nose, mouth); through nonintact skin (dermatitis/rashes, injuries, abrasions).

General Recommendations:

- *Standard precautions:* Universal precautions should be strictly observed regardless of time since death. Workers who will have direct contact with the victims, bodies, or surfaces contaminated with blood or body fluids should use universal precautions including:
  - Use heavy-duty work gloves (such as leather) to protect against injury from sharp objects.
  - Use appropriate barrier protection when handling potentially infectious materials. These barriers include latex gloves (preferably powder-free latex gloves with reduced latex protein content) and nitrile gloves. These gloves can be worn under the heavy-duty gloves. Workers should be aware that individuals can develop allergic reactions to latex gloves that can result in respiratory problems (asthma), hives, and skin rashes. Those with known latex allergies should use nitrile gloves.
  - Use eye protection (goggles or face shield) and mask covering the nose and mouth to protect the skin of the face and the mucous membranes.
  - Use protective clothing to protect exposed skin surfaces.
  - Immediately after removing gloves or other protective equipment, wash hands with soap and water.

- *Specific Recommendations*: If an injury or an exposure to blood, body fluids, or tissue were to occur, the following should be carried out:
  - Report injuries or blood/body fluid exposures to the appropriate supervisor immediately.
  - File an occupational exposure report.
  - Wash wounds and skin sites that have been in contact with blood or body fluids with soap and water; mucous membranes should be flushed with water; eyes should be rinsed with an irrigant marketed for that purpose or with clean water.
  - The application of caustic agents (e.g., bleach) or the injection of antiseptics or disinfectants into the wound is not recommended.
  - The worker should be seen by a health care professional as soon as possible for evaluation and counseling.
  - The health care professional should follow guidelines as listed in the following reference: Centers for Disease Control and Prevention. 2001. Updated US Public Health Service Guidelines for the Management of Occupational Exposures to HBV, HCV, and HIV and Recommendations for Postexposure Prophylaxis. *MMWR Recomm Rep.* 50(RR-11):1–52. In addition, the University of California, Los Angeles and CDC have developed an interactive Web site to help guide clinicians in making decisions about post-exposure care.

- Clinicians also are encouraged to consult experts via the free 24/7 National Clinicians' Needlestick Hotline for advice about assessing and managing treatment of exposures to blood and other body fluids at 888-488-4911 (toll free) or 415-469-4417 (back-up).

Source: Adapted from National Institute for Occupational Safety and Health. 2013. Guidance for Supervisors at Disaster Rescue Sites. Available at: http://www.cdc.gov/niosh/topics/emres/emhaz.html. Accessed January 25, 2017.

RESOURCES AND REFERENCES

APPENDIX Y

DISASTER MOBILE APPS

Disaster Mobile Apps for Smartphones

- ACAPS CrisisAlert: Provides phone notifications on humanitarian crises for over 40 countries. Available at:
  - Google Play: https://play.google.com/store/apps/details?id=org.acaps.acaps
- American Red Cross (Red Cross): Have developed several apps on first aid, floods, tornados, earthquakes, wildfires, hurricanes, volunteer, and Shelter Finder. Apps include warning indicators that can be customized for users living in areas prone to natural disasters. Available for Android and iOS devices at:
  - Red Cross: http://www.redcross.org/prepare/mobile-apps
- Blast Injury (Centers for Disease Control and Prevention): Provides medical and health care systems information to assist health care providers and public health professionals in the preparation, response, and management of injuries resulting from terrorist bombing events. Available at:
  - iTunes: https://itunes.apple.com/au/app/cdc-blast-injury/id890434999?mt=8&ign-mpt=uo%3D2&gt
- Disaster & Safety eGuides (QuickSeries Publishing): Library of interactive eGuides providing key information about family emergency plans, real-time weather alerts, evacuation alerts, shelters and emergency services and more. Available at:
  - EOC ready: http://eocready.com/features?gclid=CPG17sjjscoCFQEoHwod3LEPRQ
- Disaster Alert (Pacific Disaster Center): Provides monitoring of and early warning for "Active Hazards" around the globe free to the users. Available at:
  - iTunes: https://itunes.apple.com/us/app/disaster-alert-pacific-disaster/id381289235?mt=8
  - Google Play: https://play.google.com/store/apps/details?id=disasterAlert.PDC
- Emergency Medical Spanish Guide: designed for non-Spanish speaking health care professionals to quickly learn key medical information from Spanish speaking patients. Available at:
  - Mavro Inc: http://mavroinc.com/medical.html
- Federal Emergency Management Agency (FEMA): Contains disaster safety tips, an interactive emergency kit list, emergency meeting location information, and a map with open shelters and open FEMA Disaster Recovery Centers. Available at:
  - iTunes: https://itunes.apple.com/us/app/fema/id474807486?mt=8

  - Google Play: https://play.google.com/store/apps/details?id=gov.fema.mobile.android
- Flu Near You: System tracks spread of flu through the voluntary participation of individuals who report each week if they have been healthy or sick. The individual reports are mapped to generate local and national views of influenza-like illness. Symptoms for other illnesses, such as Zika, have also been added. Available at:
  - Google Play: https://play.google.com/store/apps/details?id=com.duethealth.flu&hl=en
- FluView: Information on influenza-like illness activity levels across the United States, includes trends and on-demand access to state health department Web sites for local surveillance information. Available at:
  - iTunes: https://itunes.apple.com/gb/app/fluview/id507807044?mt=8
- Humanitarian Kiosk (United Nations): Provides real time humanitarian related information from emergencies around the world. Available at:
  - iTunes: https://itunes.apple.com/us/app/humanitarian-kiosk/id546482411?mt=8
  - Google Play: https://play.google.com/store/apps/details?id=org.unocha
- Hurricane: Tracks violent storms and projects their path. Available at:
  - iTunes: https://itunes.apple.com/us/app/hurricane-by-american-red/id545689128?mt=8
- Incident Command Table: A digital board to organize command for planning missions, conduct after action reviews, and provide accountability for those responsible for managing an incident and for responders. A combination of 3 emergency management and planning apps: Tactical Police Table, Tactical Fire Table, and Tactical EMS Table. Available at:
  - Google Play: https://play.google.com/store/apps/details?id=com.tablecommand.incidentcommandtable
- Influenza for Clinicians and Health Care Professionals (CDC): Provides CDC's latest recommendations and influenza activity updates. Available at:
  - iTunes: https://itunes.apple.com/us/app/cdc-influenza-flu/id577782055
  - Google Play: https://play.google.com/store/apps/details?id=gov.cdc.topical.flu
- Laboratory Response Network Rule-Out and Refer (CDC): Helps laboratories identify potential bioterrorism agents with flowcharts, images, videos, and more. Available at:
  - iTunes: https://itunes.apple.com/WebObjects/MZStore.woa/wa/viewSoftware?id=964978618&mt=8
- Ladder Safety (National Institutes for Occupational Safety and Health): Using visual and sound signals, assists the user in positioning an extension ladder at an optimal angle. Provides graphic-oriented interactive reference materials, safety

guidelines and checklists for extension ladder selection, inspection, accessorizing, and use. Available at:
  - iTunes: https://itunes.apple.com/WebObjects/MZStore.woa/wa/viewSoftware?id=658633912&mt=8
  - Google Play: https://play.google.com/store/apps/details?id=gov.cdc.niosh.dsr.laddersafety

Local Apps

- National Library of Medicine: Includes apps on
  - CBRNE and Hazardous Substances
  - Medical and Health Information
  - Responder Support and Safety
  - Psychological Health Tools
  - U.S. Federal Organizations
  - American Red Cross Suite of Apps
  - Surveillance and Alerts
  - Family Reunification
  - Directories
  - Apps for Disasters in Libraries
  - Other Apps and Tools. Available at: disasterinfo.nlm.nih.gov/dimrc/disaster-apps.html
- Outbreaks Near Me: Tracks real-time disease outbreaks in your neighborhood, including news about H1N1 influenza ("swine flu"). Available at:
  - http://www.healthmap.org/outbreaksnearme
- Ready NYC (New York City): Aids users in making an emergency plan before disaster strikes. Available at:
  - iTunes: https://itunes.apple.com/us/app/ready-nyc/id633614907?mt=8
- ResQr: A family of First Aid and CPR apps for mobile and computer platforms that instruct you in providing first aid during an emergency, as it happens. Available at:
  - http://www.resqrfirstaid.com
- SD Emergency (San Diego County): Helps family members develop plans to contact one another, get back together, etc., in different disaster situations. Available at:
  - iTunes: https://itunes.apple.com/us/app/sd-emergency/id561733287?ls=1&mt=8
  - Google Play: https://play.google.com/store/apps/details?id=org.CountyofSanDiego.SDEmergency
- Solve the Outbreak (CDC): This application allows users to interact with and solve a disease outbreak. Available at:
  - iTunes: https://itunes.apple.com/us/app/solve-the-outbreak/id592485067?mt=8
  - Google Play: https://play.google.com/store/apps/details?id=gov.cdc.sto

- Uppsala Conflict Database (Uppsala University): Contains information on a large number of armed violence since 1975. Available at:
  - iTunes: https://itunes.apple.com/us/app/uppsala-conflict-database/id380077089?mt=8
  - Google Play: https://play.google.com/store/apps/details?id=se.uppsala.ucdp
- Weather Channel Apps: most accurate, precise weather forecast. Available at:
  - iTunes: https://itunes.apple.com/app/id295646461

APPENDIX Z

PRINCIPLES OF THE ETHICAL PRACTICE OF PUBLIC HEALTH

1. Public health should address principally the fundamental causes of disease and requirements for health, aiming to prevent adverse health outcomes.
2. Public health should achieve community health in a way that respects the rights of individuals in the community.
3. Public health policies, programs, and priorities should be developed and evaluated through processes that ensure an opportunity for input from community members.
4. Public health should advocate and work for the empowerment of disenfranchised community members, aiming to ensure that the basic resources and conditions necessary for health are accessible to all.
5. Public health should seek the information needed to implement effective policies and programs that protect and promote health.
6. Public health institutions should provide communities with the information they have that is needed for decisions on policies or programs and should obtain the community's consent for their implementation.
7. Public health institutions should act in a timely manner on the information they have within the resources and the mandate given to them by the public.
8. Public health programs and policies should incorporate a variety of approaches that anticipate and respect diverse values, beliefs, and cultures in the community.
9. Public health programs and policies should be implemented in a manner that most enhances the physical and social environment.
10. Public health institutions should protect the confidentiality of information that can bring harm to an individual or community if made public. Exceptions must be justified on the basis of the high likelihood of significant harm to the individual or others.
11. Public health institutions and their employees should engage in collaborations and affiliations in ways that build the public's trust and the institution's effectiveness.
12. Public health institutions and their employees should engage in collaborations and affiliations in ways that build the public's trust and the institution's effectiveness.

Source: Adapted from Public Health Leadership Society. 2002. *Principles of the Ethical Practice of Public Health*. Version 2.2. Washington, DC: APHA. Available at: https://www.apha.org/~/media/files/pdf/membergroups/ethics_brochure.ashx. Accessed January 25, 2017.

APPENDIX AA

LIST OF OFFICES OF THE FEDERAL EMERGENCY MANAGEMENT AGENCY

Region 1: Connecticut, Maine, Massachusetts, New Hampshire, Rhode Island, Vermont
99 High St.
Boston, MA 02110
(877) 336-2734

Region 2: New Jersey, New York, Puerto Rico, Virgin Islands
Mailing Address:
26 Federal Plaza, Suite 1307
New York, NY 10278-0002
Physical Address:
One World Trade Center
New York, NY 10007
(212) 680-3600

Region 3: Delaware, District of Columbia, Maryland, Pennsylvania, Virginia, West Virginia
One Independence Mall, 6th Floor
615 Chestnut Street
Philadelphia, PA 19106-4404
(215) 931-5500

Region 4: Alabama, Florida, Georgia, Kentucky, Mississippi, North Carolina, South Carolina, Tennessee
3003 Chamblee-Tucker Road
Atlanta, GA 30341
(770) 220-5200

Region 5: Illinois, Indiana, Michigan, Minnesota, Ohio, Wisconsin
536 S. Clark Street, 6th Floor
Chicago, IL 60605
(312) 408-5500

Region 6: Arkansas, Louisiana, New Mexico, Oklahoma, Texas
Federal Regional Center
800 N. Loop 288
Denton, TX 76209-3698
(940) 898-5104

Region 7: Iowa, Kansas, Missouri, Nebraska
9221 Ward Parkway
Kansas City, MO 64114
(816) 283-7061

Region 8: Colorado, Montana, North Dakota, South Dakota, Utah, Wyoming
Denver Federal Center
Building 710, Box 25267
Denver, CO 80225-0267
(303) 235-4800

Region 9: Arizona, California, Hawaii, Nevada, & the Pacific Islands
1111 Broadway
Suite 1200
Oakland, CA 94607-4052
(800) 621-FEMA (3362)

Region 10: Alaska, Idaho, Oregon, Washington
Federal Regional Center
130 228th Street, S.W.
Bothell, WA 98021-8627
(425) 487-4600

APPENDIX BB

USEFUL INTERNET REFERENCES AND RESOURCES

General

Agency for Healthcare Research and Quality Development of Models for Emergency Preparedness, Personal Protective Equipment, Decontamination, Isolation/Quarantine, and Laboratory Capacity

- http://www.ahrq.gov/research/devmodels
  Disaster Response Tools and Resources
  - http://www.ahrq.gov/path/katrina.htm
  Hospital Preparedness Exercises Resources
  - http://www.ahrq.gov/prep/hospex.htm
  Public Health Emergency Preparedness
  - http://www.ahrq.gov/prep
  Surge Capacity
  - http://www.ahrq.gov/prep

Agency for Toxic Substances and Disease Registry

- http://www.atsdr.cdc.gov
- http://www.atsdr.cdc.gov/risk/riskprimer/index.html
  ToxFAQs, Toxic Substances Portal
  - http://www.atsdr.cdc.gov/toxfaqs/index.asp
  Medical Management Guidelines for Acute Chemical Exposures
  - http://www.atsdr.cdc.gov/mmg/index.asp

American Academy of Child and Adolescent Psychiatry Disaster Resource Center

- http://www.aacap.org/aacap/families_and_youth/resource_centers/Disaster_Resource_Center/Home.aspx

American Academy of Experts in Traumatic Stress

- http://www.aaets.org/index.htm

American Hospital Association Emergency Readiness

- http://www.aha.org/advocacy-issues/emergreadiness/index.shtml

American Public Health Association, Get Ready

- http://www.getreadyforflu.org/newsite.htm

American Psychiatric Association, Disaster and Trauma

- https://www.psychiatry.org/psychiatrists/practice/professional-interests/disaster-and-trauma

American Radio Relay League, HAM Radio Association and Resources

- http://www.arrl.org

  Radio Amateur Civil Emergency Service Regulations

  - http://www.usraces.org

American Red Cross

- http://www.redcross.org

  Shelter Map (Web version)

  - http://app.redcross.org/nss-app

  Social Media Strategy Handbook

  - http://sites.google.com/site/wharman/social-media-strategy-handbook

  Twitter

  - http://twitter.com/redcross

American Veterinary Medical Association Disaster Preparedness

- https://www.avma.org/kb/resources/reference/disaster/pages/default.aspx?utm_source=prettyurl&utm_medium=web&utm_campaign=redirect&utm_term=disaster

  Veterinary Medical Assistance Teams

  - https://www.avma.org/ProfessionalDevelopment/TrainingAndService/VMAT/Pages/default.aspx

Armed Forces Radiobiology Research Institute

- http://www.cnic.navy.mil/regions/ndw/installations/nsa_bethesda/about/tenant_commands/afrri.html

Association for Infection Control Practitioners

- http://www.apic.org

Association of State and Territorial Health Officials

- http://www.astho.org

California Emergency Management Agency

- http://www.caloes.ca.gov

Centre for Excellence in Emergency Preparedness

- http://www.ccep.ca

CANUTEC (Canadian Transport Emergency Centre)

- https://www.tc.gc.ca/eng/canutec/menu.htm

CBS News Disaster Links

- http://www.cbsnews.com/htdocs/natural_disasters/html/framesource.html

Centers for Disease Control and Prevention, Emergency Preparedness and Response

- http://www.cdc.gov

Biosafety
  - http://www.cdc.gov/biosafety
  - http://www.cdc.gov/od/ohs/biosfty/bmbl4/bmbl4toc.htm

Bioterrorism Agents/Diseases
  - https://emergency.cdc.gov/agent/agentlist.asp

Emergency Preparedness and Response
  - http://emergency.cdc.gov

Emerging Infectious Disease Journal
  - http://wwwnc.cdc.gov/eid

Environmental Health Shelter Assessment Tool
  - https://emergency.cdc.gov/shelterassessment/index.asp

Morbidity and Mortality Weekly
  - http://www.cdc.gov/mmwr/index.html

National Center for Infectious and Zoonotic Infectious Diseases
  - http://www.cdc.gov/ncezid

Preparation and Planning
  - https://emergency.cdc.gov/planning/index.asp

Response Worker Health and Safety
  - http://www.cdc.gov/disasters/workers.html

Strategic National Stockpile
  - http://www.cdc.gov/phpr/stockpile/stockpile.htm

Center for Earthquake Research and Information at University of Memphis
- http://www.memphis.edu/ceri

Center for Food Safety and Applied Nutrition, U.S. Food and Drug Administration
- http://www.fda.gov/AboutFDA/CentersOffices/OfficeofFoods/CFSAN/WhatWeDo/ucm366279.htm

  "Bad Bug Book," Foodborne Pathogenic Microorganisms and Natural Toxins Handbook, FDA
  - http://www.fda.gov/downloads/Food/FoodSafety/FoodborneIllness/FoodborneIllnessFoodbornePathogensNaturalToxins/BadBugBook/UCM297627.pdf

(James Martin) Center for Nonproliferation Studies
- http://www.nonproliferation.org

  Chemical and Biological Weapons Resource Page
  - http://www.nonproliferation.org/?s=Chemical+and+Biological+Weapons+Resource+Page

Centre for Research on the Epidemiology of Disasters
- http://www.cred.be

Chemical Hazards Emergency Medical Management
- http://chemm.nlm.nih.gov/index.html

Climate Information and Early Warning Systems Communications Toolkit

- http://www.undp.org/content/undp/en/home/librarypage/climate-and-disaster-resilience-/climate-information-and-early-warning-systems-communications-too.html

Coast Guard Command Center

- https://www.uscg.mil/history/ops/disastersindex.asp

Counterterrorism Training and Resources for Law Enforcement

- https://www.fletc.gov/external/counterterrorism-training-and-resources-law-enforcement

Community-Based Water Resiliency Tool

- https://www.epa.gov/communitywaterresilience/community-based-water-resiliency-tool

Crisis Commons

- https://crisiscommons.org

Defense Threat Reduction Agency

- http://www.dtra.mil

DisasterAssistance.gov (portal for disaster victims)

- https://www.disasterassistance.gov/

Disaster Center

- http://www.disastercenter.com

Disaster News Network

- http://www.disasternews.net

Disaster Research Center, University of Delaware

- https://www.drc.udel.edu

Disasters Roundtable of the National Academies

- http://dels.nas.edu/dr

Earthquake Hazard Program

- http://earthquake.usgs.gov

Edwards Disaster Recovery Sourcebook

- http://www.disaster-risk-planning.com/EDRD_info.html

Emergency Management Assistance Compact

- http://www.emacweb.org

Emergency Nutrition Network

- http://www.ennonline.net

Emergency System for Advance Registration of Volunteer Health Professionals

- http://www.phe.gov/esarvhp/pages/about.aspx

Environmental Protection Agency, Emergency Response

- https://www.epa.gov/emergency-response

Federal Emergency Management Agency (FEMA)

- http://www.fema.gov

  Bibliography for Emergency Management

  - http://training.fema.gov/hiedu/docs/wayne's%20bibliography.doc

Comprehensive Preparedness Guide 101
- o https://www.fema.gov/media-library/assets/documents/25975

Federal Response Framework, Emergency Support Function #8 Public Health and Medical Services Annex
- o https://www.fema.gov/media-library-data/1470149644671-642ccad05d19449d2d13b1b0952328ed/ESF_8_Public_Health_Medical_20160705_508.pdf

FEMA for Kids
- o https://www.fema.gov/disaster/4085/updates/fema-kids-know-facts
- o https://www.ready.gov/kids

Reference and Document Library
- o https://www.fema.gov/resource-document-library

National Incident Management System
- o https://www.fema.gov/pdf/emergency/nims/NIMS_core.pdf

National Response Framework
- o https://www.fema.gov/national-response-framework

Public Assistance Guide
- o https://www.fema.gov/pdf/government/grant/pa/paguide07.pdf

Emergency Management (State) Offices and Agencies
- o https://www.fema.gov/emergency-management-agencies

Assistance to Individuals and Households
- o https://www.fema.gov/recovery-directorate/assistance-individuals-and-households

Fire Administration
- http://www.usfa.dhs.gov

Fire and Explosion Planning Matrix
- https://www.osha.gov/dep/fire-expmatrix

First Responders in the Field
- http://www.remm.nlm.gov/remm_FirstResponder.htm

FloodSmart.Gov
- https://www.floodsmart.gov/floodsmart

Food and Drug Administration Emergency Operations Plan
- http://www.fda.gov/downloads/EmergencyPreparedness/EmergencyPreparedness/UCM230973.pdf

FoodSafety.Gov
- http://www.foodsafety.gov

Gender and Disasters Network
- http://www.gdnonline.org

Geological Survey
- http://www.usgs.gov

Global Emerging Infections Surveillance and Response System

- http://www.health.mil/Military-Health-Topics/Health-Readiness/Armed-Forces-Health-Surveillance-Branch/Global-Emerging-Infections-Surveillance-and-Response

Government Emergency Telecommunications Service

- https://publicintelligence.net/u-s-government-emergency-telecommunications-service

Health Library for Disasters

- http://helid.digicollection.org/en

Hospital Incident Command System

- http://www.emsa.ca.gov/disaster_medical_services_division_hospital_incident_command_system_resources

Hurricane Watch Net

- http://www.hwn.org

Infectious Disease Society of America

- https://www.idsociety.org/Index.aspx

International Association of Emergency Managers

- http://www.iaem.com

International Critical Incident Stress Foundation

- http://www.icisf.org

International Federation of the Red Cross and Red Crescent Societies

- http://reliefweb.int/organization/ifrc

International Network of Crisis Mappers

- http://www.crisismappers.net

International Rescue Committee

- https://www.rescue.org

International Society for Traumatic Stress Studies

- https://www.istss.org/am15/home.aspx

Inventory and Assessment of Databases Relevant for Social Science Research of Terrorism

- http://www.loc.gov/rr/frd/pdf-files/inventory_04.pdf

Johns Hopkins Emergency Preparedness

- http://www.hopkinsmedicine.org/heic/emergency_preparedness.html

Defense Technical information Center (military search engine for federal laws, regulations, and documents relating to emergency management)

- http://www.dtic.mil

Lawrence Livermore National Laboratory Global Security

- https://www-gs.llnl.gov

Lessons Learned Information Sharing Program

- https://www.fema.gov/lessons-learned-information-sharing-program

Medical Reserve Corps

- https://www.ready.gov/medical-reserve-corps

Medicare and Emergency Preparedness Rule

- https://www.cms.gov/Medicare/Provider-Enrollment-and-Certification/SurveyCertEmergPrep/Emergency-Prep-Rule.html

Mental Health Field Manual

- http://store.samhsa.gov/product/Field-Manual-for-Mental-Health-and-Human-Service-Workers-in-Major-Disasters/ADM90-0537

Medical Management of Radiology Casualties Handbook, U.S. Armed Forces

- https://www.usuhs.edu/sites/default/files/media/afrri/pdf/4edmmrchandbook.pdf

Medical Management of Biological Casualties Handbook, U.S. Army Medical Research Institute of Infectious Diseases

- http://www.usamriid.army.mil/education/bluebookpdf/USAMRIID%20BlueBook%207th%20Edition%20-%20Sep%202011.pdf

Medical Management of Chemical Casualties Handbook, U.S. Army Medical Research Institute of Chemical Defense

- http://www.globalsecurity.org/wmd/library/policy/army/other/mmcc-hbk_4th-ed.pdf

National Association of Community Health Centers, Developing and Implementing an Emergency Management Plan for Your Health Center

- http://nachc.org/health-center-issues/emergency-management

National Association of County and City Health Officials, Preparedness

- http://www.naccho.org

  Public Health Preparedness

  - http://www.naccho.org/programs/public-health-preparedness

  Toolbox

  - http://www.naccho.org/resources/toolbox

National Association of School Psychologists

- http://www.nasponline.org

National Association of Social Workers

- http://www.socialworkers.org/pressroom/events/911/disasters.asp

National Center for Post-Traumatic Stress Disorder

- http://www.ptsd.va.gov

National Environmental Health Association

- http://www.neha.org

National Fire Protection Association

- http://www.nfpa.org/assets/files/AboutTheCodes/1600/1600-13-PDF.pdf

National Emergency Management Association

- https://www.nemaweb.org

National Emergency Response and Rescue Training Center

- https://teex.org/Pages/homeland-security.aspx

National Hurricane Center

- http://www.nhc.noaa.gov

National Institutes of Health

- http://www.nih.gov

  Library

  - https://nihlibrary.nih.gov/Pages/default.aspx

  National Institutes of Health Disaster Research Response

  - http://dr2.nlm.nih.gov

  National Institute on Mental Health

  - http://www.nimh.nih.gov

National Institute for Occupational Safety and Health

- http://www.cdc.gov/niosh/?

  Disaster Site Management

  - http://www.cdc.gov/niosh/topics/emres/sitemgt.html

  Pocket Guide to Chemical Hazards

  - http://www.cdc.gov/niosh/npg

  Publications and Products

  - https://www.cdc.gov/niosh/pubs/all_date_desc_nopubnumbers.html

National Library of Medicine

- http://www.nlm.nih.gov

PUBMED

- http://www.ncbi.nlm.nih.gov/pubmed

TOXNET, Toxicology Data Network

- http://toxnet.nlm.nih.gov

National Oceanic and Atmospheric Administration, Climate Prediction Center

- http://www.cpc.noaa.gov

  Advanced Hydrologic Prediction Service

  - http://water.weather.gov/ahps/about/about.php

National Weather Service

- http://www.weather.gov

  Real-Time Monitoring of Hurricane Potential for Atlantic Ocean

  - http://www.cpc.ncep.noaa.gov/products/hurricane

  Real-Time Monitoring of Hurricane Potential for East Pacific Ocean

  - http://www.cpc.ncep.noaa.gov/products/Epac_hurr

  Real-Time Tracking of Tornados

  - http://www.ustornadoes.com/tornado-tracking

  Weather Radio

  - http://www.nws.noaa.gov/nwr

  Winter Storms: The Deceptive Killers

  - http://www.nws.noaa.gov/om/winter/resources/Winter_Storms2008.pdf

National Organization for Victim Assistance

- http://www.trynova.org

National Response Center, U.S. Coast Guard

- https://www.epa.gov/emergency-response/national-response-center

National Response Team

- https://www.nrt.org

National Safety Council

- http://www.nsc.org/pages/home.aspx

National Voluntary Organizations Active in Disaster

- http://www.nvoad.org

Natural Hazards Center, University of Colorado

- https://hazards.colorado.edu
  Quick Response Research Program
  - https://hazards.colorado.edu/research/quick-response

Office of Foreign Disaster Assistance

- https://www.usaid.gov/who-we-are/organization/bureaus/bureau-democracy-conflict-and-humanitarian-assistance/office-us
- http://www.globalcorps-health.com
  Field Operations Guide, Version 4
  - https://www.usaid.gov/sites/default/files/documents/1866/fog_v4_0.pdf

Office of the Secretary of Preparedness and Response

- http://www.phe.gov/about/pages/default.aspx
  Medical Surge Capacity Handbook
  - http://www.phe.gov/Preparedness/planning/mscc/handbook/Pages/default.aspx

  National Disaster Medical System
  - http://www.phe.gov/Preparedness/responders/ndms/Pages/default.aspx

  Public Health Emergency Responders, Clinicians, and Practitioners
  - http://www.phe.gov/preparedness/responders/pages/default.aspx

  Public Health and Medical Services Support
  - http://www.phe.gov/preparedness/support/pages/default.aspx

  Public Health Emergency, Hospital Preparedness Program
  - http://www.phe.gov/Preparedness/planning/hpp/Pages/overview.aspx

  Public Health Service Act, Legal Authority and Related Guidance
  - http://www.phe.gov/preparedness/planning/authority/pages/default.aspx

Osh.net, Emergency Management—Disaster Preparedness

- http://osh.net/directory/emerg_mang/index.htm

Overview of Stafford Act Support to States

- https://www.fema.gov/pdf/emergency/nrf/nrf-stafford.pdf

Pan-American Health Organization (PAHO)

- http://paho.org/hq
- http://www.paho.org/disasters/newsletter

PAHO Humanitarian Supply Management System
  - http://www.disaster-info.net/SUMA

Presidential Directives and Executive Orders
- http://fas.org/irp/offdocs/direct.htm

Refugee Health Information Network
- https://sis.nlm.nih.gov/outreach/rhin.html

Regional Disaster Information Center Latin American and the Caribbean (CRID)
- http://itic.ioc-unesco.org/index.php?option=com_content&view=article&id=1676
- http://www.eird.org/eng/revista/No15_99/pagina25.htm

ReliefWeb, Disasters
- http://reliefweb.int/disasters

Rural EMS and Trauma Technical Assistance Center
- https://www.ruralcenter.org/tasc/resources/rural-emergency-medical-services-trauma-technical-assistance-center-ambulance-service
- https://www.ruralhealthinfo.org/topics/emergency-medical-services

State & Local Emergency Management Agencies Listing
- http://www.disasters.org/emgold/sem.htm

State Health Department Listing
- https://www.ehdp.com/links/us-shas.htm

Southern California Earthquake Center
- http://www.scec.org

Stimson Center, Pragmatic Steps for Global Security
- http://www.stimson.org

Substance Abuse and Mental Health Services Administration
- http://www.samhsa.gov/about-us/who-we-are/offices-centers/cmhs

Temblor
- http://temblor.net

Tsunami Awareness and Safety Fact Sheet
- http://nws.weather.gov/nthmp/tsunamisafety.html

United Nations High Commissioner for Refugees
- http://www.unhcr.org

U.S. Army Medicine
- https://www.army.mil/armymedicine

  Medical Research Institute of Chemical Defense
  - https://usamricd.apgea.army.mil

  Medical Research Institute of Infectious Diseases
  - http://www.usamriid.army.mil/aboutpage.htm

Public Health Command
- https://phc.amedd.army.mil/Pages/default.aspx

U.S. Coast Guard Incident Management Handbook 2014

- https://bookstore.gpo.gov/products/sku/050-012-00516-8

U.S. Department of Defense, Chemical and Biological Defense Programs

- http://www.acq.osd.mil/cp

  Dictionary of Military and Associated Terms

  - https://ratical.org/radiation/NuclearExtinction/jp1_02.pdf

U.S. Department of Health & Human Services

  - http://www.hhs.gov

  HHS Archive

  - https://archive.hhs.gov

  Disaster Information Management Research Center

  - https://disaster.nlm.nih.gov

  Public Health Services Commissioned Corps

  - http://www.usphs.gov

  Public Health Services Commissioned Corps, Emergency Response

  - http://www.usphs.gov/newsroom/features/recent/deployments.aspx

U.S. Department of Homeland Security, Preparedness, Response and Recovery

- https://www.dhs.gov/preparedness-response-recovery-committees-working-groups

  Computer Emergency Readiness Team

  - http://www.us-cert.gov

  State Contracts and Grant Award Information

  - https://www.fema.gov/grants
  - https://www.dhs.gov/how-do-i/find-and-apply-grants

U.S. Department of Transportation, Emergency Response Guidebook (First Responder's Guide for HAZMAT Operations)

- http://www.phmsa.dot.gov/hazmat/outreach-training/erg

  Developing a Hazardous Materials Exercise Program: A Handbook for State and Local Officials

  - http://ntl.bts.gov/DOCS/254.html

  HazMat Safety Community

  - http://phmsa.dot.gov/hazmat

  University of Wisconsin Disaster Management Center

  - https://epd.wisc.edu/dmc

World Health Organization (WHO)

- http://www.who.int/en

WHO Zika app

- http://www.who.int/risk-communication/zika-virus/app/en

Weekly Epidemiological Record

- http://www.who.int/wer/en

Electronic Newsletters, Periodicals, and Publications

Air University Index to Military Periodicals
- http://www.dtic.mil/dtic/aulimp

American Journal of Disaster Medicine
- http://www.pnpco.com/pn03000.html

Biosecurity and Bioterrorism
- http://online.liebertpub.com/bsp

CDC Public Health Law News
- http://www.cdc.gov/phlp/news/current.html

Clinical Infectious Disease
- http://cid.oxfordjournals.org

Digital Communities
- http://www.govtech.com

Disaster and Military Medicine
- https://disastermilitarymedicine.biomedcentral.com

Disaster Collaboratory Journal List
- http://www4.disastercollaboratory.com

Disaster Management and Response
- http://www.sciencedirect.com/science/journal/15402487

Disaster Medicine and Public Health Preparedness
- http://sdmph.org/publications/dmphp-journal

Disaster Prevention and Management
- http://www.emeraldinsight.com/journal/dpm

Disaster Recovery Journal
- http://www.drj.com

Disasters
- http://www.wiley.com/WileyCDA/WileyTitle/productCd-DISA.html

Emerging Infectious Diseases, CDC, National Center for Infectious Diseases
- http://wwwnc.cdc.gov/eid

Emergency Management
- http://www.emergencymgmt.com

Emergency Medical Services World
- http://www.emsworld.com

Environmental Hazards
- http://www.sciencedirect.com/science/journal/17477891

FEMA HAZUS News
- https://www.fema.gov/hazus

Geoenvironmental Disasters
- https://geoenvironmental-disasters.springeropen.com

Government Technology
- http://www.govtech.com

HealthNet News
- http://www.healthnet.org/e-newsletters

Homeland Defense Journal
- http://old.library.georgetown.edu/newjour/h/msg02773.html

Homeland Defense and Security Information Analysis Center Newsletter
- https://www.hdiac.org/islandora/object/hdjournal%3AcbrnJournal3

International Journal of Disaster Risk Reduction
- http://www.journals.elsevier.com/international-journal-of-disaster-risk-reduction

International Journal of Disaster Risk Science
- http://www.springer.com/earth+sciences+and+geography/natural+hazards/journal/13753

International Journal of Emergency Management
- http://www.inderscience.com/jhome.php?jcode=ijem

International Journal of Mass Emergencies and Disasters
- http://www.ijmed.org/

Journal of Geography & Natural Disasters
- http://www.omicsgroup.org/journals/geography-natural-disasters.php

The Journal of Homeland Defense
- http://www.homelanddefense.org

The Journal of Homeland Security
- http://www.homelandsecurity.org/journal/index.cfm

Medicine and Global Survival Magazine
- http://www.ippnw.org/medicine-and-global-survival.html

Morbidity and Mortality Weekly Report, CDC
- http://www.cdc.gov/mmwr

Natural Disasters Journals List
- http://www.omicsonline.org/natural-disasters-journals-list.php

Natural Hazards
- http://link.springer.com/journal/11069

Natural Hazards Center Web Resources
- https://hazards.colorado.edu/web-resources

Natural Hazards Observer
- https://hazards.colorado.edu/natural-hazards-observer/volume-xl-number-3

Natural Hazards Review
- https://hazards.colorado.edu/publications/review

The Nonproliferation Review
- http://www.nonproliferation.org/category/topics/the_nonproliferation_review

OSHA *Job Safety and Health Quarterly Magazine*
- https://www.osha.gov/html/jshq-index.html

Prehospital and Disaster Medicine

- https://www.cambridge.org/core/journals/prehospital-and-disaster-medicine

ProMED Mail

- http://www.promedmail.org

Risk Analysis

- http://onlinelibrary.wiley.com/journal/10.1111/(ISSN)1539-6924

GIS Web Sites

Community Vulnerability Assessment Tool

- http://unfccc.int/adaptation/nairobi_work_programme/knowledge_resources_and_publication s/items/5340.php

Data Sources on the Internet

- http://geo.arc.nasa.gov/sge/health/links/links.html

Duke University Library, Sites With a Variety of GIS Data

- http://guides.library.duke.edu/gisdata

ESRI, Inc.

- http://www.esri.com

FEMA Mapping and Analysis Center

- http://www.gismaps.fema.gov

Geographic Information Systems, CDC

- http://www.cdc.gov/gis
- http://www.cdc.gov/gis/gis-training.htm

Geoplace.com

- http://www.geoplace.com/ME2/Default.asp

GIS Data Depot

- http://data.geocomm.com

WHO Maps and Spatial information Technologies in Health and Environment Decision-Making

- http://www.who.int/heli/tools/maps/en

Procedures, Protocols, and Response Resources

All the Virology on the WWW

- http://www.virology.net/garryfavwebbw.html

Disaster Information Management Resource Center

- https://sis.nlm.nih.gov/dimrc/ethics.html

EPA, National Response System

- https://www.epa.gov/emergency-response/national-response-center

Incident Command System, U.S. Coast Guard

- http://www.uscg.mil/auxiliary/training/ics100.asp

Medline Plus: Disaster Preparation and Recovery

- https://medlineplus.gov/disasterpreparationandrecovery.html

Public Health Image Library

- http://phil.cdc.gov/phil/home.asp

Wildland Fire Links

- http://www.wildlandfire.com/links

Populations with Disabilities and/or Access and Functional Needs References and Resources

Children

AHRQ—Pediatric Terrorism and Disaster Preparedness

- http://archive.ahrq.gov/research/pedprep

Children and Disasters, American Academy of Pediatrics

- https://www.aap.org/en-us/advocacy-and-policy/aap-health-initiatives/Children-and-Disasters/Pages/default.aspx?nfstatus=401&nftoken=00000000-0000-0000-0000-000000000000&nfstatusdescription=ERROR:+No+local+token

Emergency Information Form

- https://www.acep.org/clinical---practice-management/emergency-information-form-for-children-with-special-health-care-needs

Emergency Preparedness Planning Guide for Child Care Centers & Child Care Homes

- http://ssom.luc.edu/media/stritchschoolofmedicine/emergencymedicine/emsforchildren/documents/disasterpreparedness/organizationalresources/childcarecenters/Emergency%20Preparedness%20Planning%20Guide%20for%20Child%20Care%20Centers.pdf

Elderly

AARP

- http://www.aarp.org

Administration on Aging, Emergency Preparedness, and Response

- http://www.acl.gov/Get_Help/Preparedness/Index.aspx

Disaster Assistance

- https://www.disasterassistance.gov/information/older-americans

Disaster Preparedness for Seniors by Seniors

- http://www.redcross.org/images/MEDIA_CustomProductCatalog/m4640086_Disaster_PreparedPrep_for_Srs-English.revised_7-09.pdf

Disaster Preparedness Guide for Elders

- http://elderaffairs.state.fl.us/doea/pubs/EU/EUdisaster2015/Disaster_Guide_2015_English_Web.pdf

Disaster Supply Guide for Elders

- http://elderaffairs.state.fl.us/doea/disaster.php

Emergency Preparedness Tips for Older Adults

- http://www.healthinaging.org/resources/resource:emergency-preparedness-for-older-adults

Just in Case: Emergency Readiness for Older Adult and Caregivers

- http://aoa.acl.gov/AoA_Programs/HCLTC/Caregiver/docs/Just_in_Case030706_links.pdf

Maintaining a Healthy State of Mind for Seniors

- https://emergency.cdc.gov/preparedness/mind/seniors

Nursing Homes Emergency Preparedness: Questions Consumers Should Ask

- https://www.in.gov/isdh/files/Questions_consumers_should_ask_Emergency-Preparedness.pdf
- https://www.agingcare.com/Articles/long-term-facility-disaster-preparedness-questions-147877.htm

Older Adult Guidebook

- http://www.naminh.org/we-support/families-friends-adults/older-adult-guidebook

Preparing Makes Sense for Older Americans

- https://www.fema.gov/media-library/assets/videos/78859

Tips for Seniors and People With Disabilities and Medical Concerns

- http://www.ilrcsf.org/wp-content/uploads/2012/09/Emergency-preparedness-for-people-with-disabilities.pdf

The Role of Long-Term Care Ombudsmen in Nursing Home Closures and Natural Disasters

- https://www.in.gov/isdh/files/NORC-Ombudsmen-in-NH-Closures.pdf

General

Access and Functional Needs Video Series

- http://ncdmph.usuhs.edu/KnowledgeLearning/2016-ComPartner.htm

Access Board

- http://www.access-board.gov

Accommodating Individuals With Disabilities in the Provision of Disaster Mass Care, Housing, and Human Services Reference Guide, FEMA

- https://www.fema.gov/news-release/2007/08/21/accommodating-people-disabilities-disasters-reference-guide-federal-law

American Association of People With Disabilities

- http://www.aapd.com/about

Americans With Disabilities Act (ADA)

- http://www.ada.gov/pubs/ada.htm

An ADA Guide for Local Governments: Making Community Emergency Preparedness and Response Programs Accessible to People With Disabilities

- http://www.ada.gov/emergencyprepguide.htm

At-Risk Populations and Pandemic Influenza, Planning Guidance for State, Territorial, Tribal, and Local Health Departments, Association of Territorial and Health Officials

- http://www.astho.org/Infectious-Disease/At-Risk-Populations/At-Risk-Populations-and-Pandemic-Influenza-Planning-Guidance

Center for Disability Issues and the Health Professions

- http://www.aahd.us/best-practice/center-for-disability-issues-and-the-health-professions-at-western-university-of-health-sciences

Disability Disaster Information

- http://www.floridadisaster.org/disability

Easter Seals S.a.f.e.t.y. First Evacuation Program

- http://www.easterseals.com/explore-resources/making-life-accessible/resources-safety-first.html

Emergency Access Rules, Federal Communications Commission (FCC)

- https://www.fcc.gov/general/access-emergency-information-television

Emergency Evacuation Planning Guide for People With Disabilities, National Fire Protection Association

- http://www.nfpa.org/public-education/by-topic/people-at-risk/people-with-disabilities

Emergency Evacuation Plans

- http://askjan.org/media/emergency.html

Emergency Power Planning for People Who Use Electricity and Battery Dependent Assistive Technology and Medical Devices

- http://www.jik.com/disaster-individ.html#Guides

Emergency Preparedness and People With Disabilities. U.S. Department of Labor, Office of Disability Employment Policy

- https://www.dol.gov/odep/topics/emergencypreparedness.htm

Emergency Preparedness, National Association of the Deaf

- http://www.nad.org/issues/emergency-preparedness

Emergency Preparedness Resources for Persons with Disabilities

- http://www.hhs.gov/civil-rights/for-individuals/special-topics/emergency-preparedness/resources-persons-disabilities/index.html

Emergency Procedures for Employees With Disabilities in Office Occupancies

- https://cws.auburn.edu/shared/content/files/1571/fire_emergency-procedures-employees-disabilities.pdf

- http://www.fire.nist.gov/bfrlpubs/fire95/art043.html

Emergency Readiness for People with Disabilities

- http://www.cdc.gov/features/emergencypreparedness

Employers' Guide to Including People With Disabilities in Emergency Evacuation Plans, Job Accommodation Network

- http://askjan.org/media/evacchecklist.html

Equal Employment Opportunity Commission (EEOC), Fact Sheet on Obtaining and Using Employee Medical Information as Part of Emergency Evacuation Procedures

- http://www.eeoc.gov/facts/evacuation.html

Family Resource Center on Disabilities

- https://frcd.org/emergency-preparedness

Functional Needs Support Services: Planning Information and Tools

- http://www.ema.ohio.gov/Documents/Plans/Functional%20Needs%20Planning%20and%20Program%20Development%20Links.pdf

Guidance on Planning for Integration of Functional Needs Support Services in General Population Shelters, FEMA

- http://www.fema.gov/pdf/about/odic/fnss_guidance.pdf

Guide to Disaster Preparedness for People With Disabilities, American Red Cross/FEMA

- http://www.redcross.org/prepare/location/home-family/disabilities

Communications Guide: Think Cultural Health

- https://www.thinkculturalhealth.hhs.gov/education/communication-guide

Inclusive Preparedness Center, Disaster Readiness

- http://www.inclusivepreparedness.org/DisasterReadiness.html

Individuals with Disabilities and Others with Access and Functional Needs

- https://www.ready.gov/individuals-access-functional-needs

June Kailes, Emergency Resources

- http://www.jik.com/disaster.html

Lift and Carries

- http://www.cert-la.com/downloads/liftcarry/Liftcarry.pdf

Lighthouse International

- http://www.lighthouse.org

Limited English Proficiency Resources

- http://www.lep.gov/resources/resources.html

Mass Care and Shelter Plan: Functional Needs Annex, California

- http://www.cdss.ca.gov/dis/res/pdf/PWDEFinalAnnex.pdf

National Council on Disability

- http://www.ncd.gov

National Institute on Disability and Rehabilitation Research

- http://www.ninds.nih.gov/find_people/government_agencies/volorg583.htm

OK WARN: Weather Alert Remote Notification for the Deaf and Hard of Hearing NOAA National Severe Storms Laboratory

- http://www.nssl.noaa.gov/education/okwarn

Persons With Disabilities, Federal Communications Commission

- https://transition.fcc.gov/pshs/clearinghouse/persons-with-disabilities.html

Planning for an Emergency: Strategies for Identifying and Engaging At-Risk Groups

- http://www.cdc.gov/nceh/hsb/disaster/atriskguidance.pdf

Prepare Now

- http://www.kidneypreparenow.org

Public Health Workbook to Define, Locate and Reach Special, Vulnerable, and At-Risk Populations in an Emergency, CDC

- https://emergency.cdc.gov/workbook/pdf/ph_workbookfinal.pdf

Ready Campaign, DHS

- http://www.ready.gov

Ready New York: Preparing for Emergencies in New York City, New York City Office of Emergency Management

- http://www.nyc.gov/html/oem/downloads/pdf/household_guide.pdf

Resources on Emergency Evacuation and Disaster Preparedness

- http://www.icdri.org/inspirational/resources_on_emergency_evacuatio.htm

Saving Lives: Including People With Disabilities in Emergency Planning, National Council on Disability

- http://www.ncd.gov/rawmedia_repository/fd66f11a_8e9a_42e6_907f_a289e54e5f94.pdf

Guidelines and Standards for Tactile Graphics, 2010

- http://brailleauthority.org/tg/web-manual

Telecommunications Relay Services

- https://www.fcc.gov/consumers/guides/telecommunications-relay-service-trs

The Pediatrician and Disaster Preparedness, Policy Paper, American Academy of Pediatrics

- http://pediatrics.aappublications.org/content/117/2/560

Visual and Tactile Alerting Devices, Hearing Loss Association of America, Albany Chapter

- https://hearinglossalbany.wordpress.com/assistive-devices

Why and How to Include People With Disabilities in Your Planning Process, Nobody Left Behind

- http://www.hpod.org/pdf/Why-and-How-to-Include.pdf

Web Accessibility Initiative Resources, W3C

- https://www.w3.org/WAI/Resources/Overview

APPENDIX CC

REFERENCES AND READINGS

Behavioral Health

American Psychiatric Association. 2014. *Diagnostic and Statistical Manual of Mental Disorders.* 5th ed. Arlington, VA: American Psychiatric Publishing.

Armenian HK. 2002. Risk factors for depression in the survivors of the 1988 earthquake in Armenia. *J Urban Health.* 79(3):373–382.

Assistant Secretary for Preparedness and Response. 2014. *Disaster Behavioral Health Capacity Assessment Tool.* Available at: http://www.phe.gov/Preparedness/planning/abc/Documents/dbh-capacity-tool.pdf. Accessed January 25, 2017.

Baum A, Fleming R, Davidson LM. 1983. Natural disaster and technological catastrophe. *Environ Behav.* 15(3):333–354.

Baxter PJ. 2002. Public health aspects of chemical catastrophes. In: Havenaar JM, Cwikel JG, Bromet EJ, eds. *Toxic Turmoil: Psychological and Societal Consequences of Ecological Disasters.* New York, NY: Kluwer Academic/Plenum.

Black D, Newman M, Harris-Hendriks J, Mezey G, eds. 1997. *Psychological Trauma: A Developmental Approach.* London, England: Royal College of Psychiatrists.

Breslau N, Davis GC, Andreski P, et al. 1991. Traumatic events and posttraumatic stress disorder in an urban population of young adults. *Arch Gen Psychiatry.* 48(3):216–222.

Bryant RA, Harvey AG. 2000. *Acute Stress Disorder: A Handbook of Theory, Assessment, and Treatment.* Washington, DC: American Psychological Association.

Department of Defense, Department of Justice, Department of Veteran Affairs, and Department of Health & Human Services. 2002. *Mental Health and Mass Violence: Evidence-Based Early Psychological Intervention for Victims/Survivors of Mass Violence. A Workshop to Reach Consensus on Best Practices.* Available at: http://files.eric.ed.gov/fulltext/ED469199.pdf. Accessed February 3, 2017.

Department of Health & Human Services. 2014. *Disaster Behavioral Health Concept of Operations.* Available at: http://www.phe.gov/Preparedness/planning/abc/Documents/dbh-conops-2014.pdf. Accessed January 25, 2017.

DeWolfe D. 2000. *Field Manual for Mental Health and Human Service Workers in Major Disasters.* Washington, DC: U.S. Department of Health & Human Services, Substance Abuse and Mental Health Services Administration.

Dodgen D, Norwood AE, Becker SM, et al. 2011. Social, psychological, and behavioral responses to a nuclear detonation in a US city: implications for health care planning and delivery. *Disaster Med Public Health Prep.* 5(Suppl 1):S54–S64.

Ehring T, Ehlers A, Cleare AJ, et al. 2008. Do acute psychological and psychobiological responses to trauma predict subsequent symptom severities of PTSD and depression? *Psychiatry Res.* 161(1):67–75.

Eisenman D, Chandra A, Fogleman S, et al. 2014. The Los Angeles county community disaster resilience project—a community-level, public health initiative to build community disaster resilience. *Int J Environ Res Public Health.* 11(8):8475–8490. Available at: http://www.ncbi.nlm.nih.gov/pmc/articles/PMC4143872/pdf/ijerph-11-08475.pdf. Accessed January 25, 2017.

Emergency Services and Disaster Relief Branch, Center for Mental Health Services. 1996. *Responding to the Needs of People With Serious and Persistent Mental Illness in Times of Disaster.* Washington, DC: Substance Abuse and Mental Health Services Administration.

Erikson K. 1995. *A New Species of Trouble: The Human Experience of Modern Disasters.* New York, NY: W.W. Norton.

Freedy JR, Hobfoll SE, eds. 1995. *Traumatic Stress: From Theory to Practice.* New York, NY: Plenum Press.

Fritz CE. 1996. *Disasters and Mental Health: Therapeutic Principles Drawn From Disaster Studies: Historical and Comparative Disaster Series #10.* Newark, DE: Disaster Research Center, University of Delaware.

Fullerton CS, Ursano RJ, eds. 1997. *Post-Traumatic Stress Disorder: Acute and Long-Term Responses to Trauma and Disaster.* Washington, DC: American Psychiatric Press.

Galea S, Ahern J, Resnick H, et al. 2002. Psychological sequelae of the September 11 terrorist attacks in New York City. *N Engl J Med.* 346(13):982–987.

Galea S, Resnick H, Ahern J, et al. 2002. Posttraumatic stress disorder in Manhattan, New York City, after the September 11th terrorist attacks. *J Urban Health.* 79(3):340–353.

Gard BA, Ruzek JI. 2006. Community mental health response to crisis. *J Clin Psychol.* 62(8): 1029–1041.

Gerrity ET, Flynn BW. 1997. Mental health consequences of disasters. In: Noji EK, ed. *Public Health Consequences of Disasters.* Oxford, England: Oxford University Press. 101–121.

Ghodse H, Galea S. 2006. Tsunami: understanding mental health consequences and the unprecedented response. *Int Rev Psychiatry.* 18(3):289–297.

Hartsough DM, Myers DG. 1995. *Disaster Work and Mental Health: Prevention and Control of Stress Among Workers.* Washington, DC: Center for Mental Health Services, Substance Abuse and Mental Health Services Administration, U.S. Public Health Service.

Havenaar JM, Cwikel JG, Bromet EJ, eds. 2002. *Toxic Turmoil: Psychological and Societal Consequences of Ecological Disasters.* New York, NY: Kluwer Academic/Plenum Publishers.

Herman D, Felton C, Susser E. 2002. Mental health needs in New York State following the September 11th attacks. *J Urban Health.* 79(3):322–331.

Hodgkinson PE, Stewart M. 1998. *Coping With Catastrophe: A Handbook of Post-Disaster Psychosocial Aftercare.* 2nd ed. London, England: Routledge.

Jack K, Glied S. 2002. The public costs of mental health response: lessons from the New York City post-9/11 needs assessment. *J Urban Health.* 79(3):332–339.

Kleber RJ, Brom D. 1992. *Coping With Trauma: Theory, Prevention and Treatment.* Amsterdam, the Netherlands: Swets & Zeitlinger.

Kliman J, Kern R, Kliman A. 1982. Natural and human-made disasters: some therapeutic and epidemiological implications for crisis intervention. In: Reuveni U, Speck RV, Speck JL, eds. *Therapeutic Intervention: Healing Strategies for Human Systems.* New York, NY: Human Sciences Press.

Lowe SR, Kwok RK, Payne J, et al. 2016. Why does disaster recovery work influence mental health? Pathways through physical health and household income. *Am J Community Psychol.* 58(3-4): 354–364. Available at: http://onlinelibrary.wiley.com/wol1/doi/10.1002/ajcp.12091/full. Accessed January 25, 2017.

Lystad M, ed. 1988. *Mental Health Response to Mass Emergencies: Theory and Practice.* New York, NY: Brunner/Mazel Publishers.

Marsella AJ, Friedman MJ, Gerrity ET, et al., eds. 1996. *Ethnocultural Aspects of Post-Traumatic Stress Disorder: Issues, Research, and Clinical Applications.* Washington, DC: American Psychological Association.

McIntyre J, Nelson Goff BS. 2011. Federal disaster mental health response and compliance with best practices. *Community Ment Health J.* 48(6):723–728.

McKnight JL, Kretzmann JP. 1990. *Mapping Community Capacity.* Evanston, IL: Center for Urban Affairs and Policy Research, Northwestern University.

Mitchell JT, Everly Jr GS. 1997. *Critical Incident Stress Debriefing: An Operations Manual for the Prevention of Traumatic Stress Among Emergency Service and Disaster Workers.* 2nd ed, revised. Ellicott City, MD: Chevron Publishing Corporation.

Myers D. 1994. *Disaster Response and Recovery: A Handbook for Mental Health Professionals.* Rockville, MD: U.S. Department of Health & Human Services, Public Health Service, Substance Abuse and Mental Health Services Administration, Center for Mental Health Services.

National Center for Post-Traumatic Stress Disorders. 2003. *Mental-Health Intervention for Disasters.* Washington, DC: Department of Veterans Affairs. Available at: http://www.georgiadisaster.info/Healthcare/HC14%20FacititatingResiliency/Link%201%20--%20NCPTSD%20Fact%20Sheet%20on%20MH%20Intervention.pdf. Accessed January 25, 2017.

Neria Y, Galea S, Norris FH, eds. 2009. *Mental Health and Disasters.* New York, NY: Cambridge University Press.

Norris FH, Alegria M. 2005. Mental health care for ethnic minority individuals and communities in the aftermath of disasters and mass violence. *CNS Spectr.* 10(2):132–140.

North CS, Pfefferbaum B. 2013. Mental health response to community disasters a systematic review. *JAMA*. 310(5):507–518.

Office of the Assistant Secretary for Preparedness and Response. 2012. Disaster behavioral health: current assets and capabilities. Available at: http://www.phe.gov/Preparedness/planning/abc/Pages/dbh-capabilities.aspx. Accessed January 25, 2017.

Pfefferbaum B, Seale TW, McDonald NB, et al. 2000. Posttraumatic stress two years after the Oklahoma City bombing in youths geographically distant from the explosion. *Psychiatry.* 63(4):358–370.

Schlenger WE, Caddell JM, Ebert L, et al. 2002. Psychological reactions to terrorist attacks: findings from the national study of Americans' reactions to September 11. *JAMA*. 288(5):581–588.

Shear K. 2016. *Managing Grief After Disaster*. U.S. Department of Veterans Affairs. Available at: http://www.ptsd.va.gov/professional/trauma/disaster-terrorism/managing-grief-after-disaster.asp. Accessed January 25, 2017.

Speckhard A. 2002. Voices from the inside: psychological response from toxic disasters. In: Havenaar JM, Cwikel JG, Bromet EJ, eds. *Toxic Turmoil: Psychological and Societal Consequences of Ecological Disasters*. New York, NY: Kluwer Academic/Plenum.

Stuber J, Fairbrother G, Galea S, et al. 2002. Determinants of counseling for children in Manhattan after the September 11 attacks. *Psychiatr Serv.* 53(7):815–822.

Substance Abuse and Mental Health Services Administration (SAMHSA). 2013. *Disaster Planning Handbook for Behavioral Health Treatment Programs*. Rockville, MD: Substance Abuse and Mental Health Services Administration. Available at: http://store.samhsa.gov/shin/content/SMA13-4779/SMA13-4779.pdf. Accessed January 25, 2017.

Substance Abuse and Mental Health Services Administration (SAMHSA). 2003. *Mental Health All-Hazards Disaster Planning Guidance*. Rockville, MD: Department of Health & Human Services. Available at: http://store.samhsa.gov/product/Mental-Health-All-Hazards-Disaster-Planning-Guidance/SMA03-3829. Accessed February 3, 2017.

Substance Abuse and Mental Health Services Administration. 2014. SAMHSA behavioral health disaster response mobile app. Available at: http://www.store.samhsa.gov/apps/disaster. Accessed January 25, 2017.

Substance Abuse and Mental Health Services Administration. 2015. *Disaster Technical Assistance Center Supplemental Research Bulletin: Disaster Behavioral Health Interventions Inventory*. Available at: http://www.samhsa.gov/sites/default/files/dtac/supplemental-research-bulletin-may-2015-disaster-behavioral-health-interventions.pdf. Accessed January 25, 2017.

Taniellan T, Stein B. 2006. Understanding and preparing for the psychological consequences of terrorism. In: Kamien D, ed. *The McGraw-Hill Homeland Security Handbook*. New York, NY: McGraw-Hill. Available at: http://www.rand.org/pubs/reprints/2006/RAND_RP1217.pdf. Accessed January 25, 2017.

Terr LC. 1992. Large-group preventive techniques for use after disaster. In: Austin LS, ed. *Responding to Disaster: A Guide for Mental Health Professionals.* Washington, DC: American Psychiatric Press. 81–99.

Ursano RJ, McCaughey BG, Fullerton CS, eds. 1994. *Individual and Community Responses to Trauma and Disaster: The Structure of Human Chaos.* Cambridge, England: Cambridge University Press.

Van der Kolk BA, McFarlane AC, Weisaeth L, eds. 1996. *Traumatic Stress: The Effects of Overwhelming Experience on Mind, Body, and Society.* New York, NY: The Guilford Press.

Van Ommeren M, Saxena S. 2004. *Mental Health of Populations Exposed to Biological and Chemical Weapons.* Geneva, Switzerland: World Health Organization.

Weisaeth L. 1993. Disasters: psychological and psychiatric aspects. In: Goldberger L, Breznitz S, eds. *Handbook of Stress: Theoretical and Clinical Aspects.* 2nd ed. New York, NY: The Free Press.

Yehuda R, ed. 1998. *Psychological Trauma.* Washington, DC: American Psychiatric Press.

Young BH, Ford JD, Ruzek JI, et al. 1998. *Disaster Mental Health Services: A Guidebook for Clinicians and Administrators.* Menlo Park, CA: National Center for Post-Traumatic Stress Disorders.

Yun K, Lurie N, Hyde PS. 2010. Moving mental health into the disaster-preparedness spotlight. *N Engl J Med.* 363(13):1193–1195.

Bioterrorism and Emerging Infections

Belluz J. 2016. Why a yellow fever outbreak in Angola is a "potential threat for the entire world." *Vox.* Available at: http://www.vox.com/2016/4/15/11432522/yellow-fever-virus-outbreak-angola. Accessed January 25, 2017.

Blank S, Moskin LC, Zucker JR. 2003. An ounce of prevention is a ton of work: mass antibiotic prophylaxis for anthrax: New York City, 2001. *Emerg Infect Dis.* 9(6):615–622.

Bravata DM, McDonald KM, Owens DK, et al. 2004. *Regionalization of bioterrorism preparedness and response. Evidence Report/Technology Assessment: Number 96.* Rockville, MD: Agency for Healthcare Research and Quality.

Burkle HM Jr, Hanfling D. 2015. Political leadership in the time of crises: primum non nocere. *PLoS Curr.* 7.

Centers for Disease Control and Prevention. 2013. Preparation and planning for bioterrorism emergencies. Available at: http://emergency.cdc.gov/bioterrorism/prep.asp. Accessed January 25, 2017.

Centers for Disease Control and Prevention. 2013. Severe acute respiratory syndrome (SARS). Available at: http://www.cdc.gov/sars. Accessed January 25, 2017.

Centers for Disease Control and Prevention. 2016. Chikungunya virus. Available at: http://www.cdc.gov/chikungunya/prevention/index.html. Accessed January 25, 2017.

Centers for Disease Control and Prevention. 2016. Middle East respiratory syndrome (MERS). Available at: http://www.cdc.gov/coronavirus/mers/index.html. Accessed February 3, 2017.

Fenner F, Henderson DA, Arita I, et al. 1988. *Smallpox and Its Eradication*. Geneva, Switzerland: World Health Organization.1–276.

Henderson DA, Inglesby TV, Bartlett JG, et al. 1999. Smallpox as a biological weapon: medical and public health management. Working Group on Civilian Devense. *JAMA*. 281(22): 2127–2137.

Henderson DA, Inglesby TV, O'Toole TO. 2002. *Bioterrorism: Guidelines for Medical and Public Health Management*. Chicago, IL: American Medical Association.

Henderson DA. 1999. Smallpox: clinical and epidemiologic features. *Emerg Infect Dis*. 5(4):537–539.

Inglesby TV, Henderson DA, Bartlett JG, et al. 1999. Anthrax as a biological weapon: medical and public health management. *JAMA*. 281(18):1735–1745.

Meehan PJ, Rosenstein NE, Gillen M, et al. 2004. Responding to detection of aerosolized Bacillus anthracis by autonomous detection systems in the workplace. *MMWR Recomm Rep*. 53(RR-7): 1–12.

Mina B, Dym J, Kuepper F, et al. 2002. Fatal inhalational anthrax with unknown source of exposure in a 61-year-old woman in New York City. *JAMA*. 287(7):858–862.

Morens DM, Fauci AS. 2012. Emerging infectious diseases in 2012: 20 years after the institute of medicine report. *MBio*. 3(6).

Murray V, ed. 1990. *Major Chemical Disasters: Medical Aspects of Management* (International Congress and Symposium Series). New York, NY: Royal Society of Medicine Services Limited.

Novick LF, Marr JS, eds. 2001. *Public Health Issues in Disaster Preparedness: Focus on Bioterrorism*. Sudbury, MA: Jones & Bartlett Learning. 1–150.

Occupational Safety and Health Administration (OSHA). 2005. *OSHA Best Practices for Hospital-Based First Receivers of Victims From Mass Casualty Incidents Involving the Release of Hazardous Substances*. Washington, DC: U.S. Department of Labor. Available at: http://www.osha.gov/dts/osta/bestpractices/html/hospital_firstreceivers.html. Accessed January 25, 2017.

O'Toole T. 1999. Smallpox: an attack scenario. *Emerg Infect Dis*. 5(4):540–546.

Occupational Safety and Health Administration. 2004. *Medical & Dental Offices: A Guide to Compliance with OSHA Standards*. Available at: https://www.osha.gov/Publications/osha3187.pdf. Accessed January 25, 2017.

Pepe PE, Rinnert KJ. 2002. Bioterrorism and medical risk management. *Int Lawyer*. 36(1):9–20.

U.S. Government Publishing Office. 2016. 49 CFR § 173.196: Category A infectious substances. Available at: http://www.ecfr.gov/cgi-bin/text-idx?SID=2a97f2935677211e1785ac643163d2a9&node=49:2.1.1.3.10.5.25.33&rgn=div8. Accessed January 25, 2017.

U.S. Department of Justice; Federal Bureau of Investigation; U.S. Army Soldier Biological Chemical Command. 2003. *Criminal and Epidemiological Investigation Handbook.* Washington, DC: Federal Bureau of Investigation; U.S. Department of Justice, Office of Justice Programs.

Wagner MM, Moore AW, Aryel RM, eds. 2006. *Handbook of Biosurveillance.* New York, NY: Elsevier.

Weinstein RS, Alibek K. 2003. *Biological and Chemical Terrorism: A Guide for Healthcare Providers and First Responders.* New York, NY: Thieme Medical.

Ebola Virus Disease *(also see "Worker Health and Safety")*

Bausch DG, Towner JS, Dowell SF, et al. 2007. Assessment of the risk of Ebola virus transmission from bodily fluids and fomites. *J Infect Dis.* 196(Suppl 2):S142–S147.

Bevington F, Kan L, Schemm K, et al. 2015. Ebola as a case study: the role of local health departments in global health security. *J Public Health Manag Pract.* 21(2):220–223.

Brosseau LM, Jones R. 2014. Commentary: Health workers need optimal respiratory protection for Ebola. Available at: http://www.cidrap.umn.edu/news-perspective/2014/09/commentary-health-workers-need-optimal-respiratory-protection-ebola. Accessed January 25, 2017.

Centers for Disease Control and Prevention. 2014. Importance of communication in outbreak response: ebola. Available at: http://www.cdc.gov/globalhealth/stories/ebola_communication.htm. Accessed January 25, 2017.

Centers for Disease Control and Prevention. 2016. Considerations for selecting protective clothing used in healthcare for protection against microorganism in blood and body fluids. Available at: https://www.cdc.gov/niosh/npptl/topics/protectiveclothing. Accessed January 25, 2017.

Centers for Disease Control and Prevention. 2015. For U.S. healthcare settings: donning and doffing personal protective equipment (PPE) for evaluating persons under investigation (puis) for Ebola who are clinically stable and do not have bleeding, vomiting, or diarrhea. Available at: http://www.cdc.gov/vhf/ebola/health care-us/ppe/guidance-clinically-stable-puis.html. Accessed January 25, 2017.

Centers for Disease Control and Prevention. 2015. Frequently asked questions for guidance on personal protective equipment to be used by healthcare workers during management of patients with confirmed Ebola or persons under investigation (PUI) for Ebola who are clinically unstable or have bleeding, vomiting or diarrhea in u.s. hospitals, including procedures for donning and doffing. Available at: http://www.cdc.gov/vhf/ebola/health care-us/ppe/faq.html. Accessed January 25, 2017.

Centers for Disease Control and Prevention. 2015. Ebola virus disease diagnosis. Available at: http://www.cdc.gov/vhf/ebola/diagnosis. Accessed January 25, 2017.

Centers for Disease Control and Prevention. 2015. Epidemiologic risk factors to consider when evaluating a person for exposure to Ebola virus. Available at: http://www.cdc.gov/vhf/ebola/exposure/risk-factors-when-evaluating-person-for-exposure.html. Accessed January 25, 2017.

Centers for Disease Control and Prevention. 2015. Guidance on personal protective equipment (PPE) to be used by healthcare workers during management of patients with confirmed Ebola or persons under investigation (PUIs) for Ebola who are clinically unstable or have bleeding, vomiting, or diarrhea in U.S. hospitals, including procedures for donning and doffing PPE. Section 1. Recommended administrative and environmental controls for healthcare facilities. Available at: http://www.cdc.gov/vhf/ebola/health care-us/ppe/guidance.html. Accessed January 25, 2017.

Centers for Disease Control and Prevention. 2015. Guidance on personal protective equipment (PPE) to be used by healthcare workers during management of patients with confirmed Ebola Virus Disease or Patients Under Investigation (PUI) for Ebola virus disease who are clinically unstable or have bleeding, vomiting or diarrhea in U.S. hospitals, including procedures for putting on (donning) and removing (doffing). Section 2. Principles of PPE. Available at: http://www.cdc.gov/vhf/ebola/health care-us/ppe/guidance.html. Accessed January 25, 2017.

Centers for Disease Control and Prevention. 2015. Guidance for Collection, Transport and Submission of Specimens for Ebola Virus Testing. Available at: http://www.cdc.gov/vhf/ebola/health care-us/laboratories/specimens.html. Accessed January 25, 2017.

Centers for Disease Control and Prevention. 2015. Preparing for Ebola—a tiered approach. Available at: http://www.cdc.gov/vhf/ebola/health care-us/preparing/index.html. Accessed January 25, 2017.

Centers for Disease Control and Prevention. 2015. Interim guidance for environmental infection control in hospitals for Ebola virus. Available at: http://www.cdc.gov/vhf/ebola/health care-us/cleaning/hospitals.html. Accessed January 25, 2017.

Centers for Disease Control and Prevention. 2015. Interim guidance for preparing Ebola assessment hospitals. Available at: http://www.cdc.gov/vhf/ebola/health care-us/preparing/assessment-hospitals.html. Accessed January 25, 2017.

Centers for Disease Control and Prevention. 2015. Interim guidance for preparing Ebola treatment centers. Available at: http://www.cdc.gov/vhf/ebola/health care-us/preparing/treatment-centers.html. Accessed January 25, 2017.

Centers for Disease Control and Prevention. 2015. Interim guidance for preparing frontline healthcare facilities for patients under investigation (PUIs) for Ebola virus disease (EVD). Available at: http://www.cdc.gov/vhf/ebola/health care-us/preparing/frontline-health care-facilities.html. Accessed January 25, 2017.

Centers for Disease Control and Prevention. 2016. 2014 Ebola outbreak in West Africa—case counts. Available at: http://www.cdc.gov/vhf/ebola/outbreaks/2014-west-africa/case-counts.html. Accessed January 25, 2017.

Centers for Disease Control and Prevention. 2016. 2014 West Africa Ebola outbreak communication resources. Available at: http://www.cdc.gov/vhf/ebola/outbreaks/2014-west-africa/communication-resources. Accessed January 25, 2017.

Dowell SF, Mukunu R, Ksiazek TG, et al. 1999. Transmission of Ebola hemorrhagic fever: a study of risk factors in family members, Kikwit, Democratic Republic of the Congo, 1995. Commission de Lutte contre les Epidemies a Kikwit. *J Infect Dis.* 179(Suppl 1):S87–S91.

Formenty P, Leroy EM, Epelboin A, et al. 2006. Detection of Ebola virus in oral fluid specimens during outbreaks of Ebola virus hemorrhagic fever in the Republic of Congo. *Clin Infect Dis.* 42(11):1521–1526.

Francesconi P, Yoti Z, Declich S, et al. 2003. Ebola hemorrhagic fever transmission and risk factors of contacts, Uganda. *Emerg Infect Dis.* 9(11):1430–1437.

Frieden TR, Damon IK. 2015. Ebola in West Africa—CDC's role in epidemic detection, control, and prevention. *Emerg Infect Dis.* 21(11):1897–1905.

Gilbert GL, Kerridge I. 2015. Communication and communicable disease control: lessons from Ebola virus disease. *Am J Bioeth.* 15(4):62–65.

Goldberg AB, Ratzan SC, Jacobson KL, et al. 2015. Addressing Ebola and other outbreaks: a communication checklist for global health leaders, policymakers, and practitioners. *J Health Commun.* 20(2):121–122.

Killanski A, Evans NG. 2015. Effectively communicating the uncertainties surrounding Ebola virus transmission. *PLoS Pathog.* 11(10):e1005097.

National Association of County and City Health Officers. 2016. What local health departments need to know about Ebola. Available at: http://nacchopreparedness.org/what-local-health-departments-need-to-know-about-ebola. Accessed January 25, 2017.

Nishiura H, Chowell G. 2015. Theoretical perspectives on the infectiousness of Ebola virus disease. *Theor Biol Med Model.* 12:1.

Occupational Safety and Health Administration. 2014. *PPE Selection Matrix for Occupational Exposure to Ebola Virus: Guidance for Common Exposure Scenarios.* Available at: https://www.osha.gov/Publications/OSHA3761.pdf. Accessed January 25, 2017.

Oyeyemi SO, Gabarron E, Wynn R. 2014. Ebola, Twitter, and misinformation: a dangerous combination? *BMJ.* 4(349):g6178.

Pan American Health Organization, World Health Organization. 2014. *Ebola Risk Communication Action Plan.* Washington, DC: Pan American Health Organization.

Roels TH, Bloom AS, Buffington J, et al. 1999. Ebola hemorrhagic fever, Kikwit, Democratic Republic of the Congo, 1995: risk factors for patients without a reported exposure. *J Infect Dis.* 179(Suppl 1):S92–S97.

Rosenbaum L. 2015. Communicating uncertainty—Ebola, public health, and the scientific process. *New Engl J Med.* 372(1):7–9.

Santibanez S, Siegel V, O'Sullivan M, et al. 2015. Health communications and community mobilization during an Ebola response: partnerships with community and faith-based organizations. *Public Health Rep.* 130(2):128–133.

U.S. Department of Health & Human Services. 2015. Ebola information for healthcare professionals and healthcare settings. Available at: http://www.phe.gov/Preparedness/responders/ebola/Pages/default.aspx. Accessed February 3, 2017.

Pandemic Influenza

Agency for Healthcare Research and Quality (AHRQ). 2004. *Community-Based Mass Prophylaxis: A Planning Guide for Public Health Preparedness*. Rockville, MD: AHRQ. Available at: http://archive.ahrq.gov/downloads/pub/biotertools/cbmprophyl.pdf. Accessed February 3, 2017.

American College of Emergency Physicians. 2009. *National Strategic Plan for Emergency Department Management of Outbreaks of Novel H1N1 Influenza*. Washington, DC: U.S. Department of Health & Human Services. Available at: http://www.acep.org/workarea/DownloadAsset.aspx?id=45781. Accessed February 3, 2017.

Association of Public Health Laboratories (APHL). 2010. *Public Health Laboratories: Diminishing Resources in an Era of Evolving Threats*. Silver Spring, MD: APHL. Available at: https://www.aphl.org/aboutAPHL/publications/Documents/PHPR_2010_Public-Health-Laboratories-Diminishing-Resources-in-an-Era-of-Evolving-Threats.pdf#search=Association%20of%20Public%20Health%20Laboratories%20%28APHL%29%2E%202010%2E%20Public%20Health%20Laboratories%3A%20Diminishing%20Resources%20in%20an%20Era%20of%20Evolving%20Threats. Accessed February 3, 2017.

Association of State and Territorial Health Officers. 2008. *At-Risk Populations in Pandemic Influenza: Planning Guidance for State, Territorial, Tribal, and Local Health Departments*. Falls Church, VA: International Association of Emergency Managers. Available at: http://www.astho.org/Infectious-Disease/At-Risk-Populations/At-Risk-Populations-and-Pandemic-Influenza-Planning-Guidance. Accessed February 3, 2017.

Barrios LC, Koonin LM, Kohl KS, et al. 2012. Selecting nonpharmaceutical strategies to minimize influenza spread: the 2009 influenza A (H1N1) pandemic and beyond. *Public Health Rep*. 127(6):565–571.

Centers for Disease Control and Prevention. 2001. Considerations for distinguishing influenza-like illness from inhalational anthrax. *MMWR Morb Mortal Wkly Rep*. 50(44):985–986.

Centers for Disease Control and Prevention. 2003. Notice to readers: guidelines for maintaining and managing the vaccine cold chain. *MMWR Mord Mortal Wkly Rep*. 52(42):1023–1025.

Centers for Disease Control and Prevention (CDC). 2009. *Abbreviated Pandemic Influenza Plan Template for Primary Care Provider Offices: Guidance From Stakeholders*. Atlanta, GA: CDC. Available at: http://www.cdc.gov/h1n1flu/guidance/pdf/abb_pandemic_influenza_plan.pdf. Accessed February 3, 2017.

Centers for Disease Control and Prevention. 2009. Interim biosafety guidance for all individuals handling clinical specimens or isolates containing 2009–H1N1 influenza A virus novel H1N1, including vaccine strains. Available at: http://www.cdc.gov/h1n1flu/guidelines_labworkers.htm. Accessed February 3, 2017.

Centers for Disease Control and Prevention. 2009. Interim guidance on specimen collection, processing, and testing for patients with suspected novel influenza A H1N1 virus infection. Available at: http://www.cdc.gov/h1n1flu/specimencollection.htm. Accessed February 3, 2017.

Centers for Disease Control and Prevention. 2010. Interim guidance on infection control measures for 2009 H1N1 influenza in healthcare settings, including protection of healthcare personnel. Available at: http://www.cdc.gov/h1n1flu/guidelines_infection_control.htm. Accessed February 3, 2017.

Centers for Disease Control and Prevention. 2016. Influenza risk assessment tool (IRAT). Available at: http://www.cdc.gov/flu/pandemic-resources/tools/risk-assessment.htm. Accessed February 3, 2017.

Centers for Disease Control and Prevention. 2007. *Interim Pre-Pandemic Planning Guidance: Community Strategy for Pandemic Influenza Mitigation in the United States—Early, Targeted, Layered Use of Nonpharmaceutical Interventions*. Available at: https://www.cdc.gov/flu/pandemic-resources/pdf/community_mitigation-sm.pdf. Accessed February 3, 2017.

Centers for Disease Control and Prevention. 2016. Seasonal influenza-associated hospitalizations in the United States. Available at: http://www.cdc.gov/flu/about/qa/hospital.htm. Accessed February 3, 2017.

ESRI. 2009. *Geographic Information Systems and Pandemic Influenza Planning and Response*. Redlands, CA: ESRI. Available at: http://www.esri.com/library/whitepapers/pdfs/gis-and-pandemic-planning.pdf. Accessed February 3, 2017.

Ethics Subcommittee of the Advisory Committee to the Director, Centers for Disease Control and Prevention. 2007. *Ethical Guidelines in Pandemic Influenza*. Available at: http://www.cdc.gov/od/science/integrity/phethics/panFlu_Ethic_Guidelines.pdf. Accessed February 3, 2017.

Holloway R, Rasmussen SA, Zaza S, et al. 2014. Updated preparedness and response framework for influenza pandemics. *MMWR Recomm Rep*. 63(RR-06):1–18.

Knebel A, Phillips SJ, eds. 2008. *Home Health Care During an Influenza Pandemic: Issues and Resources*. Rockville, MD: Agency for Healthcare Research and Quality. Available at: http://citeseerx.ist.psu.edu/viewdoc/download?doi=10.1.1.168.6497&rep=rep1&type=pdf. Accessed February 3, 2017.

Lister SA, Redhead CS. 2009. *The 2009 Influenza Pandemic: An Overview*. Washington, DC: Congressional Research Service. Available at: http://handle.dtic.mil/100.2/ADA501479. Accessed February 3, 2017.

Occupational Safety and Health Administration. 2009. *Pandemic Influenza Preparedness and Response Guidance for Healthcare Workers*. Washington, DC: U.S. Department of Labor. Available at: http://www.osha.gov/Publications/OSHA_pandemic_health.pdf. Accessed February 3, 2017.

Public Health Emergency, Office of the Assistant Secretary for Preparedness and Response. 2007. *Public Health Emergency Response: A Guide for Leaders and Responders*. Washington, DC: U.S. Department of Health & Human Services. Available at: https://www.hsdl.org/?view&did=481394. Accessed February 3, 2017.

Reed C, Biggerstaff M, Finelli L, et al. 2013. Novel framework for assessing epidemiologic effects of influenza epidemics and pandemics. *Emerg Infect Dis*. 19(1):85–91.

Thompson MG, Shay SK, Zhou H, et al. 2010. Estimates of deaths associated with seasonal influenza—United States, 1976-2007. *MMWR Morb Mortal Wkly Rep*. 59(33):1057–1062.

Trock SC, Burke SA, Cox NJ. 2012. Development of an influenza virologic risk assessment tool. *Avian Dis*. 56(4 Suppl):1058–1061.

Trock SC, Burke SA, Cox NJ. 2015. Development of framework for assessing influenza virus pandemic risk. *Emerg Infect Dis*. 21(8):1372–1378.

U.S. Department of Health & Human Services (HHS). 2008. *Federal Guidance to Assist States in Improving State-Level Pandemic Influenza Operating Plans*. Washington, DC: HHS.

U.S. Department of Health & Human Services (HHS). 2007. *Interim Pre-pandemic Planning Guidance: Community Strategy for Pandemic Influenza Mitigation in the United States—Early, Targeted, Layered Use of Nonpharmaceutical Interventions*. Washington, DC: HHS. Available at: https://stacks.cdc.gov/view/cdc/11425. Accessed February 3, 2017.

U.S. Government Accountability Office. 2011. *Influenza Pandemic: Lessons From the H1N1 Pandemic Should Be Incorporated into Future Planning*. Available at: http://www.gao.gov/assets/330/320187.pdf. Accessed February 3, 2017.

U.S. Department of Health & Human Services. 2016. Influenza (flu): past pandemic. Available at: https://www.cdc.gov/flu/pandemic-resources/basics/past-pandemics.html. Accessed February 3, 2017.

U.S. Department of Health & Human Services (HHS). 2016. Influenza (flu). Washington, DC: HHS. Available at: https://www.cdc.gov/flu. Accessed February 3, 2017.

World Health Organization (WHO). 2005. *Avian Influenza: Assessing the Pandemic Threat*. Geneva, Switzerland: WHO. Available at: http://www.who.int/influenza/resources/documents/h5n1_assessing_pandemic_threat/en. Accessed February 3, 2017.

World Health Organization (WHO). 2008. *Outbreak Communication Planning Guide*. Geneva, Switzerland: WHO. Available at: http://www.who.int/ihr/publications/outbreak-communication-guide/en. Accessed February 3, 2017.

World Health Organization (WHO). 2009. *Interim Planning Considerations for Mass Gatherings in the Context of Pandemic (H1N1) 2009 Influenza*. Geneva, Switzerland: WHO. Available at: http://www.who.int/csr/resources/publications/swineflu/cp002_2009-0511_planning_considerations_for_mass_gatherings.pdf. Accessed February 3, 2017.

World Health Organization (WHO). 2013. *Pandemic Influenza Risk Management WHO Interim Guidance*. Geneva, Switzerland: WHO. Available at: http://www.who.int/influenza/preparedness/pandemic/GIP_PandemicInfluenzaRiskManagementInterimGuidance_Jun2013.pdf?ua=1. Accessed February 3, 2017.

Zika

Centers for Disease Control and Prevention. 2016. Announcement: guidance for U.S. laboratory testing for Zika virus infection: implications for health care providers. *MMWR Morb Mortal Wkly Rep*. 65(46):1304.

Hayden EC. 2016. Spectre of Ebola haunts Zika response. *Nature.* 531(7592):19.

Petersen EE, Meaney-Delman D, Neblett-Fanfair R, et al. 2016. Update: interim guidance for preconception counseling and prevention of sexual transmission of Zika virus for persons with possible Zika virus exposure—United States, September 2016. *MMWR Morb Mortal Wkly Rep.* 65(39):1077–1081.

Russell K, Oliver SE, Lewis L, et al. 2016. Update: interim guidance for the evaluation and management of infants with possible congenital Zika virus infection—United States, August 2016. *MMWR Morb Mortal Wkly Rep.* 65(33):870–878.

U.S. Department of Health & Human Services, FDA. 2016. *Donor Screening Recommendations to Reduce the Risk of Transmission of Zika Virus by Human Cells, Tissues, and Cellular and Tissue-Based Products.* Available at: http://www.fda.gov/downloads/BiologicsBloodVaccines/GuidanceComplianceRegulatoryInformation/Guidances/Tissue/UCM488582.pdf. Accessed February 3, 2017.

U.S. Department of Health & Human Services, FDA. 2016. *Questions and Answers Regarding "Recommendations for Donor Screening, Deferral, and Product Management to Reduce the Risk of Transfusion-Transmission of Zika Virus: Guidance for Industry."* Available at: http://www.fda.gov/downloads/BiologicsBloodVaccines/GuidanceComplianceRegulatoryInformation/Guidances/Blood/UCM490435.pdf. Accessed February 3, 2017.

U.S. Department of Health & Human Services, FDA. 2016. *Recommendations for Donor Screening, Deferral, and Product Management to Reduce the Risk of Transfusion Transmission of Zika Virus.* Available at: http://www.fda.gov/downloads/BiologicsBloodVaccines/GuidanceCompliance RegulatoryInformation/Guidances/Blood/UCM486360.pdf. Accessed February 3, 2017.

U.S. Department of Health & Human Services, FDA. 2016. Emergency use authorization: Zika virus EUA information. Available at: http://www.fda.gov/EmergencyPreparedness/Counterterrorism/MedicalCountermeasures/MCMLegalRegulatoryandPolicyFramework/ucm182568.htm#zika. Accessed February 3, 2017.

Care Guidelines and Standards

Assistant Secretary for Preparedness and Response. [n.d.]. *Disaster Response Guidance for Health Care Providers: Identifying and Understanding the Health Care Needs of Individuals Experiencing Homelessness.* Available at: http://www.phe.gov/Preparedness/planning/abc/Documents/clinical-guidance-toolkit060615.pdf. Accessed February 3, 2017.

Center for Health Policy, Columbia University School of Nursing. 2008. *Adapting Standards of Care Under Extreme Conditions: Guidance For Professionals During Disasters, Pandemics and Other Extreme Emergencies.* Silver Spring, MD: American Nurses Association. Available at: http://nursingworld.org/MainMenuCategories/WorkplaceSafety/Healthy-Work-Environment/DPR/TheLawEthicsof DisasterResponse/AdaptingStandardsofCare.pdf. Accessed February 3, 2017.

Centers for Medicare and Medicaid Services. 2002. *Preparing for Emergencies: A Guide for People on Dialysis*. Available at: https://www.cms.gov/Outreach-and-Education/Medicare-Learning-Network-MLN/MLNProducts/downloads/10150.pdf. Washington, DC: U.S. Department of Health & Human Services. Accessed February 3, 2017.

Hanfling D. 2012. *Crisis Standards of Care: a Systems Framework for Catastrophic Disaster Response*. Washington, DC: National Academies Press.

Institute of Medicine. 2009. *Guidance for Establishing Crisis Standards of Care for Use in Disaster Situations*. Washington, DC: Institute of Medicine. Available at: http://www.nap.edu/catalog/12749/guidance-for-establishing-crisis-standards-of-care-for-use-in-disaster-situations. Accessed February 3, 2017.

Nolte KB, Hanzlick RL, Payne DC, et al. 2004. Medical examiners, coroners, and biologic terrorism: a guidebook for surveillance and case management. *MMWR Recomm Rep.* 53(RR-8):1–27.

Occupational Safety and Health Administration (OSHA). 2005. *OSHA Best Practices for Hospital-Based First Receivers of Victims From Mass Casualty Incidents Involving the Release of Hazardous Substances*. Washington, DC: U.S. Department of Labor. Available at: http://www.osha.gov/dts/osta/bestpractices/html/hospital_firstreceivers.html. Accessed February 3, 2017.

Phillips S, Knebel A. 2007. *Mass Medical Care With Scarce Resources: A Community Planning Guide*. Rockville, MD: Agency for Healthcare Research and Quality. Publication No. 07-0001. Available at: http://archive.ahrq.gov/research/mce/mceguide.pdf. Accessed February 3, 2017.

Sasser SM, Hunt RC, Sullivent EE, et al. 2009. Guidelines for field triage of injured patients recommendations of the national expert panel on field triage. *MMWR Recomm Rep.* 58(RR-1):1–35.

The Joint Commission. 2006. *Surge Hospitals: Providing Safe Care in Emergencies*. Available at: https://www.jointcommission.org/assets/1/18/surge_hospital.pdf. Accessed February 3, 2017.

U.S. Food and Drug Administration. 2014. Disposal of contaminated devices. Available at: http://www.fda.gov/MedicalDevices/Safety/EmergencySituations/ucm055974.htm. Accessed February 3, 2017.

U.S. Food and Drug Administration. 2015. Medical devices requiring refrigeration. Available at: http://www.fda.gov/MedicalDevices/Safety/EmergencySituations/ucm056075.htm. Accessed February 3, 2017.

U.S. Food and Drug Administration. 2014. Medical Devices that have been exposed to heat and humidity. Available at: http://www.fda.gov/MedicalDevices/Safety/EmergencySituations/ucm056086.htm. Accessed February 3, 2017.

U.S. Food and Drug Administration. 2009. Tips for mammography facilities following natural disasters or severe weather conditions. Available at: http://www.fda.gov/Radiation-EmittingProducts/MammographyQualityStandardsActandProgram/FacilityCertificationandInspection/ucm127723.htm. Accessed February 3, 2017.

U.S. Food and Drug Administration. 2015. Safe drug use after a natural disaster. Available at: http://www.fda.gov/Drugs/EmergencyPreparedness/ucm085200.htm. Accessed February 3, 2017.

Case Studies

Emerging Infections

Aldridge C, Shah UA, Kim-Farley R. 2015. Local health department preparedness and response to Ebola in the United States. National Association of County and City Health Officers Preparedness Brief. Available at: http://nacchopreparedness.org/local-health-department-preparedness-and-response-to-ebola-in-the-united-states. Accessed September 23, 2016.

Centers for Disease Control and Prevention. 2016. CDC's response to the 2014–2016 Ebola epidemic—West Africa and United States. *MMWR Morb Mortal Wkly Rep*. 65(3 Suppl):1–106. Available at: http://www.cdc.gov/mmwr/volumes/65/su/pdfs/su6503.pdf. Accessed February 3, 2017.

Koonin LM, Jamieson DJ, Jernigan JA, et al. 2015. Systems for rapidly detecting and treating persons with Ebola virus disease—United States. *MMWR Morb Mortal Wkly Rep*. 64(8):222–225. Available at: http://www.cdc.gov/mmwr/preview/mmwrhtml/mm6408a5.htm?s_cid=mm6408a5_w. Accessed February 3, 2017.

Kuehnert MJ, Basavaraju SV, Moseley RR, et al. 2016. Screening of blood donations for Zika virus infection—Puerto Rico, April 3–June 11, 2016. *MMWR Morb Mortal Wkly Rep*. 65(24):627–628. Available at: http://www.cdc.gov/mmwr/volumes/65/wr/mm6524e2.htm?s_cid=mm6524e2_w. Accessed February 3, 2017.

Lee CT, Vora NM, Bajwa W, et al. 2016. Zika virus surveillance and preparedness—New York City, 2015–2016. *MMWR Morb Mortal Wkly Rep*. 65(24):629–635. Available at: http://www.cdc.gov/mmwr/volumes/65/wr/mm6524e3.htm?s_cid=mm6524e3_w. Accessed February 3, 2017.

Levine R, Ghiselli M, Conteh A, et al. 2016. Notes from the field: development of a contact tracing system for Ebola virus disease—Kambia District, Sierra Leone, January–February 2015. *MMWR Morb Mortal Wkly Rep*. 65(15):402 Available at: http://www.cdc.gov/mmwr/volumes/65/wr/mm6515a4.htm?s_cid=mm6515a4_w. Accessed February 3, 2017.

Mangal CN, Bean CL, Becker SJ. 2014. Gastrointestinal anthrax associated with a drumming circle in New Hampshire. In: Landesman LY, Weisfuse IB, eds. *Case Studies in Public Health Preparedness and Response to Disasters*. Burlington, MA: Jones and Bartlett. 251–270.

Millman AJ, Chamany S, Guthartz S, et al. 2016. Active monitoring of travelers arriving from Ebola-affected countries—New York City, October 2014–April 2015. *MMWR Morb Mortal Wkly Rep*. 65(3):51–54. Available at: http://www.cdc.gov/mmwr/volumes/65/wr/mm6503a3.htm?s_cid=mm6503a3_w. Accessed February 3, 2017.

Parham M, Edison L, Soetebier K, et al. 2015. Ebola active monitoring system for travelers returning from West Africa—Georgia, 2014–2015. *MMWR Morb Mortal Wkly Rep*. 64(13):347–350. Available at: http://www.cdc.gov/mmwr/preview/mmwrhtml/mm6413a3.htm?s_cid=mm6413a3_w. Accessed February 3, 2017.

Simeone RM, Shapiro-Mendoza CK, Meaney-Delman D, et al. 2016. Possible Zika virus infection among pregnant women—United States and territories, May 2016. *MMWR Morb Mortal Wkly*

Rep. 65(20):514–519. Available at: http://www.cdc.gov/mmwr/volumes/65/wr/mm6520e1.htm?s_cid=mm6520e1_w. Accessed February 3, 2017.

Influenza

Higdon MA, Stoto MA. 2014. The Martha's Vineyard public health system response to 2009 H1N1. In: Landesman LY, Weisfuse IB, eds. *Case Studies in Public Health Preparedness and Response to Disasters*. Burlington, MA: Jones and Bartlett. 346–358.

Jhung M. 2014. Surveillance in emergency preparedness: the 2009 H1N1 preparedness response. In: Landesman LY, Weisfuse IB, eds. *Case Studies in Public Health Preparedness and Response to Disasters*. Burlington, MA: Jones and Bartlett. 271–310.

Terry A, Atchison C, Pentella M. 2014. 2009 H1N1 influenza epidemic in Iowa. In: Landesman LY, Weisfuse IB, eds. *Case Studies in Public Health Preparedness and Response to Disasters*. Burlington, MA: Jones and Bartlett. 332–344.

Varlese DR, and Chason K. 2014. Mandatory Vaccination and H1N1: A Large Urban Hospital's Response. In: Landesman LY and Weisfuse IB eds. *Case Studies in Public Health Preparedness and Response to Disasters*. Burlington, MA: Jones and Bartlett. 312–329.

Natural Events

Babaie J, Moslehi S, Ardalan A. 2014. Rapid health needs assessment experience in 11 August 2012 East Azerbaijan Earthquakes: a qualitative study. *PloS Curr*. 6. Available at: http://www.ncbi.nlm.nih.gov/pmc/articles/PMC4096797. Accessed February 3, 2017.

Bernstein RS, Baxter PJ, Falk H, et al. 1986. Immediate public health concerns and actions in volcanic eruptions: lessons from Mount St. Helens eruptions, May 18–October 18, 1980. *Am J Public Health*. 76(3 Suppl):25–37.

Carr SJ, Leahy SM, London S, et al. 1996. The public health response to the Los Angeles, 1994 earthquake. *Am J Public Health*. 86(4):589–590.

Centers for Disease Control and Prevention. 1992. Rapid health needs assessment following Hurricane Andrew—Florida and Louisiana, 1992. *MMWR Morb Mortal Wkly Rep*. 41(37):685–688.

Centers for Disease Control and Prevention. 1993. Comprehensive assessment of health needs 2 months after Hurricane Andrew—Dade County, Florida. *MMWR Morb Mortal Wkly Rep*. 42(22):434–437.

Centers for Disease Control and Prevention. 1993. Injuries and illnesses related to Hurricane Andrew—Louisiana, 1992. *MMWR Morb Mortal Wkly Rep*. 42(13):242–244, 249–251.

Centers for Disease Control and Prevention. 1993. Morbidity surveillance following the Midwest flood—Missouri, 1993. *MMWR Morb Mortal Wkly Rep*. 42(41):797–798.

Centers for Disease Control and Prevention. 1993. Public health consequences of a flood disaster—Iowa, 1993. *MMWR Morb Mortal Wkly Rep.* 42(34):653–656.

Centers for Disease Control and Prevention. 1994. Rapid assessment of vectorborne diseases during the Midwest flood, United States, 1993. *MMWR Morb Mortal Wkly Rep.* 43(26):481–483.

Centers for Disease Control and Prevention. 2002. Morbidity and mortality associated with Hurricane Floyd—North Carolina, September-October 1999. *MMWR Morb Mortal Wkly Rep.* 49(17):369–372.

Centers for Disease Control and Prevention. 2004. Rapid assessment of the needs and health status of older adults after Hurricane Charley—Charlotte, DeSoto, and Hardee Counties, Florida, August 27–31, 2004. *MMWR Morb Mortal Wkly Rep.* 53(36):837–840.

Centers for Disease Control and Prevention. 2004. Rapid community health and needs assessments after Hurricanes Isabel and Charley—North Carolina, 2003–2004. *MMWR Morb Mortal Wkly Rep.* 53(36):840–842.

Centers for Disease Control and Prevention. 2005. Carbon monoxide poisoning after Hurricane Katrina—Alabama, Louisiana, and Mississippi, August-September 2005. *MMWR Morb Mortal Wkly Rep.* 54(39):996–998.

Centers for Disease Control and Prevention. 2005. Health concerns associated with disaster victim identification after a tsunami—Thailand, December 26, 2004–March 31, 2005. *MMWR Morb Mortal Wkly Rep.* 54(14):349–352.

Centers for Disease Control and Prevention. 2005. Hurricane Katrina response and guidance for health-care providers, relief workers, and shelter operators. *MMWR Morb Mortal Wkly Rep.* 54(35):877.

Centers for Disease Control and Prevention. 2005. Infectious disease and dermatologic conditions in evacuees and rescue workers after Hurricane Katrina—multiple states, August–September 2005. *MMWR Morb Mortal Wkly Rep.* 54(38):961–964.

Centers for Disease Control and Prevention. 2005. Rapid health response, assessment, and surveillance after a tsunami—Thailand, 2004–2005. *MMWR Morb Mortal Wkly Rep.* 54(3):61–64.

Centers for Disease Control and Prevention. 2005. Vibrio illnesses after Hurricane Katrina—multiple states, August–September 2005. *MMWR Morb Mortal Wkly Rep.* 54(37):928–931.

Centers for Disease Control and Prevention. 2006. Assessment of health-related needs after Hurricanes Katrina and Rita—Orleans and Jefferson Parishes, New Orleans Area, Louisiana, October 17–22, 2005. *MMWR Morb Mortal Wkly Rep.* 55(2):38–41.

Centers for Disease Control and Prevention. 2006. Health concerns associated with mold in water-damaged homes after Hurricanes Katrina and Rita—New Orleans Area, Louisiana, October 2005. *MMWR Morb Mortal Wkly Rep.* 55(2):41–44.

Centers for Disease Control and Prevention. 2006. Health hazard evaluation of police officers and firefighters after Hurricane Katrina—New Orleans, Louisiana, October 17–28 and November 30–December 5, 2005. *MMWR Morb Mortal Wkly Rep.* 55(16):456–458.

Centers for Disease Control and Prevention. 2006. Heat-related deaths—United States, 1999–2003. *MMWR Morb Mortal Wkly Rep.* 55(29):796–798.

Centers for Disease Control and Prevention. 2006. Monitoring poison control center data to detect health hazards during hurricane season—Florida, 2003-2005. *MMWR Morb Mortal Wkly Rep.* 55(15):426–428.

Centers for Disease Control and Prevention. 2006. Public health response to Hurricanes Katrina and Rita—Louisiana, 2005. *MMWR Morb Mortal Wkly Rep.* 55(2):29–30.

Centers for Disease Control and Prevention. 2006. Rapid assessment of health needs and resettlement plans among Hurricane Katrina evacuees—San Antonio, Texas, September 2005. *MMWR Morb Mortal Wkly Rep.* 55(9):242–244.

Centers for Disease Control and Prevention. 2006. Rapid community needs assessment after Hurricane Katrina—Hancock County, Mississippi, September 14–15, 2005. *MMWR Morb Mortal Wkly Rep.* 55(9):234–236.

Centers for Disease Control and Prevention. 2006. Rapid needs assessment of two rural communities after Hurricane Wilma—Hendry County, Florida, November 1–2, 2005. *MMWR Morb Mortal Wkly Rep.* 55(15):429–431.

Centers for Disease Control and Prevention. 2006. Surveillance for illness and injury after Hurricane Katrina—three counties, Mississippi, September 5–October 11, 2005. *MMWR Morb Mortal Wkly Rep.* 55(9):231–234.

Centers for Disease Control and Prevention. 2006. Surveillance in hurricane evacuation centers—Louisiana, September–October 2005. *MMWR Morb Mortal Wkly Rep.* 55(2):32–35.

Centers for Disease Control and Prevention. 2006. Tuberculosis control activities after Hurricane Katrina—New Orleans, Louisiana, 2005. *MMWR Morb Mortal Wkly Rep.* 55(12):332–335.

Centers for Disease Control and Prevention. 2007. Wildfire-related deaths—Texas, March 12–20, 2006. *MMWR Morb Mortal Wkly Rep.* 56(30):757–760.

Centers for Disease Control and Prevention. 2008. Carbon monoxide exposures after Hurricane Ike—Texas, September 2008. *MMWR Morb Mortal Wkly Rep.* 58(31):845–849.

Centers for Disease Control and Prevention. 2008. Monitoring health effects of wildfires using the biosense system—San Diego County, California, October 2007. *MMWR Morb Mortal Wkly Rep.* 57(27):741–747.

Centers for Disease Control and Prevention. 2009. Hurricane Ike rapid needs assessment—Houston, Texas, September 2008. *MMWR Morb Mortal Wkly Rep.* 58(38):1066–1071.

Centers for Disease Control and Prevention. 2010. Rapid establishment of an internally displaced persons disease surveillance system after an earthquake—Haiti, 2010. *MMWR Morb Mortal Wkly Rep.* 59(30):939–945.

Centers for Disease Control and Prevention. 2013. Tuberculosis control activities before and after Hurricane Sandy—Northeast and Mid-Atlantic States, 2012. *MMWR Morb Mortal Wkly Rep.*

62(11):206–208. Available at: http://www.cdc.gov/mmwr/preview/mmwrhtml/mm6211a3.htm. Accessed February 3, 2017.

Clinton JJ, Hagebak BR, Sirmons JG, et al. 1995. Lessons from the Georgia floods. *Public Health Rep*. 110(6):684–688.

Combs DL, Parrish RG, McNabb SJ, et al. 1996. Deaths related to Hurricane Andrew in Florida and Louisiana, 1992. *Int J Epidemiol*. 25(3):537–544.

Doran R, Sato M, Kamigaki T, et al. 2014. Public health recovery after the great east Japan earthquake: experience in selected areas of Miyagi Prefecture. In: Landesman LY, Weisfuse IB, eds. *Case Studies in Public Health Preparedness and Response to Disasters*. Burlington, MA: Jones and Bartlett.

Durkin ME, Thiel CC Jr, Schneider JE, et al. 1991. Injuries and emergency medical response in the Loma Prieta earthquake. *Bull Seismological Soc Am*. 81:2143–2166.

Erikson K. 1976. *Everything in Its Path: Destruction of Community in the Buffalo Creek Flood*. New York, NY: Simon & Schuster.

Glassman KS. 2014. The evacuation of NYU Langone Medical Center during Hurricane Sandy: lessons learned. In: Landesman LY, Weisfuse, IB eds. *Case Studies in Public Health Preparedness and Response to Disasters*. Burlington, MA: Jones and Bartlett.

Grace MC, Green BL, Lindy JD, et al. 1993. The Buffalo Creek Disaster: a 14-year follow-up. In: Wilson JP, Raphael B, eds. *The International Handbook of Traumatic Stress Syndromes*. New York, NY: Plenum Press. 441–449.

Green BL, Grace MC, Lindy JD, et al. 1990. Buffalo Creek survivors in the second decade: comparison with unexposed and non-litigant groups. *J Appl Soc Psychol*. 20(13):1033–1050.

Haynes BE, Freeman C, Rubin JL, et al. 1992. Medical response to catastrophic events: California's planning and the Loma Prieta earthquake. *Ann Emerg Med*. 21(4):368–374.

Hogan DE, Waeckerle JF, Dire DJ, et al. 1999. Emergency department impact of the Oklahoma City terrorist bombing. *Ann EmergMed*. 34(2):160–167.

Klaiman T, Twersky-Bumgardner S. 2014. Residential facilities and functional needs: preparing for and responding to emergencies in Pennsylvania. In: Landesman LY, Weisfuse IB, eds. *Case Studies in Public Health Preparedness and Response to Disasters*. Burlington, MA: Jones and Bartlett. 61–72.

Landesman LY. 2001. A department of health learns about its role in emergency public health. In: Rowitz L, ed. *Public Health Leadership: Putting Principles Into Practice*. Gaithersburg, MD: Aspen Publishers. 150–153.

Marcellino JA. 2014. Hurricane Irene: Evacuation of Coney Island Hospital. In: Landesman LY, Weisfuse IB, eds. *Case Studies in Public Health Preparedness and Response to Disasters*. Burlington, MA: Jones and Bartlett. 73–96.

McBride DA. 2014. The 1999 North Carolina Floyd Flood. In: Landesman LY, Weisfuse IB, eds. *Case Studies in Public Health Preparedness and Response to Disasters*. Burlington, MA: Jones and Bartlett. 39–60.

McNabb SJ, Kelso KY, Wilson SA, et al. 1995. Hurricane Andrew related injuries and illnesses, Louisiana. 1992. *South Med J*. 88(6):615–618.

Noji EK. 2014. The great east Japan earthquake of 2011. In: Landesman LY, Weisfuse IB, eds. *Case Studies in Public Health Preparedness and Response to Disasters*. Burlington, MA: Jones and Bartlett. 3–19.

Rosen M, Gotsch AR, Caravanos J. 2014. Hurricane Sandy: training to improve response and recovery. In: Landesman LY, Weisfuse IB, eds. *Case Studies in Public Health Preparedness and Response to Disasters*. Burlington, MA: Jones and Bartlett.

Sasser SM, Hunt RC, Sullivent EE, et al. 2009. Guidelines for field triage of injured patients recommendations of the national expert panel on field triage. *MMWR Recomm Rep*. 58(RR01):1–35.

Siddiqui N, Andrulis D, Pacheco G. 2014. Southern California wildfires of 2007: preparing and responding to culturally & linguistically diverse communities. In: Landesman LY, Weisfuse IB, eds. *Case Studies in Public Health Preparedness and Response to Disasters*. Burlington, MA: Jones and Bartlett. 21–38.

Whitman S, Good G, Donoghue ER, et al. 1997. Mortality in Chicago attributed to the July 1995 heat wave. *Am J Public Health*. 87(9):1515–1518.

Man-Made or Technological

Chamany S. 2014. Planning for the Republican National Convention 2004: Findings from the New York City Department of Health and Mental Hygiene. In: Landesman LY, Weisfuse IB, eds. *Case Studies in Public Health Preparedness and Response to Disasters*. Burlington, MA: Jones and Bartlett. 195–208.

Diaz JH. 2014. The Deepwater Horizon Gulf oil spill disaster. In: Landesman LY, Weisfuse IB, eds. *Case Studies in Public Health Preparedness and Response to Disasters*. Burlington, MA: Jones and Bartlett. 149–193.

Federal Communications Commission (FCC). 2008. *Emergency Communications During the Minneapolis Bridge Disaster: A Technical Case Study*. Washington, DC: FCC. Available at: https://www.fcc.gov/general/emergency-communications-during-minneapolis-bridge-disaster. Accessed January 25, 2017.

Leonard HB, Howitt AM. 2013. *Preliminary Thoughts and Observations on the Boston Marathon Bombings*. Cambridge, MA: Program on Crisis Leadership, John F. Kennedy School of Government, Harvard University. Available at: https://www.hks.harvard.edu/content/download/67375/1242310/version/1/file/Leonard+and+Howitt_Boston+Marathon_Preliminary+Thoughts+HBL+AMH+2013+04+22+v3.pdf. Accessed January 25, 2017.

Marghella P, Ashkenazi I. 2014. The lessons of tragedy: the 2004 Madrid train bombings. In: Landesman LY, Weisfuse IB, eds. *Case Studies in Public Health Preparedness and Response to Disasters.* Burlington, MA: Jones and Bartlett. 135–148.

Nolte KB, Hanzlick RL, Payne DC, et al. 2004. Medical examiners, coroners, and biologic terrorism: a guidebook for surveillance and case management. *MMWR Recomm Rep.* 53(RR08): 1–27.

Ramírez de Arellano AB. 2014. Rescue following a mine collapse in Chile, 2010. In: Landesman LY, Weisfuse, IB eds. *Case Studies in Public Health Preparedness and Response to Disasters.* Burlington, MA: Jones and Bartlett. 99–134.

World Trade Center

Centers for Disease Control and Prevention. 2001. Injury and illness among New York City Fire Department rescue workers after responding to the World Trade Center attacks. *MMWR Morb Mortal Wkly Rep Special Issue.* 51 Spec No:1–5.

Centers for Disease Control and Prevention. 2002. Community needs assessment of Lower Manhattan residents following the World Trade Center attacks—Manhattan, New York City, 2001. *MMWR Morb Mortal Wkly Rep.* 51 Spec No:10–13.

Centers for Disease Control and Prevention. 2002. Impact of September 11 attacks on workers in the vicinity of the World Trade Center—New York City. *MMWR Morb Mortal Wkly Rep.* 51 Spec No:8–10.

Centers for Disease Control and Prevention. 2002. Notice to readers: New York City Department of Health response to terrorist attack, September 11, 2001. *MMWR Morb Mortal Wkly Rep.* 50(38):821.

Centers for Disease Control and Prevention. 2002. Psychological and emotional effects of the September 11 attacks on the World Trade Center—Connecticut, New Jersey, and New York, 2001. *MMWR Morb Mortal Wkly Rep.* 51(35):784–786.

Centers for Disease Control and Prevention. 2002. Rapid assessment of injuries among survivors of the terrorist attack on the World Trade Center—New York City, September 2001. *MMWR Morb Mortal Wkly Rep.* 51(1):1–5.

Centers for Disease Control and Prevention. 2002. Use of respiratory protection among responders at the World Trade Center site—New York City, September 2001. *MMWR Morb Mortal Wkly Rep.* 51 Spec No:6–8.

Centers for Disease Control and Prevention. 2004. Preliminary results from the World Trade Center Evacuation Study—New York City, 2003. *MMWR Morb Mortal Wkly Rep.* 53(35):815–817.

Chapman LE, Sullivent EE, Grohskopf LA, et al. 2008. Recommendations for postexposure interventions to prevent infection with Hepatitis B virus, Hepatitis C virus, or human immunodeficiency virus, and tetanus in persons wounded during bombings and other mass-casualty events—United States, 2008. *MMWR Recomm Rep.* 57(RR-6):1–21.

Cohen N. 2014. Addressing the mental well-being of New Yorkers in the aftermath of the 9/11 and bioterror attacks. In: Landesman LY, Weisfuse IB, eds. *Case Studies in Public Health Preparedness and Response to Disasters.* Burlington, MA: Jones and Bartlett. 233–247.

Gershon R. 2014. World Trade Center attack on Sept 11, 2011. In: Landesman LY, Weisfuse IB, eds. *Case Studies in Public Health Preparedness and Response to Disasters.* Burlington, MA: Jones and Bartlett. 209–232.

Zika

Brent C, Dunn A, Savage H, et al. 2016. Preliminary findings from an investigation of Zika virus infection in a patient with no known risk factors—Utah, 2016. *MMWR Morb Mortal Wkly Rep.* 65(36):981–982.

Brooks RB, Carlos MP, Myers R, et al. 2016. Likely sexual transmission of Zika virus from a man with no symptoms of infection—Maryland, 2016. *MMWR Morb Mortal Wkly Rep.* 65(34):915–916.

Dirlikov E, Major CG, Mayshack M, et al. 2016. Guillain-Barre syndrome during ongoing Zika virus transmission—Puerto Rico, January 1-July 31, 2016. *MMWR Morb Mortal Wkly Rep.* 65(34):910–914.

Leal MC, Muniz LF, Ferreira TS, et al. 2016. Hearing loss in infants with microcephaly and evidence of congenital Zika virus infection—Brazil, November 2015–May 2016. *MMWR Morb Mortal Wkly Rep.* 65(34):917–919.

Madad SS, Masci J, Cagliuso NV Sr, et al. 2016. Preparedness for Zika virus disease—New York City, 2016. *MMWR Morb Mortal Wkly Rep.* 65(42):1161–1165.

Goodman, AB, Dziuban EJ, Powell K, et al. 2016. Characteristics of children aged <18 years with Zika virus disease acquired postnatally—U.S. States, January 2015–July 2016. *MMWR Morb Mortal Wkly Rep.* 65(39):1082–1085.

van der Linden V, Pessoa A, Dobyns W, et al. 2016. Description of 13 infants born during October 2015–January 2016 with congenital Zika virus infection without microcephaly at birth—Brazil. *MMWR Morb Mortal Wkly Rep.* 65(47):1343–1348.

Chemical Accidents

Chemical Casualty Care Division, U.S. Army Medical Research Institute of Chemical Defense (USAMRICD). 2007. *Medical Management of Chemical Casualties Handbook.* 4th ed. Aberdeen Proving Ground, MD: USAMRICD. Available at: http://www.globalsecurity.org/wmd/library/policy/army/other/mmcc-hbk_4th-ed.pdf. Accessed January 25, 2017.

InterAgency Board. Interactive standardized equipment list. Available at: https://iab.gov/SEL.aspx. Accessed January 25, 2017.

Cibulsky SM, Kirk MA, Ignacio JS, et al. 2014. *Patient Decontamination in a Mass Chemical Exposure Incident: National Planning Guidance for Communities.* Washington, DC: U.S. Department of Homeland Security, Department of Health & Human Services. Available at: http://www.dhs.gov/sites/default/files/publications/Patient%20Decon%20National%20Planning%20Guidance_Final_December%202014.pdf. Accessed January 25, 2017.

World Health Organization (WHO). 2009. *Manual for the Public Health Management of Chemical Accidents.* Geneva, Switzerland: WHO. Available at: http://www.who.int/environmental_health_emergencies/publications/Manual_Chemical_Incidents/en. Accessed January 25, 2017.

Communication

AnyLogic. 2016. AnyLogic: multimethod simulation software. Available at: http://www.anylogic.com. Accessed February 3, 2017.

Association of State and Territorial Health Officials (ASTHO). 2016. *Communication Toolkit, Promoting the Impact and Importance of the Public Health Emergency Preparedness Program.* Arlington, VA: ASTHO. Available at: https://pheptoolkit.files.wordpress.com/2016/04/phep-communications-toolkit-final-web.pdf. Accessed February 3, 2017.

Balachandran K, Budka KC, Chu TP, et al. 2006. Mobile responder communication networks for public safety. *IEEE Commun Mag.* 44(1):56–64.

Baseman JG, Revere D, Painter I, et al. 2013. Public health communications and alert fatigue. *BMC Health Servs Res.* 13:295.

Calhoun R, Young D, Meischke H, et al. 2009. Practice, more practice, best practice: improving our service to limited-English callers. *Wash State J Public Health Prac.* 2(1):34–37.

Carroll LN, Calhoun RE, Subido CC, et al. 2013. Serving limited English proficient callers: a survey of 9-1-1 police telecommunicators. *Prehosp Disaster Med.* 28(3):286–291.

Cates AL, Arnold BW, Cooper GP, et al. 2013. Impact of dual-polarization radar technology and Twitter on the Hattiesburg, Mississippi tornado. *Disaster Med Public Health Prep.* 7(6):585–592.

Centers for Disease Control and Prevention. 2015. CDC social media tools, guidelines & best practices. Atlanta, GA: CDC. Available at: http://www.cdc.gov/socialmedia/tools/guidelines. Accessed January 25, 2017.

Chamberlain AT, Seib K, Wells K, et al. 2012. Perspectives of immunization program managers on 2009-10 H1N1 vaccination in the United States: a national survey. *Biosecur Bioterror.* 10(1):142–150.

Cool CT, Claravall MC, Hall JL, et al. 2015. Social media as a risk communication tool following Typhoon Haiyan. *Western Pac Surveill Response J.* 6(Suppl 1):86–90.

Culleton E. 2013. How a "whole community" approach to social media in times of crisis increases its effectiveness. Emergency 2.0 Wiki. Available at: http://emergency20wiki.org/20130413/how-a-whole-of-community-approach-to-using-social-media-in-times-of-crisis-increases-its-effectiveness. Accessed January 25, 2017.

Daugherty JD, Eiring H, Blake S, et al. 2012. Disaster preparedness in home health and personal-care agencies: are they ready? *Gerontology*. 58(4):322–330.

Department of Homeland Security. 2016. *SAFECOM: Land Mobile Radio (LMR) 101*. Available at: https://www.dhs.gov/sites/default/files/publications/LMR%20101_508FINAL.pdf. Accessed February 3, 2017.

Evidence Aid Priority Setting Group EA. 2013. Prioritization of themes and research questions for health outcomes in natural disasters, humanitarian crises or other major healthcare emergencies. *PLoS Curr.* 5. Available at: http://www.ncbi.nlm.nih.gov/pmc/articles/PMC3805831/?report=classic. Accessed February 3, 2017.

Federal Communications Commission (FCC). 2010. *Amendment of Part 97 of the Commission's Rules Regarding Amateur Radio Service Communications During Government Disaster Drills.* Washington, DC: FCC. Available at: http://www.arrl.org/files/file/Regulatory/FCC-10-124A1.pdf. Accessed January 25, 2017.

Federal Emergency Management Agency. 2011. Integrated public alert & warning systems. Available at: http://www.fema.gov/integrated-public-alert-warning-system. Accessed January 25, 2017.

Federal Emergency Management Agency. 2015. Common alerting protocol. Available at: https://www.fema.gov/common-alerting-protocol. Accessed February 3, 2017.

First Responders Group, Department of Homeland Security. 2015. Advanced Communications Video Over LTE: Efficient Network Utilization Research. Available at: https://www.dhs.gov/sites/default/files/publications/VQiPS_T3X3_2%206%209%202_EfficientUtilization_MemorandumReport_Final_Draft_v4-508.pdf. Accessed February 3, 2017.

Fischhoff B, Lichtenstein S, Slovic P, et al. 1981. *Acceptable Risk.* Cambridge, MA: Cambridge University Press.

Galarce EM, Viswanath K. 2012. Crisis communication: an inequalities perspective on the 2010 Boston water crisis. *Disaster Med Public Health Prep.* 6(4):349–356.

Houston JB, Hawthorne J, Perreault MF, et al. 2015. Social media and disasters: a functional framework for social media use in disaster planning, response, and research. *Disasters.* 39(1):1–22.

Ivey SL, Tseng W, Dahrouge D, et al. 2014. Assessment of state- and territorial-level preparedness capacity for serving deaf and hard-of-hearing populations in disasters. *Public Health Rep.* 129(2):148–155.

Karasz H, Bogan S. 2011. What 2 know b4 u text: short message service opportunities for local health departments. *Wash State J Public Health Prac.* 4(1):20–27.

Karasz H, Bogan S. 2012. Investing in a text messaging system: a comparison of three solutions. *Northwest Public Health.* 29(1):20–21.

Karasz HN, Bogan S, Bosslet L. 2014. Communicating with the workforce during emergencies: developing an employee text messaging program in a local public health setting. *Public Health Rep.* 129(Suppl 4):61–66.

Karasz HN, Eiden A, Bogan S. 2013. Text messaging to communicate with public health audiences: how the HIPAA Security Rule affects practice. *Am J Public Health.* 103(4):617–622.

Kierkegaard P, Kaushal R, Vest JR. 2014. Applications of health information exchange information to public health practice. *AMIA Annu Symp Proc.* 2014:795–804.

Kim TJ, Arrieta MI, Eastburn SL, et al. 2013. Post-disaster Gulf Coast recovery using telehealth. *Telemed J E Health.* 19(3):200–210.

Kirchhoff K, Turner AM, Axelrod A, et al. 2011. Application of statistical machine translation to public health information: a feasibility study. *J Am Med Inform Assoc.* 18(4):473–478.

Kittler AF, Hobbs J, Volk LA, et al. 2004. The Internet as a vehicle to communicate health information during a public health emergency: a survey analysis involving the anthrax scare of 2001. *J Med Internet Res.* 6(1):e8.

Kryvasheyeu Y, Chen H, Obradovich N, et al. 2016. Rapid assessment of disaster damage using social media activity. *Sci Adv.* 2(3):e1500779.

Lagasse LP, Rimal RN, Smith KC, et al. 2011. How accessible was information about H1N1 flu? literacy assessments of CDC guidance documents for different audiences. *PLoS One.* 6(10):e23583.

Lien YN, Hung-Chin Jang HC, Tsai TC. 2009. A MANET based emergency communication and information system for catastrophic natural disasters. Paper presented at the 29th IEEE International Conference on Distributed Computing Systems Workshops. Available at: http://140.119.162.51/~lien/Pub/c76sahns.pdf. Accessed February 3, 2017.

Lin L, Jung M, McCloud R, et al. 2014. *Media Use and Communication Inequalities in a Public Health Emergency: A Case Study of 2009-2010 Pandemic Influenza A Virus Subtype H1N1.* Public Health Reports. Available at: http://www.ncbi.nlm.nih.gov/pmc/articles/PMC4187307/pdf/phr129s40049.pdf. Accessed February 3, 2017.

Lin L, Minsoo J, McCloud RF, et al. 2014. Media use and communication inequalities in a public health emergency: a case study of 2009–2010 pandemic influenza a virus subtype H1N1. *Public Health Rep.* 129(Suppl 4):49–60.

Magee M, Isakov A, Paradise HT, et al. 2011. Mobile phones and short message service texts to collect situational awareness data during simulated public health critical events. *Am J Disaster Med.* 6(6):379–386.

Mayo Clinic. 2016. Mayo Clinic Social Media Network. Available at: https://socialmedia.mayoclinic.org. Accessed February 3, 2017.

Meischke HW, Calhoun RE, Yip M-P, et al. 2013. The effect of language barriers on dispatching EMS response. *Prehospital Emergency Care*. 17(4):475–480.

Meranus D, Stergachis A, Arnold J, et al. 2012. Assessing vaccine safety communication with health care providers in a large urban county. *Pharmacoepidemiol Drug Saf.* 21(3):269–275.

Offenbecher W. 2012. *What Community Members Want from Public Health Text Messages.* NACCHO Preparedness Brief.

Ong BN, Yip MP, Feng S, et al. 2012. Barriers and facilitators to using 9-1-1 and emergency medical services in a limited English proficiency Chinese community. *J Immigr Minority Health*. 14(2):307–313.

Pollard W. 2003. Public perceptions of information sources concerning bioterrorism before and after anthrax attacks: an analysis of national survey data. *J Health Commun.* 8(Suppl 1):93–103.

Preis T, Moat HS, Bishop SR, et al. 2013. Quantifying the digital traces of Hurricane Sandy on Flickr. *Sci Rep*. 3:3141.

Researchgate. 2016. Is there a labelled dataset readily available for training classifiers to categorize text/tweets into one of the four (many) disaster phases? https://www.researchgate.net/post/Is_there_a_labelled_dataset_readily_available_for_training_classifiers_to_categorize_text_tweets_into_one_of_the_fourmany_disaster_phases. Accessed February 3, 2017.

Reeder B, Turner AM. 2011. Scenario-based design: A method for connecting information system design with public health operations and emergency management. *J Biomed Inform*. 44(6):978–988.

Revere D, Nelson K, Thiede H, et al. 2011. Public health emergency preparedness and response communications with health care providers: a literature review. *BMC Public Health*. 11:337.

Revere D, Painter I, Oberle M, et al. 2014. Health-care provider preferences for time-sensitive communications from public health agencies. *Public Health Rep*. 129(Suppl 4):67–76.

Revere D, Schwartz MR, Baseman J. 2014. How 2 txt: an exploration of crafting public health messages in SMS. *BMC Research Notes*. 7(1):514.

Rouil R, Izquierdo A, Gentile C, et al. 2015. *Nationwide Public Safety Broadband Network Deployment: Network Parameter Sensitivity Analysis.* Gaithersburg, MD: National Institute of Standards and Technology. Available at: http://nvlpubs.nist.gov/nistpubs/ir/2015/NIST.IR.8039.pdf. Accessed February 3, 2017.

Rubin S, Bouri N, Jolani N, et al. 2014. The adoption of social media and mobile health technologies for emergency preparedness by local health departments: a joint perspective from NACCHO and the UPMC center for health security. *J Public Health Manag Pract*. 20(2):259–263.

Savoia E, Stoto MA, Gupta R, et al. 2015. Public response to the 2014 chemical spill in West Virginia: knowledge, opinions and behaviours. *BMC Public Health*. 15:790.

Siskey A, Islam T. 2016. Social media best practices in emergency management. *J Emerg Manag.* 14(2):113–125.

Stokes C, Senkbeil JC. 2016. Facebook and Twitter, communication and shelter, and the 2011 Tuscaloosa tornado. *Disasters*. 41(1):194–208.

Sutton J. 2009. The public uses social networking during disasters to verify facts, coordinate information analysis, social; media package part 1 of 2. *Emerg Manage*. Available at: http://www.govtech.com/em/safety/The-Public-Uses-Social-Networking.html. Accessed February 3, 2017.

Tierney TF. 2014. Crowdsourcing disaster response: mobilizing social media for urban resilience. *Europ Bus Rev*. Available at: http://www.europeanbusinessreview.com/?p=4911. Accessed February 3, 2017.

U.S. Department of Homeland Security (DHS). 2005. *The System of Systems Approach for Interoperable Communications*. Washington, DC: DHS. Available at: http://www.npstc.org/download.jsp?tableId=37&column=217&id=2458&file=SOSApproachforInteroperableCommunications_02.pdf. Accessed January 25, 2017.

Vander M. 2010. How to: prepare for disasters using social media. *Mashable*. Available at: http://mashable.com/2010/03/09/prepare-disaster-social-media. Accessed January 25, 2017.

Veil S, Buehner T, Palenchar MJ. 2011. A work-in-process literature review: incoporating social media in risk and crisis communication. *J Contingencies Crisis Manag*. 19(2):110–122.

Williams R, Burton D. 2012. *The Use of Social Media for Disaster Recovery*. Available at: http://extension.missouri.edu/greene/documents/PlansReports/socia_media_in_disasters.pdf. Accessed February 3, 2017.

Wray RJ, Kreuter MW, Jacobsen J, et al. 2004. Theoretical perspectives on public communication preparedness for terrorist attacks. *Fam Commun Health*. 27(3):232–241.

Yasin R. 2010. 5 ways to use social media for better emergency response. *FCW*. Available at: https://fcw.com/articles/2010/09/06/social-media-emergency-management.aspx. Accessed February 3, 2017.

Yip MP, Ong B, Painter I, et al. 2008. Information-seeking behaviors and response to the H1N1 outbreak in Chinese limited-English proficient individuals living in King County, Washington. *Am J Disaster Med*. 4(6):353–360.

Yip MP, Ong BN, Meischke HW, et al. 2013. The role of self-efficacy in communication and emergency response in Chinese limited English proficiency (LEP) populations. Health promotion practice. 14(3):400–407.

Cultural Considerations

Athey J, Moody-Williams J. 2003. *Developing Cultural Competence in Disaster Mental Health Programs. Washington, DC: U.S. Department of Health & Human Services, Substance Abuse and Mental Health Service Administration*. Available at: http://calmhsa.org/wp-content/uploads/2011/11/Developing-Cultural-Competence-in-Disaster-MH-Prog.pdf. Accessed January 25, 2017.

Betancourt JR, Green AR, Carrillo JE, et al. 2003. Defining cultural competence: a practical framework for addressing racial/ethnic disparities in health and health care. *Public Health Rep.* 118(4):293–302.

Davidson TM, Price M, McCauley JL, et al. 2013. Disaster impact across cultural groups: comparison of whites, African Americans, and Latinos. *Am J Community Psychol.* 52(1-2):97–105.

Montgomery County Advanced Practice Center. 2008. Emergency preparedness training curriculum for Latino health promoters. Available at: http://www.cidrap.umn.edu/practice/emergency-preparedness-training-curriculum-latino-promoters-md. Accessed January 25, 2017.

Moore T. 2010. *Institutional Barriers to Resilience in Minority Communities.* Durham, NC: Institute for Homeland Security Solutions. Available at: https://sites.duke.edu/ihss/files/2011/12/IHSS_Moore.pdf. Accessed January 25, 2017.

Nunez A, Robertson C. 2006. Cultural competence. In: Satcher D, Primes RJ, eds. *Multicultural Medicine and Health Disparities.* New York, NY: McGraw Hill.

Shiu-Thornton S, Balabis J, Senturia K, et al. 2007. Disaster preparedness for Limited English Proficient (LEP) communities: medical interpreters as cultural brokers and gatekeepers. *Public Health Rep.* 122(4):466–471.

Curriculum

Gebbie KM. 1999. The public health workforce: key to public health infrastructure. *Am J Public Health.* 89(5):660–661.

Landesman LY. 1993. The availability of disaster preparation courses at US schools of public health. *Am J Public Health.* 83(10):1494–1495.

Landesman LY, ed. 2001. *Disaster Preparedness in Schools of Public Health: A Curriculum for the New Century.* Washington, DC: Association of Schools of Public Health.

Qureshi KA, Gershon RRM, Merrill JA, et al. 2004. Effectiveness of an emergency preparedness training program for public health nurses in New York City. *Fam Commun Health.* 27(3):242–249.

Cyclone

Malilay J. 1997. Tropical cyclones. In: Noji EK, ed. *The Public Health Consequences of Disasters.* New York, NY: Oxford University Press. 287–301.

General Disasters

Dynes RR, Tierney KJ, eds. 1994. *Disasters, Collective Behavior, and Social Organization.* Newark, NJ: University of Delaware Press.

Disabilities, Access and Functional Needs

Association of Schools of Public Health (ASPH); Centers for Disease Control and Prevention (CDC). 2006. *ASPH/CDC Collaboration Group on Emergency Preparedness and Vulnerable Populations: Educational Resources*. Atlanta, GA: CDC. Available at: http://lms.southcentralpartnership.org/AdditionalCourseMaterial/P227/P227_module2matrix.pdf. Accessed February 3, 2017.

Centers for Disease Control and Prevention (CDC). 2010. *Public Health Workbook to Define, Locate, and Reach Special, Vulnerable, and At-Risk Populations in an Emergency*. Atlanta, GA: CDC. Available at: http://emergency.cdc.gov/workbook/pdf/ph_workbookfinal.pdf. Accessed February 3, 2017.

Centers for Disease Control and Prevention (CDC). 2015. Planning for an Emergency:

Strategies for Identifying and Engaging At-Risk Groups. Atlanta, GA: CDC. Available at: http://www.cdc.gov/nceh/hsb/disaster/atriskguidance.pdf. Accessed February 3, 2017.

Cutter SL, Boruff BJ, Shirley WL. 2003. Social vulnerability to environmental hazards. *Soc Sci Q*. 84(2):242–261.

Americans with Disabilities Act. 2008. An ADA guide for local governments: making community emergency preparedness and response programs accessible to people with disabilities. Available at: https://www.ada.gov/emergencyprepguide.htm. Accessed February 3, 2017.

Ringel JS, Chandra A, Williams M, et al. 2009. *Enhancing Public Health Emergency Preparedness for Special Needs Populations: A Toolkit for State and Local Planning and Response*. Santa Monica, CA: RAND. Available at: http://www.rand.org/pubs/technical_reports/TR681. Accessed February 3, 2017.

Children

Centers for Bioterrorism Preparedness Planning Pediatric Task Force; New York City Department of Health and Mental Health Pediatric Disaster Advisory Group. 2006. *Hospital Guidelines for Pediatrics in Disasters*. 2nd ed. Available at: https://www.omh.ny.gov/omhweb/disaster_resources/pandemic_influenza/hospitals/bhpp_focus_ped_toolkit.pdf. Accessed February 3, 2017.

Markenson D, Redlener I. 2003. *Pediatric Preparedness for Disasters and Terrorism: A National Consensus Conference. Executive Summary*. New York, NY: National Center for Disaster Preparedness. Available at: https://www.aap.org/en-us/advocacy-and-policy/aap-health-initiatives/Children-and-Disasters/Documents/execsumm03.pdf. Accessed February 3, 2017.

Norris FH, Friedman MJ, Watson PJ, et al. 2002. 60,000 disaster victims speak: part I: an empirical review of the empirical literature, 1981–2001. *Psychiatry*. 65(3):207–239.

Weiner DL. 2009. Lessons learned from disasters affecting children. *Ped Emerg Med*. 10(3): 149–152.

Dementia

Alzheimer's Association, RTI International. *Disaster Preparedness: Home and Community-Based Services for People With Dementia and Their Caregivers.* Research Triangle Park, NC: RTI International. Available at: http://www.une.edu/sites/default/files/Toolkit_2_Disaster_Preparedness.pdf. Accessed February 3, 2017.

Dialysis

Centers for Medicare and Medicaid Services. 2007. *Preparing for Emergencies: A Guide for People on Dialysis.* Available at: https://www.cms.gov/Outreach-and-Education/Medicare-Learning-Network-MLN/MLNProducts/downloads/10150.pdf. Accessed February 3, 2017.

Disabilities

Commonwealth of Massachusetts. 2016. *Access and Functional Needs Resource Guide.* Available at: http://www.mass.gov/eohhs/docs/dph/emergency-prep/dph-afn-resource-guide.pdf. Accessed February 3, 2017.

Disability Rights Section, Civil Rights Division. 2007. *Americans With Disabilities Act: ADA Checklist for Emergency Shelters.* Washington, DC: U.S. Department of Justice. Available at: https://www.ada.gov/pcatoolkit/chap7shelterchk.htm. Accessed February 3, 2017.

Fernandez LS, Byard D, Lin CC. 2002. Frail elderly as disaster victims: emergency management strategies. *Prehosp Disaster Med.* 17(2):67–74.

Kailes JI, Enders A. 2007. Moving beyond special needs: a function–based framework for emergency management and planning. *J Disability Policy Stud.* 17(4):230–237.

Kailes JI. 2016. Individual emergency preparedness for people with disabilities, their families and support networks. Playa del Rey, CA: June Isaacson Kailes. Available at: http://www.jik.com/disaster-individ.html. Accessed February 3, 2017.

Kailes JI. 2002. *Emergency Evacuation Preparedness: Taking Responsibility for Your Safety: A Guide for People With Disabilities and Other Activity Limitations.* Pomona, CA: Center for Disability Issues and the Health Professions, Western University of Health Sciences. Available at: https://und.edu/affirmative-action/_files/docs/emergencyevacuation.pdf. Accessed February 3, 2017.

U.S. Access Board. 2001. Resources on emergency evacuation and disaster preparedness. Available at: http://www.icdri.org/inspirational/resources_on_emergency_evacuatio.htm. Accessed March 30, 2017.

Ethnic Communities

Andrulis DP, Siddiqui NJ, Gantner JL. 2007. Preparing racially and ethnically diverse communities for public health emergencies. *Health Aff (Millwood).* 26(5):1269–1279.

Carter-Pokras O, Zambrana RE, Mora SE, et al. 2007. Emergency preparedness: knowledge and perceptions of Latin American immigrants. *J Health Care Poor Underserved.* 18(2): 465–481.

Home Health Agencies

National Association for Home Care and Hospice (NAHCH). 2008. *Emergency Preparedness Packet for Home Health Agencies.* Washington, DC: NAHCH. Available at: http://www.nahc.org/assets/1/7/EP_Binder.pdf. Accessed February 3, 2017.

Older Adults

Aldrich N, Benson W. 2008. Disaster preparedness and the chronic disease needs of vulnerable older adults. *Prev Chronic Dis.* 5(1):A27.

Centers for Disease Control and Prevention (CDC) Healthy Aging Program. 2006. *Disaster Planning Tips for Older Adults and Their Families.* Atlanta, GA: CDC. Available at: https://www.cdc.gov/aging/pdf/disaster_planning_tips.pdf. Accessed February 3, 2017.

Fernandez LS, Byard D, Lin CC, et al. 2002. Frail elderly as disaster victims: emergency management strategies. *Prehosp Disaster Med.* 17(2):67–74.

Gibson MJ. 2006. *We Can Do Better: Lessons Learned for Protecting Older Persons in Disasters.* Washington, DC: AARP. Available at: http://assets.aarp.org/rgcenter/il/better.pdf. Accessed February 3, 2017.

Wilken CS, Gillen M. 2012. *Preparing for a Disaster: Strategies for Older Adults.* Gainesville, FL: University of Florida Institute of Food and Agricultural Sciences Extension Electronic Data Information Source. Available at: http://edis.ifas.ufl.edu/fy750. Accessed February 3, 2017.

Pandemics

Bouye K, Truman B, Hutchins S, et al. 2009. Pandemic influenza preparedness and response among public-housing residents, single parent families, and low-income populations. *Am J Public Health.* 99(Suppl 2):S287–S293.

Groom A, Jim C, LaRoque M, et al. 2009. Pandemic influenza preparedness and vulnerable populations in tribal communities. *Am J Public Health.* 99(Suppl 2):S271–S278.

Hutchins S, Truman B, Merlin T, et al. 2009. Protecting vulnerable populations from pandemic influenza in the United States: a strategic imperative. *Am J Public Health.* 99(Suppl 2): S243–S248.

Truman B, Tinker T, Vaughn E, et al. 2009. Pandemic influenza preparedness and response among immigrants and refugees. *Am J Public Health.* 99(Suppl 2):S278–S286.

Vaughn E, Tinker T. 2009. Effective health risk communication about pandemic influenza for vulnerable populations. *Am J Public Health.* 99(Suppl 2):S324–S332.

Planning

National Council on Disability (NCD). 2005. Saving Lives: Including People With Disabilities in Emergency Planning. Washington, DC: NCD. Available at: http://www.ncd.gov/publications/2005/saving-lives-including-people-disabilities-emergency-planning. Accessed January 25, 2017.

Earthquake

Bissell RA, Pinet P, Nelson M, et al. 2004. Evidence of the effectiveness of health sector preparedness in disaster response: the example of four earthquakes. *Fam Community Health.* 27(3):193–203.

Guha-Sapir D. 1991. Rapid assessment of health needs in mass emergencies: review of current concepts and methods. *World Health Stat Q.* 44(3):171–181.

Guha-Sapir D. 1993. Health effects of earthquakes and volcanoes: epidemiological and policy issues. *Disasters.* 17(3):255–262.

Noji EK. 1997. Earthquakes. In: Noji EK, ed. *The Public Health Consequences of Disasters.* New York, NY: Oxford University Press. 135–178.

Environmental Control

Berry MA, Bishop J, Blackburn C, et al. 2009. *Suggested Guidelines for Remediation of Damage from Sewage Backflow into Buildings*. Research Triangle Park, NC: U.S. Environmental Protection Agency. Available at: http://inspectapedia.com/hazmat/Sewage_Remediatin_EPA_Berry.pdf. Accessed January 25, 2017.

Boyce JM, Pittet D, eds. 2002. *Guideline for Hand Hygiene in Health-Care Settings: Recommendations of the Healthcare Infection Control Practice Advisory Committee of the HICPA/SHEA/APIC/Hand Hygiene Task Force.* Atlanta, GA: Centers for Disease Control and Prevention. Available at: http://www.cdc.gov/mmwr/PDF/rr/rr5116.pdf. Accessed January 25, 2017.

California Conference of Directors of Environmental Health. 2012. *Disaster Field Manual for Environmental Health Specialists.* Cameron Park, CA: California Association of Environmental Health Administrators. Available at: http://www.ccdeh.com/resources/products-for-sale/disaster-field-manual. Accessed January 30, 2017.

Centers for Disease Control and Prevention. 2016. Hand hygiene in healthcare settings. Available at: https://www.cdc.gov/handhygiene. Accessed January 30, 2017.

Centers for Disease Control and Prevention (CDC). 2009. *Fact Sheet for Healthy Drinking Water: Drinking Water Treatment Methods for Backcountry and Travel Use.* Atlanta, GA: CDC. Available at: http://www.cdc.gov/healthywater/pdf/drinking/Backcountry_Water_Treatment.pdf. Accessed January 30, 2017.

Centers for Disease Control and Prevention. 2014. Disinfecting wells after a disaster. Table 1: Approximate amount of bleach for disinfection of a bored or dug well. Available at: https://www.cdc.gov/disasters/wellsdisinfect.html. Accessed January 30, 2017.

Claudio L, Garg A, Landrigan PJ. 2003. Addressing environmental health concerns. In: *Terrorism and Public Health.* Levy BS, Sidel VW, eds. New York, NY: Oxford University Press.

Diaz JH. 2004. The public health impact of global climate change. *Fam Community Health.* 27(3):218–229.

Disaster Preparedness Technical Advisory Committee, Community Health Technical Advisory Committee. 2006. *Environmental Health Disaster Preparedness Model Planning Guide.* Carmichael, CA: California Association of Environmental Health Administrators. Available at: http://www.ccdeh.com/resources/documents/products-1/67-ccdeh-environmental-health-disaster-preparedness-model-planning-guide-2006-1/file. Accessed January 30, 2017.

Esrey SA, Potash JB, Roberts L, et al. 1991. Effects of improved water supply and sanitation on ascariasis, diarrhoea, dracunculiasis, hookworm infection, schistosomiasis, and trachoma. *Bull World Health Organ.* 69(5):609–621.

Golob BR. 2007. *Environmental Health Emergency Response Guide.* Hopkins, MN: Twin Cities Metro Advanced Practice Center. Available at: http://www.cdc.gov/nceh/ehs/Docs/EH_Emergency_Response_Guide.pdf. Accessed January 30, 2017.

Hatch D, Waldman RJ, Lungu GW, et al. 1994. Epidemic cholera during refugee resettlement in Malawi. *Int J Epidemiol.* 23(6):1292–1299.

Houston Department of Health & Human Services, City of Houston. 2005. Food surveillance and salvage following disasters. Available at: http://www.houstontx.gov/health/Food/food-surv.htm. Accessed January 30, 2017.

National Fire Protection Association (NFPA). 2016. *NFPA 1600 Standard on Disaster/Emergency Management and Business Continuity Programs.* 2016 ed. Quincy, MA: NFPA. Available at: http://www.nfpa.org/codes-and-standards/all-codes-and-standards/list-of-codes-and-standards?mode=code&code=1600. Accessed January 25, 2017.

National Institute for Occupational Safety and Health. 2003. *Guidance for Filtration and Air-Cleaning Systems to Protect Building Environments From Airborne Chemical, Biological, or Radiological Attacks.* Washington, DC: Department of Health & Human Services. Available at: https://www.cdc.gov/niosh/docs/2003-136/pdfs/2003-136.pdf. Accessed January 25, 2017.

Occupational Safety and Health Administration. 2016. Evacuation plans and procedures eTool. Available at: https://www.osha.gov/SLTC/etools/evacuation/eap.html. Accessed January 30, 2017.

Occupational Safety and Health Administration. 2006. Hazardous waste operations and emergency response standard. Available at: https://www.osha.gov/pls/oshaweb/owadisp.show_document?p_table=STANDARDS&p_id=9765. Accessed January 25, 2017.

Peterson AE, Roberts L, Toole M, et al. 1998. Soap use effect on diarrhea: Nyamithuthu refugee camp. *Int J Epidemiol.* 27(3):520–524.

Spears MC, Gregoire M, Spears M. 2007. *Foodservice Organizations: A Managerial and Systems Approach.* 6th ed. New York, NY: Pearson Education.

U.S. Environmental Protection Agency. 2012. *2012 Edition of the Drinking Water Standards and Health Advisories.* Microbiology table, page 11. Washington, DC: EPA. Available at: https://www.epa.gov/sites/production/files/2015-09/documents/dwstandards2012.pdf. Accessed January 30, 2017.

U.S. Environmental Protection Agency (EPA). 2012. Particulate matter (PM) standards—table of historical PM national ambient air quality standards (NAAQS). Washington, DC: EPA. Available at: http://www3.epa.gov/ttn/naaqs/standards/pm/s_pm_history.html. Accessed January 30, 2017.

Washington State Department of Health. 2013. Purifying water during an emergency. 2013. Available at: http://www.doh.wa.gov/Emergencies/EmergencyPreparednessandResponse/Factsheets/WaterPurification. Accessed January 30, 2017.

Wisner B, Adams J, eds. 2002. *Control Measures for Ensuring Food Safety From Environmental Health in Emergencies and Disasters.* Geneva, Switzerland: World Health Organization.

Mold

Brandt M, Brown C, Burkhart J, et al. 2006. Mold prevention strategies and possible health effects in the aftermath of hurricanes and major floods. *MMWR Recomm Rep.* 55(RR-1):1–27.

Centers for Disease Control and Prevention, Environmental Protection Agency, Federal Emergency Management Agency, Department of Housing and Urban Development, and National Institutes of Health. 2015. *Homeowner's and Renter's Guide to Mold Cleanup After Disasters.* Available at: http://www.cdc.gov/mold/pdfs/homeowners_and_renters_guide.pdf. Accessed January 30, 2017.

Chew GL, Horner WE, Kennedy K, et al. 2016. Procedures to assist health care providers to determine when home assessments for potential mold exposure are warranted. *J Allergy Clin Immunol Pract.* 4(3):417–422.

Environmental Protection Agency. 2010. A brief guide to mold, moisture, and your home. Available at: https://www.epa.gov/mold/brief-guide-mold-moisture-and-your-home. Accessed January 30, 2017.

Environmental Protection Agency. 2008. *Mold Remediation in Schools and Commercial Buildings.* Available at: https://www.epa.gov/sites/production/files/2014-08/documents/moldremediation.pdf. Accessed January 30, 2017.

New York City Department of Health and Mental Hygiene. 2008. *Guidelines on Assessment and Remediation of Fungi in Indoor Environments.* Available at: https://www1.nyc.gov/assets/doh/downloads/pdf/epi/epi-mold-guidelines.pdf. Accessed January 30, 2017.

UConn Health. Center for Indoor Environments and Health. 2013. *Mold and Moisture Clean-up After the Storm: A Guide for Your Safety.* Available at: http://hurricane-weather-health.doem.uconn.edu/wp-content/uploads/sites/807/2014/07/5.29.-15-UCONN-Guide-for-your-safety-logo-on-front-_website-update.png. Accessed January 30, 2017.

World Health Organization. 2009. *Guidelines for Indoor Air Quality Dampness and Mold.* Available at: http://www.euro.who.int/__data/assets/pdf_file/0017/43325/E92645.pdf. Accessed January 25, 2017.

Epidemic

Connolly, MA, ed. *A Field Manual: Communicable Disease Control in Emergencies.* 2005. Geneva, Switzerland: World Health Organization. Available at: http://whqlibdoc.who.int/publications/2005/9241546166_eng.pdf. Accessed January 30, 2017.

Manderson L, Aaby P. 1992. An epidemic in the field? Rapid assessment procedures and health research. *Soc Sci Med.* 35(7):839–850.

Toole MJ. 1994. The rapid assessment of health problems in refugee and displaced populations. *Med Global Survival.* 1(4):200–207.

Toole MJ. 1997. Communicable diseases and disease control. In: Noji EK, ed. *The Public Health Consequences of Disasters.* New York, NY: Oxford University Press: 79–100.

Toole MJ, Waldman R. 1993. Refugees and displaced persons: war, hunger, and public health. *JAMA.* 270(5):600–605.

World Health Organization (WHO). 1999. *Rapid Health Assessment Protocols for Emergencies.* Geneva, Switzerland: WHO.

Ethics

Bayer R, Gostin LO, Jennings B, et al, eds. 2007. *Public Health Ethics: Theory, Policy and Practice.* New York, NY: Oxford University Press.

Centers for Disease Control and Prevention. *Ethical Guidelines in Pandemic Influenza.* 2007. Available at: http://www.cdc.gov/od/science/integrity/phethics/panFlu_Ethic_Guidelines.pdf. Accessed January 30, 2017.

Centers for Disease Control and Prevention. *Public Health Law 101: A CDC* Foundational course for public health practitioners. Available at: http://www.cdc.gov/phlp/publications/phl_101.html. Accessed January 25, 2017.

Gostin L. 2006. Public health strategies for pandemic influenza: ethics and the law. *JAMA*. 295(14):1700–1704.

Hick JL, Hanfling D, Cantrill SV. 2012. Allocating scarce resources in disasters: emergency department principles. *Ann Emerg Med*. 59(3):177–187.

Jennings B. 2008. *Disaster Planning and Public Health*. Garrison, NY: The Hastings Center.

Jennings B, Arras J. *Ethical Guidance for Public Health Emergency Preparedness and Response: Highlighting Ethics and Values in a Vital Public Health Service*. 2008. Atlanta, GA: Centers for Disease Control and Prevention. Available at: http://www.cdc.gov/od/science/integrity/phethics/docs/White_Paper_Final_for_Website_2012_4_6_12_final_for_web_508_compliant.pdf. Accessed January 30, 2017.

Pandemic Influenza Working Group. 2005. *Stand on Guard for Thee: Ethical Considerations in Preparedness Planning for Pandemic Influenza*. Toronto, Ontario: University of Toronto Joint Centre for Bioethics. Available at: http://www.jointcentreforbioethics.ca/people/documents/upshur_stand_guard.pdf. Accessed January 25, 2017.

Phillips SJ, Knebel A, eds. 2007. *Mass Medical Care with Scarce Resources: A Community Planning Guide*. Rockville, MD: Agency for Healthcare Research and Quality. Available at: http://archive.ahrq.gov/research/mce/mceguide.pdf. Accessed January 30, 2017.

Pou A. 2013. Ethical and legal challenges in disaster medicine are you ready? *South Med J*. 106(1):27–30.

Presidential Commission for the Study of Bioethical Issues. 2015. *Ethics and Ebola: Public Health Planning and Response*. Available at: http://bioethics.gov/sites/default/files/Ethics-and-Ebola_PCSBI_508.pdf. Accessed January 30, 2017.

The Sphere Project. 2011. Humanitarian charter and minimum standards in humanitarian response. Available at: http://www.sphereproject.org. Accessed January 25, 2017.

Thompson AK, Faith K, Gibson JL, et al. 2006. Pandemic influenza preparedness: an ethical framework to guide decision-making. *BMC Med Ethics*. 7:E12.

Venkat A, Asher SL, Wolf L, et al. 2015. Ethical issues in the response to ebola virus disease in united states emergency departments: a position paper of the american college of emergency physicians, the emergency nurses association, and the society for academic emergency medicine. *Acad Emerg Med*. 22(5):605–615.

Wisconsin State Expert Panel on the Ethics of Disaster Preparedness, Wisconsin Division of Public Health, and the Wisconsin Hospital Association. 2008. *Ethics of Health Care Disaster Preparedness*. Available at: http://pandemic.wisconsin.gov/docview.asp?docid=14447. Accessed January 30, 2017.

World Health Organization. 2015. *Ethics in Epidemics, Emergencies and Disasters: Research, Surveillance and Patient Care, Training Manual*. Available at: http://apps.who.int/iris/bitstream/10665/196326/1/9789241549349_eng.pdf. Accessed January 30, 2017.

Evaluation Methods Applied to Emergencies and Disasters

Bissell R, Pretto E, Angus D, et al. 1994. Post-preparedness medical disaster response in Costa Rica. *Prehosp Disaster Med.* 9(2):96–106.

De Boer J. 1997. Tools for evaluating disasters: preliminary results of some hundreds of disasters. *Eur J Emerg Med.* 4(2):107–110.

Institute of Medicine. 2015. *Enabling Rapid and Sustainable Public Health Research During Disasters: Summary of a Joint Workshop by the Institute of Medicine and the U.S. Department of Health & Human Services.* Washington, DC: Institute of Medicine.

Leinhos M, Qari SH, Williams-Johnson M. 2014. Preparedness and emergency response research centers: using a public health systems approach to improve all-hazards preparedness and response. *Public Health Rep.* 129(Suppl 4):8–18.

Ricci E. 1985. A model for evaluation of disaster management. *Prehosp Disaster Med.* Suppl 1.

Thorpe LE, Assari S, Deppen S, et al. 2015. The role of epidemiology in disaster response policy development. *Ann Epidemiol.* 25(5):377–386.

Flood

Malilay J. 1997. Floods. In: Noji EK, ed. *The Public Health Consequences of Disasters.* New York, NY: Oxford University Press. 287–301.

Geographic Information Systems

Amdahl G. 2001. *Disaster Response: GIS for Public Safety.* Redlands, CA: ESRI Press.

Cromley EK, McLafferty SL. 2002. *GIS and Public Health.* New York, NY: The Guilford Press.

Enders A, Brandt Z. 2007. Using geographic information system technology to improve emergency management and disaster response for people with disabilities. *J Disability Policy Stud.* 17(4):223–229.

ESRI. 2008. *Geographic Information Systems Providing the Platform for Comprehensive Emergency Management.* Redlands, CA: ESRI. Available at: http://www.esri.com/library/whitepapers/pdfs/gis-platform-emergency-management.pdf. Accessed January 30, 2017.

Greene RW. 2002. *Confronting Catastrophe: A GIS Handbook.* Redlands, CA: ESRI Press.

Kennedy H, ed. 2001. *Dictionary of GIS Terminology.* Redlands, CA: ESRI Press.

Lang L. 2000. *GIS for Health Organizations.* Redlands, CA: ESRI Press.

McLeod J. 2010. *A Risk Too Great: Using Unmanaged GIS Data For Emergency Notification*. Nashville, TN: Infocode. Available at: http://www.infocode.com/whitepaper.php. Accessed January 30, 2017.

Skinner R. 2011. Integrating location into hospital and healthcare facility emergency management. *J Healthcare Prot Manage*. 27(1):31–35.

Handling Dead Bodies

Jenson PA, Lambert LA, Iademarco MF, et al. 2005. Guidelines for preventing the transmission of Mycobacterium tuberculosis in health-care settings, 2005. *MMWR Recomm Rep*. 54(RR-17):1–141. Available at: http://www.cdc.gov/mmwr/pdf/rr/rr5417.pdf. Accessed January 30, 2017.

Demiryurek D, Bayramoglu A, Ustacelebi S. 2002. Infective agents in fixed human cadavers: a brief review and suggested guidelines. *Anat Rec*. 269(4):194–197.

Gershon RR, Vlahov D, Escamilla JA, et al. 1998. Tuberculosis risk in funeral home employees. *J Occup Environ Med*. 40(5):497–503.

Healing TD, Hoffman PN, Young SEE. 1995. The infectious hazards of human cadavers. *Commun Dis Rep CDR Rev*. 5(5):R61–R68.

Pan American Health Organization (PAHO). 2004. *Management of Dead Bodies in Disaster Situations*. Washington, DC: PAHO. Available at: http://www.who.int/hac/techguidance/management_of_dead_bodies.pdf. Accessed January 30, 2017.

World Health Organization. 2008. *Disposal of Dead Bodies in Emergency Conditions*. Available at: http://www.who.int/water_sanitation_health/publications/2011/WHO_TN_08_Disposal_of_dead_bodies.pdf. Accessed January 30, 2017.

Health Care Coalitions

Acosta J, Howard S, Chandra A, et al. 2015. Contributions of health care coalitions to preparedness and resilience: perspectives from hospital preparedness program and health care preparedness coalitions. *Disaster Med Public Health Prep*. 9(6):690–697.

Assistant Secretary of Preparedness (ASPR). 2016. *TRACIE: Coalition Models and Functions*. Washington, DC: ASPR. Available at: https://asprtracie.hhs.gov/Documents/coalition-models-and-functions.pdf. Accessed January 30, 2017.

Barr P. 2012. Coming together: coalitions offer cooperative approach to disasters. *Mod Healthc*. 42(45):14.

Carrier, Yee T, Cross D, et al. 2012. Emergency preparedness and community coalitions: opportunities and challenges. *Res Brief*. (24):1-9.

Cormier S, Wargo M, Winslow W. 2015. Transforming health care coalitions from hospitals to whole of community: lessons learned from two large health care organizations. *Disaster Med Public Health Prep.* 9(6):712–716.

Courtney B, Toner E, Waldhorn R, et al. 2009. Healthcare coalitions: the new foundation for national healthcare preparedness and response for catastrophic health emergencies. *Biosecur Bioterror.* 7(2):153–163.

Dobalian A. 2015. The US Department of Veterans Affairs and Sustainable Health Care Coalitions. *Disaster Med Public Health Prep.* 9(6):726–727.

Dornauer ME. 2015. In preparation or response: examining health care coalitions amid a changing economic and political landscape. *Disaster Med Public Health Prep.* 9(6):698–703.

Einav S, Hick JL, Hanfling D, et al. 2014. Surge capacity logistics: care of the critically ill and injured during pandemics and disasters: CHEST consensus statement. *Chest.* 146(4 Suppl):e17S–e43S.

Harris C. 2015. Health care coalitions: The Georgia approach. *Disaster Med Public Health Prep.* 9(6):599.

Hinton CF, Griese SE, Anderson MR, et al. 2015. CDC grand rounds: addressing preparedness challenges for children in public health emergencies. *MMWR Morb Mortal Wkly Rep.* 64(35):972–974.

Hupert N, Biala K, Holland T, et al. 2015. Optimizing health care coalitions: conceptual frameworks and a research agenda. *Disaster Med Public Health Prep.* 9(6):717–723.

Kenningham K, Koelemay K, King MA. 2014. Pediatric disaster triage education and skills assessment: a coalition approach. *J Emerg Manag.* 12(2):141–151.

Leonhardt KK, Keuler M, Safdar N, et al. 2015. Ebola preparedness planning and collaboration by two health systems in Wisconsin, September to December 2014. *Disaster Med Public Health Prep.* 10(4):691–697.

U.S. Department of Health & Human Services. *The Next Challenge in Healthcare Preparedness: Catastrophic Health Events.* 2010. Baltimore, MD: Center for Biosecurity of UPMC. Available at: http://www.upmchealthsecurity.org/our-work/pubs_archive/pubs-pdfs/2010/2010-01-29-prepreport.pdf. Accessed January 30, 2017.

Priest C, Stryckman B. 2015. Identifying indirect benefits of federal health care emergency preparedness grant funding to coalitions: a content analysis. *Disaster Med Public Health Prep.* 9(6):704–711.

Rambhia KJ, Waldhorn RE, Selck F, et al. 2012. A survey of hospitals to determine the prevalence and characteristics of health care coalitions for emergency preparedness and response. *Biosecur Bioterror.* 10(3):304–313.

U.S. Department of Health & Human Services. 2007. *Medical Surge Capacity Handbook.* Available at: http://www.phe.gov/preparedness/planning/mscc/handbook/pages/default.aspx. Accessed January 30, 2017.

U.S. Department of Health & Human Services. 2009. *MSCC: The Healthcare Coalition in Emergency Response and Recovery.* Available at: http://www.phe.gov/Preparedness/planning/mscc/health carecoalition/Pages/default.aspx. Accessed January 30, 2017.

Walsh J, Swan AG. 2016. Utilization of health care coalitions and resiliency forums in the united states and united kingdom: different approaches to strengthen emergency preparedness. *Disaster Med Public Health Prep.* 10(1):161–164.

Walsh L, Craddock H, Gulley K, et al. 2015. Building health care system capacity: training health care professionals in disaster preparedness health care coalitions. *Prehosp Disaster Med.* 30(2):123–130.

Walsh L, Craddock H, Gulley K, et al. 2016. Building health care system capacity to respond to disasters: successes and challenges of disaster preparedness health care coalitions. *Prehosp Disaster Med.* 30(2):112-122.

Hospital Preparedness

Centers for Disease Control and Prevention. 2015. Immediate need for healthcare facilities to review procedures for cleaning, disinfecting, and sterilizing reusable medical devices. Available at: http://emergency.cdc.gov/han/han00382.asp. Accessed January 25, 2017.

Delaney KA. 2002. Impact of the threat of biological and chemical terrorism on public safety-net hospitals. *Int Lawyer.* 36(1):21–28.

Joint Commission on Accreditation of Healthcare Organizations. 2003. *Health Care at the Crossroads: Strategies for Creating and Sustaining Community-wide Emergency Preparedness Systems.* Oakbrook Terrace, IL: The Joint Commission. Available at: http://www.jointcommission.org/assets/1/18/emergency_preparedness.pdf. Accessed January 30, 2017.

Henderson T, Campbell S. 2015. Laboratory preparedness: Ebola and other emerging infectious diseases. Now that the immediate crisis has passed, what have hospitals in the United States learned? *MLO Med Lab Obs.* 47(3):8–9.

Landesman LY, ed. 1997. *Emergency Preparedness in the Healthcare Environment.* Oakbrook, IL: Joint Commission on Accreditation of Healthcare Organizations.

Landesman LY, Leonard R. 1993. SARA three years later: physician knowledge and actions in hospital preparedness. *Prehosp Disaster Med.* 8(1):39–44.

Landesman LY, Markowitz SB, Rosenberg SN. 1994. Hospital preparedness for chemical accidents: the effect of environmental legislation on health care services. *Prehosp Disaster Med.* 9(3):154–159.

Landesman LY. 1994. *Hospital Preparedness for Chemical Accidents: Plant, Technology and Safety Management Series.* Oakbrook, IL: Joint Commission on Accreditation of Healthcare Organizations.

Osgood R, Scanlon C, Jotwani R, et al. 2015. Shaken but prepared: Analysis of disaster response at an academic medical centre following the Boston Marathon bombings. *J Bus Contin Emer Plan.* 9(2):177–184.

Peters MS. 1996. Hospitals respond to water loss during the Midwest floods of 1993: preparedness and improvisation. *J Emerg Med.* 14(3):345–350.

Salinas C, Salinas C, Kurata J. 1998. The effects of the Northridge earthquake on the pattern of emergency department care. *Am J Emerg Med.* 16(3):254–256.

Simon HK, Stegelman M, Button T. 1998. A prospective evaluation of pediatric emergency care during the 1996 Summer Olympic Games in Atlanta, Georgia. *Pediatr Emerg Care.* 14(1):1–3.

Information Systems

Federal Communications Commission. 2015. Disaster information reporting system (DIRS). Available at: http://www.fcc.gov/pshs/services/cip/dirs/dirs.html. Accessed January 30, 2017.

O'Carroll PW, Friede A, Noji EK, et al. 1995. The rapid implementation of a statewide emergency health information system during the 1993 Iowa flood. *Am J Public Health.* 85(4):564–567.

Van Bemmel JH, Musen MA, eds. 1997. *Handbook of Medical Informatics.* Houten, the Netherlands: Bohn Stafleu Van Loghum.

Legal

ABA Center on Children and the Law. 2008. *Children, Law, and Disasters: What We Learned From Katrina and the Hurricanes of 2005.* Houston, TX: University of Houston's Center for Children, Law and Policy.

Centers for Disease Control and Prevention. 2014. *Selected Federal Legal Authorities Pertinent to Public Health Emergencies.* Available at: https://www.cdc.gov/phlp/docs/ph-emergencies.pdf. Accessed January 30, 2017.

Centers for Medicare and Medicaid Services. 2013. *Provider survey and Certification Frequently Asked Questions: Declared Public Health Emergencies—All Hazards Health Standards and Quality Issues.* Available at: https://www.cms.gov/About-CMS/Agency-Information/Emergency/Downloads/Provider-Survey-and-Certification-Frequently-Asked-Questions.pdf. Accessed January 30, 2017.

Farber D, Chen J. 2006. *Disasters and the Law: Katrina and Beyond.* New York, NY: Aspen Publishers.

Federal Emergency Management Agency (FEMA). 2016. *Public Assistance Program and Policy Guide.* Washington, DC: FEMA. Available at: http://www.fema.gov/media-library-data/1456167739485-75a028890345c6921d8d6ae473fbc8b3/PA_Program_and_Policy_Guide_2-21-2016_Fixes.pdf. Accessed January 30, 2017.

Gostin LO, Wiley LW. 2016. *Public Health Law: Power, Duty, Restraint.* 3rd ed. Berkeley: University of California Press.

Gostin LO. 2002. Public health law in an age of terrorism: rethinking individual rights and common goods. *Health Aff (Milwood).* 21(6):79–93.

Johns Hopkins Public Health Preparedness Programs, Center for Law, Science and Innovation, and Arizona State University. 2011. *Frequently Asked Questions about Legal Preparedness for Health Care Providers and Administrators, Public Health Officials, Emergency Planners, and Others Regarding Mental and Behavioral Health.* Available at: http://www.jhsph.edu/research/centers-and-institutes/center-for-law-and-the-publics-health/research/FAQ_LegalPreparedness.pdf. Accessed January 30, 2017.

Martin W. 2004. Legal and public policy responses of states to bioterrorism. *Am J Public Health.* 94(7):1093–1096.

McCormick E, ed. 2009. *Frequently Asked Questions About Federal Public Health Emergency Law.* Atlanta, GA: Centers for Disease Control and Prevention. Available at: http://archived.naccho.org/topics/infrastructure/PHLaw/upload/Microsoft-Word-FINAL-Public-Health-Emergency-Law-FAQ.pdf. Accessed January 30, 2017.

Misrahi JJ, Foster JA, Shaw FE, et al. 2004. HHS/CDC legal response to SARS outbreak. *Emerg Infect Dis.* 10(2):353–355.

Man-Made Disasters

Baum A. 1987. Toxins, technology, disasters. In: VandenBos GR, Bryant BK, eds. *Cataclysms, Crises, and Catastrophes: Psychology in Action.* Washington, DC: American Psychological Association.

Becker SM. 1997. Psychosocial assistance after environmental accidents: a policy perspective. *Environ Health Perspect.* 105(Suppl 6):1557–1563.

Bromet EJ, Parkinson DK, Dunn LO. 1990. Long-term mental health consequences of the accident at Three Mile Island. *Int J Mental Health.* 19(2):48–60.

Cuthbertson BH, Nigg JM. 1987. Technological disaster and the nontherapeutic community: a question of true victimization. *Environ Behav.* 19(4):462–483.

Edelstein MR, Wandersman A. 1987. Community dynamics in coping with toxic contaminants. In: Altman I, Wandersman A, eds. *Neighborhood and Community Environments.* Vol 9, Series Human Behavior and Environment: Advances in Theory and Research. New York, NY: Plenum Press.

Edelstein MR. 1988. *Contaminated Communities: The Social and Psychological Impacts of Residential Toxic Exposure.* Boulder, CO: Westview.

Haavenaar JM, Rumyantzeva GM, van den Brink W, et al. 1997. Long-term mental health effects of the Chernobyl disaster: an epidemiologic survey of two former Soviet regions. *Am J Psychiatry.* 154(11):1605–1607.

Kroll-Smith JS, Couch SR. 1993. Technological hazards: social responses as traumatic stressors. In: Wilson JP, Raphael B, eds. *The International Handbook of Traumatic Stress Syndromes.* New York, NY: Plenum Press. 79–91.

Lillibridge SR. 1997. Industrial disasters. In: Noji EK, ed. *The Public Health Consequences of Disasters.* New York, NY: Oxford University Press. 354–372.

Quarantelli EL. 1993. The environmental disasters of the future will be more and worse but the prospect is not hopeless. *Disaster Prev Manage.* 2(1):11–25.

Medical Care Delivery

Ciottone GR, Biddinger PD, Darling RG, et al. 2016. *Ciottone's Disaster Medicine.* 2nd ed. Amsterdam, Netherlands: Elsevier.

Institute for Clinical Systems Improvement. 2011. *Health Care Protocol: Rapid Response Team.* Available at: https://www.icsi.org/_asset/8snj28/RRT.pdf. Accessed January 30, 2017.

Hogue MD, Hogue HB, Lander RD, et al. 2009. The nontraditional role of pharmacists after Hurricane Katrina: process description and lessons learned. *Public Health Rep.* 124(2): 217–223.

Koenig KL, Schultz CH, eds. 2009. *Koenig and Schultz's Disaster Medicine: Comprehensive Principles and Practices.* New York, NY: Cambridge University Press.

Leach LS, Mayo AM. 2013. Rapid response teams: qualitative analysis of their effectiveness. *Am J Crit Care.* 22(3):198–210.

Lemonick DM. 2011. Epidemics after natural disasters. *Am J Clin Med.* 8(3):144–152.

Pointer JE, Michaelis J, Saunders C, et al. 1992. The 1989 Loma Prieta earthquake: impact on hospital patient care. *Ann Emerg Med.* 21(10):1228–1233.

Quinn B, Baker R, Pratt J. 1994. Hurricane Andrew and a pediatric emergency department. *Ann Emerg Med.* 23(4):737–741.

Rashid MF, Imran M, Javeri Y, et al. 2014. Evaluation of rapid response team implementation in medical emergencies: A gallant evidence based medicine initiative in developing countries for serious adverse events. *Int J Crit Illn Inj Sci.* 4(1):3–9.

Sabatino F. 1992. Stories of survival. Hurricane Andrew. South Florida hospitals shared resources and energy to cope with the storm's devastation. *Hospitals.* 66(24):26–28, 30.

Villanueva-Reiakvam S. *Do Rapid Response Teams Work?* Available at: http://www.zoll.com/codecommunicationsnewsletter/ccnl10_13/Do-RRTs-Work.pdf. Accessed January 30, 2017.

Yeck WL, Shaheen AF, Benz HM, et al. 2016. Rapid response, monitoring, and mitigation of induced seismicity near Greeley, Colorado. *Seismological Res Lett.* 87(4):1–11. Available at: https://www.researchgate.net/publication/304153797_Rapid_Response_Monitoring_and_Mitigation_of_Induced_Seismicity_near_Greeley_Colorado. Accessed January 30, 2017.

Morbidity and Mortality

McNabb SJ, Kelso KY, Wilson SA, et al. 1995. Hurricane Andrew-related injuries and illnesses, Louisiana 1992. *South Med J.* 88(6):615–618.

Noji EK, Armenian HK, Oganessian A. 1993. Issues of rescue and medical care following the 1988 Armenian earthquake. *Int J Epidemiol.* 22(6):1070–1076.

Noji EK. 1993. Analysis of medical needs during disasters caused by tropical cyclones: anticipated injury patterns. *J Trop Med Hyg.* 96(6):370–376.

Natural Hazards

Global Facility for Disaster Reduction and Recovery (GFDRR). 2016. *The Making of a Riskier Future: How Our Decisions Are Shaping Future Disaster Risk.* Washington, DC: GFDRR. Available at: https://www.gfdrr.org/sites/default/files/publication/Riskier%20Future.pdf. Accessed January 30, 2017.

National Oceanic and Atmospheric Administration (NOAA). 2016. NOAA weather radio all hazards. Available at: http://www.weather.gov/nwr. Accessed January 30, 2017.

White GF, Haas JE. 1975. *Assessment of Research on Natural Hazards.* Cambridge, MA: The MIT Press.

White GF. 1974. *Natural Hazards: Local, National, Global.* New York, NY: Oxford University Press.

Zebrowski Jr E. 1997. *Perils of a Restless Planet: Scientific Perspectives on Natural Disasters.* Cambridge, England: Cambridge University Press.

Nutrition

Food and Drug Administration. 2015. Food emergency and salvage information. Available at: http://www.fda.gov/training/forstatelocaltribalregulators/ucm121777.htm. Accessed January 30, 2017.

National Voluntary Organizations Active in Disaster (NVOAD). 2015. *Multi-Agency Feeding Support Plan Template.* Arlington, VA: NVOAD. Available at: http://www.fns.usda.gov/sites/default/files/Multi-Agency_Feeding_Plan_v2_June2015.pdf. Accessed January 30, 2017.

World Health Organization (WHO). 2000. *The Management of Nutrition in Major Emergencies.* Geneva, Switzerland: International Federation of Red Cross and Red Crescent Societies, United Nations High Commissioner for Refugees, WHO.

Organization of Response

Agency for Healthcare Research and Quality (AHRQ). 2005. Development of models for emergency preparedness: personal protective equipment, decontamination, isolation/quarantine, and laboratory capacity. Available at: https://archive.ahrq.gov/research/devmodels. Accessed January 30, 2017.

Agency for Healthcare Research and Quality (AHRQ). 2011. Disaster response tools and resources. Available at: http://archive.ahrq.gov/path/katrina.htm. Accessed January 30, 2017.

California Emergency Medical Services Authority. 2014. *Hospital Incident Command System Guidebook*. 5th ed. Available at: http://www.emsa.ca.gov/disaster_medical_services_division_hospital_incident_command_system. Accessed January 30, 2017.

California Emergency Medical Services Authority. Hospital Incident Command System—Forms. Available at: http://www.emsa.ca.gov/hospital_incident_command_system_forms_2014. Accessed January 30, 2017.

Centers for Disease Control and Prevention. Emergency preparedness and response. Available at: http://emergency.cdc.gov. Accessed January 30, 2017.

Centers for Disease Control and Prevention. Strategic national stockpile. Available at: http://www.cdc.gov/phpr/stockpile/stockpile.htm. Accessed January 30, 2017.

Emergency Management Assistant Compact. 2015. Nationally adopted interstate mutual aid agreement. Available at: http://www.emacweb.org/?305. Accessed January 30, 2017.

Federal Emergency Management Agency. Public assistance: resources and tools. Available at: http://www.fema.gov/public-assistance-resources-and-tools. Accessed January 30, 2017.

Federal Emergency Management Agency (FEMA). 2010. *Developing and Maintaining Emergency Operations Plans Comprehensive Preparedness Guide (CPG) 101*. Version 2.0. Washington, DC: FEMA. Available at: https://www.fema.gov/media-library-data/20130726-1828-25045-0014/cpg_101_comprehensive_preparedness_guide_developing_and_maintaining_emergency_operations_plans_2010.pdf. Accessed January 30, 2017.

Federal Emergency Management Agency (FEMA). 2016. *Working Draft: National Incident Management System Refresh Review Package*. Washington, DC: FEMA. Available at: http://www.fema.gov/media-library-data/1467113975990-09cb03e2669b06b91a9a25cc5f97bc46/NE_DRAFT_NIMS_20160407.pdf. Accessed January 30, 2017.

Federal Emergency Management Agency (FEMA). 2008. *Overview of Stafford Act Support to States*. Washington, DC: FEMA. Available at: http://www.fema.gov/pdf/emergency/nrf/nrf-stafford.pdf. Accessed January 30, 2017.

Federal Emergency Management Agency (FEMA). 2015. *Stafford Act Declaration Process Fact Sheet*. Washington, DC: FEMA. Available at: http://www.dhsem.wv.gov/Documents/Declaraton%20Process/Fact%20Sheet-Declaration%20Process%20093015.pdf. Accessed January 30, 2017.

Hodge JG, Gostin LO, Vernick JS. 2007. The Pandemic and All-Hazards Preparedness Act. *JAMA*. 299(15):1708–1711. Available at: http://jama.ama-assn.org/content/297/15/1708.full. Accessed January 30, 2017.

Lister S. 2008. *Public Health and Medical Preparedness and Response: Issues in the 110th Congress*. Washington, DC: Congressional Research Service.

National Fire Protection Association (NFPA). 2016. *NFPA 1600: Standard on Disaster/Emergency Management and Business Continuity/Continuity of Operations Programs*. 2016 ed. Quincy,

MA: NFPA. Available at: http://www.nfpa.org/codes-and-standards/all-codes-and-standards/list-of-codes-and-standards?mode=code&code=1600. Accessed January 30, 2017.

National Response Framework. Emergency Support Function #8: Public Health and Medical Services Annex. Available at: https://www.fema.gov/media-library-data/1470149644671-642ccad05d19449d2d13b1b0952328ed/ESF_8_Public_Health_Medical_20160705_508.pdf. Accessed January 30, 2017.

Office of the Assistant Secretary for Preparedness and Response. 2016. Guidance, reports, and research: hospital preparedness program. Available at: http://phe.gov/Preparedness/planning/hpp/reports/Pages/default.aspx. Accessed January 30, 2017.

Office of the Assistant Secretary for Preparedness and Response. 2016. National health security strategy. Available at: http://www.phe.gov/Preparedness/planning/authority/nhss/Pages/default.aspx. Accessed January 30, 2017.

Office of the Assistant Secretary for Preparedness and Response. 2016. Responders, clinicians and practitioners. Washington, DC: U.S. Department of Health & Human Services. Available at: http://www.phe.gov/preparedness/responders/pages/default.aspx. Accessed January 30, 2017.

Office of the Assistant Secretary for Preparedness and Response. 2015. Public health and medical services support. Available at: http://www.phe.gov/preparedness/support/Pages/default.aspx. Accessed January 30, 2017.

Office of the Assistant Secretary for Preparedness and Response. 2015. Legal authority. Available at: http://www.phe.gov/preparedness/planning/authority/pages/default.aspx. Accessed January 30, 2017.

Office of the Assistant Secretary for Preparedness and Response. 2013. Medical surge capacity capability. Available at: http://www.phe.gov/Preparedness/planning/mscc/Pages/default.aspx. Accessed January 30, 2017.

Office of the Civilian Volunteer Medical Reserve Corps. 2016. Contacting and starting an MRC unit. Available at: https://mrc.hhs.gov/partnerFldr/QuestionsAnswers/ContactingStarting. Accessed January 30, 2017.

GovTrack. H.R. 307 (113th): Pandemic and All Hazards Preparedness Act of 2013. Available at: https://www.govtrack.us/congress/bills/113/hr307. Accessed January 30, 2017.

U.S. Agency for International Development, Bureau for Humanitarian Response, Office of Foreign Disaster Assistance. 2005. *Field Operations Guide for Disaster Assessment and Response*. Available at: https://scms.usaid.gov/sites/default/files/documents/1866/fog_v4_0.pdf. Accessed January 30, 2017.

U.S. Department of Health & Human Services. 2014. Commissioned corps deployments: public health emergency responders. Available at: http://www.usphs.gov/newsroom/features/action/deployments.aspx. Accessed January 30, 2017.

U.S. Department of Health & Human Services. 2016. The Emergency system for advance registration of volunteer health professionals (ESAR-VHP). About ESAR-VHP. Available at: http://www.phe.gov/esarvhp/Pages/about.aspx. Accessed January 30, 2017.

U.S. Department of Homeland Security. 2016. Incident management. Available at: https://www.ready.gov/business/implementation/incident. Accessed January 30, 2017.

U.S. Department of Homeland Security. 2016. Core capabilities. Available at: http://www.fema.gov/core-capabilities. Accessed January 30, 2017.

U.S. Department of Homeland Security (DHS). 2016. *National Response Framework*. 3rd ed. Washington, DC: DHS. Available at: http://www.fema.gov/media-library-data/1466014682982-9bcf8245ba4c60c120aa915abe74e15d/National_Response_Framework3rd.pdf. Accessed January 30, 2017.

U.S. Department of Homeland Security. 2015. National preparedness guidelines. Available at: https://www.dhs.gov/national-preparedness-guidelines. Accessed January 30, 2017.

Planning

Auf der Heide E. 1996. *Community Medical Disaster Planning and Evaluation Guide*. Dallas, TX: American College of Emergency Physicians.

Auf der Heide E. 1996. Disaster planning, part II: disaster problems, issues, and challenges identified in the research literature. *Emerg Med Clin North Am*. 14(2):453–480.

Auf der Heide E. 2004. Common misconceptions about disasters: panic, the disaster syndrome, and looting. In: O'Leary M, ed. *The First 72 Hours: A Community Approach to Disaster Preparedness*. Lincoln, NE: iUniverse Publishing.

Auf der Heide E. 2006. The importance of evidence-based disaster planning. *Ann Emerg Med*. 47(1):34–49.

Dynes RR. 1994. Community emergency planning: false assumptions and inappropriate analogies. *Int J Mass Emerg Disasters*. 12(2):141–158.

Federal Emergency Management Agency. 2016. PPD-8 news, updates & announcements. http://www.fema.gov/ppd-8-news-updates-announcements. Accessed January 30, 2017.

Federal Emergency Management Agency. 2016. National planning frameworks. Available at: http://www.fema.gov/national-planning-frameworks. Accessed January 30, 2017.

Federal Emergency Management Agency. 2016. National preparedness resource library. Available at: http://www.fema.gov/national-preparedness-resource-library. Accessed January 30, 2017.

Fong F, Schrader DC. 1996. Radiation disasters and emergency department preparedness. *Emerg Med Clin North Am*. 14(2):349–370.

Gibbs M, Lachenmeyer JR, et al. 1996. Effects of the AVIANCA aircrash on disaster workers. *Int J Mass Emerg Disasters*. 14(1):23–32.

Landesman LY. 2004. Forward: does preparedness make a difference? *Fam Community Health*. 27(3):186–187.

Lindell MK, Perry RW. 1992. *Behavioral Foundations of Community Emergency Planning.* Philadelphia, PA: Hemisphere Publishing.

U.S. Department of Health & Human Services. ASPR playbooks. Available at: http://www.phe.gov/Preparedness/planning/playbooks/Pages/default.aspx. Accessed January 30, 2017.

U.S. Department of Health & Human Services. FEMA's functional needs support services guidance. Available at: http://www.phe.gov/Preparedness/planning/abc/Pages/funcitonal-needs.aspx. Accessed January 30, 2017.

U.S. Department of Health & Human Services. Pandemic and All-Hazards Preparedness Reauthorization Act. http://www.phe.gov/Preparedness/legal/pahpa/Pages/pahpra.aspx. Accessed January 30, 2017.

U.S. Department of Homeland Security. 2016. *National Planning System.* Available at: http://www.fema.gov/media-library-data/1454504745569-c5234d4556a00eb7b86342c869531ea0/National_Planning_System_20151029.pdf. Accessed January 30, 2017.

U.S. Department of Homeland Security. 2016. *National Preparedness System.* Available at: https://www.fema.gov/national-preparedness-system. Accessed January 30, 2017.

U.S. Department of Homeland Security. Homeland security exercise and evaluation program (HSEEP). Available at: http://www.globalsecurity.org/security/systems/hseep.htm. Accessed January 30, 2017.

Wright KS, Thomas MW, Durham DP Jr, et al. 2010. A public health academic-practice partnership to develop capacity for exercise evaluation and improvement planning. *Public Health Rep.* 125(Suppl 5):107–116.

Public Health

Lechat MF. 1979. Disasters and public health. *Bull World Health Organ.* 57(1):11–17.

Noji E, ed. 1997. *The Public Health Consequences of Disaster.* New York, NY: Oxford University Press.

Rosen G. 1993. *A History of Public Health.* Baltimore, MD: Johns Hopkins University Press.

Radiation

American College of Radiology. Radiation disasters: preparedness and response for radiology. Available at: http://www.acr.org/membership/legal-business-practices/disaster-preparedness. Accessed January 25, 2017.

Armed Forces Radiobiology Research Institute. 2013. *Medical Management Of Radiological Casualties.* 4th ed. Available at: https://www.usuhs.edu/sites/default/files/media/afrri/pdf/4edmmrchandbook.pdf. Accessed January 25, 2017.

Centers for Disease Control and Prevention. 2013. Acute radiation syndrome: a fact sheet for clinicians. Available at: http://emergency.cdc.gov/radiation/arsphysicianfactsheet.asp. Accessed January 30, 2017.

Centers for Disease Control and Prevention. 2014. Acute radiation syndrome (ARS): a fact sheet for the public. Available at: http://emergency.cdc.gov/radiation/ars.asp. Accessed January 30, 2017.

Centers for Disease Control and Prevention; Public Health Law Program. 2014. *Public Health Preparedness: Examination of Legal Language Authorizing Responses to Incidents Involving Contamination with Radioactive Material.* Available at: http://www.cdc.gov/phlp/docs/php-radioactive.pdf. Accessed January 30, 2017.

Fukushima Booklet Publication Committee. 2016. *10 Lessons From Fukushima: Reducing Risks and Protecting Communities From Nuclear Disasters*. 2nd ed. Available at: http://fukushimalessons.jp/en-booklet.html. Accessed January 30, 2017.

National Academies of Sciences, Engineering, and Medicine. 2014. *Lessons Learned from the Fukushima Nuclear Accident for Improving Safety and Security of U.S. Nuclear Plants: Phase 2.* Washington, DC: National Academies Press.

New York State Department of Health. 2011. Potassium iodide (KI) and radiation emergencies: fact sheet. Available at: https://www.health.ny.gov/environmental/radiological/potassium_iodide/fact_sheet.htm. Accessed January 30, 2017.

Radiation Emergency Medical Management. Nuclear detonation: weapons, improvised nuclear devices. Available at: http://www.remm.nlm.gov/nuclearexplosion.htm#categories. Accessed January 30, 2017.

Oak Ridge Institute for Science and Education. 2011. Radiation emergency assistance center/training site (REAC/TS). Available at: http://www.orau.gov/reacts. Accessed January 30, 2017.

Office of the Assistant Secretary for Preparedness and Response. Radiation emergencies. Available at: http://www.phe.gov/emergency/radiation/Pages/default.aspx. Accessed January 30, 2017.

U.S. Food and Drug Administration (FDA). 2001. *Guidance: Potassium Iodide as a Thyroid Blocking Agent in Radiation Emergencies*. Rockville, MD: FDA. Available at: http://www.fda.gov/downloads/Drugs/GuidanceComplianceRegulatoryInformation/Guidances/ucm080542.pdf. Accessed January 30, 2017.

Williams JD. 2015. Apples and oranges—understanding curies and REM in radiation sources. *Domestic Preparedness J.* Available at: http://www.domesticpreparedness.com/First_Responder/Fire_HAZMAT/Apples_%26_Oranges_-_Understanding_Curies_%26_REM_in_Radiation_Sources. Accessed January 30, 2017.

Zablotska LB. 2016. 30 Years after the Chernobyl nuclear accident: time for reflection and re-evaluation of current disaster preparedness plans. *J Urban Health.* 93(3):407–413.

Rapid Needs Assessment

Brown V, Jacquier G, Coulombier D, et al. 2001. Rapid assessment of population size by area sampling in disaster situations. *Disasters*. 25(2):164–171.

Centers for Disease Control and Prevention. 2016. Community Assessment for Public Health Emergency Response (CASPER). Available at: https://www.cdc.gov/nceh/hsb/disaster/casper. Accessed January 30, 2017.

Centers for Disease Control and Prevention (CDC). 2012. *Community Assessment for Public Health Emergency Response (CASPER) Toolkit*. 2nd ed. Chamblee, GA: CDC Division of Environmental Hazards and Health Effects. Available at: https://www.cdc.gov/nceh/hsb/disaster/casper/docs/cleared_casper_toolkit.pdf. Accessed January 30, 2017.

Guha-Sapir D. 1991. Rapid assessment of health needs in mass emergencies: review of current concepts and methods. *World Health Stat Q*. 44(3):171–181.

Hlady WG, Quenemoen LE, Armenia-Cope RR, et al. 1994. Use of a modified cluster sampling method to perform rapid needs assessment after Hurricane Andrew. *Ann Emerg Med*. 23(4):719–725.

Lillibridge SR, Noji EK, Burkle FM Jr. 1993. Disaster assessment: the emergency health evaluation of a population affected by a disaster. *Ann Emerg Med*. 22(11):1715–1720.

Malilay J, Flanders WD, Brogan D. 1996. A modified cluster-sampling method for post-disaster rapid assessment of needs. *Bull World Health Organ*. 74(4):399–405.

World Health Organization (WHO). 1999. *Rapid Health Assessment Protocols for Emergencies*. Geneva, Switzerland: WHO.

World Health Organization (WHO). 2001. *Rapid Assessment of Mental Health Needs of Refugees, Displaced and Other Populations Affected by Conflict and Post-Conflict Situations*. Geneva, Switzerland: WHO.

Recovery

Berke PR, Kartez J, Wenger D. 1993. Recovery after disaster: achieving sustainable development, mitigation and equity. *Disasters*. 17(2):93–109.

Cohen R. 1995. *Refugee and Internally Displaced Women: A Development Perspective*. Washington, DC: Brookings Institution.

Cuny F. 1983. *Disasters and Development*. New York, NY: Oxford University Press.

Federal Emergency Management Agency. 2013. *Commonly Used Sheltering Items & Services Listing Catalog*. Available at: http://www.nationalmasscarestrategy.org/wp-content/uploads/2014/07/cusi-catalog-as-of-march-2013-v2.pdf. Accessed January 30, 2017.

Federal Emergency Management Agency. 2016. Individual assistance program tools frequently asked questions. Available at: http://www.fema.gov/individual-assistance-program-tools-frequently-asked-questions. Accessed January 30, 2017.

Federal Emergency Management Agency (FEMA). 2010. *Guidance on Planning for Integration of Functional Needs Support Services in General Population Shelters*. Washington, DC: FEMA. Available at: http://www.fema.gov/pdf/about/odic/fnss_guidance.pdf. Accessed January 30, 2017.

Federal Emergency Management Agency. National disaster recovery framework. 2016. Available at: http://www.fema.gov/national-disaster-recovery-framework. Accessed January 30, 2017.

Federal Emergency Management Agency. 2016. Public assistance: local, state, tribal, and non-profit. Available at: http://www.fema.gov/public-assistance-local-state-tribal-and-non-profit. Accessed January 30, 2017.

Federal Emergency Management Agency (FEMA), American Red Cross. 2015. *Shelter Field Guide FEMA P-785*. Washington, DC: FEMA. Available at: http://www.nationalmasscarestrategy.org/wp-content/uploads/2015/10/Shelter-Field-Guide-508_f3.pdf. Accessed January 30, 2017.

Felton C. 2002. Project Liberty: a public health response to New Yorkers' mental health needs arising from the World Trade Center terrorist attacks. *J Urban Health*. 79(3):429–433.

Grefenstette JJ, Brown ST, Rosenfeld R, et al. 2013. FRED (A Framework for Reconstructing Epidemic Dynamics): An open-source software system for modeling infectious diseases and control strategies using census-based populations. *BMC Public Health*. 13(1):940.

Hughes J. 2013. Tracking System Prepares New York to Evacuate Patients in Emergencies. *Emerg Manag*. Available at: http://www.govtech.com/health/Tracking-System-Prepares-New-York-to-Evacuate-Patients-in-Emergencies.html. Accessed January 30, 2017.

Institute of Medicine. 2015. *Enabling Rapid and Sustainable Public Health Research During Disasters: Summary of a Joint Workshop by the Institute of Medicine and the U.S. Department of Health & Human Services*. Washington, DC: Institute of Medicine.

Leinhos M, Qari SH, Williams-Johnson M. 2014. Preparedness and emergency response research centers: using a public health systems approach to improve all-hazards preparedness and response. *Public Health Rep*. 129(Suppl 4):8–18.

McDonnell S, Troiano RP, Barker N, et al. 1995. Evaluation of long-term community recovery from Hurricane Andrew: sources of assistance received by population sub-groups. *Disasters*. 19(4): 338–347.

Moore S, Daniel M, Linnan L, et al. 2004. After Hurricane Floyd passed: investigating the social determinants of disaster preparedness and recovery. *Fam Community Health*. 27(3):204–217.

National Governors Association. 2014. *Governors' Guide to Mass Evacuation*. Available at: http://www.nga.org/files/live/sites/NGA/files/pdf/GovGuideMassEvacuation.pdf. Accessed January 30, 2017.

National Centers for Environmental Health, Division of Environmental Hazards and Health Effects. 2015. *A Guide to Operating Public Shelters in a Radiation Emergency*. Atlanta, GA: Centers for Disease Control and Prevention. Available at: http://emergency.cdc.gov/radiation/pdf/operating-public-shelters.pdf. Accessed January 30, 2017.

National Mass Care Strategy. 2016. Available at: http://nationalmasscarestrategy.org. Accessed January 30, 2017.

National Response Framework. *Emergency Support Function #6: Mass Care, Emergency Assistance, Temporary Housing, and Human Services Annex.* Available at: https://www.fema.gov/media-library-data/1470149820826-7bcf80b5dbabc158953058a6b5108e98/ESF_6_MassCare_20160705_508.pdf. Accessed January 30, 2017.

Occupational Safety and Health Administration. Evacuation planning matrix. Available at: http://www.osha.gov/dep/evacmatrix/index.html. Accessed January 30, 2017.

Occupational Safety and Health Administration. Evacuation plans and procedures eTool. Available at: http://www.osha.gov/SLTC/etools/evacuation/index.html. Accessed January 30, 2017.

Shrivastava P. 1996. Long-term recovery from the Bhopal Crisis. In: Mitchell JK, ed. *The Long Road to Recovery: Community Responses to Industrial Disaster.* Tokyo, Japan: United Nations University Press. 121–147.

Thorpe LE, Assari S, Deppen S, et al. 2015. The role of epidemiology in disaster response policy development. *Ann Epidemiol.* 25(5):377–386.

U.S. Department of Justice, Civil Rights Division; Americans with Disabilities Act (ADA). ADA best practices tool kit for state and local governments: the ADA and emergency shelters: access for all in emergencies and disasters. Available at: http://www.ada.gov/pcatoolkit/chap7shelterprog.htm. Accessed January 30, 2017.

Resilience

Bach R, Doran R, Gibb L, et al. 2010. Policy challenges in supporting community resilience. Paper presented at: the London Workshop of the Multinational Community Resilience Policy Group; November 4–5; London, England.

International Risk Governance Council. 2016. IRGC resource guide on resilience. Available at: https://www.irgc.org/irgc-resource-guide-on-resilience. Accessed January 30, 2017.

Kaminsky M, McCabe OL, Langlieb AM, et al. 2007. An evidence-informed model of human resistance, resilience, and recovery: the Johns Hopkins' outcome-driven paradigm for disaster mental health services. *Brief Treatment Crisis Intervent.* 7(1):1–11.

Madrid PA, Grant R, Reilly MJ, et al. 2006. Challenges in meeting immediate emotional needs: short-term impact of a major disaster on children's mental health: building resiliency in the aftermath of Hurricane Katrina. *Pediatrics.* 117(5 Pt 3):S448–S453.

Masten AS, ObradovicJ. 2007. Disaster preparation and recovery: lessons from research on resilience in human development. *Ecology Soc.* 13(1):9.

Norris FH, Stevens SP. 2007. Community resilience and the principles of mass trauma intervention. *Psychiatry.* 70(4):320–328.

Norris FH, Stevens SP, Pfefferbaum B, et al. 2008. Community resilience as a metaphor, theory, set of capacities, and strategy for disaster readiness. *Am J Community Psychol.* 41(1-2): 127–150.

Wulff K, Donato D, Lurie N. 2015. What is health resilience and how can we build it? *Annu Rev Public Health.* 36:361–374.

Risk Assessment

Emanuel K, Ravela S, Vivant E, et al. 2006. A statistical deterministic approach to hurricane risk assessment. *Bull Am Meteorol Soc.* 87(3):299–314.

Greiving S, Fleischhauer M, Lückenkötter J. 2007. A methodology for an integrated risk assessment of spatially relevant hazards. *J Environ Plan Manage.* 49(1):1–19.

Malilay J, Henderson A, McGeehin M, et al. 1997. Estimating health risks from natural hazards using risk assessment and epidemiology. *Risk Anal.* 17(3):353–358.

Smith K. 2013. *Environmental Hazards: Assessing Risk and Reducing Disaster.* 6th ed. New York, NY: Routledge.

U.S. Department of Homeland Security. *Threat and Hazard Identification and Risk Assessment Guide, Comprehensive Preparedness Guide (CPG) 201.* 2nd ed. 2013. Available at: http://www.fema.gov/media-library-data/8ca0a9e54dc8b037a55b402b2a269e94/CPG201_htirag_2nd_edition.pdf. Accessed January 30, 2017.

Wisner B, Blaikie P, Cannon T, et al. 2014. *At Risk: Natural Hazards, People's Vulnerability and Disasters.* 2nd ed. New York, NY: Routledge.

Social Distancing

Baum NM, Jacobson PD, Goold SD. 2009. "Listen to the people": public deliberation about social distancing measures in a pandemic. *Am J Bioeth.* 9(11):4–14.

Berkman BE. 2008. Mitigating pandemic influenza: the ethics of implementing a school closure policy. *J Public Health Manag Pract.* 14(4):372–378.

Blake KD, Blendon RJ, Viswanath K. 2010. Employment and compliance with pandemic influenza mitigation recommendations. *Emerg Infect Dis.* 16(2):212–218.

Booy R, Ward J. 2014. *Social Distancing: Evidence Summary.* Westmead, New South Wales: National Centre for Immunisation Research and Surveillance; Australian Government Department of Health and Ageing. Available at: http://www.health.gov.au/internet/main/publishing.nsf/Content/519F9392797E2DDCCA257D47001B9948/$File/Social.pdf. Accessed January 30, 2017.

Borse RH, Behravesh CB, Dumanovsky T, et al. 2011. Closing schools in response to the 2009 pandemic influenza A H1N1 virus in New York City: economic impact on households. *Clin Infect Dis.* 52(Suppl 1):S168–S172.

Centers for Disease Control and Prevention. 2009. Impact of seasonal influenza-related school closures on families—Southeastern Kentucky, February 2008. *MMWR Morb Mortal Wkly Rep.* 58(50):1405–1409.

Centers for Disease Control and Prevention. 2010. Parental attitudes and experiences during school dismissals related to 2009 influenza A (H1N1)—United States, 2009. *MMWR Morb Mortal Wkly Rep.* 59(35):1131–1134.

Dalton CB, Durrheim DN, Conroy MA. 2008. Likely impact of school and childcare closures on public health workforce during an influenza pandemic: a survey. *Communicable Dis Intell Q Rep.* 32(2):261–262.

Earn DJ, He D, Loeb MB, et al. 2012. Effects of school closure on incidence of pandemic influenza in Alberta, Canada. *Ann Intern Med.* 156(3):173–181.

Egger JR, Konty KJ, Wilson E, et al. 2012. The effect of school dismissal on rates of influenza-like illness in New York City schools during the spring 2009 novel H1N1 outbreak. *J Sch Health.* 82(3):123–130.

European Centre for Disease Prevention and Control. 2009. *Guide to Public Health Measures to Reduce the Impact of Influenza Pandemics in Europe: "The ECDC Menu."* Stockholm, Sweden: European Centre for Disease Prevention and Control. Available at: http://www.ecdc.europa.eu/en/publications/Publications/0906_TER_Public_Health_Measures_for_Influenza_Pandemics.pdf. Accessed January 30, 2017.

Gift TL, Palekar RS, Sodha SV, et al. 2010. Household effects of school closure during pandemic (H1N1) 2009, Pennsylvania, USA. *Emerg Infect Dis.*16(8):1315–1317.

Halder N, Kelso JK, Milne GJ. 2010. Developing guidelines for school closure interventions to be used during a future influenza pandemic. *BMC Infect Dis.* 10:221.

Heymann AD, Hoch I, Valinsky L, et al. 2009. School closure may be effective in reducing transmission of respiratory viruses in the community. *Epidemiol Infect.* 137(10):1369–1376.

Jarquin VG, Callahan DB, Cohen NJ, et al. 2011. Effect of school closure from pandemic (H1N1) 2009, Chicago, Illinois, USA. *Emerg Infect Dis.* 17(4):751–753.

Miyaki K, Sakurazawa H, Mikurube H, et al. 2011. An effective quarantine measure reduced the total incidence of influenza A H1N1 in the workplace: another way to control the H1N1 flu pandemic. *J Occup Health.* 53(4):287–292.

Rodriguez CV, Rietberg K, Baer A, Kwan-Gett T, Duchin J. 2009. Association between school closure and subsequent absenteeism during a seasonal influenza epidemic. *Epidemiology.* 20(6):787–792.

Yu H, Cauchemez S, Donnelly CA, et al. 2012. Transmission dynamics, border entry screening, and school holidays during the 2009 influenza A (H1N1) pandemic, China. *Emerg Infect Dis.* 18(5):758–766.

Wheeler CC, Erhart LM, Jehn ML. 2010. Effect of school closure on the incidence of influenza among school-age children in Arizona. *Public Health Rep.* 125(6):851–859.

Surveillance

Disaster Surveillance

Council for State and Territorial Epidemiologists. 2014. Environmental health: disaster epidemiology. Available at: http://www.cste.org/group/DisasterEpi. Accessed January 30, 2017.

Glass RI, Noji EK. 1992. Epidemiologic surveillance following disasters. In: Halperin W, Baker EL, eds. *Public Health Surveillance.* New York, NY: Van Nostrand Reinhold. 195–205.

Heffernan R, Mostashari F, Das D, et al. 2004. Syndromic surveillance in public health practice, New York City. *Emerg Infect Dis.* 10(5):858–864.

Lechat MF. 1993. Accident and disaster epidemiology. *Public Health Rev.* 21(3-4):243–253.

Legome E, Robbins A, Rund A. 1995. Injuries associated with floods: the need for an international reporting scheme. *Disasters.* 19(1):50–54.

Lore EL, Fonseca V, Brett KM, et al. 1993. Active morbidity surveillance after Hurricane Andrew–Florida, 1992. *JAMA.* 270(5):591–594.

Noji EK. 1997. The use of epidemiologic methods in disasters. In: Noji EK, ed. *The Public Health Consequences of Disasters.* New York, NY: Oxford University Press. 21–36.

O'Connell EK, Zhang G, Legeun F, et al. 2010. Innovative uses for syndromic surveillance. *Emerg Infect Dis.* 16(4):669–671.

Office of the Assistant Secretary for Preparedness and Response. 2007. Public health response. In: *Public Health Emergency Response: A Guide for Leaders and Responders.* Washington, DC: U.S. Department of Health & Human Services. Available at: https://www.hsdl.org/?view&did=481394. Accessed January 30, 2017.

Western KA.1982. *Epidemiologic Surveillance after Natural Disasters.* Washington, DC: Pan American Health Organization.

Wetterhall SF, Noji EK. 1997. Surveillance and epidemiology. In: Noji EK, ed. *The Public Health Consequences of Disasters.* New York, NY: Oxford University Press. 37–64.

Malilay J, Heumann M, Perrotta D, et al. 2014. The role of applied epidemiology methods in the disaster management cycle. *Am J Public Health.* 104(11):2092–2102.

Environmental Public Health Surveillance

Deutsch PV, Adler J, Richter ED. 1992. Sentinel markers for industrial disasters. *Isr J Med Sci.* 28(8-9):526–533.

Thacker SB, Stroup DF. 1994. Future directions of comprehensive public health surveillance and health information systems in the United States. *Am J Epidemiol.* 140(5):383–397.

Thacker SB, Stroup DF, Parrish RG, et al. 1996. Surveillance in environmental public health: issues, systems, and sources. *Am J Public Health.* 86(5):633–638.

General Surveillance

Angulo JJ. 1987. Interdisciplinary approaches in epidemic studies—II: Four geographic models of the flow of contagious disease. *Soc Sci Med.* 24(1):57–69.

Brooker S, Hotez PJ, Bundy DA. 2010. The global atlas of helminth infection: mapping the way forward in neglected tropical disease control. *PLoS Negl Trop Dis.* 4(7):e779.

Brown ST, Tai JH, Bailey RR, et al. 2011. Would school closure for the 2009 H1N1 influenza epidemic have been worth the cost?: a computational simulation of Pennsylvania. *BMC Public Health.* 11:353.

Buczak AL, Baugher B, Babin SM, et al. 2014. Prediction of high incidence of dengue in the Philippines. *PLoS Negl Trop Dis.* 8(4):e2771.

Bush RM, Bender CA, Subbarao K, et al. 1999. Predicting the evolution of human influenza A. *Science.* 286(5446):1921–1925.

Campbell TC, Hodanics CJ, Babin SM, et al. 2012. Developing open source, self-contained disease surveillance software applications for use in resource-limited settings. *BMC Med Inform Decis Mak.* 12:99.

Carnevale RJ, Talbot TR, Schaffner W, et al. 2011. Evaluating the utility of syndromic surveillance algorithms for screening to detect potentially clonal hospital infection outbreaks. *J Am Med Inform Assoc.* 18(4):466–472.

Centers for Disease Control and Prevention (CDC). 2016. *A Primer for Understanding the Principles and Practices of Disaster Surveillance in the United States.* Atlanta, GA: CDC. Available at: http://www.cdc.gov/nceh/hsb/disaster/Disaster_Surveillance_508.pdf. Accessed January 30, 2017.

Chan EH, Sahai V, Conrad C, et al. 2011. Using web search query data to monitor dengue epidemics: a new model for neglected tropical disease surveillance. *PLoS Negl Trop Dis.* 5(5):e1206.

Chaudet H, Meynard JB, Texier G, et al. 2005. Distributed and mobile collaboration for real time epidemiological surveillance during forces deployments. *Stud Health Technol Inform.* 116:983–988.

Constantin de Magny G, Murtugudde R, Sapiano MR, et al. 2008. Environmental signatures associated with cholera epidemics. *Proc Natl Acad Sci U S A.* 105(46):17676–17681.

Corley CD, Pullum LL, Hartley DM, et al. 2014. Disease prediction models and operational readiness. *PLoS One.* 9(3):e91989.

Daszak P. 2009. A call for "Smart Surveillance": a lesson learned from H1N1. *Ecohealth.* 6(1):1–2.

Dorea FC, McEwen BJ, McNab WB, et al. 2013. Syndromic surveillance using veterinary laboratory data: algorithm combination and customization of alerts. *PLoS One*. 8(12):e82183.

Eisen L, Eisen RJ. 2011. Using geographic information systems and decision support systems for the prediction, prevention, and control of vector-borne diseases. *Annu Rev Entomol.* 56:41–61.

Estrada-Pena A, Zatansever Z, Gargili A, et al. 2007. Modeling the spatial distribution of crimean-congo hemorrhagic fever outbreaks in Turkey. *Vector Borne Zoonotic Dis*. 7(4):667–678.

Ford TE, Colwell RR, Rose JB, et al. 2009. Using satellite images of environmental changes to predict infectious disease outbreaks. *Emerg Infect Dis*. 15(9):1341–1346.

Gesteland PH, Gardner RM, Tsui FC, et al. 2003. Automated syndromic surveillance for the 2002 Winter Olympics. *J Am Med Inform Assoc*. 10(6):547–554.

Grigg OA, Farewell VT, Spiegelhalter DJ. 2003. Use of risk-adjusted CUSUM and RSPRT charts for monitoring in medical contexts. *Stat Methods Med Res*. 12(2):147–170.

Halperin W, Baker EL Jr, Monson RR, eds. 1992. *Public Health Surveillance.* New York, NY: Van Nostrand Reinhold.

Hashimoto S, Murakami Y, Taniguchi K, et al. 2000. Detection of epidemics in their early stage through infectious disease surveillance. *Int J Epidemiol.* 29(5):905–910.

Hu PJ, Zeng D, Chen H, et al. 2007. System for infectious disease information sharing and analysis: design and evaluation. *IEEE Trans Inf Technol Biomed*. 11(4):483–492.

Jackson C, Vynnycky E, Hawker J, et al. 2013. School closures and influenza: systematic review of epidemiological studies. *BMJ Open*. 3(2).

Kawaguchi R, Miyazono M, Noda T, et al. 2009. Influenza (H1N1) 2009 outbreak and school closure, Osaka Prefecture, Japan. *Emerg Infect Dis*. 15(10):1685.

Keller M, Blench M, Tolentino H, et al. 2009. Use of unstructured event-based reports for global infectious disease surveillance. *Emerg Infect Dis*. 15(5):689–695.

Kleinman K, Lazarus R, Platt R. 2004. A generalized linear mixed models approach for detecting incident clusters of disease in small areas, with an application to biological terrorism. *Am J Epidemiol.* 159(3):217–224.

Klauke DN, Buehler JW, Thacker SB, et al. 1988. Guidelines for evaluating surveillance systems. *MMWR Morbid Mortal Wkly Rep.* 37(5):1–18.

Knorr-Held L, Besag J. 1998. Modelling risk from a disease in time and space. *Stat Med.* 17(18):2045–2060.

Langmuir AD. 1971. Evolution of the concept of surveillance in the United States. *Proc R Soc Med.* 64(6):681–684.

Liao YC, Lee MS, Ko CY, et al. 2008. Bioinformatics models for predicting antigenic variants of influenza A/H3N2 virus. *Bioinformatics.* 24(4):505–512.

Liccardo A, Fierro A. 2015. Multiple lattice model for influenza spreading. *PLoS One.* 10(10):e0141065.

Lloyd-Smith JO, George D, Pepin KM, et al. 2009. Epidemic dynamics at the human-animal interface. *Science.* 326(5958):1362–1367.

Lombardo J, Buckeridge D. 2007. *Disease Surveillance: A Public Health Informatics Approach.* New York, NY: Wiley-Interscience.

Lombardo J, Burkom H, Elbert E, et al. 2003. A systems overview of the Electronic Surveillance System for the Early Notification of Community-Based Epidemics (ESSENCE II). *J Urban Health.* 80(2 Suppl 1):i32–i42.

Lombardo JS, Burkom H, Pavlin J. 2004. ESSENCE II and the framework for evaluating syndromic surveillance systems. *MMWR Suppl.* 53:159–165.

Lucero C, Oda G, Cox K, et al. 2011. Enhanced health event detection and influenza surveillance using a joint Veterans Affairs and Department of Defense biosurveillance application. *BMC Med Inform Decis Mak.* 11:56.

Matsuda F, Ishimura S, Wagatsuma Y, et al. 2008. Prediction of epidemic cholera due to Vibrio cholerae O1 in children younger than 10 years using climate data in Bangladesh. *Epidemiol Infect.* 136(1):73–79.

Meynard JB, Chaudet H, Green AD, et al. 2008. Proposal of a framework for evaluating military surveillance systems for early detection of outbreaks on duty areas. *BMC Public Health.* 8:146.

Miller JC, Slim AC, Volz EM. 2012. Edge-based compartmental modelling for infectious disease spread. *J R Soc Interface.* 9(70):890–906.

National Capital Region Geospatial Data Exchange. Available at: https://ncrgdx.maps.arcgis.com/home/index.html. Accessed January 30, 2017.

Perez L, Dragicevic S. 2009. An agent-based approach for modeling dynamics of contagious disease spread. *Int J Health Geogr.* 8:50.

Planning Committee on Information-Sharing Models and Guidelines for Collaboration: Applications to an Integrated One Health Biosurveillance Strategy—A Workshop. *Information Sharing and Collaboration: Applications to Integrated Biosurveillance: Workshop Summary.* 2012. Washington, DC: Board on Health Sciences Policy; Institute of Medicine.

Riley S. 2007. Large-scale spatial-transmission models of infectious disease. *Science.* 316(5829): 1298–1301.

Rosewell A, Ropa B, Randall H, et al. 2013. Mobile phone-based syndromic surveillance system, Papua New Guinea. *Emerg Infect Dis.* 19(11):1811–1818.

Siettos CI, Russo L. 2013. Mathematical modeling of infectious disease dynamics. *Virulence.* 4(4):295–306.

Stigi K, Baer A, Duchin JS, et al. 2014. Evaluation of electronic ambulatory care data for influenza-like illness surveillance, Washington State. *J Public Health Manag Pract.* 20(6):580–582.

Takla A, Velasco E, Benzler J. 2012. The FIFA Women's World Cup in Germany 2011—a practical example for tailoring an event-specific enhanced infectious disease surveillance system. *BMC Public Health*. 12:576.

Tatem AJ, Hay SI, Rogers DJ. 2006. Global traffic and disease vector dispersal. *Proc Natl Acad Sci U S A*. 103(16):6242–6247.

Van den Broeck W, Gioannini C, Goncalves B, et al. 2011. The GLEaMviz computational tool, a publicly available software to explore realistic epidemic spreading scenarios at the global scale. *BMC Infect Dis*. 11:37.

Vazquez-Prokopec GM, Bisanzio D, Stoddard ST, et al. 2013. Using GPS technology to quantify human mobility, dynamic contacts and infectious disease dynamics in a resource-poor urban environment. *PLoS One*. 8(4):e58802.

Wong WK, Moore A, Cooper G, et al. 2003. WSARE: What's Strange About Recent Events? *J Urban Health*. 80(2 Suppl 1):i66–i75.

Zelicoff A, Brillman J, Forslund DW, et al. 2001. The rapid syndrome validation project (RSVP). *Proc AMIA Symp*. 2001:771–775.

Zikos D, Diomidous M. 2012. Integration of data analysis methods in syndromic surveillance systems. *Stud Health Technol Inform*. 180:1114–1116.

Surveillance After Specific Disasters

Centers for Disease Control and Prevention. 1990. Surveillance of shelters after Hurricane Hugo. *MMWR Morb Mortal Wkly Rep*. 39(3):41–42, 47.

Centers for Disease Control and Prevention. 1992. Rapid health needs assessment following Hurricane Andrew—Florida and Louisiana, 1992. *MMWR Morb Mortal Wkly Rep*. 41(37):685–688.

Centers for Disease Control and Prevention. 1993. Rapid assessment of vector-borne diseases during the Midwest flood—United States. *MMWR Morb Mortal Wkly Rep*. 43:481–483.

Centers for Disease Control and Prevention. 1994. Coccidioidomycosis following the Northridge earthquake, California, 1994. *MMWR Morb Mortal Wkly Rep*. 43(10):194–195.

Centers for Disease Control and Prevention. 1996. Surveillance for injuries and illnesses and rapid health-needs assessment following Hurricanes Marilyn and Opal, September–October 1995. *MMWR Morb Mortal Wkly Rep*. 45(4):81–85.

Centers for Disease Control and Prevention. 1997. Tornado-associated fatalities in Arkansas, 1997. *MMWR Morb Mortal Wkly Rep*. 46(19):412–416.

Centers for Disease Control and Prevention. 1998. Community needs assessment and morbidity surveillance following an ice storm, Maine, January 1998. *MMWR Morb Mortal Wkly Rep*. 47(17):351–354.

Centers for Disease Control and Prevention. 2006. Morbidity surveillance after Hurricane Katrina—Arkansas, Louisiana, Mississippi, and Texas, September 2005. *MMWR Morb Mortal Wkly Rep*. 55(26):727–731.

Centers for Disease Control and Prevention. 2006. Surveillance for illness and injury after Hurricane Katrina—Three Counties, Mississippi, September 5–October 11, 2005. *MMWR Morb Mortal Wkly Rep*. 55(9):231–234.

Centers for Disease Control and Prevention. 2006. Surveillance in hurricane evacuation centers—Louisiana, September–October 2005. *MMWR Morb Mortal Wkly Rep*. 55(2):32–35.

Centers for Disease Control and Prevention. 2010. Launching a National Surveillance System After an Earthquake—Haiti, 2010. *MMWR Morb Mortal Wkly Rep*. 59(30):933–938.

Centers for Disease Control and Prevention. 2012. Notes from the field: carbon monoxide exposures reported to poison centers and related to Hurricane Sandy—Northeastern United States, 2012. *MMWR Morb Mortal Wkly Rep*. 61(44):905–905.

Malilay J, Guido MR, Ramirez AV, et al. 1996. Public health surveillance after a volcanic eruption: lessons from Cerro Negro, Nicaragua, 1992. *Bulletin PAHO*. 30(3):218–226.

O'Carroll PW, Friede A, Noji EK, et al. 1995. The rapid implementation of a statewide emergency health information system during the 1993 Iowa flood. *Am J Public Health*. 85(4): 564–567.

Veterinary Management

American Veterinary Medical Association. Disaster preparedness for veterinarians. Available at: https://www.avma.org/KB/Resources/Reference/disaster/Pages/default.aspx. Accessed January 30, 2017.

Volcanic Eruption

Annenberg Learner. Volcanoes: can we predict volcanic eruptions? Available at: http://www.learner.org/exhibits/volcanoes/entry.html. Accessed January 30, 2017.

Baxter PJ. 1997. Volcanoes. In: Noji EK, ed. *The Public Health Consequences of Disasters*. New York, NY: Oxford University Press.

U.S. Geological Survey. 1999. The nature of volcanoes. Available at: http://pubs.usgs.gov/gip/volc/nature.html. Accessed January 30, 2017.

U.S. Geological Survey. Volcano hazards program. Available at: http://volcanoes.usgs.gov/index.html. Accessed January 30, 2017.

Worker Health and Safety

Centers for Disease Control and Prevention. 2014. Interim health recommendations for workers who handle human remains after a disaster. Available at: https://www.cdc.gov/disasters/handleremains.html. Accessed January 30, 2017.

Centers for Disease Control and Prevention. 2015. Emergency response resources: medical recommendations for relief workers and emergency responders. Available at: http://www.cdc.gov/niosh/topics/emres/flood.html. Accessed January 30, 2017.

Centers for Disease Control and Prevention. 2013. Eye Safety for emergency response and disaster recovery. Available at: http://www.cdc.gov/niosh/topics/eye/eyesafe.html. Accessed January 30, 2017.

Centers for Disease Control and Prevention. 2016. NIOSH noise and hearing loss prevention. Available at: http://www.cdc.gov/niosh/topics/noise/default.html. Accessed January 30, 2017.

Centers for Disease Control and Prevention. 2016. NIOSH Pocket guide to chemical hazards. Available at: http://www.cdc.gov/niosh/npg. Accessed January 30, 2017.

Centers for Disease Control and Prevention. 2012. Skin exposures & effects. Available at: http://www.cdc.gov/niosh/topics/skin. Accessed January 30, 2017.

Centers for Disease Control and Prevention. 2012. Worker safety during fire cleanup. Available at: http://www.cdc.gov/disasters/wildfires/cleanupworkers.html. Accessed January 30, 2017.

Centers for Disease Control and Prevention. 2013. Emergency response resources. Available at: http://www.cdc.gov/niosh/topics/emres/ppe.html. Accessed January 30, 2017.

Golob BR. 2007. *Environmental Health Emergency Response Guide*. Hopkins, MN: Twin Cities Metro Advanced Practice Center. Available at: http://www.cdc.gov/nceh/ehs/Docs/EH_Emergency_Response_Guide.pdf. Accessed January 30, 2017.

Jackson BA, Peterson DJ, Bartis JT, et al. 2002. *Protecting Emergency Responders: Lessons Learned From Terrorist Attacks*. Santa Monica, CA: RAND Science and Technology Policy Institute. Available at: http://www.rand.org/pubs/conf_proceedings/2006/CF176.pdf. Accessed January 30, 2017.

Liverman CT, Domnitz SB, McCoy MA; Institute of Medicine. 2015. *The Use and Effectiveness of Powered Air Purifying Respirators in Health Care: Workshop Summary*. Washington, DC: National Academies Press. Available at: http://books.nap.edu/openbook.php?record_id=18990&page=R1. Accessed January 30, 2017.

National Institute of Environmental Health Sciences. 2007. Hurricane Response Orientation, *Safety Awareness for Responders to Hurricanes: Protecting Yourself by Helping Others*. Available at: http://www.asse.org/assets/1/7/NIEHS-ProtectingYourselfWhileHelpingOthers.pdf. Accessed January 30, 2017.

National Institute for Occupational Safety and Health. 2015. *Hospital Respiratory Protection Program Toolkit*. Available at: http://www.cdc.gov/niosh/docs/2015-117/pdfs/2015-117.pdf. Accessed January 30, 2017.

National Institute for Occupational Safety and Health. 2004. *Protecting Emergency Responders,* Vol 3. Safety Management in Disaster and Terrorism Response. Washington, DC: U.S. Department of Health & Human Services. Available at: http://www.cdc.gov/niosh/docs/2004-144/pdfs/2004-144.pdf. Accessed January 30, 2017.

National Institute of Occupational Safety and Health. 2009. Recommendations for the selection and use of respirators and protective clothing for protection against biological agents. Available at: http://www.cdc.gov/niosh/docs/2009-132. Accessed January 30, 2017.

National Institute for Occupational Safety and Health. 2016. Guidance for supervisors at disaster rescue sites. Available at: http://www.cdc.gov/niosh/topics/emres/emhaz.html. Accessed January 30, 2017.

National Institute of Environmental Health Sciences. National clearinghouse for worker safety and health training. Available at: https://tools.niehs.nih.gov/wetp/index.cfm. Accessed January 30, 2017.

National Institute of Environmental Health Sciences. Safety awareness for responders to hurricanes: protecting yourself while helping others. Available at: https://tools.niehs.nih.gov/wetp/index.cfm?id=2472. Accessed January 30, 2017.

National Institute of Environmental Health Sciences. 2007. Hurricane Response Orientation, *Safety Awareness for Responders to Hurricanes: Protecting Yourself While Helping Others.* Available at: http://www.asse.org/assets/1/7/NIEHS-ProtectingYourselfWhileHelpingOthers.pdf. Accessed January 30, 2017.

National Institute of Environmental Health Sciences. Hurricanes & floods. Available at: http://tools.niehs.nih.gov/wetp/index.cfm?id=2472. Accessed January 30, 2017.

National Institute of Environmental Health and the National Clearinghouse for Worker Safety and Health Training. 2005. *Guidelines for the Protection and Training of Workers Engaged in Maintenance and Remediation Work Associated with Mold.*

Occupational Safety and Health Administration. 1994. OSHA regulation standard 29 CFR 1926.65. Appendix B. General description and discussion of the levels of protection and protective gear. Washington, DC. Available at: http://www.osha.gov/pls/oshaweb/owadisp.show_document?p_table=STANDARDS&p_id=10653. Accessed January 30, 2017.

Occupational Safety and Health Administration. Personal protective equipment. Available at: https://www.osha.gov/SLTC/personalprotectiveequipment. Accessed January 30, 2017.

Occupational Safety and Health Administration. 2004. *Principal Emergency Response and Preparedness: Requirements and Guidance.* Washington, DC: U.S. Department of Labor. Available at: https://www.osha.gov/Publications/osha3122.pdf. Accessed January 30, 2017.

Occupational Safety and Health Administration. 2005. *OSHA Best Practices for Hospital-Based First Receivers of Victims from Mass Casualty Incidents Involving the Release of Hazardous Sub-*

stances. Washington, DC: U.S. Department of Labor. Available at: https://www.osha.gov/dts/osta/bestpractices/html/hospital_firstreceivers.html. Accessed January 30, 2017.

Occupational Safety and Health Administration. Occupational Safety and Health Standards. 29 CFR § 1910. Available at: http://www.osha.gov/pls/oshaweb/owastand.display_standard_group?p_toc_level=1&p_part_number=1910. Accessed January 30, 2017.

Occupational Safety and Health Administration. Emergency preparedness and response: getting started. general business preparedness for general, construction and maritime industries. Available at: https://www.osha.gov/SLTC/emergencypreparedness/gettingstarted.html. Accessed January 30, 2017.

Occupational Safety and Health Administration. Occupational safety and health standards. 29 CFR § 1910, Subpart I, Appendix B to Subpart I of Part 1910—nonmandatory compliance guidelines for hazard assessment and personal protective equipment selection. Available at: https://www.osha.gov/pls/oshaweb/owadisp.show_document?p_table=STANDARDS&p_id=9696. Accessed January 30, 2017.

INDEX

A

B

C

F

G

H

I

N

O

P

Q

R

S

T

U

V

W

Y

Z